Edited by
Felix Kratz, Peter Senter,
and Henning Steinhagen

Drug Delivery in Oncology

Related Titles

Fialho, A., Chakrabarty, A. (eds.)

Emerging Cancer Therapy
Microbial Approaches and Biotechnological Tools

2010
ISBN: 978-0-470-44467-2

Jorgenson, L., Nielson, H. M. (eds.)

Delivery Technologies for Biopharmaceuticals
Peptides, Proteins, Nucleic Acids and Vaccines

2009
ISBN: 978-0-470-72338-8

Airley, R.

Cancer Chemotherapy
Basic Science to the Clinic

2009
ISBN: 978-0-470-09254-5

Missailidis, S.

Anticancer Therapeutics

2009
ISBN: 978-0-470-72303-6

Dübel, S. (ed.)

Handbook of Therapeutic Antibodies

2007
ISBN: 978-3-527-31453-9

Knäblein, J. (ed.)

Modern Biopharmaceuticals
Design, Development and Optimization

2005
ISBN: 978-3-527-31184-2

Edited by Felix Kratz, Peter Senter, and Henning Steinhagen

Drug Delivery in Oncology

From Basic Research to Cancer Therapy

Volume 3

WILEY-VCH

WILEY-VCH Verlag GmbH & Co. KGaA

The Editors

Dr. Felix Kratz
Head of the Division of
Macromolecular Prodrugs
Tumor Biology Center
Breisacherstrasse 117
D-79106 Freiburg
Germany

Dr. Peter Senter
Vice President Chemistry
Seattle Genetics, Inc.
218, Drive S.E. Bothell
Seattle, WA 98021
USA

Dr. Henning Steinhagen
Vice President
Head of Global Drug Discovery
Grünenthal GmbH
Zieglerstr. 6
52078 Aachen
Germany

Library of Congress Card No.: applied for

British Library Cataloguing-in-Publication Data
A catalogue record for this book is available from the British Library.

Bibliographic information published by the Deutsche Nationalbibliothek
The Deutsche Nationalbibliothek lists this publication in the Deutsche Nationalbibliografie; detailed bibliographic data are available on the Internet at <http://dnb.d-nb.de>.

Composition Laserwords Private Ltd., Chennai
Printing and Binding betz-druck GmbH, Darmstadt
Cover Design Schulz Grafik-Design, Fußgönheim

Printed in the Federal Republic of Germany
Printed on acid-free paper

ISBN: 978-3-527-32823-9
oBook ISBN: 978-3-527-63405-7

Foreword

It is highly likely that the reason our therapies so often fail our patients with cancer is that either (i) those therapies actually never get to their intended targets or (ii) those therapies are "intercepted" by similar targets on normal cells. If we want to understand why many of our therapies fail our patients, and what we can do to possibly remedy those failures, this book *Drug Delivery in Oncology* can help all of us achieve that understanding – and with this book it will be a state-of-the-art understanding.

Drs. Kratz, Senter, and Steinhagen have assembled a respectable breadth of both seasoned and precocious investigators to put together this very special treatise (49 chapters in all). The chapters are well written with basic science, preclinical, and clinical perspectives.

The book begins with a history and the limitations of conventional chemotherapy. Expert discussions of the vascular physiology of tumors that affect drug delivery (and how to defeat those issues) then follow. There are excellent discussions of the neonatal Fc receptor, development of cancer targeted ligands, and antibody-directed enzyme prodrug therapy (ADEPT).

A very special part of this book is the emphasis on tumor imaging. Again, the authors are major experts in this field, which undoubtedly will continue to mature to enable us to document whether or not our therapeutics actually make it to their intended target(s) – and if not, why not.

There are impressive chapters on macromolecular drug delivery systems, including biospecific antibodies, antibody–drug conjugates, and antibody–radionuclide conjugates. Up-to-date discussions of polymer-based drug delivery systems including PEGylation, thermoresponsive polysaccharide-based and even low-density lipoprotein–drug complexes are also presented.

Those with an interest in learning about nano- and microparticulate drug delivery systems can study liposomes to immunoliposomes, to hydrogels, micelles, albumin–drug nanoparticles, and even carbon nanotubes, which are all covered in this book.

Other special delivery systems covered include peptides–drug conjugates, vitamin–drug conjugates, and growth factor–drug conjugates, conjugates of drugs with fatty acids, RNA and RNA interference delivery, and specific targeted organ drug delivery.

As investigators who want to more effectively treat and indeed cure cancer we have many worries. The first of these is that many of our therapeutics just do not make it into the targets in the tumors. This book gives the reader a comprehensive insight into multiple ways to address this problem. A second major worry is that we are losing our pharmacologists who can solve those drug delivery issues. The editors and the authors of this incredible treatise give us comfort that these pharmacologists are alive and well, and thinking as to how they can contribute to getting control of this awful disease.

Daniel D. Von Hoff, MD, FACP
Physician in Chief and Distinguished Professor,
Translational Genomics Research Institute (TGen)
Professor of Medicine, Mayo Clinic
Chief Scientific Officer, Scottsdale Healthcare and US Oncology

Contents to Volume 1

Part I Principles of Tumor Targeting *1*

1 **Limits of Conventional Cancer Chemotherapy** *3*
Klaus Mross and Felix Kratz

2 **Pathophysiological and Vascular Characteristics of Solid Tumors in Relation to Drug Delivery** *33*
Peter Vaupel

3 **Enhanced Permeability and Retention Effect in Relation to Tumor Targeting** *65*
Hiroshi Maeda

4 **Pharmacokinetics of Immunoglobulin G and Serum Albumin: Impact of the Neonatal Fc Receptor on Drug Design** *85*
Jan Terje Andersen and Inger Sandlie

5 **Development of Cancer-Targeting Ligands and Ligand–Drug Conjugates** *121*
Ruiwu Liu, Kai Xiao, Juntao Luo, and Kit S. Lam

6 **Antibody-Directed Enzyme Prodrug Therapy (ADEPT) – Basic Principles and its Practice So Far** *169*
Kenneth D. Bagshawe

Part II Tumor Imaging *187*

7 **Imaging Techniques in Drug Development and Clinical Practice** *189*
John C. Chang, Sanjiv S. Gambhir, and Jürgen K. Willmann

8 **Magnetic Nanoparticles in Magnetic Resonance Imaging and Drug Delivery** *225*
Patrick D. Sutphin, Efrén J. Flores, and Mukesh Harisinghani

9 **Preclinical and Clinical Tumor Imaging with SPECT/CT and PET/CT** *247*
Andreas K. Buck, Florian Gärtner, Ambros Beer, Ken Herrmann, Sibylle Ziegler, and Markus Schwaiger

Contents to Volume 2

Part III Macromolecular Drug Delivery Systems *289*

Antibody-Based Systems *289*

10 **Empowered Antibodies for Cancer Therapy** *291*
Stephen C. Alley, Simone Jeger, Robert P. Lyon, Django Sussman, and Peter D. Senter

11 **Mapping Accessible Vascular Targets to Penetrate Organs and Solid Tumors** *325*
Kerri A. Massey and Jan E. Schnitzer

12 **Considerations of Linker Technologies** *355*
Laurent Ducry

13 **Antibody–Maytansinoid Conjugates: From the Bench to the Clinic** *375*
Hans Erickson

14 **Calicheamicin Antibody–Drug Conjugates and Beyond** *395*
Puja Sapra, John DiJoseph, and Hans-Peter Gerber

15 **Antibodies for the Delivery of Radionuclides** *411*
Anna M. Wu

16 **Bispecific Antibodies and Immune Therapy Targeting** *441*
Sergej M. Kiprijanov

Polymer-Based Systems *483*

17 **Design of Polymer–Drug Conjugates** *485*
Jindřich Kopeček and Pavla Kopečková

18 **Dendritic Polymers in Oncology: Facts, Features, and Applications** *513*
Mohiuddin Abdul Quadir, Marcelo Calderón, and Rainer Haag

19 **Site-Specific Prodrug Activation and the Concept of Self-Immolation** *553*
André Warnecke

20 **Ligand-Assisted Vascular Targeting of Polymer Therapeutics** *591*
Anat Eldar-Boock, Dina Polyak, and Ronit Satchi-Fainaro

21 **Drug Conjugates with Poly(Ethylene Glycol)** *627*
Hong Zhao, Lee M. Greenberger, and Ivan D. Horak

22 **Thermo-Responsive Polymers** *667*
Drazen Raucher and Shama Moktan

23 **Polysaccharide-Based Drug Conjugates for Tumor Targeting** *701*
Gurusamy Saravanakumar, Jae Hyung Park, Kwangmeyung Kim, and Ick Chan Kwon

24 **Serum Proteins as Drug Carriers of Anticancer Agents** *747*
Felix Kratz, Andreas Wunder, and Bakheet Elsadek

25 **Future Trends, Challenges, and Opportunities with Polymer-Based Combination Therapy in Cancer** *805*
Coralie Deladriere, Rut Lucas, and María J. Vicent

26 **Clinical Experience with Drug–Polymer Conjugates** *839*
Khalid Abu Ajaj and Felix Kratz

Part IV Nano- and Microparticulate Drug Delivery Systems *885*

Lipid-Based Systems *885*

27 **Overview on Nanocarriers as Delivery Systems** *887*
Haifa Shen, Elvin Blanco, Biana Godin, Rita E. Serda, Agathe K. Streiff, and Mauro Ferrari

28 **Development of PEGylated Liposomes** *907*
I. Craig Henderson

29 **Immunoliposomes** *951*
Vladimir P. Torchilin

30 **Responsive Liposomes (for Solid Tumor Therapy)** *989*
Stavroula Sofou

31 **Nanoscale Delivery Systems for Combination Chemotherapy** *1013*
Barry D. Liboiron, Paul G. Tardi, Troy O. Harasym, and Lawrence, D. Mayer

Polymer-Based Systems *1051*

32 **Micellar Structures as Drug Delivery Systems** *1053*
Nobuhiro Nishiyama, Horacio Cabral, and Kazunori Kataoka

33 **Tailor-Made Hydrogels for Tumor Delivery** *1071*
Sungwon Kim and Kinam Park

34 **pH-Triggered Micelles for Tumor Delivery** *1099*
Haiqing Yin and You Han Bae

35 **Albumin–Drug Nanoparticles** *1133*
Neil Desai

36 **Carbon Nanotubes** *1163*
David A. Scheinberg, Carlos H. Villa, Freddy Escorcia, and Michael R. McDevitt

Contents to Volume 3

Foreword *V*
Preface *XXI*

Part V **Ligand-Based Drug Delivery Systems** *1187*

37 **Cell-Penetrating Peptides in Cancer Targeting** *1189*
Kaido Kurrikoff, Julia Suhorutšenko, and Ülo Langel
37.1 Introduction *1189*
37.2 Applications of CPPs *1190*
37.2.1 Modifying Classical Anticancer Drugs *1191*
37.2.2 Inherent Antineoplastic Activity of CPPs *1195*
37.2.3 Delivery of Nucleic Acids and Oligonucleotides *1195*
37.2.4 CPP Application in Oncogenic Signaling and Cell Cycle Modulation in Tumors *1198*
37.2.4.1 Oncoproteins *1199*
37.2.4.2 Tumor Suppressor p53 *1200*
37.2.4.3 Tumor Suppressor p16 *1201*

37.2.4.4 Tumor Suppressors p21 and p27 *1202*
37.3 Tumor Targeting of CPPs *1202*
37.3.1 Passive Targeting of CPPs *1203*
37.3.1.1 EPR Effect *1203*
37.3.1.2 Matrix Metalloproteases *1204*
37.3.1.3 pH- and O_2-Sensitive CPP Systems *1204*
37.3.2 Active Targeting of CPPs *1205*
37.3.2.1 Antibodies as a Targeting Moiety *1205*
37.3.2.2 Radioimmunotherapy *1206*
37.3.2.3 Homing Peptides *1207*
37.4 Advantages and Considerations of CPPs as Delivery Vectors *1208*
37.5 Conclusions *1209*
Acknowledgments *1210*
References *1210*

38 Targeting to Peptide Receptors *1219*
Andrew V. Schally and Gabor Halmos
38.1 Introduction *1219*
38.2 Rationale for the Concept of Delivery to Peptide Receptors *1220*
38.3 Example 1: Cytotoxic Analogs of LHRH1 *1221*
38.3.1 Preclinical Considerations and Development *1221*
38.3.1.1 LHRH1 and its Receptors *1221*
38.3.1.2 Design and Synthesis of Targeted Cytotoxic Analogs of LHRH1 *1223*
38.3.1.3 Mechanism of Action of Cytotoxic LHRH1 Analogs: Targeting to LHRH1 Receptors on Tumors *1225*
38.3.1.4 Responses of Human Experimental Cancers Expressing Receptors for LHRH1 to Targeted Cytotoxic Analogs of LHRH1 *1228*
38.3.1.5 Side-Effects of Cytotoxic LHRH1 Analogs *1234*
38.3.2 Clinical Development *1235*
38.3.2.1 Clinical Phase I and Phase II Trials of Cytotoxic LHRH1 Analog AN-152 (AEZS-108) in Women with Ovarian and Endometrial Cancers *1235*
38.4 Example 2: Targeted Cytotoxic Somatostatin Analogs *1236*
38.4.1 Preclinical Considerations and Development *1236*
38.4.1.1 Somatostatin and its Receptors *1236*
38.4.1.2 Synthesis of Cytotoxic Analogs of Somatostatin *1238*
38.4.1.3 Side-Effects of Cytotoxic Somatostatin Analogs *1243*
38.4.2 Clinical Development *1244*
38.5 Example 3: Cytotoxic Analogs of Bombesin/Gastrin-Releasing Peptide *1244*
38.5.1 Preclinical Considerations and Development *1244*
38.5.1.1 Bombesin/Gastrin-Releasing Peptide and their Receptors *1244*
38.5.1.2 Radiolabeled and Cytotoxic Bombesin Analogs *1245*
38.5.2 Clinical Development *1246*
38.6 Example 4: Antagonists of GHRH *1247*

38.6.1 Preclinical Considerations and Development *1247*
38.6.1.1 GHRH and GHRH Receptors in Tumors *1247*
38.6.1.2 Antagonistic Analogs of GHRH *1249*
38.6.2 Clinical Developments *1251*
38.7 Conclusions and Perspectives *1251*
Acknowledgments *1252*
References *1252*

39 Aptamer Conjugates: Emerging Delivery Platforms for Targeted Cancer Therapy *1263*
Zeyu Xiao, Jillian Frieder, Benjamin A. Teply, and Omid C. Farokhzad
39.1 Introduction *1263*
39.2 Isolating Aptamers for Targeted Delivery *1265*
39.2.1 SELEX Against Purified Proteins *1265*
39.2.2 SELEX Against Living Cells *1265*
39.3 Applications of Aptamer Conjugates for Targeted Cancer Therapy *1269*
39.3.1 Small-Molecule Delivery via Aptamer Conjugates *1270*
39.3.2 Nanoparticle Delivery via Aptamer Conjugate *1271*
39.3.3 siRNA Delivery via Aptamer Conjugates *1273*
39.4 Considerations of Aptamer Characteristics for *In Vivo* Applications *1275*
39.4.1 Nuclease Resistance *1275*
39.4.2 Optimal Circulating Half-Life *1275*
39.4.3 Rapid Penetration and Longer Retention Time in Target Tissue *1276*
39.4.4 Toxicology *1276*
39.5 Conclusions and Perspectives *1277*
Acknowledgments *1278*
References *1278*

40 Design and Synthesis of Drug Conjugates of Vitamins and Growth Factors *1283*
Iontcho R. Vlahov, Paul J. Kleindl, and Fei You
40.1 Introduction *1283*
40.2 Chemical Aspects of FA–Drug Conjugate Design *1284*
40.2.1 Folate Receptor-Mediated Endocytosis for Targeted Drug Delivery *1284*
40.2.2 General Criteria for the Design of FA–Drug Conjugates and their Intracellular Release Mechanisms *1286*
40.2.3 Synthesis of FA–Cancer Drug Conjugates Containing Disulfide-Based Linker Systems *1288*
40.2.3.1 Exploiting Peptide-Based Spacers *1288*
40.2.3.2 Exploiting Carbohydrate-Based Spacers *1293*
40.2.3.3 Introduction of a Second Unsymmetrical Disulfide Bond: Synthesis of Releasable Dual-Drug Conjugates *1295*

40.2.4 Application of pH-Responsive Linker Systems for the Synthesis of FA–Drug Conjugates *1298*
40.2.5 FR-Targeted Immunotherapy *1298*
40.3 Chemical Aspects of Vitamin B_{12}–Drug Conjugate Design *1300*
40.3.1 Vitamin B_{12}-Binding Proteins and Cellular Transport *1300*
40.3.2 Structural Considerations in Vitamin B_{12} Conjugate Design *1301*
40.3.3 Synthesis of Vitamin B_{12}–Drug Conjugates *1301*
40.3.3.1 Releasable β-Ligand Conjugates *1301*
40.3.3.2 Other Vitamin B_{12}–Drug Conjugates *1303*
40.4 Chemical Aspects of Biotin–Drug Conjugate Design *1304*
40.4.1 Biotin and Biotin Conjugate Targeting in Cancer Therapy *1304*
40.4.2 Synthesis of Biotin–Drug Conjugates *1305*
40.5 Other Vitamin–Drug Conjugates *1307*
40.5.1 Conjugates of Vitamin E *1307*
40.5.2 Conjugates of Vitamin B_6 *1307*
40.6 Concluding Remarks on Vitamin Targeting *1308*
40.7 Growth Factor Conjugates for Tumor Targeting *1308*
40.7.1 Growth Factors and Growth Factor Receptors *1308*
40.7.2 Growth Factor Targeted Delivery of Protein Toxin *1310*
40.7.3 Growth Factor Targeted Delivery of Chemotherapeutics *1311*
40.7.4 Growth Factor Targeted Delivery in Radiotherapy and Photodynamic Therapy *1311*
40.7.5 Peptides Targeting Growth Factor Receptor *1312*
40.7.6 Concluding Remarks on Growth Factor Targeting *1313*
Acknowledgments *1313*
References *1313*

41 Drug Conjugates with Polyunsaturated Fatty Acids *1323*
Joshua Seitz and Iwao Ojima
41.1 Introduction *1323*
41.2 Rationale for the Potential Benefits of PUFA Conjugation to Chemotherapeutic Drugs *1323*
41.2.1 PUFAs in Cancer Progression and Control *1324*
41.2.2 Effects of PUFA Internalization on Membrane Composition and Signaling *1325*
41.2.3 Suppression of Tumor-Promoting Eicosanoid Biosynthesis by PUFAs *1326*
41.2.4 Influences of PUFAs on Signal Transduction Pathways and Gene Expression *1328*
41.2.5 PUFA Peroxidation and ROS *1331*
41.2.6 Synergy of Cytotoxic Drugs and PUFAs for the Treatment of Cancer Cell Lines *1331*
41.3 Drug Conjugates with PUFAs *1332*
41.3.1 DHA–Paclitaxel and PUFA–Second-Generation Taxoid Conjugates (1) *1332*

41.3.2 DHA–10-Hydroxycamptothecin (2) *1334*
41.3.3 DHA/LNA–DOX (3/4) *1334*
41.3.4 DHA/EPA–Propofol (5a/b) *1335*
41.3.5 DHA–Illudin M (6) *1336*
41.3.6 PUFA–Chlorambucil (7) *1336*
41.3.7 PUFA–Mitomycin C (8) *1336*
41.3.8 PUFA–2′-Deoxy-5-fluorouridine (9) and PUFA–Tegafur (10 and 11) *1337*
41.3.9 DHA–Methotrexate (11) *1338*
41.4 Case Study in PUFA Conjugation: TXP (DHA–Paclitaxel) *1338*
41.4.1 Preclinical Evaluations *1338*
41.4.2 Pharmacokinetics *1339*
41.4.3 Phase I Trials *1342*
41.4.4 Phase II/III Trials *1343*
41.5 PUFA Conjugates of Second-Generation Taxoids *1345*
41.5.1 Preclinical Study of PUFA–Second-Generation Taxoid Conjugates *1345*
41.5.1.1 DLD-1 (P-gp$^+$ Colon) Tumor Xenograft *1346*
41.5.1.2 A121 (P-gp$^-$ Ovarian) Tumor Xenograft *1348*
41.5.1.3 Panc-1 (Pancreatic) Tumor Xenograft *1348*
41.5.1.4 CFPAC-1 (Pancreatic) Tumor Xenograft *1348*
41.5.1.5 H460 (NSCLC) Tumor Xenograft *1349*
41.5.1.6 LNA– and LA–Second-Generation Taxoids *1349*
41.5.2 Cytochrome P450 Screening for Assessment of Potential Drug–Drug Interaction *1349*
41.6 Conclusions and Perspectives *1350*
Acknowledgments *1350*
References *1350*

Part VI Special Topics *1359*

42 RNA Drug Delivery Approaches *1361*
Yuan Zhang and Leaf Huang
42.1 Introduction *1361*
42.2 RNA Molecules with Potential for Cancer Treatment *1361*
42.3 Chemical Modification Strategies *1362*
42.3.1 Sugar Modification *1364*
42.3.2 Nucleobase Modification *1364*
42.3.3 Terminal Modification *1365*
42.4 Challenges in RNA Delivery *1365*
42.4.1 Chemical Stability and Structure Modification *1365*
42.4.2 Extracellular Delivery Stage *1366*
42.4.3 Target Cell Specificity and Uptake via Targeting Ligands *1366*
42.4.4 Endosomal Release *1367*
42.5 Potential Adverse Effects of RNA Therapy *1367*

42.5.1 Induction of Immune Responses *1367*
42.5.2 Off-Target Effect *1368*
42.5.3 Saturation of Endogenous Silencing Pathway *1368*
42.6 RNA Delivery *1368*
42.6.1 Physical Methods *1369*
42.6.1.1 Hydrodynamic Injection *1369*
42.6.1.2 Electroporation *1370*
42.6.1.3 Particle Bombardment *1371*
42.6.2 Chemical Vectors for RNA Delivery *1371*
42.6.2.1 Cationic Lipids/Liposomes and Cationic Lipid Nanoparticles (Lipoplexes) *1371*
42.6.2.2 Ionizable Lipids *1372*
42.6.2.3 Lipid-Like Delivery Molecules (Lipidoids) *1373*
42.6.2.4 Cationic Polymers (Polyplexes) *1373*
42.6.2.5 Core/Membrane Lipid-Based Nanoparticles (Lipopolyplexes) *1376*
42.6.2.6 Aptamer–siRNA Chimeras *1379*
42.7 Targeting Ligands *1381*
42.7.1 Aptamers *1381*
42.7.2 CPPs *1381*
42.7.3 Antibodies *1381*
42.7.4 Peptides and Proteins *1382*
42.7.5 Small-Molecular-Weight Ligands *1382*
42.8 Therapeutic Application for Treatment of Cancer *1383*
42.8.1 siRNA Therapeutic Mechanisms *1383*
42.8.2 Examples in Cancer Treatment of RNA Delivery Technology *1383*
42.9 Conclusions *1385*
Acknowledgments *1385*
References *1385*

43 Local Gene Delivery for Therapy of Solid Tumors *1391*
Wolfgang Walther, Peter M. Schlag, and Ulrike Stein
43.1 Introduction *1391*
43.2 Gene Therapeutic Strategies for Cancer Treatment *1391*
43.2.1 Gene Correction Therapy *1392*
43.2.2 Immunogene Therapy *1394*
43.2.3 Suicide Gene Therapy *1397*
43.2.4 Virotherapy *1397*
43.2.5 Gene Suppression *1397*
43.3 Vectors for Cancer Gene Therapy *1398*
43.3.1 Viral Vectors *1399*
43.3.2 Nonviral Vectors *1400*
43.3.3 Bacterial Vectors *1401*
43.4 Local Application of Gene Therapy *1401*
43.4.1 Specific Strategies for Local Gene Delivery *1402*
43.4.2 Technologies for Local Gene Delivery *1404*

43.4.3 Jet-Injection Technology for Local Cancer Gene Therapy *1406*
43.4.4 Clinical Application of Local Jet-Injection Gene Therapy *1406*
43.5 Conclusions *1407*
References *1408*

44 Viral Vectors for RNA Interference Applications in Cancer Research and Therapy *1415*
Henry Fechner and Jens Kurreck
44.1 Introduction *1415*
44.2 Plasmid Expression of Short Hairpin RNAs *1418*
44.3 Conditional RNAi Systems *1422*
44.3.1 Irreversible Conditional Systems *1423*
44.3.2 Reversible Systems *1423*
44.4 Viral Vectors for shRNA Delivery *1426*
44.4.1 Retroviral Vectors *1428*
44.4.2 Adenoviral Vectors and Oncolytic Adenoviruses *1431*
44.4.3 Vectors Based on AAVs *1433*
44.5 Outlook *1435*
Acknowledgments *1436*
References *1436*

45 Design of Targeted Protein Toxins *1443*
Hendrik Fuchs and Christopher Bachran
45.1 Introduction *1443*
45.1.1 Basic Idea *1443*
45.1.2 Cell Death *1445*
45.1.3 Combination with Other Therapy Strategies *1445*
45.2 Rationale for the Respective Drug Delivery Concept *1446*
45.2.1 Design *1446*
45.2.1.1 Domains *1446*
45.2.1.2 Targeting Moieties *1448*
45.2.1.3 Toxins *1448*
45.2.1.4 Toxin Delivery *1455*
45.2.2 Obstacles and Circumvention *1458*
45.2.2.1 Production *1458*
45.2.2.2 Biological Half-Life *1459*
45.2.2.3 Immunogenicity *1460*
45.2.2.4 Tumor Penetration *1461*
45.2.2.5 Undesirable Effects *1461*
45.3 Examples *1462*
45.3.1 Preclinical Development *1462*
45.3.1.1 Drugs Based on Bacterial Toxins *1462*
45.3.1.2 Drugs Based on Plant Toxins *1466*
45.3.1.3 Drugs Based on Human Proteins *1468*
45.3.2 Clinical Development *1472*

45.3.2.1 Denileukin Diftitox *1472*
45.3.2.2 BL22/HA22 *1477*
45.3.2.3 SS1P *1479*
45.3.2.4 Cintredekin Besudotox *1479*
45.3.2.5 Combotox *1480*
45.3.2.6 Ranpirnase *1480*
45.4 Conclusions and Perspectives *1480*
Acknowledgments *1481*
References *1481*

46 Drug Targeting to the Central Nervous System *1489*
Gert Fricker, Anne Mahringer, Melanie Ott, and Valeska Reichel
46.1 Introduction *1489*
46.2 Anatomy of the BBB *1490*
46.3 Alterations of the BBB in Brain Tumors *1495*
46.4 Relevance of the BBB for Drug Delivery *1495*
46.4.1 Prodrug Approaches to Overcome the BBB *1495*
46.4.2 Inhibition of ABC Export Proteins *1497*
46.4.3 Intrathecal or Intraventricular Injection *1498*
46.4.4 Infusion of Hyperosmotic Solutions *1499*
46.4.5 Focused Ultrasound Treatment *1499*
46.4.6 Vector-Coupled Drugs *1499*
46.4.7 Liposomal Drug Delivery to the CNS *1502*
46.4.8 CNS Drug Delivery by Polymer Nanoparticles *1505*
46.4.9 Magnetically Controlled CNS Drug Delivery *1507*
46.4.10 Polymeric Micelles and Dendrimers *1508*
46.4.11 Solid Lipid Nanoparticles *1508*
46.5 Intranasal Delivery to Bypass the BBB *1509*
46.6 Conclusion and Perspectives *1509*
References *1510*

47 Liver Tumor Targeting *1519*
Katrin Hochdörffer, Giuseppina Di Stefano, Hiroshi Maeda, and Felix Kratz
47.1 Introduction *1519*
47.1.1 Epidemiology and Incidence of HCC *1519*
47.1.2 Therapeutic Options for Treating Liver Cancer *1520*
47.1.2.1 Liver Resection *1521*
47.1.2.2 Local Ablative Therapy *1521*
47.1.2.3 Transarterial Chemoembolization *1521*
47.1.2.4 Chemotherapy/Targeted Therapy *1522*
47.2 Rationale for Drug Delivery Concepts for Treating Liver Cancer *1522*
47.2.1 Receptor for ASGPs: A Target for Delivering Drugs to Hepatocytes *1524*

47.2.2 Designing Drug-Encapsulated Nanoparticles for Liver Tumor Uptake by the RES *1527*
47.2.3 Liver Tumor Targeting Using HepDirect Prodrugs *1527*
47.3 Preclinical Development of Hepatotropic Drug Delivery Systems *1528*
47.3.1 HepDirect Prodrugs *1529*
47.3.2 Drug–Polymer Conjugates *1529*
47.3.2.1 PK2: A HPMA-Based Copolymer with *N*-Galactosamine *1529*
47.3.2.2 Lactosaminated Albumin: A Safe and Efficient Hepatotropic Carrier for Treating Liver Tumors *1532*
47.3.2.3 SMANCS: A Conjugate of Poly(Styrene-*co*-Maleic Acid) and the Antitumor Agent Neocarzinostatin *1543*
47.3.3 Development of Nanoparticles for Treating Liver Tumors *1546*
47.3.3.1 Doxorubicin Transdrug *1546*
47.3.3.2 Mitoxantrone-Loaded Nanoparticles *1547*
47.3.3.3 YCC-DOX: A Multifunctional DOX-Loaded Superparamagnetic Iron Oxide Nanoparticle *1548*
47.4 Clinical Development *1550*
47.4.1 Phase I Study with PK2: A HPMA-Based Copolymer with *N*-Galactosamine *1551*
47.4.2 Doxorubicin Transdrug: A DOX Nanoparticle with PIHCA that Advanced to Phase II/III Trials *1553*
47.4.3 Phase I/II Trials of Mitoxantrone-Loaded PBCA Nanoparticles *1553*
47.4.4 ThermoDox®: A Heat-Sensitive Liposomal Formulation of DOX in Phase II Trials *1554*
47.4.5 SMANCS: A Conjugate of SMA and the Antitumor Agent NCS *1555*
47.5 Conclusions and Perspectives *1559*
References *1560*

48 Photodynamic Therapy: Photosensitizer Targeting and Delivery *1569*
Pawel Mroz, Sulbha K. Sharma, Timur Zhiyentayev, Ying-Ying Huang, and Michael R. Hamblin
48.1 Introduction *1569*
48.2 Photochemistry and Photophysics *1569*
48.3 Photosensitizers *1571*
48.4 Subcellular Localization *1573*
48.5 Targeting in PDT *1573*
48.6 Preclinical Developments *1573*
48.6.1 Drug Delivery Vehicles: Liposomes Micelles and Nanoparticles *1573*
48.6.2 Photosensitizer Targeting via Antibodies *1575*
48.6.2.1 Direct Photosensitizer–mAab Conjugates *1578*
48.6.2.2 Photosensitizer Linked to mAab via Polymers or Other Macromolecular Linkers *1578*
48.6.3 Peptide or Growth Factor Conjugates *1579*
48.6.4 Conjugates between Photosensitizer and Nonantibody Proteins *1580*

48.6.5 Polymer–Photosensitizer Conjugates *1584*
48.6.6 Enzyme-Cleavable Photosensitizer Conjugates *1586*
48.6.7 Small-Molecule–Photosensitizer Conjugates *1588*
48.6.8 Photochemical Internalization *1589*
48.7 Clinical Developments *1591*
48.8 Conclusions and Perspectives *1592*
Acknowledgments *1592*
References *1593*

49 Tumor-Targeting Strategies with Anticancer Platinum Complexes *1605*
Markus Galanski and Bernhard K. Keppler
49.1 Introduction *1605*
49.2 Mode of Action of Platinum-Based Anticancer Drugs and Rationale for the Respective Drug Delivery Concept *1607*
49.3 Examples *1611*
49.3.1 Active and Organ-Specific Targeting *1612*
49.3.2 Passive Targeting *1616*
49.3.2.1 Liposomal Drug Delivery –LipoPlatin and LipOxal *1616*
49.3.2.2 Polymeric Delivery Systems –ProLindac *1619*
49.4 Clinical Development *1622*
49.4.1 LipoPlatin *1622*
49.4.2 LipOxal *1624*
49.4.3 ProLindac *1625*
49.5 Conclusions and Perspectives *1626*
Acknowledgments *1627*
References *1627*

Index *1631*

Preface

Modern oncology research is highly multidisciplinary, involving scientists from a wide array of specialties focused on both basic and applied areas of research. While significant therapeutic advancements have been made, there remains a great need for further progress in treating almost all of the most prevalent forms of cancer. Unlike many other diseases, cancer is commonly characterized by barriers to penetration, heterogeneity, genetic instability, and drug resistance. Coupled with the fact that successful treatment requires elimination of malignant cells that are very closely related to normal cells within the body, cancer therapy remains one of the greatest challenges in modern medicine.

Early on, chemotherapeutic drugs were renowned for their systemic toxicities, since they poorly distinguished tumor cells from normal cells. It became apparent to scientists within the field that further advancements in cancer medicine would require new-generation drugs that ideally targeted critical pathways, unique markers, and distinguishing physiological traits that were selectively found within the malignant cells and solid tumor masses. Several new areas of research evolved from this realization, including macromolecular-based therapies that exploit impaired lymphatic drainage often associated with solid tumors, antiangiogenesis research to cut the blood supply off from growing tumors, antibody-based strategies that allow for selective targeting to tumor-associated antigens, and new drug classes that attack uniquely critical pathways that promote and sustain tumor growth. A large proportion of both recently approved and clinically advanced anticancer drugs fall within these categories.

Beyond the generation of such drug classes, it has also been recognized that approved cancer drugs could be made more effective and less toxic through delivery and transport technologies that maximize tumor exposure while sparing normal tissues from chemotherapeutic damage. By doing so, existing or highly potent cytotoxic drugs may display improved therapeutic indices. This has attracted considerable attention and has spawned the area of macromolecular-based delivery strategies.

There are few places where those actively engaged in drug delivery or who may wish to enter the field can find the major advancements consolidated in one place. This prompted us to organize the series of books entitled *Drug Delivery in Oncology* comprised of 49 chapters written by 121 internationally recognized leaders in the field. The work within the book series overviews many of the major breakthroughs in cancer medicine made in the last 10–15 years and features many of the chemotherapeutics of the future. Included among them are recombinant antibodies, antibody fragments, and antibody fusion proteins as well as tumor-seeking ligands for selective drug delivery and tumor imaging, and passive targeting strategies using macromolecules and nano- and microparticulate systems.

One of the special distinguishing features of this series is that the chapters are written for novices and experts alike. Each chapter is written in a style that allows interested readers to not only to find out about the most recent advancements within the field being discussed, but to actually see the data in numerous illustrations, photos, graphs, and tables that accompany each chapter.

None of this would have been possible without the devoted efforts of the contributing authors, all of whom shared the common goal of creating a new series of books that would provide an important cornerstone in the modern chemotherapeutic treatment of cancer. We are all very thankful for their efforts.

We also wish to thank the publishing team at Wiley-VCH in Weinheim, Germany. In particular, we want to give our wholehearted thanks and kind acknowledgments to Frank Weinreich, Gudrun Walter, Bernadette Gmeiner, Claudia Nußbeck, Hans-Jochen Schmitt, and Ina Wiedemann, who were always helpful and supportive during the 2 years it took to put all this together. It is our hope that this series will provide readers with inspired ideas and new directions for research in drug delivery in oncology.

July 2011

Felix Kratz
Peter Senter
Henning Steinhagen

Part V
Ligand-Based Drug Delivery Systems

Drug Delivery in Oncology: From Basic Research to Cancer Therapy, First Edition.
Edited by Felix Kratz, Peter Senter, and Henning Steinhagen.

37
Cell-Penetrating Peptides in Cancer Targeting

Kaido Kurrikoff, Julia Suhorutšenko, and Ülo Langel

37.1
Introduction

In 1998, it was noted that the transactivating transcriptional activator protein (TAT) of HIV-1 was easily taken up by cells in tissue culture [1]. Later, cell-penetrating domains of HIV TAT and penetratin, a peptide derived from the homeodomain of the Antennapedia protein of *Drosophila*, were described [2, 3]. These were the first characterized cell-penetrating peptides (CPPs; sometimes referred to as protein transduction domains (PTDs)). The first breakthrough in the field showed that the cell-penetrating capability of these proteins was largely mediated by short domains of the proteins and that these peptides were able not only to translocate through the cell membrane, but also to take cargo along. This property makes CPPs promising candidates for drug delivery, since permeabilizing the bioactive drugs to cell membranes permits using lower clinical doses. Considering the difficulties of reaching intracellular or nuclear targets by conventional methods, CPPs hold great promise for the delivery of nucleic acids and other nonpermeable molecules.

Another major breakthrough came from the first demonstration of the *in vivo* application of CPPs, by the groups of Langel [4] and Dowdy [5], for the delivery of peptide nucleic acidss (PNAs), small peptides, and large proteins. Since then, numerous *in vivo* applications of CPPs have been described. When analyzing these works, it could be said that CPPs currently represent a major approach in developing delivery systems that mediate noninvasive and nontoxic transport of problematic cargos into cells.

The mechanism of cell penetration was first suggested to be energy-independent membrane translocation (Figure 37.1), but over the last few years evidence favors endocytosis as a preferred mechanism of entry for CPPs [6], at least when attached to bioactive cargo. Most likely, different CPPs and CPP–cargo conjugates utilize multiple internalization mechanisms in combination [7, 8]. The number of known CPP sequences has grown rapidly since the first reports, with dozens of new

Drug Delivery in Oncology: From Basic Research to Cancer Therapy, First Edition.
Edited by Felix Kratz, Peter Senter, and Henning Steinhagen.

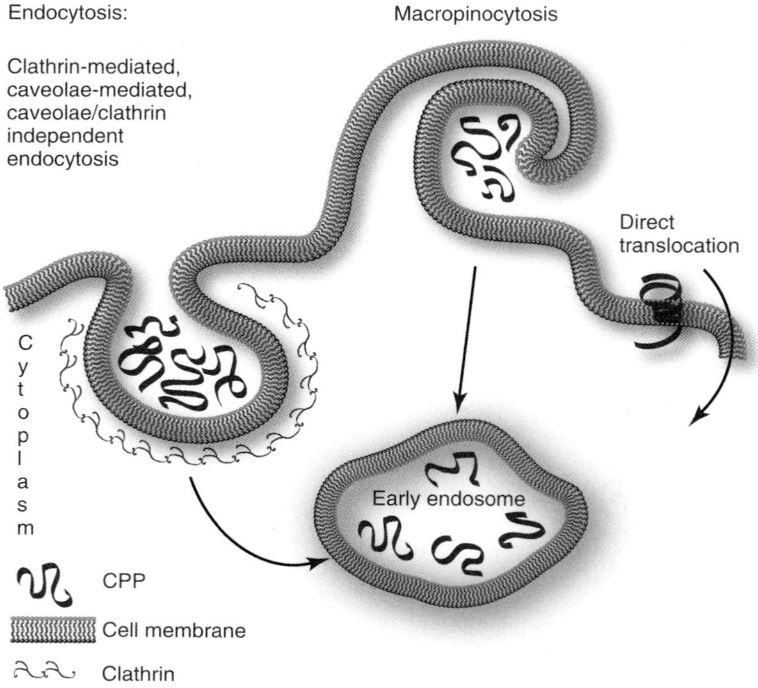

Figure 37.1 Overview of different internalization routes of CPPs. Both endocytosis and direct membrane translocation account for CPP uptake. Depending on the CPP and cargo, all endocytosis types can be included: clathrin-dependent, caveolae-mediated, and caveolae/clathrin-independent endocytosis, as well as macropinocytosis. Moreover, for several CPP–cargo types, energy-independent membrane translocation has been described.

peptide sequences added to the existing ones every year. These novel CPPs are very often derived from well-established proteins and optimized to be the shortest possible peptide sequences still capable of penetrating the plasma membrane and preferably also carrying the desired payload (an overview of different types of cargo is presented in Figure 37.2) [9]. A small selection of frequently used CPPs is presented in Table 37.1.

37.2
Applications of CPPs

CPPs have been widely tested as delivery vectors for different types of bioactive cargo (Figure 37.2). Among the widely used cargos are cytotoxic or cytostatic drugs, antibodies and peptides modifying cell division/apoptosis, as well as oligonucleotides and their analogs. A selection of different cargos delivered by CPPs and obtained antitumor effects are summarized in Table 37.2.

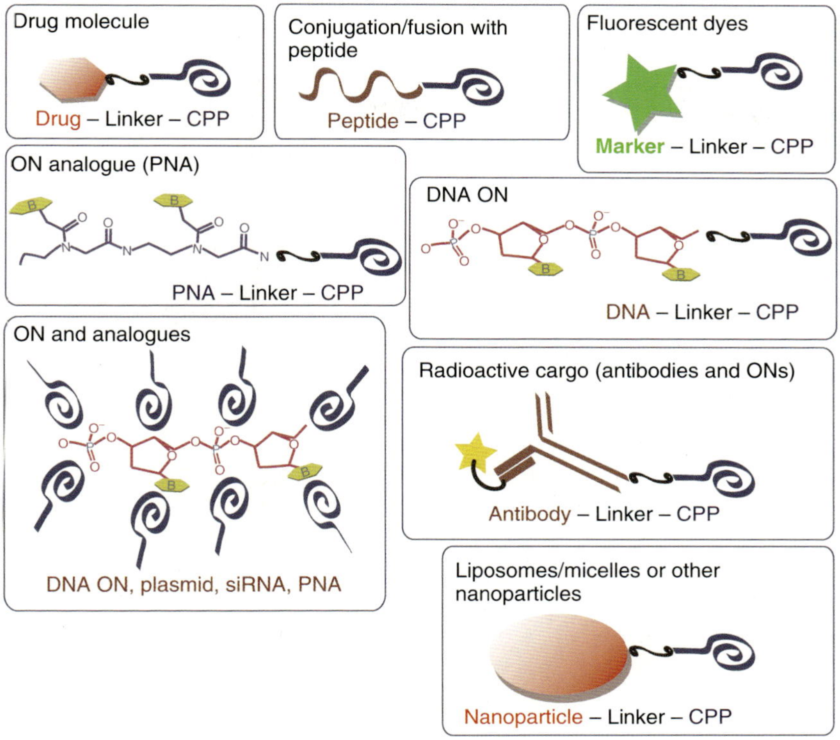

Figure 37.2 Selection of frequently used CPP–cargo types.

Table 37.1 Selected CPPs and their sequences.

CPP	Sequence	References
Penetratin	RQIKIWFQNRRMKWKK-NH_2	[10]
TAT (48–60)	GRKKRRQRRRPPQ	[2]
Transportan	GWTLNSAGYLLGKINLKALAALAKKIL-NH_2	[4]
TP10	AGYLLGKINLKALAALAKKIL-NH_2	[11]
Oligoarginine	$(RRR)_n$	[12]
Pep-1	KETWWETWWTEWSQPKKKRKV-Cya	[13]
MPG	GALFLGFLGAAGSTMGA-Cya	[14]

37.2.1
Modifying Classical Anticancer Drugs

One of the extensively studied fields of utilizing CPPs in oncologic research is through conjugation with classical chemotherapeutic agents. It has been shown that such an approach can modify several properties of the drug, such

Table 37.2 Examples of *in vivo* delivery of antineoplastic cargo or tumor-labeling markers by CPPs.

CPP	Cargo	Targeting mechanism	Effect	References
Penetratin SynB1	chemotherapeutic drug	–	delivery of otherwise nonpermeable chemotherapeutic drug into brain parenchyma in mice	[15, 16]
Pep-3	antisense PNA, targeting cell division	–	inhibition of tumor growth in mice	[17]
MPG-cholesterol	siRNA, targeting cell division	–	inhibition of tumor growth in mice	[18]
TAT	inhibitor of tumor-associated transcription factor	breast cancer-specific antibody mimetic	inhibition of tumor growth in mice	[19, 20]
Penetratin TAT	radiolabeled scFv against tumor-associated glycoprotein	cargo is also a targeting moiety	Increased tumor retention of scFvs in mice	[21]
TAT	radiolabeled antisense oligonucleotide	breast cancer-specific antibody	delivery of radionuclides to the tumor cell nuclei in mice	[22]
Oligoarginine	fluorescent label	activation of delivery vector by tumor-associated extracellular enzymes	accumulation of fluorescence into a wide variety of tumors and metastases in mice	[23]
pVEC	chemotherapeutic drug	tumor-homing peptide	increased antitumor efficacy of chemotherapeutic drugs in mice	[24]

as biodistribution, plasma half-life, drug internalization into the cell, and biological effect. Notably, a number of works have demonstrated that conjugation to CPPs helps overcome drug resistance, frequently accompanying serious hindrance with chemotherapy.

The advantage of peptide vectors is pronounced when delivery into "hard-to-reach" organs (like the brain) is necessary. The potential of CPPs as delivery vectors able to carry bioactive molecules through the blood–brain barrier (BBB) without eliciting any toxic reactions was demonstrated by Schwarze, who showed the ability of TAT to deliver large cargo, a 120-kDa β-galactosidase (β-Gal) protein, to all tissues in mice, including the brain, after systemic administration [5]. Central nervous system delivery by CPPs has been demonstrated on numerous occasions with different CPPs [25]. One of the first applications of CPPs in conjunction with chemotherapeutic drugs was demonstrated by Rouselle *et al.*, who conjugated doxorubicin with two different CPPs, penetratin and SynB1 (Figure 37.3) [15, 16]. Strikingly, vectors with either CPP were shown to penetrate the BBB and effectively carry doxorubicin into the brain parenchyma (free doxorubicin levels in

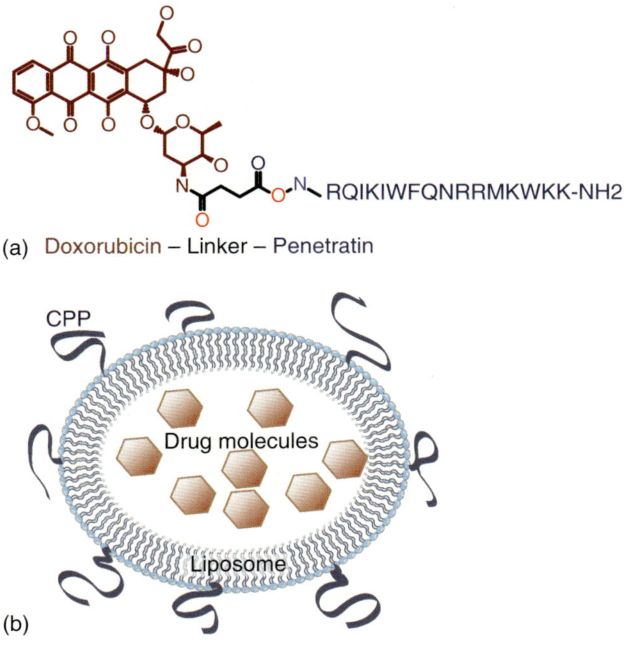

Figure 37.3 Schematic representation of two different approaches to designing a vector for the CPP-assisted delivery of antineoplastic agents into tumors. (a) Covalent conjugation of the anticancer drug (doxorubicin as an illustrating case) and the CPP (penetratin, in this case). CPP transports the drug into the cell and, depending on the design of the linker, liberates the drug. (b) Anticancer drug is encapsulated into liposomes, modified with CPP. Each liposome encapsulates many drug molecules and liberates them over time; CPP grants cell entry.

brain are negligible upon intravenous administration). The authors showed that CPP–doxorubicin was present in brain parenchyma at 20-fold higher levels than free doxorubicin.

Another advantage of CPPs conjugated to classical chemotherapeutics is their ability to overcome multidrug resistance (MDR). One of the mechanisms of MDR is overexpression of P-glycoprotein (P-gp), a drug efflux "pump," at tumor cell membranes [26]. Interestingly, the BBB also contains P-gp. Thus, the therapeutic potential of cerebral antineoplastic agents is particularly limited, as a result of the action of P-gp both at the BBB and tumor cells [27].

As a follow-up to the previously described work by Rouselle, where effective CPP–doxorubicin penetration into the brain was demonstrated [16], the same vectorized doxorubicin was tested *in vitro* for antitumor efficacy, using human doxorubicin-resistant cells. The conjugate showed more potent dose-dependent inhibition of cell growth, compared with about 20-fold higher IC_{50} for the free doxorubicin [15]. Doxorubicin resistance has also been effectively overcome when conjugating the drug with other CPPs, like TAT, penetratin, and maurocalcine [28–31].

Enhanced antitumor effects of the CPP–drug conjugates have been shown in several other works, with different classical chemotherapeutics and different CPPs. For example, enhanced efficacy of oligoarginine–Taxol® [32], as well as conjugates of CPPs YTA2 and YTA4 with methotrexate [33], and pVEC with chlorambucil [24, 34] against drug-resistant human cancer cell lines *in vitro* and *in vivo* has been shown. The conjugate can be designed in a way that the drug release can be controlled (for example the cargo is liberated only upon cleavage of the disulfide linker). This results in a more favorable pharmacokinetics, where the drug levels remain more sustained during longer periods of time, avoiding the bolus effect of the free drug.

One of the advantages of CPPs is that different cargo can be transported through the cell membrane. Accordingly, CPPs have been conjugated not only to classical chemotherapeutics, but also to other impermeable cytotoxic molecules. For example, *de novo* synthesized antimicrobial amphipathic peptide $(KLAKLAK)_2$, fused to a CPP, PTD5, inhibited the growth of tumors *in vitro* and in a mouse model [35]. Similarly, the chicken anemia virus-derived protein apoptin and TAT conjugate has been shown to selectively induce apoptosis in cancer cells *in vitro* [36].

There are other essentially similar vectors that are able to modify pharmacological properties of the drugs, besides CPPs. As of today, liposomes are probably the most widely used carriers of all kinds of small-molecular drugs, including classical chemotherapeutics (Doxil®). However, in spite of their advantages, most notably increasing metabolic stability and plasma half-life, using liposomes is accompanied by difficulties. One of these is related to biodistribution and tissue/cell penetration of this kind of delivery. Liposomes (and all larger-molecular-weight molecules and particles) accumulate in tumor tissues due to the enhanced permeability and retention (EPR) effect, but this will not guarantee cellular uptake. It has been demonstrated in many works that the cellular uptake efficacy of the liposomes can be greatly increased by conjugating them with a CPP (Figure 37.3b) [37–39]. Several groups are pursuing this approach, as it combines the advantages of both CPPs and liposomes, offering packing of drug molecules into complexes and high cellular uptake.

37.2.2 Inherent Antineoplastic Activity of CPPs

Among the large number of different peptides with cell-penetrating properties that have been found [40], some CPPs with inherent "special" properties have also been described. For example, some CPPs have inherent targeting properties, internalizing only into certain types of cells. Along the same line, some CPPs exert cytotoxic properties. The approach of finding these CPPs has attracted interest in tumor research [41]. For the peptides described in this section, it would be more correct to state that there are some peptides that exert cell-penetrating properties, because these are not generally used as CPPs (i.e., carrying different cargo into the cell).

An interesting paper by Laakonen *et al.* identified a peptide LyP-1 with inherent tumor lymphatic homing properties. LyP-1 was identified using phage-display as a peptide that binds to tumor, but not to normal cells. Fluorescein-labeled LyP-1 was shown to bind tumor-associated lymphatic vessels and tumor cells in MDA-MB-435 xenografts. Intriguingly, this peptide effectively internalized into certain tumor cells and exerted cytotoxic effects, inducing apoptosis *in vitro* and inhibiting tumor growth *in vivo* upon intravenous administration. In agreement with the binding properties of LyP-1, the tumors of the treated animals showed reduced numbers of lymphatic vessels, compared to the tumors from untreated animals [42].

One of the first described CPPs with cytotoxic properties was a peptide derived from $p14^{ARF}$, a peptide often deregulated in cancers. It has been shown that a shorter N-terminal fragment of $p14^{ARF}$ is capable of mimicking the function of the intact $p14^{ARF}$ protein [43]. Interestingly, it was discovered that this fragment had cell-penetrating properties, exerting similar cell internalization efficacies as a known CPP, TP10, and effectively inhibiting the growth of MCF-7 and MDA-MB-231 cells, resulting in significant decrease in proliferation in both cell lines [44]. Another example is a recent work that described cytotoxic CPP L-2, derived from antilipopolysaccharide factor of a horseshoe crab *Limulus*. Apparently, this peptide has CPP capacity and antineoplastic effects, both *in vitro* and *in vivo*, although the tumor-specific apoptotic mechanism is not known [45].

37.2.3 Delivery of Nucleic Acids and Oligonucleotides

Oligonucleotides are increasingly recognized for their potential as therapeutic agents against a variety of diseases. Unfortunately, for delivery vectors like liposomes, the delivery is restricted only to certain organs. Consequently, it is not surprising that the most popular clinical targets have been related to drug delivery into liver, spleen, kidneys, and lungs, and it is no coincidence that much of the successful oligonucleotide delivery seen in recent years has targeted disease within these organs [46]. Fortunately, using oligonucleotides in oncology seems a fairly promising prospect, because of the EPR effect in tumor tissue [47], rendering the tumor blood vessels "leaky." This results in higher possibilities of delivering any vector into tumors.

There are numerous examples of delivering oligonucleotides, as well as oligonucleotide analogs and plasmids, using CPPs. The classical way of delivering cargo with CPPs is to attach the payload via a covalent bond (Figure 37.4). This approach has the advantage of allowing selective "activation" of the cargo after the drug

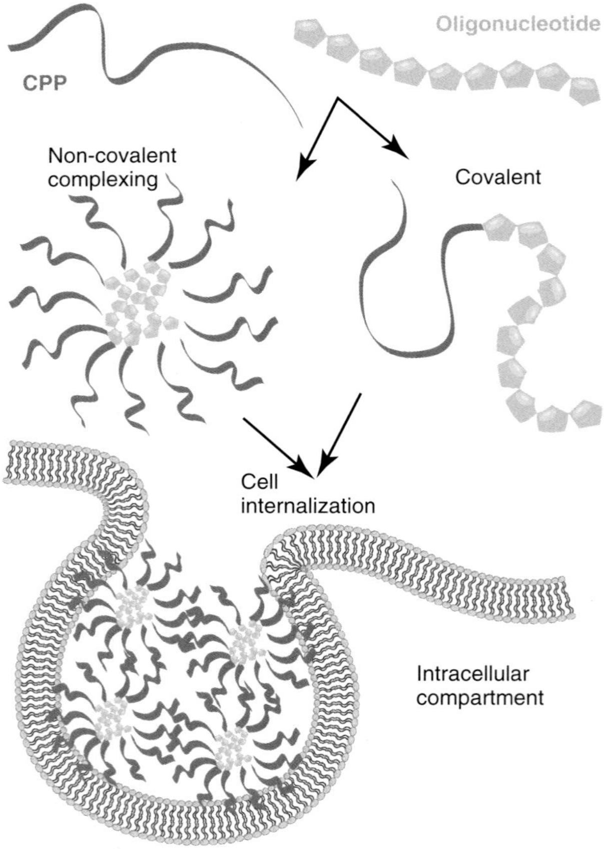

Figure 37.4 Strategies for the vectorization of oligonucleotides with CPPs. Oligonucleotides can be vectorized via a covalent conjugation of the nucleic acid and the peptide carrier. Alternatively, noncovalent complexing of the cationic CPP moiety and anionic nucleic acids can be performed.

molecule has been delivered into the cell and released. However, for the delivery of oligonucleotides, the noncovalent strategy offers the advantage of simplification of vector preparation and flexibility, as the same vector (CPP) can be used for the delivery of different oligonucleotides, by simply mixing the two together (Figure 37.4). Nevertheless, both covalent and noncovalent strategies have been successfully used.

Henke *et al.* conjugated a CPP with an antisense oligonucleotide to the gene Id1, a transcription factor required for tumor invasiveness, metastasis, and angiogenesis. For this, an antisense oligonucleotide delivery vector was constructed, based on a CPP, F3, that homes specifically to tumor neovessels. The CPP F3 is a 31-amino-acid fragment of human high mobility group protein 2, that has been shown to internalize into the nuclei of lung carcinoma and breast cancer cells [48]. Due to the inherent tumor-targeting properties of the CPP, Id1 was effectively downregulated in tumor endothelial cells *in vitro* and *in vivo*. Moreover, the group demonstrated *in vivo* enhanced hemorrhage, hypoxia, and inhibition of primary tumor growth and metastasis in two different tumor models – breast cancer and lung carcinoma – after systemic (intravenous) administration of the vector [49].

Most effort, however, has been invested in noncovalent strategies (Figure 37.4) for the delivery of oligonucleotides or their analogs. For example, a short amphipathic peptide Pep-3 is a vector designed for the noncovalent delivery of PNA. Pep-3, in complex with cyclin B1 antisense PNA, has been shown to block tumor growth *in vivo* upon intravenous injection [17]. MPG is a TAT-derived CPP vector, designed for the noncovalent delivery of single- and double-stranded oligonucleotides [14]. MPG complex with antisense oligonucleotide targeting MDR1, a gene encoding the MDR P-gp drug efflux "pump," reversed the drug resistance in leukemia cells [50]. In addition, MPG, complexed with the telomerase antisense oligonucleotide effectively decreased the IC_{50}, of the unvectorized oligonucleotide, inhibiting the expression of telomerase in renal carcinoma cells [51].

The newest field of the oligonucleotide applications is RNA interference (RNAi). The first clinical results of using small interfering RNA (siRNA) in humans are just beginning to appear. Very recently, the first example of using siRNA to inhibit the growth of solid tumors in humans was published [52]. Considering that application of RNAi is only starting to develop and that utilizing CPPs for oligonucleotide delivery as a very recent advance in the field, promising applications may be expected in the future.

One of the first examples of using RNAi against tumor activity with CPP-mediated delivery was described in 2006 [53]. In this work, siRNA against Mdm2 (Figure 37.5), a p53-associated oncogene, was encapsulated into oligoarginine-liposomes. This siRNA vector demonstrated high transfection efficiency in SK-MES-1 lung tumor cells, resistant for the regular liposome, Lipofectamine 2000-mediated transfection. As a result, the expression of the Mdm2 was knocked down and *in vitro* proliferation of cancer cells was inhibited.

More importantly, many works have demonstrated the usefulness of CPPs in siRNA delivery *in vivo*. For example, cholesterol-modified oligoarginine was shown to complex with siRNA and effectively silence the vascular endothelial growth factor (VEGF) gene, inhibiting tumor growth in a mouse model upon local administration [54]. In another study, Crombez *et al.* modified the CPP peptide MPG with cholesterol and demonstrated that this was an effective vector, capable of delivering siRNA upon intravenous administration, without any toxic effects [18]. Indeed, the vector, in complex with cyclin B1 siRNA, inhibited tumor growth *in vivo*. An interesting approach was taken by Dowdy's group, who developed a TAT-derived siRNA delivery vector (PTD-DRBD) [55]. This group performed combinatorial targeting of two known oncogenes, simultaneously knocking down both epidermal growth factor receptor (EGFR) and Akt2 [56]. This approach increased the survival of the animals bearing intracerebral glioblastoma, upon intratumoral injection of the CPP–siRNA complexes. Similar peptide carrier and siRNA complexes have also been designed using CPPs derived from protamine. For example, siRNA against VEGF was complexed with protamine-derived CPP and it was shown that, upon systemic (intraperitoneal) administration, this effectively suppressed tumor growth *in vivo* [57], without any toxic side-effects. TAT, in comparison, worked with identical efficacy [57].

Several other promising strategies utilizing noncovalent complexation of negatively charged oligo- or polynucleotides (steric block oligonucleotide, siRNA, plasmid DNA) with CPPs have been described recently. For example, stearylated TP10 as an efficient vector for splice-correction assay [58] and stearylated $(RxR)_4$ as plasmid and splice-correcting oligonucleotide delivery vehicle [59] have been described. Another promising strategy involves using CPP-modified liposomes (Figure 37.3b), pioneered by the group of Torchilin. Efficient *in vivo* transfection with a model plasmid, Green Fluorescent Protein (GFP), has been demonstrated via intratumoral injection of TAT–liposome–plasmid complexes, resulting in production of GFP protein by Lewis lung carcinoma tumor cells. In contrast, no fluorescence was seen with liposome–plasmid complexes without TAT [60]. The same group has also shown that a TAT–liposome delivery vector, in complex with GFP plasmid, is capable of selectively transfecting U87 glioblastoma cells in a mouse intracranial tumor model, after intratumoral injection. Transfection selectivity was seen, because no signal was detected from adjacent normal brain tissue [61].

37.2.4
CPP Application in Oncogenic Signaling and Cell Cycle Modulation in Tumors

Oncogenic signaling as a result of cancer-dependent protein–protein interactions can induce oncogenesis, through cell cycle progression, inhibition of apoptosis, and insensitivity to antigrowth signals. Increases in oncoprotein nuclear translocation are often observed in cancer cells, and can further promote transformation and metastases. Significant progress has been made in the identification of tumor-specific cellular pathways, which can be strategically blocked *in vitro* and *in vivo*. Recently, a growing number of studies have demonstrated successful application of CPPs in the modulation of tumor biology, and in the induction of cancer cell apoptosis *in vitro* as well as in preclinical animal models.

37.2.4.1 **Oncoproteins**

Oncoproteins are normal proteins that can become oncogenic due to mutations or increased expression. Normally, they help to regulate cell growth and differentiation, and are often involved in signal transduction and execution of mitogenic signals, but once overactivated can become tumor-inducing agents. A number of these oncoprotein pathways have been targeted with CPP-based delivery vectors (see Figure 37.5 for an overview).

One of such oncoproteins is MUC1, displaying deregulated expression in many types of cancers [62]. Interactions of MUC1 with other oncogenes (Src, glycogen synthase kinase 3β, EGFR, β-catenin) are important for cancer progression. This interaction was targeted by Bitler *et al.*, who designed a MUC1-inhibiting

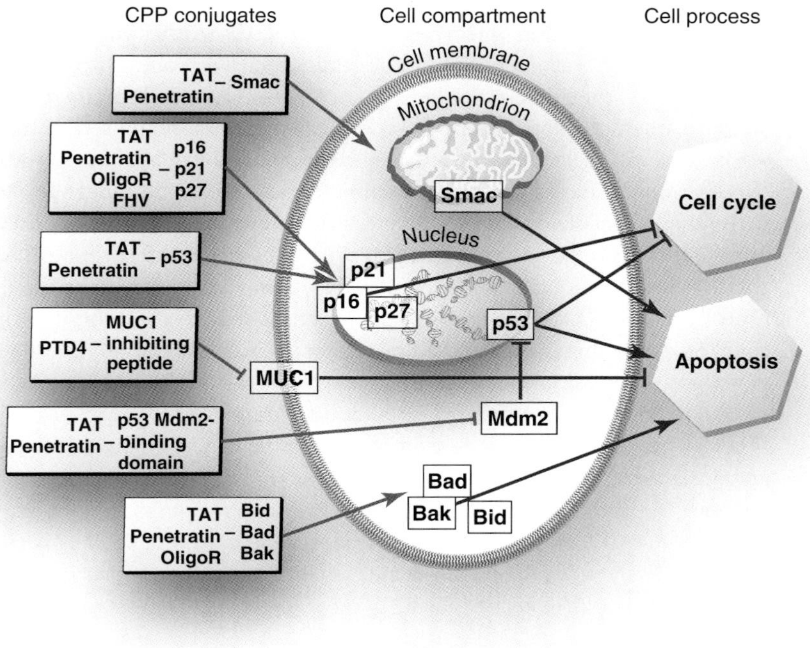

Figure 37.5 Overview of interactions between selected oncogenes and cell growth/death processes. The middle part depicts oncogenes that are discussed in the text and their schematic localization in the cell. The left part lists CPP-conjugated oncogenes and their enhancing or inhibiting interactions with cell division or apoptosis are shown on the right part.

peptide that blocked the intracellular interaction of MUC1 with other oncogenes. Linking this inhibitor peptide to a CPP, PTD4, resulted in effective inhibition of breast cancer cell growth *in vitro* and *in vivo* in a mouse model upon systemic administration [63].

Another frequently studied oncogene is the mitochondrial protein Smac that can inactivate the inhibitor of apoptosis proteins (IAPs). Several studies have shown that Smac, linked to either TAT or penetratin, sensitized cells to proapoptotic stimuli. For example, Fulda *et al.* tested the function of the Smac–TAT peptide in an intracranial glioblastoma xenograft model. The authors showed that coadministration of tumor necrosis factor-related apoptosis-inducing ligand (TRAIL) and Smac–TAT provided a synergistic effect on tumor volume reduction and consequent increase in mouse survival. Furthermore, histological analysis revealed no evidence of remaining tumor in the brain [64]. Another group has produced a Smac–penetratin fusion peptide, and showed that treatment of human breast cancer cells with this fusion peptide significantly enhanced induction of apoptosis and long-term antiproliferative effects of different antineoplastic agents, including paclitaxel, etoposide, and doxorubicin [65]. Similar disruption of apoptosis inhibition was also seen when melanoma IAP (melanoma inhibitor of apoptosis protein ML-IAP) was conjugated to penetratin [66]. In yet another study, linking the N-terminal domain of Smac to oligoarginine enhanced chemotherapy-induced suppression of non-small-cell lung cancer cell growth in mouse xenografts [67].

The proteins of Bcl-2 family are important regulators of apoptosis. Thus, death suppressors such as Bcl-X_L have been found to play a role in cancer development by inhibiting normal cell death, whereas other homologs like Bak and Bax have opposing functions and promote apoptosis. Cancer cells often show altered balance between these proapoptotic and antiapoptotic proteins. Consequently, the expression of truncated Bak could be sufficient to induce cell death in transfected cells. This hypothesis was tested by Holinger *et al.*, who showed that delivery of penetratin–Bak conjugate into the cytosol of intact HeLa cells resulted in the induction of a caspase-dependent apoptotic program [68].

Letai *et al.* refined these observations further by exploring the ability to induce apoptosis in cancer cells by transduction of the BH3 domains of the Bcl-2-derived peptides Bid and Bad [69]. Utilization of conjugates containing the proapoptotic peptides with CPP oligoarginine was more efficient than with CPPs penetratin and TAT, effectively inducing apoptosis and sensitizing to killing *in vitro* [69], and in a neuroblastoma model *in vivo* [70].

37.2.4.2 **Tumor Suppressor p53**

Cell proliferation is an ordered, tightly regulated process involving multiple checkpoints that assess extracellular growth signals, cell size, and DNA integrity. Processes that govern cell cycle entrance/exit also play an important role in tumor growth. The function of the tumor suppressor gene p53 is severed in more than 50% of human tumors. Consequently, regulation of apoptosis, DNA repair, and cell cycle is impaired. Reconstitution of p53 restores the link between proapoptotic stimuli and apoptotic execution machinery, resulting in cell death in a DNA damage dependent manner.

Selivanova *et al.* linked CPP penetratin to the C-terminal of p53 peptide, and found that the fusion peptide could activate specific DNA binding of wild-type p53 *in vitro* and could restore the transcriptional transactivating function of mutant p53 proteins in living cells [71]. Moreover, penetratin–p53 fusion caused apoptosis in mutant as well as in wild-type p53-carrying human tumor cell lines of different origin, whereas normal cells were not affected [72]. These findings raised for the first time the possibility of developing a CPP-based drug that restored the tumor suppressor function of mutant p53, thus selectively eliminating tumor cells. Similar results were later obtained by Araki *et al.*, who developed fusion peptides using different CPPs like TAT, oligoarginine, and FHV, and linked them to the C-terminal domain of p53. Their results showed that a single application of oligoarginine–p53 and FHV–p53 significantly inhibited the growth of bladder cancer cells, decreasing tumor burden and increasing survival in a model of bladder cancer [73].

Several reports have demonstrated application of CPPs in the suppression of Mdm2, a protein inducing degradation of p53, overexpressed in many cancers. For instance, Kanovsky *et al.* prepared a series of peptides derived from the p53 Mdm2-binding region and additionally attached to the CPP penetratin to permit cellular internalization. The idea was to produce competitive binding to p53-degrading Mdm2 and subsequent preservation of cellular p53 activity. Indeed, blockage of the binding of p53 to Mdm2 in transformed pancreatic cells increased the half-life of p53, resulting in cell cycle arrest and apoptosis. Such treatment did not have any effect on the growth of normal cells. Interestingly, cancer cell death could be induced even in p53-mutant or-null cancer cells [74]. These results were further tested *in vivo* by Harbour *et al.*, who developed a TAT fusion peptide with the Mdm2-inhibiting construct and tested this in a rabbit xenograft model of retinoblastoma. They demonstrated accumulation of p53 and preferential apoptosis of tumor cells, with no effect on normal cells and no histological damage of the retina upon intravitreal injection [75]. Similar results have also been demonstrated with penetratin fusion with Mdm2-binding residues [76].

37.2.4.3 **Tumor Suppressor p16**

Tumor suppressor protein p16, encoded by the CDKN2A (cyclin-dependent kinase inhibitor 2A) gene plays an important role in cell cycle regulation by preventing the formation of active cyclin D–CDK4/6 complexes and providing G_0/G_1 phase cell cycle arrest. Deletions and mutations in p16 increase the risk of developing a variety of cancers. In accordance with this, several studies have demonstrated that wild-type p16, covalently linked to a CPP (penetratin–p16, TAT–p16), rapidly transduces into cells and retains its properties of eliciting an early G_1 phase cell cycle arrest by subsequent inhibition of cyclin D–CDK4/6 activity [77–79]. The TAT-mediated protein transduction method was also used to introduce p16 into primary peripheral blood lymphocytes, and highlighted the role of p16 and cyclin D–CDK4/6 in regulating the reversible transition from G_0 to early G_1. In addition, deregulation of cyclin D–CDK4/6 complexes in human malignancy prevents cells from exiting early G_1/G_0 and only additional mutational events can inappropriately activate cyclin E–CDK2 complexes and drive cells across the irreversible restriction point into G_1/S phase [80].

Finally, in experiments performed by Hosotani *et al.*, intraperitoneal delivery of a penetratin–p16 fusion peptide inhibited the growth of pancreatic cancer cells, growing as peritoneal or subcutaneous tumors in nude mice. The authors found that penetratin–p16 slowed tumor growth by inducing apoptosis in cancer cells [81]. At the same time no toxicity to normal tissues was observed, indicating that cancer cells may be much more sensitive to the effects of transducible tumor suppressor peptides than nontransformed cells.

37.2.4.4 **Tumor Suppressors p21 and p27**

Recent developments have shown that the reactivation of the p53 pathway in tumors can be achieved also by restoration or mimicry of the p21 protein, which is capable of mediating cell growth suppression by inhibition of the G_1 cyclin–CDK complexes. Treatment of tumor cells with p21-derived peptide, coupled to CPPs penetratin or TAT, was able to induce strong G_1 phase cell cycle arrest [82–84] and showed that p21 can also function in different cells with wild-type p53. In another report, Chen *et al.* introduced short peptides that can block the interaction of cyclin A–CDK2 with the transcription factor E2F1 substrates. Thus, E2F1-derived peptide and p21-derived peptide were introduced into the cells as chimeras containing either TAT or penetratin. These peptides preferentially induced transformed cells to undergo apoptosis relative to nontransformed cells, demonstrating that short peptides can block the interaction of cyclin A–CDK2 and cyclin E–CDK2 complexes with their substrates and selectively kill transformed cells [85].

p27, encoded by the CDKN1B gene, is a CDK inhibitor, often deregulated in tumors. p27 is capable of preventing the activation of cyclin E–CDK2 or cyclin D–CDK4 complexes and thus controls the cell cycle progression at G_1, inhibiting cell division. In order to reconstitute the tumor suppressor function of p27 in cancer cells, Nagahara *et al.* synthesized TAT–p27 fusion peptide and demonstrated its transduction ability into a variety of cell types, resulting in a substantial G_1 phase cell cycle arrest [86]. Similar results with TAT–p27 were obtained by Parada *et al.*, showing the antitumor potential of such constructs [87].

37.3
Tumor Targeting of CPPs

Use of CPPs as therapeutic delivery vectors has the disadvantage of a lack of an inherent targeting mechanism, as most CPPs are able to transduce all cells, without any regard to the cell type, proliferative state, and so on. On the other hand, this high transduction efficacy is needed to be able to deliver cargo to hard-to-reach tissues (like the brain) or into the tissue parenchyma, beyond blood vessels. Unfortunately, tumor cells themselves can be considered as a difficult target. Accordingly, poor tissue penetration of classical chemotherapeutics [88] and antibodies [89] has been shown. Moreover, if drug resistance has developed [26], the drug uptake is usually seriously compromised. Both of these problems have been overcome by using CPPs.

There are two broad approaches to the targeting problem. Some delivery vectors rely on inherent differences in the tumor environment (e.g., differences in extracellular physicochemical characteristics such as pH). These vectors – *passive targeting* vectors – do not actively seek tumor cells, but release the drug when blood flow carries them into this different environment. Other targeting mechanisms – *active targeting* – include an element that binds to a specific oncogene, such as a ligand binding to a receptor, or monoclonal antibody (mAb), targeted against a tumor-specific antigene. Although active targeting also relies on (passive) blood flow into the tumor area, the interaction between delivery vector and tumor cells is active binding in nature. Both classes of targeting have been extensively utilized with CPP delivery vectors, and have their own advantages and disadvantages. An overview of CPP-related tumor-targeting systems is presented in Figure 37.6.

37.3.1 Passive Targeting of CPPs

37.3.1.1 EPR Effect

The EPR effect [47] is a result of increased permeability of the tumor vasculature to circulating macromolecules due to defects in the endothelium. As a result, low-molecular-weight drugs coupled with high-molecular-weight carriers tend to

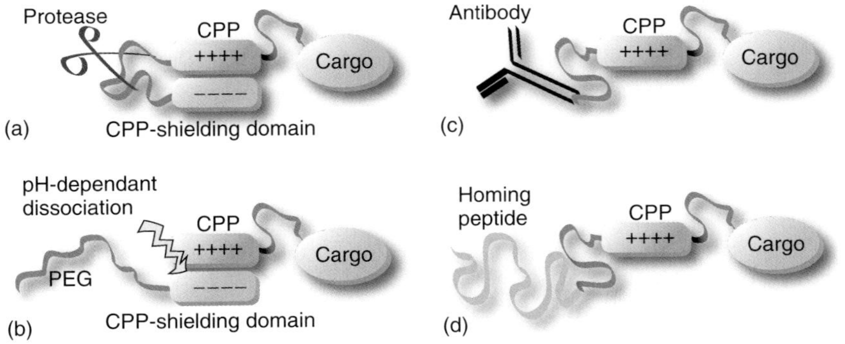

Figure 37.6 Schematic representation of selected tumor-targeting mechanisms applied to CPP-based drug delivery vectors. (a and b) Passive targeting mechanisms; these systems rely on different extracellular properties of the tumor tissue, such as high levels of certain proteases or lower pH. (c and d) Frequently used active targeting vector systems. (a) Protease-dependent activation of the CPP [90]. CPP and cargo can internalize into the cell after tumor-specific extracellular enzymes cleave the CPP-shielding domain, exposing the CPP. (b) pH-dependent deshielding of the CPP [91]. CPP is exposed upon entering a lower pH environment, such as in tumors, after which the cargo can be internalized into nearby cells. (c) Antibody-dependent binding of the vector [92]. CPP–cargo internalization occurs after tumor-specific binding of the antibody. (d) Tumor targeting by homing peptides [93]. Selective tumor targeting is achieved through high-affinity binding of the homing peptide.

accumulate into tumors. In theory, any CPP-based delivery vector (or any other type of delivery vector, in this context) should concentrate in tumors as a result of the EPR effect, even without an active targeting mechanism. This should also be considered when analyzing the treatment results with various novel delivery vectors; for example, it is often demonstrated that the targeted delivery vector, conjugated to an antineoplastic drug, shows superior accumulation into tumors, compared to the free drug. Theoretically, this could be not because of the targeting mechanism, but at least partly because of the enhanced retention, as the drug delivery vector is simply a larger molecule than the free drug and its renal clearance has been altered, resulting in increased plasma half-life and enhanced tumor retention. In essence, discovery of the EPR and taking advantage of this effect in anticancer therapies is of course excellent, but it may somewhat diminish the value of other targeting mechanisms, as it is not easy to determine which mechanism underlies the tumor accumulation.

37.3.1.2 Matrix Metalloproteases

Several reports have utilized extracellular enzymatic activity, involved in angiogenesis and cell migration processes, as a targeting mechanism, as these enzymes are essential in tumor growth, neovascularization, and metastases. CPPs have been used with tumor-related proteases such as matrix metalloproteinases (MMPs) – a family of enzymes responsible for the breakdown of the extracellular matrix. This process is important in normal cell migration and proliferation. The MMP peptides have been shown to be upregulated in many tumors [94], mediating tissue invasion and metastasis.

Aguilera *et al.* designed a vector where tumor-specific MMP activity cleaves inactive prodrug, resulting in release of the activated CPP vector (Figure 37.6a). The vector consisted of three domains: an oligoarginine-based CPP, a negatively charged polyglutamate (CPP-shielding) domain, and, connecting them, an MMP enzyme-cleavable linker. In the native, prodrug state, the negatively charged polyglutamate domain shields the oligoarginine domain by electrostatic interaction. In the presence of MMP, however, the connecting linker is cleaved and the CPP deshielded, allowing cell entry [90]. This model has been shown to be efficient in selective *in vivo* labeling of a wide variety of different tumors and metastases upon intravenous administration [23]. The approach was very recently broadened by the same group. In order to find new tumor-specific protease substrate sequences they did not use a rational design, but parallel *in vivo* and *in vitro* phage-display selection. As a result, a unique sequence was described that was cleaved by plasmin and elastases, both of which have been shown to be overexpressed in tumors. A similar fluorescently tagged oligoarginine vector, but now containing the new linker domain, selectively labeled mammary tumors and metastases *in vivo* after intravenous injection [95].

37.3.1.3 pH- and O_2-Sensitive CPP Systems

Another possibility to target the delivery is to take advantage of the lower pH in the extracellular matrix of the tumors and design a drug-releasing mechanism, dependent on certain pH values (Figure 37.6). Sethuraman *et al.* have designed a delivery system this way, consisting of a CPP–drug core and a pH-dependent shielding shell. The core was a poly(ethylene glycol) (PEG)–TAT conjugated polymeric micelle, capable of incorporating antineoplastic agent. The shielding shell, constructed from a pH-sensitive copolymer of sulfonamide and PEG, detaches from the main particle at lower pH values, deshielding the TAT. Accordingly, significantly higher *in vitro* cellular uptake of TAT micelles was observed at pH 6.6 compared to a normal pH [96].

A similar approach was also tested *in vivo* by Kale *et al.*, who used pegylated CPP–liposomes as drug carriers [97]. The PEG-shielding was attached through pH-dependent hydrazone bond, which is degraded in lower pH environments, deshielding and exposing the underlying TAT peptide. This system was tested both in tumor and ischemic cells, both characterized by lower extracellular pH, *in vitro* and *in vivo*. As a result, the pH-targeted fluorescent vector showed higher internalization into lung carcinoma xenografts upon intratumoral injection *in vivo*, compared to the pH-insensitive vector [91].

Unregulated proliferation and high metabolic demands of tumor cells lead to development of hypoxia in solid tumors. Harada has designed a delivery vector that is in stable conformation only in hypoxic environments, using an oxygen-dependent degradation domain (ODD) of the hypoxia-inducible factor-1α, coupled to TAT. This vector is degraded in the presence of higher levels of oxygen (i.e., in normoxic conditions). The efficacy and specificity of the vector was tested both *in vitro* and *in vivo* using β-Gal as a marker and caspase-3 as an apoptotic agent. As expected, TAT–ODD–β-Gal was detected from the tumors but not in normal tissues in a mouse model after intraperitoneal injection. When delivering apoptotic agent, TAT–ODD–caspase-3 effectively inhibited the growth of the tumor without causing toxic side-effects that would be expected from delivering active caspase-3 to an entire mouse [98].

37.3.2 Active Targeting of CPPs

37.3.2.1 Antibodies as a Targeting Moiety

Owing to their ability to specifically recognize their respective antigens, antibodies are probably the most logical choice of targeting agent for the delivery vehicle (Figure 37.6). Moreover, in some cases, antibodies can inhibit the functional activity of the target antigen (oncogene, in this case); these kind of antibodies are also being used as unarmed therapeutics (such as anti-VEGF or anti-HER2 antibodies), or, when in combination with delivery vehicle, dual antineoplastic effect can be obtained [19]. Antibodies represent one of most often used targeting mechanisms with numerous examples for *in vivo* use.

As an early attempt, Anderson *et al.* designed a conjugation strategy between antitumor mAbs and a synthetic amphipathic peptide GALA, as well as with TAT. It was shown that peptide conjugation enhanced the retention and internalization of the antigen-binding Fab fragments of the antimelanoma and pan-carcinoma antibodies *in vitro* [99, 100].

In addition to the CPP and antibody, another cytotoxic entity or cargo can be added to the delivery vehicle. For example, Song *et al.* have designed a protamine–antibody fusion protein to deliver siRNA to specific cell types [92], targeting one of the most widely used oncogenes, EGFR ErbB2, as this receptor is overexpressed in many breast cancer cells. Accordingly, anti-ErbB2 single-chain variable fragment (scFV) antibody fused with protamine effectively delivered siRNA *in vitro* and silenced Ku70 (involved in DNA repair) specifically in ErbB2-expressing breast cancer cells, but not in ErbB2-negative cells. The antibody–CPP conjugate vectors have proved their tumor selectivity and antitumor efficacy also *in vivo*. For example, TAT conjugated to the anti-HER2/*neu* peptide mimetic AHNP specifically targeted ErbB2-overexpressing breast cancer cells *in vitro* and *in vivo* [19]. Moreover, when additionally conjugated to an inhibitor of STAT3, a transcription factor that is often constitutively active in tumors, the vector effectively inhibited tumor cell growth *in vitro* and *in vivo* (upon intraperitoneal injection) more readily in ErbB2 overexpressing cells, compared to ErbB2 low-expressing cancer cells [19].

Sawant *et al.* have described an even more complicated system, where cancer-specific antinucleosome mAb 2C5 is attached to long-circulating PEGylated liposomes, additionally modified with TAT. This system includes double targeting: in addition to the cancer-specific antibody, there is a pH-sensitive control mechanism, shielding TAT with the hydrazone-PEG moiety (as described in the previous section). The pH sensitive hydrazone-PEG unshields TAT at lower pH values. The advantage of this system is that the nonspecific activity of the CPP is blocked until it reaches its target. Thus, although the liposomes demonstrated binding with antibody substrates at normal pH, no cellular internalization occurred. When U87 glioblastoma cells were incubated at lower pH, the nanocarriers were effectively internalized [101].

37.3.2.2 **Radioimmunotherapy**

CPPs have also been successfully applied in a related field, in radioimmunotherapy (i.e., the use of an antibody labeled with a radionuclide to deliver cytotoxic radiation into tumor cells). Currently, radiolabeled antibodies, such as Bexxar® and Zevalin® (directed against CD20), have been approved by the US Food and Drug Administration (FDA) for the therapy of non-Hodgkin's lymphoma. Unfortunately, only modest success has been achieved with tumor-antigen-targeted intact antibodies as vehicles to deliver diagnostic and therapeutic agents to solid tumors [102]. The main obstacles include long circulation times and poor penetration, as a result of the large molecular mass of the IgG. The expected role of CPPs is to improve the uptake and tissue penetration of the antibodies, and thus increase the efficacy of this kind of therapeutic.

To improve the pharmacokinetics and biodistribution of the mAbs, antibody fragments (scFVs) could be used instead. Due to their smaller size, improved biodistribution could be expected. However, scFVs are rapidly eliminated from the circulation and the resultant accumulation into tumors is poor. Jain *et al.*

coadministered therapeutic scFVs with the CPP penetratin, and achieved improved tumor uptake and more homogeneous tumor distribution [21], without any increase in the uptake by normal tissues. However, it yet remains to be elucidated if this strategy can be extrapolated for the delivery of other antibodies.

An interesting work was reported by Hu *et al.*, who used an antibody directed against an intracellular target p21 [103]. p21 is a CDK inhibitor, a key cell cycle regulator and a protein predominantly found in the nucleus. The underlying idea was delivering a radiolabeled mAb into the tumor cell nuclei. Indeed, it was shown that the CPP activity of the TAT peptide resulted in a significant increase in the accumulation of radioactivity into the nuclei of tumor cells. Although these results are most interesting, suggesting an effective intracellularly directed radioimmunotherapy, the drawback of the current work may be the lack of a tumor-targeting mechanism, as the antibody was targeted against an intracellular factor (and thus would not aid in recognizing tumor cells).

In this regard, an advanced study was conducted by Liu *et al.*, who also designed a tumor-specific radionuclide delivery vector, but instead of radioactive antibodies, they used radioactive antisense technology [22]. This work used the observation that antisense oligonucleotides, once intracellular, are retained in the cell nucleus and therefore are a good moiety to carry radionuclides [22]. Thus, they have used an antisense oligonucleotide directed against the mRNA of an oncogene RIa, overexpressed in many tumor types. To achieve tumor cell targeting, anti-HER2 antibody trastuzumab was linked to TAT via biotin–streptavidin linking. Interestingly, *in vivo* tumor and normal tissue levels of the TAT–trastuzumab–oligonucleotide nanoparticles were comparable to those of the free trastuzumab (confirming the intactness of the mAb), but the nanoparticles showed nuclear accumulation only in tumor tissue – a result attributable to the antisense oligonucleotide binding against an oncogene mRNA.

37.3.2.3 **Homing Peptides**

Utilizing tumor-homing peptides is a widely used strategy to achieve tumor targeting. The "homing" research was pioneered by Ruoslahti, who has extensively screened for peptide sequences that bind selectively to tumor tissues, but not to normal tissues. Ruoslahti *et al.* has concentrated on finding homing sequences that also exert cell-penetrating properties and has characterized several such homing CPPs [41].

The first report of combining homing domains and CPPs (Figure 37.6) conjugated a homing peptide, PEGA, previously shown to accumulate in breast tumor vasculature [93], and a CPP, pVEC [24]. PEGA peptide did not cross the plasma membrane *per se*; however, when attached to the CPP, the conjugate was efficiently taken up by different breast cancer cells *in vitro* and *in vivo*. Furthermore, the efficacy of a chemotherapeutic drug, chlorambucil, was increased upon conjugation to the pVEC. In another work, Mäe *et al.* designed a similar delivery construct, based on yet another homing sequence from Ruoslahti's group, CREKA [104]. An enhanced *in vitro* cell growth-inhibiting effect of chlorambucil was reported [34].

It is also possible to find homing sequences to tumor lymphatic vessels. Thus, a homing sequence LyP-1 was characterized. Quite interestingly, this homing peptide also has cell-penetrating properties and induced apoptosis upon internalization into the cell, effectively inhibiting tumor growth *in vivo* [42]. A similar example is a peptide derived from azurin, a cupredoxin secreted by *Pseudomonas aeruginosa*. It was shown that this peptide, termed p28, preferentially penetrates human cancer cells and exerts cytotoxic effects with no apparent activity on nontumor cells. Interestingly, very recently, peptide p28 entered phase I clinical trials to determine the safety of the potential anticancer peptide.

37.4
Advantages and Considerations of CPPs as Delivery Vectors

The main interest for developing CPP-based vectors is due to their potential for broad biodistribution and low cytotoxicity. It is important that peptide-based vectors are generally much less toxic than other types of delivery vehicles. Broad biodistribution of the CPP vectors is reflected by large number of CPP-based research papers that do not target liver, lung, or kidneys [25]. While not essentially a prerequisite for cancer therapy in general, BBB penetration is a necessary property for targeting brain tumors, as the ineffectiveness of classical chemotherapy for gliomas is well known. Although lipid carriers and the PEGylation strategy have been shown to improve brain penetration [105], the improvement in treatment efficacy in humans is questionable [106]. The examples presented in previous sections show the advantage of adding a CPP moiety to the drug vector and resultant increase in cellular uptake of the drug, antibody-targeted drug, or liposomes.

Nevertheless, CPP-based vectors are a newer field, compared to more traditional viral vectors and liposomes, and it will be yet proved if these potential advantages can be realized in the clinic. To date, many applications have utilized the most elementary TAT or oligoarginine-based peptides. In the future, more advanced peptide systems will probably be available that exert more potential to be developed as a universal vector system. This would also boost the clinical utilization of CPPs as oligonucleotide vectors.

As already discussed in Section 37.3, an advantage of CPPs – broad biodistribution capacity – is paradoxically also a disadvantage of these vectors. The reason is that adding a targeting moiety to a delivery vector also means additional optimization of the targeted delivery. Unfortunately, this aspect is rarely addressed. The potential problem is that the targeting activity is usually absolutely independent from the cell-penetrating activity, which means that adding a targeting property will not eliminate the ability to penetrate into nontarget cells and concomitantly deliver the cytotoxic drug also into normal tissues. The target/nontarget delivery efficacy as a function of the CPP/targeting moiety ratio has been demonstrated in earlier studies. Thus, higher CPP/targeting moiety ratios result in higher nontarget internalization [21, 99, 100]. This is a factor that should be considered when developing a targeted CPP vector.

One simple way of eliminating the need to target the drug vector to tumors is using a local administration procedure. Local administration has an advantage of eliminating a large part of toxicity to normal tissues. However, this can be applied only to certain tumors and this approach does not influence metastasis. Therefore, there is no clinical demand for a delivery vector that could be used only locally. Unfortunately, a large number of research papers have used "intratumoral" administration of the drug vector, even if the authors have developed a tumor-targeting mechanism that is supposed to discriminate normal and tumor cells. One cannot help but wonder, would the vector be effective if a systemic route of administration had been used?

Surprisingly, after years of investigation, some aspects of controversy still persist in the field of CPPs. First, there is uncertainty about the cell penetration mechanism of CPPs [107]. The prevalent theory of internalization seems to be endocytosis, but many papers argue against this and some CPP-based vectors claim to penetrate independent of the endocytotic pathway, at least when these CPPs carry only very small cargo molecules. Furthermore, contradicting results have been obtained even with the same CPP. Thus, some works describe cargo delivery by TAT as being mediated (and hindered) by endocytotic process [108], while others demonstrate the transduction being independent of endocytosis [2, 31]. Similarly, some works have shown that TAT delivers its cargo into the cell nucleus [2, 31], while others have not seen this [36]. These discrepancies could at least partially be explained by different cargo molecules, modifying the uptake of CPPs differently. For example, the route of cell penetration may depend on the size of the cargo. Clarification of these aspects is quite important, as it determines in which cell compartment the cargo ends up being transported. Moreover, if the cargo is trapped within the endosomes, it may not be able to exert its biological function at all, although being effectively internalized into the cell [38].

37.5 Conclusions

Although traditional tumor therapies have shown great progress over the last decade, drug delivery still suffers from poor delivery efficacy and specificity, resulting in gross toxicity in normal tissues. The ability of CPPs to deliver cargo of different type and size effectively into virtually every cell *in vivo* has opened a new approach of developing novel cancer therapies. It is even possible to deliver cargo such as oligonucleotides, which were not considered among potential therapeutics 10 years ago. As a result of new delivery methods (CPPs among them), the therapeutic potential of RNAi is today considered to be vast. The first example of using siRNA to inhibit the growth of solid tumors in humans was published only very recently [52]. Considering that developing CPP-based vectors is still a relatively new field, its application in the clinic is only beginning to expand.

In this chapter, we have summarized the potential of using CPPs as carriers of classical chemotherapeutics and other cytotoxic/cytostatic agents for tumor treatment. Of particular interest is the ability of CPPs to negate MDR against classical chemotherapeutics, to deliver oligonucleotides, and to intervene with tumor growth through modification of gene expression. There are also numerous examples of using CPPs in conjunction with oncogenic peptides, proteins, and antibodies – all of these showing great potential for delivering impermeable molecules into tumor cells.

Numerous preclinical and clinical applications of CPP-based delivery approaches are currently under evaluation [109]. The first CPP-based clinical trial was initiated a few years ago for the delivery of cyclosporine linked to polyarginine [110]. Very recently, the anticancer CPP peptide p28 entered phase I clinical trials to determine the safety of the potential drug. Moreover, several companies are working on the clinical development of CPPs for topical and systemic administration of different therapeutic molecules. For example, Traversa (www.traversathera.com) is currently developing a CPP-based noncovalent siRNA delivery vector usable for the treatment of cancer.

Characterization of many potent therapeutic molecules that are not permeable to cells or with low bioavailability has determined that development of delivery vehicles is at least as important as development of the therapeutic agent itself. Peptide-derived vectors have clearly proved their value in preclinical studies, showing advantages hardly comparable to other types of vectors. Accordingly, carrier peptides avoid the bioavailability problem encountered with many types of therapeutic molecules and offer an efficient way to deliver the cargo into target cells, without causing toxic reactions.

Acknowledgments

The work presented in this article was supported by the Swedish Research Council (VR-NT); by the Center for Biomembrane Research, Stockholm; by Knut and Alice Wallenberg Foundation; by the Cancer Foundation, Stockholm; by the EU through the European Regional Development Fund through the Center of Excellence in Chemical Biology, Estonia; and by the targeted financing **SF0180027s08** from the Estonian Government.

References

1. Frankel, A.D. and Pabo, C.O. (1988) Cellular uptake of the tat protein from human immunodeficiency virus. *Cell*, **55**, 1189–1193.
2. Vivès, E., Brodin, P., and Lebleu, B. (1997) A truncated HIV-1 Tat protein basic domain rapidly translocates through the plasma membrane and accumulates in the cell nucleus. *J. Biol. Chem.*, **272**, 16010–16017.
3. Joliot, A., Pernelle, C., Deagostinibazin, H., and Prochiantz, A. (1991) Antennapedia homeobox peptide regulates neural morphogenesis. *Proc. Natl. Acad. Sci. USA*, **88**, 1864–1868.
4. Pooga, M., Soomets, U., Hällbrink, M., Valkna, A., Saar, K., Rezaei, K., Kahl, U., Hao, J.X., Xu, X.J., Wiesenfeld-Hallin, Z., Hökfelt, T., Bartfai, T., and Langel, Ü. (1998) Cell

penetrating PNA constructs regulate galanin receptor levels and modify pain transmission *in vivo*. *Nat. Biotechnol.*, **16**, 857–861.

5. Schwarze, S.R., Ho, A., Vocero-Akbani, A., and Dowdy, S.F. (1999) *In vivo* protein transduction: delivery of a biologically active protein into the mouse. *Science*, **285**, 1569–1572.
6. Richard, J.P., Melikov, K., Vivès, E., Ramos, C., Verbeure, B., Gait, M.J., Chernomordik, L.V., and Lebleu, B. (2003) Cell-penetrating peptides – a reevaluation of the mechanism of cellular uptake. *J. Biol. Chem.*, **278**, 585–590.
7. Lundin, P., Johansson, H., Guterstam, P., Holm, T., Hansen, M., Langel, Ü., and EL Andaloussi, S. (2008) Distinct uptake routes of cell-penetrating peptide conjugates. *Bioconjug. Chem.*, **19**, 2535–2542.
8. Duchardt, F., Fotin-Mleczek, M., Schwarz, H., Fischer, R., and Brock, R. (2007) A comprehensive model for the cellular uptake of cationic cell-penetrating peptides. *Traffic*, **8**, 848–866.
9. Hansen, M., Kilk, K., and Langel, Ü. (2008) Predicting cell-penetrating peptides. *Adv. Drug Deliv. Rev.*, **60**, 572–579.
10. Derossi, D., Joliot, A., Chassaing, G., and Prochiantz, A. (1994) The third helix of the Antennapedia homeodomain translocates through biological membranes. *J. Biol. Chem.*, **269**, 10444–10450.
11. Soomets, U., Lindgren, M., Gallet, X., Hällbrink, M., Elmquist, A., Balaspiri, L., Zorko, M., Pooga, M., Brasseur, R., and Langel, Ü. (2000) Deletion analogues of transportan. *Biochim. Biophys. Acta*, **1467**, 165–176.
12. Futaki, S., Suzuki, T., Ohashi, W., Yagami, T., Tanaka, S., Ueda, K., and Sugiura, Y. (2001) Arginine-rich peptides. An abundant source of membrane-permeable peptides having potential as carriers for intracellular protein delivery. *J. Biol. Chem.*, **276**, 5836–5840.
13. Morris, M.C., Depollier, J., Mery, J., Heitz, F., and Divita, G. (2001) A peptide carrier for the delivery of biologically active proteins into mammalian cells. *Nat. Biotechnol.*, **19**, 1173–1176.
14. Morris, M.C., Vidal, P., Chaloin, L., Heitz, F., and Divita, G. (1997) A new peptide vector for efficient delivery of oligonucleotides into mammalian cells. *Nucleic Acids Res.*, **25**, 2730–2736.
15. Mazel, M., Clair, P., Rousselle, C., Vidal, P., Scherrmann, J.M., Mathieu, D., and Temsamani, J. (2001) Doxorubicin–peptide conjugates overcome multidrug resistance. *Anti-Cancer Drugs*, **12**, 107–116.
16. Rousselle, C., Clair, P., Lefauconnier, J.M., Kaczorek, M., Scherrmann, J.M., and Temsamani, J. (2000) New advances in the transport of doxorubicin through the blood–brain barrier by a peptide vector-mediated strategy. *Mol. Pharmacol.*, **57**, 679–686.
17. Morris, M.C., Gros, E., Aldrian-Herrada, G., Choob, M., Archdeacon, J., Heitz, F., and Divita, G. (2007) A non-covalent peptide-based carrier for *in vivo* delivery of DNA mimics. *Nucleic Acids Res.*, **35**, e49.
18. Crombez, L., Morris, M.C., Dufort, S., Aldrian-Herrada, G., Nguyen, Q., Mc Master, G., Coll, J.L., Heitz, F., and Divita, G. (2009) Targeting cyclin B1 through peptide-based delivery of siRNA prevents tumour growth. *Nucleic Acids Res.*, **37**, 4559–4569.
19. Tan, M., Lan, K.H., Yao, J., Lu, C.H., Sun, M.H., Neal, C.L., Lu, J., and Yu, D.H. (2006) Selective inhibition of ErbB2-overexpressing breast cancer *in vivo* by a novel TAT-based ErbB2-targeting signal transducers and activators of transcription 3-blocking peptide. *Cancer Res.*, **66**, 3764–3772.
20. Bromberg, J.F., Wrzeszczynska, M.H., Devgan, G., Zhao, Y.X., Pestell, R.G., Albanese, C., and Darnell, J.E. (1999) Stat3 as an oncogene. *Cell*, **98**, 295–303.
21. Jain, M., Chauhan, S.C., Singh, A.P., Venkatraman, G., Colcher, D., and Batra, S.K. (2005) Penetratin improves tumor retention of single-chain antibodies: a novel step toward optimization of radioimmunotherapy

of solid tumors. *Cancer Res.*, **65**, 7840–7846.

22. Liu, X.R., Wang, Y., Nakamura, K., Kawauchi, S., Akalin, A., Cheng, D.F., Chen, L., Rusckowski, M., and Hnatowich, D.J. (2009) Auger radiation-induced, antisense-mediated cytotoxicity of tumor cells using a 3-component streptavidin-delivery nanoparticle with In-111. *J. Nucl. Med.*, **50**, 582–590.
23. Olson, E.S., Aguilera, T.A., Jiang, T., Ellies, L.G., Nguyen, Q.T., Wong, E.H., Gross, L.A., and Tsien, R.Y. (2009) *In vivo* characterization of activatable cell penetrating peptides for targeting protease activity in cancer. *Integr. Biol.*, **1**, 382–393.
24. Myrberg, H., Zhang, L.L., Mäe, M., and Langel, Ü. (2008) Design of a tumor-homing cell-penetrating peptide. *Bioconjug. Chem.*, **19**, 70–75.
25. Chen, L. and Harrison, S. (2007) Cell-penetrating peptides in drug development: enabling intracellular targets. *Biochem. Soc. Trans.*, **35**, 821–825.
26. Tsuji, A. (1998) P-glycoprotein-mediated efflux transport of anticancer drugs at the blood–brain barrier. *Ther. Drug Monit.*, **20**, 588–590.
27. Dean, M., Fojo, T., and Bates, S. (2005) Tumour stem cells and drug resistance. *Nat. Rev. Cancer*, **5**, 275–284.
28. Aroui, S., Ram, N., Appaix, F., Ronjat, M., Kenani, A., Pirollet, F., and De Waard, M. (2009) Maurocalcine as a non toxic drug carrier overcomes doxorubicin resistance in the cancer cell line MDA-MB 231. *Pharm. Res.*, **26**, 836–845.
29. Aroui, S., Brahim, S., De Waard, M., and Kenani, A. (2010) Cytotoxicity, intracellular distribution and uptake of doxorubicin and doxorubicin coupled to cell-penetrating peptides in different cell lines: a comparative study. *Biochem. Biophys. Res. Commun.*, **391**, 419–425.
30. Castex, C., Merida, P., Blanc, E., Clair, P., Rees, A.R., and Temsamani, J. (2004) 2-Pyrrolinodoxorubicin and its peptide-vectorized form bypass multidrug resistance. *Anti-Cancer Drugs*, **15**, 609–617.
31. Nori, A., Jensen, K.D., Tijerina, M., Kopeckova, P., and Kopecek, J. (2003) Tat-conjugated synthetic macromolecules facilitate cytoplasmic drug delivery to human ovarian carcinoma cells. *Bioconjug. Chem.*, **14**, 44–50.
32. Dubikovskaya, E.A., Thorne, S.H., Pillow, T.H., Contag, C.H., and Wender, P.A. (2008) Overcoming multidrug resistance of small-molecule therapeutics through conjugation with releasable octaarginine transporters. *Proc. Natl. Acad. Sci. USA*, **105**, 12128–12133.
33. Lindgren, M., Rosenthal-Aizman, K., Saar, K., Eiriksdóttir, E., Jiang, Y., Sassian, M., Ostlund, P., Hällbrink, M., and Langel, Ü. (2006) Overcoming methotrexate resistance in breast cancer tumour cells by the use of a new cell-penetrating peptide. *Biochem. Pharmacol.*, **71**, 416–425.
34. Mäe, M., Myrberg, H., El-Andaloussi, S., and Langel, Ü. (2009) Design of a tumor homing cell-penetrating peptide for drug delivery. *Int. J. Pept. Res. Ther.*, **15**, 11–15.
35. Mai, J.C., Mi, Z.B., Kim, S.H., Ng, B., and Robbins, P.D. (2001) A proapoptotic peptide for the treatment of solid tumors. *Cancer Res.*, **61**, 7709–7712.
36. Guelen, L., Paterson, H., Gaken, J., Meyers, M., Farzaneh, F., and Tavassoli, M. (2004) TAT–apoptin is efficiently delivered and induces apoptosis in cancer cells. *Oncogene*, **23**, 1153–1165.
37. Marty, C., Meylan, C., Schott, H., Ballmer-Hofer, K., and Schwendener, R.A. (2004) Enhanced heparan sulfate proteoglycan-mediated uptake of cell-penetrating peptide-modified liposomes. *Cell. Mol. Life Sci.*, **61**, 1785–1794.
38. Tseng, Y.L., Liu, J.J., and Hong, R.L. (2002) Translocation of liposomes into cancer cells by cell-penetrating peptides penetratin and TAT: a kinetic and efficacy study. *Mol. Pharmacol.*, **62**, 864–872.
39. Torchilin, V.P., Rammohan, R., Weissig, V., and Levchenko, T.S. (2001) TAT peptide on the surface of liposomes affords their efficient

intracellular delivery even at low temperature and in the presence of metabolic inhibitors. *Proc. Natl. Acad. Sci. USA*, **98**, 8786–8791.

40. Ezzat, K., El Andaloussi, S., Abdo, R., and Langel, Ü. (2010) Peptide-based matrices as drug delivery vehicles. *Curr. Pharm. Des.*, **16**, 1167–1178.
41. Ruoslahti, E., Duza, T., and Zhang, L. (2005) Vascular homing peptides with cell-penetrating properties. *Curr. Pharm. Des.*, **11**, 3655–3660.
42. Laakkonen, P., Akerman, M.E., Biliran, H., Yang, M., Ferrer, F., Karpanen, T., Hoffman, R.M., and Ruoslahti, E. (2004) Antitumor activity of a homing peptide that targets tumor lymphatics and tumor cells. *Proc. Natl. Acad. Sci. USA*, **101**, 9381–9386.
43. Midgley, C.A., Desterro, J.M.P., Saville, M.K., Howard, S., Sparks, A., Hay, R.T., and Lane, D.P. (2000) An N-terminal $p14^{ARF}$ peptide blocks Mdm2-dependent ubiquitination *in vitro* and can activate p53 *in vivo*. *Oncogene*, **19**, 2312–2323.
44. Johansson, H.J., El-Andaloussi, S., Holm, T., Mäe, M., Jänes, J., Maimets, T., and Langel, Ü. (2008) Characterization of a novel cytotoxic cell-penetrating peptide derived from $p14^{ARF}$ protein. *Mol. Ther.*, **16**, 115–123.
45. Vallespi, M.G., Fernandez, J.R., Torrens, I., Garcia, I., Garay, H., Mendoza, O., Granadillo, M., Falcon, V., Acevedo, B., Ubieta, R., Guillen, G.E., and Reyes, O. (2010) Identification of a novel antitumor peptide based on the screening of an Ala-library derived from the LALF(32–51) region. *J. Pept. Sci.*, **16**, 40–47.
46. Whitehead, K., Langer, R., and Anderson, D. (2009) Knocking down barriers: advances in siRNA delivery. *Nat. Rev. Drug Discov.*, **8**, 129–138.
47. Matsumura, Y. and Maeda, H. (1986) A new concept for macromolecular therapeutics in cancer chemotherapy: mechanism of tumoritropic accumulation of proteins and the antitumor agent smancs. *Cancer Res.*, **46**, 6387–6392.
48. Porkka, K., Laakkonen, P., Hoffman, J.A., Bernasconi, M., and Ruoslahti, E. (2002) A fragment of the HMGN2 protein homes to the nuclei of tumor cells and tumor endothelial cells *in vivo*. *Proc. Natl. Acad. Sci. USA*, **99**, 7444–7449.
49. Henke, E., Perk, J., Vider, J., de Candia, P., Chin, Y., Solit, D.B., Ponomarev, V., Cartegni, L., Manova, K., Rosen, N., and Benezra, R. (2008) Peptide-conjugated antisense oligonucleotides for targeted inhibition of a transcriptional regulator *in vivo*. *Nat. Biotechnol.*, **26**, 91–100.
50. Marthinet, E., Divita, G., Bernaud, J., Rigal, D., and Baggetto, L.G. (2000) Modulation of the typical multidrug resistance phenotype by targeting the MED-1 region of human MDR1 promoter. *Gene Ther.*, **7**, 1224–1233.
51. Asai, A., Oshima, Y., Yamamoto, Y., Uochi, T., Kusaka, H., Akinaga, S., Yamashita, Y., Pongracz, K., Pruzan, R., Wunder, E., Piatyszek, M., Li, S.H., Chin, A.C., Harley, C.B., and Gryaznov, S. (2003) A novel telomerase template antagonist (GRN163) as a potential anticancer agent. *Cancer Res.*, **63**, 3931–3939.
52. Davis, M.E., Zuckerman, J.E., Choi, C.H.J., Seligson, D., Tolcher, A., Alabi, C.A., Yen, Y., Heidel, J.D., and Ribas, A. (2010) Evidence of RNAi in humans from systemically administered siRNA via targeted nanoparticles. *Nature*, **464**, 1067–U140.
53. Zhang, C.L., Tang, N., Liu, X.J., Liang, W., Xu, W., and Torchilin, V.P. (2006) siRNA-containing liposomes modified with polyarginine effectively silence the targeted gene. *J. Control. Release*, **112**, 229–239.
54. Kim, W.L., Christensen, L.V., Jo, S., Yockman, J.W., Jeong, J.H., Kim, Y.H., and Kim, S.W. (2006) Cholesteryl oligoarginine delivering vascular endothelial growth factor siRNA effectively inhibits tumor growth in colon adenocarcinoma. *Mol. Ther.*, **14**, 343–350.
55. Eguchi, A., Meade, B.R., Chang, Y.C., Fredrickson, C.T., Willert, K., Puri, N., and Dowdy, S.F. (2009) Efficient siRNA delivery into primary cells by a peptide transduction domain–dsRNA binding

domain fusion protein. *Nat. Biotechnol.*, **27**, 567–U110.
56. Michiue, H., Eguchi, A., Scadeng, M., and Dowdy, S.F. (2009) Induction of *in vivo* synthetic lethal RNAi responses to treat glioblastoma. *Cancer Biol. Ther.*, **8**, 2306–2313.
57. Choi, Y.S., Lee, J.Y., Suh, J.S., Kwon, Y.M., Lee, S.J., Chung, J.K., Lee, D.S., Yang, V.C., Chung, C.P., and Park, Y.J. (2010) The systemic delivery of siRNAs by a cell penetrating peptide, low molecular weight protamine. *Biomaterials*, **31**, 1429–1443.
58. Mäe, M., El Andaloussi, S., Lundin, P., Oskolkov, N., Johansson, H.J., Guterstam, P., and Langel, Ü. (2009) A stearylated CPP for delivery of splice correcting oligonucleotides using a non-covalent co-incubation strategy. *J. Control. Release*, **134**, 221–227.
59. Lehto, T., Abes, R., Oskolkov, N., Suhorutšenko, J., Copolovici, D.M., Mäger, I., Viola, J.R., Simonson, O.E., Ezzat, K., Guterstam, P., Eriste, E., Smith, C.I.E., Lebleu, B., El Andaloussi, S., and Langel, Ü. (2010) Delivery of nucleic acids with a stearylated $(RxR)_4$ peptide using a non-covalent co-incubation strategy. *J. Control. Release*, **141**, 42–51.
60. Torchilin, V.P., Levchenko, T.S., Rammohan, R., Volodina, N., Papahadjopoulos-Sternberg, B., and D'Souza, G.G.M. (2003) Cell transfection *in vitro* and *in vivo* with nontoxic TAT peptide–liposome–DNA complexes. *Proc. Natl. Acad. Sci. USA*, **100**, 1972–1977.
61. Gupta, B., Levchenko, T.S., and Torchilin, V.P. (2007) TAT peptide-modified liposomes provide enhanced gene delivery to intracranial human brain tumor xenografts in nude mice. *Oncol. Res.*, **16**, 351–359.
62. Byrd, J.C. and Bresalier, R.S. (2004) Mucins and mucin binding proteins in colorectal cancer. *Cancer Metastasis Rev.*, **23**, 77–99.
63. Bitler, B.G., Menzl, I., Huerta, C.L., Sands, B., Knowlton, W., Chang, A., and Schroeder, J.A. (2009) Intracellular MUC1 peptides inhibit cancer progression. *Clin. Cancer Res.*, **15**, 100–109.
64. Fulda, S., Wick, W., Weller, M., and Debatin, K.M. (2002) Smac agonists sensitize for Apo2L/TRAIL- or anticancer drug-induced apoptosis and induce regression of malignant glioma *in vivo*. *Nat. Med.*, **8**, 808–815.
65. Arnt, C.R., Chiorean, M.V., Heldebrant, M.V., Gores, G.J., and Kaufmann, S.H. (2002) Synthetic Smac/DIABLO peptides enhance the effects of chemotherapeutic agents by binding XIAP and cIAP1 *in situ*. *J. Biol. Chem.*, **277**, 44236–44243.
66. Vucic, D., Deshayes, K., Ackerly, H., Pisabarro, M.T., Kadkhodayan, S., Fairbrother, W.J., and Dixit, V.M. (2002) SMAC negatively regulates the anti-apoptotic activity of melanoma inhibitor of apoptosis (ML-IAP). *J. Biol. Chem.*, **277**, 12275–12279.
67. Yang, L.L., Mashima, T., Sato, S., Mochizuki, M., Sakamoto, H., Yamori, T., Oh-hara, T., and Tsuruo, T. (2003) Predominant suppression of apoptosome by inhibitor of apoptosis protein in non-small cell lung cancer H460 cells: therapeutic effect of a novel polyarginine-conjugated Smac peptide. *Cancer Res.*, **63**, 831–837.
68. Holinger, E.P., Chittenden, T., and Lutz, R.J. (1999) Bak BH3 peptides antagonize Bcl-x_L function and induce apoptosis through cytochrome *c*-independent activation of caspases. *J. Biol. Chem.*, **274**, 13298–13304.
69. Letai, A., Bassik, M.C., Walensky, L.D., Sorcinelli, M.D., Weiler, S., and Korsmeyer, S.J. (2002) Distinct BH3 domains either sensitize or activate mitochondrial apoptosis, serving as prototype cancer therapeutics. *Cancer Cell*, **2**, 183–192.
70. Goldsmith, K.C., Liu, X., Dam, V., Morgan, B.T., Shabbout, M., Cnaan, A., Letai, A., Korsmeyer, S.J., and Hogarty, M.D. (2006) BH3 peptidomimetics potently activate apoptosis and demonstrate single agent efficacy in neuroblastoma. *Oncogene*, **25**, 4525–4533.
71. Selivanova, G., Iotsova, V., Okan, I., Fritsche, M., Strom, M., Groner, B.,

Grafstrom, R.C., and Wiman, K.G. (1997) Restoration of the growth suppression function of mutant p53 by a synthetic peptide derived from the p53 C-terminal domain. *Nat. Med.*, **3**, 632–638.

72. Snyder, E.L. and Dowdy, S.F. (2004) Cell penetrating peptides in drug delivery. *Pharm. Res.*, **21**, 389–393.
73. Araki, D., Takayama, K., Inoue, M., Watanabe, T., Kumon, H., Futaki, S., Matsui, H., and Tomizawa, K. (2010) Cell-penetrating D-isomer peptides of p53 C-terminus: long-term inhibitory effect on the growth of bladder cancer. *Urology*, **75**, 813–819.
74. Kanovsky, M., Raffo, A., Drew, L., Rosal, R., Do, T., Friedman, F.K., Rubinstein, P., Visser, J., Robinson, R., Brandt-Rauf, P.W., Michl, J., Fine, R.L., and Pincus, M.R. (2001) Peptides from the amino terminal mdm-2-binding domain of p53, designed from conformational analysis, are selectively cytotoxic to transformed cells. *Proc. Natl. Acad. Sci. USA*, **98**, 12438–12443.
75. Harbour, J.W., Worley, L., Ma, D.D., and Cohen, M. (2002) Transducible peptide therapy for uveal melanoma and retinoblastoma. *Arch. Ophthalmol.*, **120**, 1341–1346.
76. Do, T.N., Rosal, R.V., Drew, L., Raffo, A.J., Michl, J., Pincus, M.R., Friedman, F.K., Petrylak, D.P., Cassai, N., Szmulewicz, J., Sidhu, G., Fine, R.L., and Brandt-Rauf, P.W. (2003) Preferential induction of necrosis in human breast cancer cells by a p53 peptide derived from the MDM2 binding site. *Oncogene*, **22**, 1431–1444.
77. Gius, D.R., Ezhevsky, S.A., Becker-Hapak, M., Nagahara, H., Wei, M.C., and Dowdy, S.F. (1999) Transduced $p16^{INK4a}$ peptides inhibit hypophosphorylation of the retinoblastoma protein and cell cycle progression prior to activation of Cdk2 complexes in late G_1. *Cancer Res.*, **59**, 2577–2580.
78. Fahraeus, R., Paramio, J.M., Ball, K.L., Lain, S., and Lane, D.P. (1996) Inhibition of pRb phosphorylation and cell-cycle progression by a 20-residue peptide derived from $p16^{CDKN2/INK4A}$. *Curr. Biol.*, **6**, 84–91.
79. Frizelle, S.P., Kratzke, M.G., Carreon, R.R., Engel, S.C., Youngquist, L., Klein, M.A., Fourre, L., Shekels, L.L., and Kratzke, R.A. (2008) Inhibition of both mesothelioma cell growth and Cdk4 activity following treatment with a $TATp16^{INK4a}$ peptide. *Anticancer Res.*, **28**, 1–7.
80. Ezhevsky, S.A., Ho, A., Becker-Hapak, M., Davis, P.K., and Dowdy, S.F. (2001) Differential regulation of retinoblastoma tumor suppressor protein by G_1 cyclin-dependent kinase complexes *in vivo*. *Mol. Cell. Biol.*, **21**, 4773–4784.
81. Hosotani, R., Miyamoto, Y., Fujimoto, K., Doi, R., Otaka, A., Fujii, N., and Imamura, M. (2002) Trojan p16 peptide suppresses pancreatic cancer growth and prolongs survival in mice. *Clin. Cancer Res.*, **8**, 1271–1276.
82. Baker, R.D., Howl, J., and Nicholl, I.D. (2007) A sychnological cell penetrating peptide mimic of $p21^{WAF1/CIP1}$ is pro-apoptogenic. *Peptides*, **28**, 731–740.
83. Bonfanti, M., Taverna, S., Salmona, M., Dincalci, M., and Broggini, M. (1997) $p21^{WAF1}$-derived peptides linked to an internalization peptide inhibit human cancer cell growth. *Cancer Res.*, **57**, 1442–1446.
84. Ball, K.L., Lain, S., Fahraeus, R., Smythe, C., and Lane, D.P. (1997) Cell-cycle arrest and inhibition of Cdk4 activity by small peptides based on the carboxy-terminal domain of $p21^{WAF1}$. *Curr. Biol.*, **7**, 71–80.
85. Chen, Y.N.P., Sharma, S.K., Ramsey, T.M., Jiang, L., Martin, M.S., Baker, K., Adams, P.D., Bair, K.W., and Kaelin, W.G. (1999) Selective killing of transformed cells by cyclin/cyclin-dependent kinase 2 antagonists. *Proc. Natl. Acad. Sci. USA*, **96**, 4325–4329.
86. Nagahara, H., Vocero-Akbani, A.M., Snyder, E.L., Ho, A., Latham, D.G., Lissy, N.A., Becker-Hapak, M., Ezhevsky, S.A., and Dowdy, S.F. (1998) Transduction of full-length TAT fusion proteins into mammalian cells: $TAT\text{-}p27^{Kip1}$ induces cell migration. *Nat. Med.*, **4**, 1449–1452.

87. Parada, Y., Banerji, L., Glassford, J., Lea, N.C., Collado, M., Rivas, C., Lewis, J.L., Gordon, M.Y., Thomas, N.S., and Lam, E.W. (2001) BCR-ABL and interleukin 3 promote haematopoietic cell proliferation and survival through modulation of cyclin D2 and $p27^{Kip1}$ expression. *J. Biol. Chem.*, **276**, 23572–23580.
88. Minchinton, A.I. and Tannock, I.F. (2006) Drug penetration in solid tumours. *Nat. Rev. Cancer*, **6**, 583–592.
89. Thurber, G.M., Schmidt, M.M., and Wittrup, K.D. (2008) Antibody tumor penetration: transport opposed by systemic and antigen-mediated clearance. *Adv. Drug Deliv. Rev.*, **60**, 1421–1434.
90. Aguilera, T.A., Olson, E.S., Timmers, M.M., Jiang, T., and Tsien, R.Y. (2009) Systemic *in vivo* distribution of activatable cell penetrating peptides is superior to that of cell penetrating peptides. *Integr. Biol.*, **1**, 371–381.
91. Kale, A.A. and Torchilin, V.P. (2007) "Smart" drug carriers: PEGylated TATp-modified pH-sensitive liposomes. *J. Liposome Res.*, **17**, 197–203.
92. Song, E.W., Zhu, P.C., Lee, S.K., Chowdhury, D., Kussman, S., Dykxhoorn, D.M., Feng, Y., Palliser, D., Weiner, D.B., Shankar, P., Marasco, W.A., and Lieberman, J. (2005) Antibody mediated *in vivo* delivery of small interfering RNAs via cell-surface receptors. *Nat. Biotechnol.*, **23**, 709–717.
93. Essler, M. and Ruoslahti, E. (2002) Molecular specialization of breast vasculature: a breast-homing phage-displayed peptide binds to aminopeptidase P in breast vasculature. *Proc. Natl. Acad. Sci. USA*, **99**, 2252–2257.
94. Trudel, D., Fradet, Y., Meyer, F., Harel, F., and Tetu, B. (2003) Significance of MMP-2 expression in prostate cancer: an immunohistochemical study. *Cancer Res.*, **63**, 8511–8515.
95. Whitney, M., Crisp, J.L., Olson, E.S., Aguilera, T.A., Gross, L.A., Ellies, L.G., and Tsien, R.Y. (2010) Parallel *in vivo* and *in vitro* selection using phage display identifies protease dependent tumor targeting peptides. *J. Biol. Chem.*, **285**, 22532–22541.
96. Sethuraman, V.A. and Bae, Y.H. (2007) TAT peptide-based micelle system for potential active targeting of anti-cancer agents to acidic solid tumors. *J. Control. Release*, **118**, 216–224.
97. Kale, A.A. and Torchilin, V.P. (2007) Enhanced transfection of tumor cells *in vivo* using "Smart" pH-sensitive TAT-modified pegylated liposomes. *J. Drug Target.*, **15**, 538–545.
98. Harada, H., Hiraoka, M., and Kizaka-Kondoh, S. (2002) Antitumor effect of TAT-oxygen-dependent degradation–caspase-3 fusion protein specifically stabilized and activated in hypoxic tumor cells. *Cancer Res.*, **62**, 2013–2018.
99. Anderson, D.C., Manger, R., Schroeder, J., Woodle, D., Barry, M., Morgan, A.C., and Fritzberg, A.R. (1993) Enhanced *in vitro* tumor cell retention and internalization of antibody derivatized with synthetic peptides. *Bioconjug. Chem.*, **4**, 10–18.
100. Anderson, D.C., Nichols, E., Manger, R., Woodle, D., Barry, M., and Fritzberg, A.R. (1993) Tumor cell retention of antibody fab fragments is enhanced by an attached HIV TAT protein-derived peptide. *Biochem. Biophys. Res. Commun.*, **194**, 876–884.
101. Sawant, R.M., Hurley, J.P., Salmaso, S., Kale, A., Tolcheva, E., Levchenko, T.S., and Torchilin, V.P. (2006) "SMART" drug delivery systems: double-targeted pH-responsive pharmaceutical nanocarriers. *Bioconjug. Chem.*, **17**, 943–949.
102. Imam, S.K. (2001) Status of radioimmunotherapy in the new millennium. *Cancer Biother. Radiopharm.*, **16**, 237–256.
103. Hu, M.D., Chen, P., Wang, J., Scollard, D.A., Vallis, K.A., and Reilly, R.M. (2007) I-123-labeled HIV-1 tat peptide radioimmunoconjugates are imported into the nucleus of human breast cancer cells and functionally interact *in vitro* and *in vivo* with the cyclin-dependent kinase inhibitor, $p21^{WAF-1/Cip-1}$. *Eur. J. Nucl. Med. Mol. Imaging*, **34**, 368–377.
104. Simberg, D., Duza, T., Park, J.H., Essler, M., Pilch, J., Zhang, L.L., Derfus, A.M., Yang, M.,

Hoffman, R.M., Bhatia, S., Sailor, M.J., and Ruoslahti, E. (2007) Biomimetic amplification of nanoparticle homing to tumors. *Proc. Natl. Acad. Sci. USA*, **104**, 932–936.

105. Siegal, T., Horowitz, A., and Gabizon, A. (1995) Doxorubicin encapsulated in sterically stabilized liposomes for the treatment of a brain tumor model: biodistribution and therapeutic efficacy. *J. Neurosurg.*, **83**, 1029–1037.

106. Beier, C.P., Schmid, C., Gorlia, T., Kleinletzenberger, C., Beier, D., Grauer, O., Steinbrecher, A., Hirschmann, B., Brawanski, A., Dietmaier, C., Jauch-Worley, T., Kolbl, O., Pietsch, T., Proescholdt, M., Rummele, P., Muigg, A., Stockhammer, G., Hegi, M., Bogdahn, U., and Hau, P. (2009) RNOP-09: pegylated liposomal doxorubicine and prolonged temozolomide in addition to radiotherapy in newly diagnosed glioblastoma – a phase II study. *BMC Cancer*, **9**, 308.

107. Dietz, G.P.H. and Bahr, M. (2005) Peptide-enhanced cellular internalization of proteins in neuroscience. *Brain Res. Bull.*, **68**, 103–114.

108. Kameyama, S., Horie, M., Kikuchi, T., Omura, T., Tadokoro, A., Takeuchi, T., Nakase, I., Sugiura, Y., and Futaki, S. (2007) Acid wash in determining cellular uptake of fab/cell-permeating peptide conjugates. *Biopolymers*, **88**, 98–107.

109. Heitz, F., Morris, M., and Divita, G. (2009) Twenty years of cell-penetrating peptides: from molecular mechanisms to therapeutics. *Br. J. Pharmacol.*, **157**, 195–206.

110. Rothbard, J., Jessop, T., Lewis, R., Murray, B., and Wender, P. (2004) Role of membrane potential and hydrogen bonding in the mechanism of translocation of guanidinium-rich peptides into cells. *J. Am. Chem. Soc.*, **126**, 9506–9507.

38
Targeting to Peptide Receptors

Andrew V. Schally and Gabor Halmos

38.1
Introduction

The introduction into clinical practice of new therapeutic strategies based on molecular targeting and the development of several new drugs capable thereof have revolutionized our approach to cancer treatment over the past 30 years [1–7]. The concept of drug targeting was created by Paul Ehrlich more than 100 years ago [8]. He conceived the idea of a molecule with specific affinity for a certain organ, and which could be linked to a therapeutically active group and then selectively delivered to the organ in question, thus eradicating the disease [8] (reviewed in [6]). The vision of a "magic bullet" was thereby born [6]. However, there was no concept of how to create "magic bullets" and, therefore, they remained unexplored for many decades.

Great progress in targeted cancer therapy was made with the discovery of receptors and the development of monoclonal antibodies (mAbs) [1–7]. Several mAbs are now approved for clinical use and are very effective against appropriate types of cancer [3–5]. These include Erbitux® (cetuximab), a derivative of the mAb 225, which binds to the epidermal growth factor receptor (EGFR) and inhibits metastatic colorectal cancer [3], Herceptin® (trastuzumab), a humanized mAb against EGFR2 (HER2) that is very successfully used against metastatic breast cancers overexpressing HER2 [4], and Avastin® (bevacizumab) [5], a recombinant mAb targeting vascular endothelial growth factor (VEGF). Many cancers are resistant to treatment with mAbs alone, but can be killed when a cytotoxic agent is attached to that antibody [1, 2]. Immunoconjugates of this kind are made by linking chemotherapeutic drugs, radioisotopes, enzymes, or toxins to the antibody [1, 2]. Several recombinant immunotoxins exist, composed of antibody fragments fused to powerful bacterial toxins [2]. In addition, various low-molecular-weight inhibitors of EGFR tyrosine kinase, exemplified by gefitinib (Iressa®) and erlotonib (Tarceva®), have been developed and can be used orally. However, tyrosine kinase inhibitors of this type are targeted only passively and not actively, as they are not attached to a carrier that binds to a specific target [9]. These advances are chronicled in other chapters of this volume.

Drug Delivery in Oncology: From Basic Research to Cancer Therapy, First Edition.
Edited by Felix Kratz, Peter Senter, and Henning Steinhagen.

38.2
Rationale for the Concept of Delivery to Peptide Receptors

This chapter focuses on the concepts, descriptions, and experimental and clinical evaluation of chemotherapeutic compounds linked to various hormonal peptides, developed for targeting (homing) to tumors expressing receptors for these peptides [6, 7]. Thus, one of the many possible approaches to targeted cancer therapy is based on the finding that receptors for certain peptide hormones, such as somatostatin, bombesin, growth hormone-releasing hormone (GHRH), and luteinizing hormone-releasing hormone-1 (LHRH1; now also known in genome and microarray databases as gonadotropin-releasing hormone-1 (GnRH-1)), are expressed on various tumors in higher concentrations than on most corresponding normal cells [6, 7, 9]. Consequently, these peptide hormones and their analogs can be used as carrier vectors to deliver cytotoxic agents such as anthracycline derivatives directly to malignant cells [6, 7] (Figure 38.1). Although cytotoxic hybrids of GHRH antagonists are not yet developed, the targeting of GHRH antagonists themselves to cancers that express GHRH receptors would nevertheless be effective and therapeutically functional because binding to these receptors can exert inhibitory effects on tumors without the delivery of a cytotoxic radical [9]. Various radionuclides can be also conjugated to the analogs of these diverse hormonal peptides.

These hybrid peptides conjugated to a cytotoxic agent bind to the receptors on the cell surface, are internalized by receptor-mediated endocytosis, and upon delivery to the cytoplasm, mediate cell death [6, 7]. The presence of peptide receptors on various tumors (reviewed in [6, 7]) can serve as a target for peptide ligands and permit the implementation of the targeted therapy proposed by Paul Ehrlich more than 100 years ago [8]. These specific approaches will be reviewed below in the sections designated for each individual receptor type.

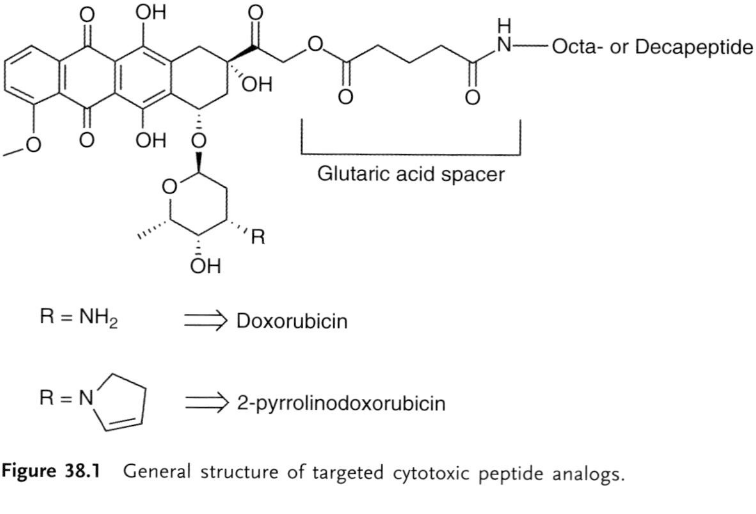

Figure 38.1 General structure of targeted cytotoxic peptide analogs.

Most endocrine (hormonal) approaches to target cytotoxic agents and radionuclides to tumors are based on peptides [10]. Antibodies are subject to nonspecific uptake by the liver and reticuloendothelial system, whereas peptides are not. Liver and bone marrow toxicities are thus also dose-limiting factors. Peptides are easier to design and synthesize, and are much smaller than mAbs, which because of their size may not reach the interior of large tumors [7]. Thus, peptides may be superior to mAbs as targeting agents [10].

Targeted chemotherapy, which can be homed directly to tumor cells, represents a modern oncological strategy designed to improve the effectiveness of cytotoxic drugs while decreasing toxicity. This targeted approach increases the concentration of the drugs in tumor tissue and spares normal, noncancerous cells from unnecessary exposure to the toxic effects of systemic chemotherapy [7]. It is well documented that chemotherapeutic agents produce toxic effects. Various chemotherapeutic agents can cause myelosuppression, and can also have gastrointestinal, cardiac, pulmonary, hepatic, renal, neurologic, and other types of toxicities [11]. The efficacy of systemic chemotherapy can also be restricted by multidrug resistance (MDR) of tumor cells. Some cancers, such as ovarian cancers, may quickly become refractory to further therapy [11] and other neoplasias such as non-small-cell lung cancer (NSCLC), are intrinsically resistant to most chemotherapeutic agents [11]. Dose escalations also may be limited by toxicity.

A more selective delivery of the chemotherapeutic agents to the primary tumors and their metastases, based on targeted chemotherapy, can potentially allow significant dose escalation while reducing the systemic toxicity. Targeting chemotherapeutic drugs directly to tumor cells could overcome MDR based on transmembrane efflux [12]. Various findings indicate that targeted chemotherapy with cytotoxic peptide analogs can delay or suppress chemoresistance mediated by the gene *MDR-1* and MDR-1 protein (MRP-1) efflux pumps [13, 14]. Collectively, the advances in the past 20 years have placed the concept of "magic bullets" on a firm foundation. The information accumulated on cytotoxic peptide analogs from studies in our laboratory and selected findings by others are herein reviewed.

38.3 Example 1: Cytotoxic Analogs of LHRH1

38.3.1 Preclinical Considerations and Development

38.3.1.1 LHRH1 and its Receptors

Hypothalamic LHRH1 is the primary link between the brain and the pituitary in the regulation of gonadal functions, and plays a critical role in vertebrate reproduction [15]. In addition, LHRH1 may be a growth factor in various tumors. Several LHRH1 agonists, such as triptorelin (Decapeptyl®), leuprolide (Lupron®), and goserelin (Zoladex®), have various important clinical applications in gynecology, urology, and oncology [15–17]. In addition, potent antagonists of LHRH1 such as Cetrorelix®

have also been synthesized for clinical use. The actions of LHRH1 and its analogs are mediated by high-affinity receptors for LHRH1 found on the membranes of the pituitary gonadotrophs and of multiple cancers [15–17]. LHRH1 receptors are members of the rhodopsin-like family of seven-transmembrane-domain G-protein-coupled receptors (GPCRs) [18–20]. Both LHRH1 receptor subtypes (LHRH1 and LHRH2) couple to the $G_{q/11}$ family of G-proteins, which activates phospholipase C (PLC), and stimulates production of inositol triphosphate (IP_3) and diacylglycerol [18–20]. In the pituitary this process induces Ca^{2+} mobilization and activation of protein kinase C (PKC) resulting in the release of luteinizing hormone (LH) and follicle-stimulating hormone (FSH) [15]. Type I LHRH1 receptor has high affinity for LHRH1 and lower affinity for LHRH2. The mammalian type I LHRH1 receptors are atypical among the rhodopsin-like GPCR superfamily because they completely lack a cytoplasmic C-terminal tail [18–20]. Mammalian type II and nonmammalian LHRH1 receptors all have a cytoplasmic C-terminal tail, a potential site for phosphorylation by GPCR kinases and/or second messenger-regulated kinases [18–20]. There are major functional differences between LHRH1 receptors in pituitary and in tumors, in spite of the expression of identical receptor transcripts. Classical LHRH1 receptor signal transduction mechanisms for tumors appear to be different from those for the pituitary. Pituitary LHRH1 receptors have high affinity for agonists, but most tumoral LHRH1 receptors have low affinity. In the pituitary, LHRH1 receptors are coupled via $G_{q/11}$ to PLC causing an IP_3-mediated mobilization of Ca^{2+} and a PKC-mediated activation of mitogen-activated protein kinases (MAPKs) [20]. However, components of the pituitary LHRH1 system such as $G_{\alpha q}$-protein [21], PLC, and PKC [22] are not involved in the mediation of antimitogenic effects of LHRH1 in gynecological and breast cancers. In the case of tumoral LHRH1 receptors no PLC activation occurs; however, instead, G_i-mediated activation of protein phosphatase and inhibition of MAPK activity takes place as part of the antiproliferative effects mediated by these LHRH1 receptors. After binding of its ligand, the LHRH1 receptor in cancers couples to $G_{\alpha i}$-protein and activates a phosphotyrosine phosphatase [21, 22]. This phosphotyrosine phosphatase then dephosphorylates the receptors for EGF [21]. As a result, mitogenic signaling induced by binding of EGF to its receptor is nullified, leading to a suppression of EGF-induced activation of MAPK, c-*fos* expression, and EGF-induced proliferation [21, 22].

38.3.1.1.1 Receptors for LHRH1 on Tumors Tumoral receptors for LHRH1 have been detected on human breast, prostatic, ovarian, endometrial, and pancreatic cancers [23–27]. The expression of LHRH1 receptor genes in human breast, endometrial, ovarian, and prostate tumors, and respective cancer cell lines was also demonstrated by reverse transcription polymerase chain reaction (RT-PCR) [15, 17]. Thus, high-affinity binding sites for LHRH1 were found on 52% of surgical specimens of human breast cancer and also in various human breast cancer cell lines [24]. LHRH1 receptors and expression of mRNA for LHRH1 receptors were also demonstrated in about 86% of surgical samples of human prostate cancer and in several human prostate cancer lines [26]. Similarly, receptors for LHRH1 were detected in 78% of human epithelial ovarian cancer specimens [27] and ovarian cancer cell lines, as well as in 80% of human endometrial carcinomas and many endometrial cancer cell lines [21, 25]. More recently they have been detected in melanomas [28], non-Hodgkin's lymphomas (NHLs) [29], and renal cell carcinomas (RCCs) [30]. The evidence for the production of an LHRH1-like peptide and/or the expression of mRNA for LHRH1 was also demonstrated in human breast, prostatic, ovarian, and endometrial cancer cell lines (for reviews, see [15, 31]). These findings suggest that locally produced LHRH1 may be involved in the growth of these tumors and may form an autocrine/paracrine regulatory loop with tumoral LHRH1 receptors. LHRH1 agonists and antagonists could inhibit proliferation *in vitro* of human mammary, prostatic, ovarian, and endometrial cancer cell lines through downregulation or blocking of LHRH1 receptors on tumor cells [15, 16]. In some cancers, however, locally produced LHRH1 may actually stimulate proliferation rather than inhibit it. Some investigators postulate that LHRH1 produced by tumor cells might have an inhibitory function; however, inhibitory effects of LHRH1 agonists can be best explained by receptor downregulation [15]. Additional investigations are necessary to clarify the role and action of these endogenous LHRH1-like peptides produced by various tumors.

38.3.1.1.2 Targeting of LHRH1 Conjugates to Tumors The expression of LHRH1 receptors in tumors [32–39] has been exploited for an approach to targeted cancer therapy. Various toxins conjugated to LHRH1 and other chimeric proteins have been used for targeting to the LHRH1 receptors on tumors [33–39]. Thus, LHRH1 and its analogs have been fused with or linked to bacterial and plant toxins to target and kill cancer cells expressing LHRH1 receptors [32, 33, 37–39]. Qi *et al.* [34] and Schlick *et al.* [39] demonstrated that conjugated or recombinant fusion proteins composed of pokeweed antiviral protein linked to analogs of LHRH1 can inhibit various cancer cells expressing LHRH1 receptors, such as prostate and breast. Ben-Yehuda *et al.* [37, 38] reported that a chimeric protein composed of LHRH1 analog and *Pseudomonas* exotoxin suppressed the growth of a colonic adenocarcinoma cell line xenografted into nude mice. Human proapoptotic BLC-2 proteins, BIK, BAK, and BAX, as well as the caspase-activated DNase, DFF40, have also been coupled to LHRH1 by protein fusion [32]. These chimeric proteins induced apoptosis, and inhibited proliferation of colorectal and renal cancers [32]. It was also reported that bovine RNase A conjugated to LHRH1 can inhibit growth of prostate and breast cancers [35].

Lueschner *et al.* [33] developed a targeted cytotoxic LHRH1 analog consisting of hecate, a lytic peptide, conjugated to LHRH1. This conjugate was highly cytotoxic *in vitro* for prostate cancer cells such as LNCaP, PC-3, and DU-145 expressing LHRH1 receptors. The LHRH1–hecate conjugate also inhibited growth of PC-3 prostatic cancer in nude mice *in vivo* [33]. Thus, various compounds with anticancer activity can be produced by targeting to LHRH1 receptors.

38.3.1.2 Design and Synthesis of Targeted Cytotoxic Analogs of LHRH1

The design of cytotoxic LHRH1 analogs was based on the use of agonists or antagonists of LHRH1 as carrier molecules that were then linked to cytotoxic agents

[6, 7, 15, 17]. As the replacement of the Gly residue at position 6 of LHRH1 by various D-amino acids increases the stability of the analog to enzymatic degradation, and results in potent analogs of LHRH1 with high binding affinity and biological activity [6, 7, 15, 17], a D-Lys moiety at position 6 has been used for attachment of various cytotoxic compounds. It was found that even bulky molecules could be linked to the ε-amino group of the D-Lys^6 moiety without loss of the binding affinity to receptors of LHRH1. Thus, we synthesized cytotoxic LHRH1 hybrids in which diverse cytotoxic radicals were attached covalently to the D-Lys side-chain of the LHRH1 carrier [6]. These cytotoxic compounds initially included cisplatin, methotrexate, and 2-(hydroxymethyl)anthraquinone. D-Melphalan – an alkylating nitrogen mustard derivative of D-phenylalanine – has also been incorporated at position 6 of LHRH1 [6]. Some of these compounds had high binding affinity to receptors and showed cytotoxic activity *in vitro* [6]. Early conjugates with [D-Lys^6]LHRH1 also included the DNA intercalating antibiotic doxorubicin (DOX) – a widely used anticancer agents with a broad spectrum of antitumor activity [6]. The antiproliferative activity of DOX is due mainly to its ability to intercalate into DNA and break the strands of the double helix by inhibiting topoisomerase II. At first, DOX was linked to LHRH1 analogs through a glutaric acid spacer to form a carboxamide bond between the daunosamine nitrogen of DOX and the ε-amino group of D-Lys^6 moiety of the carrier [6]. Regrettably, the neutralization of the daunosamine nitrogen of DOX in these analogs resulted in great loss of cytotoxic activity [7]. However, several years later, procedures for the formation of LHRH1–DOX hybrids with preservation of antitumoral activity were developed. In view of the findings that 14-*O* ester bonds of DOX are stable at acidic and neutral pH and have similar antitumor activity as DOX, *N*-Fmoc-DOX-14-*O*-hemiglutarate was linked to the D-Lys^6 side-chain of the LHRH1 analogs [40]. Thus, [D-Lys^6]LHRH1 (Glp-His-Trp-Ser-Tyr-D-Lys-Leu-Arg-Pro-Gly-NH_2) was selected as the agonistic LHRH1 carrier and Ac-D-Nal(2)- D-Phe(4C1)-D-Pal(3)-Ser-Tyr-D-Lys-Leu-Arg-Pro-D-Ala-NH_2 as the antagonistic LHRH1 carrier. N-Fmoc-DOX-14-*O*-hemiglutarate was coupled covalently to the ε-amino group of the D-Lys residue of the respective peptide sequences. The cytotoxic agonistic analog AN-152 obtained after deprotection (Figure 38.2) thus fully preserved the cytotoxicity of DOX and the binding affinity of the LHRH1 carrier. Several daunosamine-modified derivatives of DOX

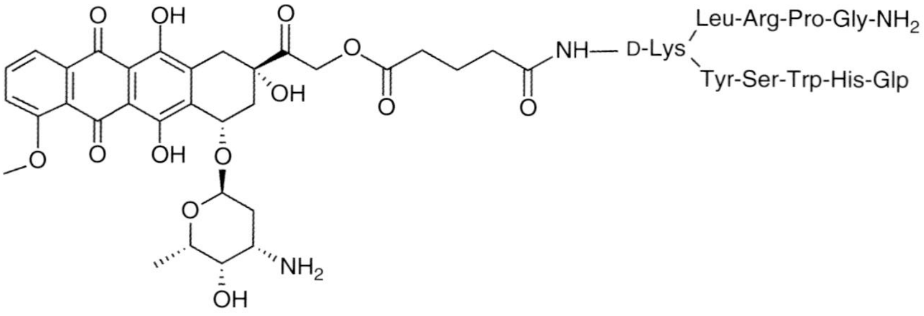

Figure 38.2 Structure of targeted cytotoxic LHRH1 analog AN-152 linked to doxorubicin.

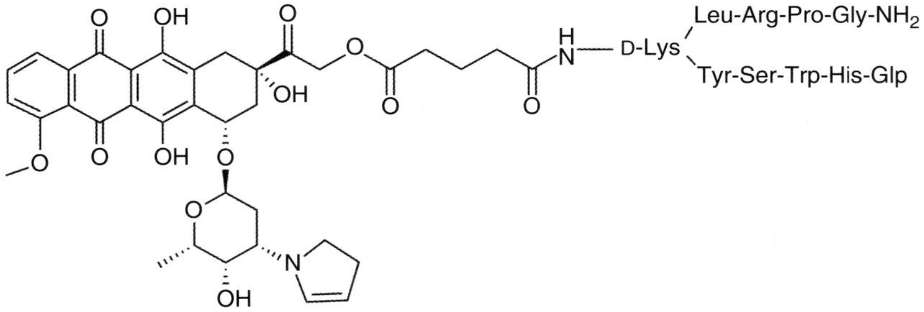

Figure 38.3 Structure of targeted cytotoxic LHRH1 analog AN-207 linked to 2-pyrrolino-DOX.

that could be coupled to the carriers were also developed. The most active was 3′-deamino-3′-(2″-pyrroline-1″-yl (2-pyrrolino)-DOX, designated as AN-201, which is up to 500 times more active *in vitro* than DOX [40]. AN-201 was noncardiotoxic and non-cross-resistant with DOX [7, 40]. AN-152, in which DOX is linked to [D-Lys^6]LHRH1, is easily converted chemically, in a high yield, to superactive analog AN-207, containing 2-pyrrolino-DOX (Figure 38.3). Cytotoxic LHRH1 antagonist analog with DOX (AN-241) was converted similarly to a derivative containing 2-pyrrolino-DOX (AN-243). The antiproliferative activity of the cytotoxic radical and the high binding affinity of the carrier to LHRH1 receptors were fully preserved in the cytotoxic LHRH1 analog AN-207 [7, 40]. The mechanism of action of cytotoxic LHRH1 analog AN-207, containing AN-201 is similar to that of AN-152. A major difference between the two cytotoxic LHRH1 analogs AN-152 and AN-207 is the fact that the effective dose of AN-207 is about 100 times lower than that of AN-152. Therefore, AN-207 should be useful for targeting tumors with a low receptor concentration. The production of free oxygen radicals by DOX has been linked to its cardiotoxicity, which is its dose-limiting toxicity (DLT). In contrast, AN-201, the cytotoxic radical in AN-207, is noncardiotoxic. Nevertheless, as a powerful DNA intercalator, AN-201 can be toxic to all types of rapidly proliferating cells. The binding affinities of cytotoxic LHRH1 analogs to receptors for LHRH1 on membrane preparations of rat anterior pituitaries were determined in competitive binding assays. Radioiodinated [D-Trp^6]LHRH1 was used as radioligand. The binding affinities were expressed as IC_{50} values (i.e., the concentration of unlabeled analog required to displace 50% of the binding of the radioligand). Thus, the IC_{50} values for AN-152, AN-207, and the carrier [D-Lys^6]LHRH1 were found to be similar, being 2.29, 5.59, and 2.26 nM, respectively, indicating that the binding activity was fully preserved [7, 40].

38.3.1.3 Mechanism of Action of Cytotoxic LHRH1 Analogs: Targeting to LHRH1 Receptors on Tumors

The binding of cytotoxic LHRH1 analogs to receptors for LHRH1 on cancerous cells is followed by cellular internalization of the hybrid molecule and the release of the cytotoxic agent in the lysosomes. As the internalization of LHRH1 agonists

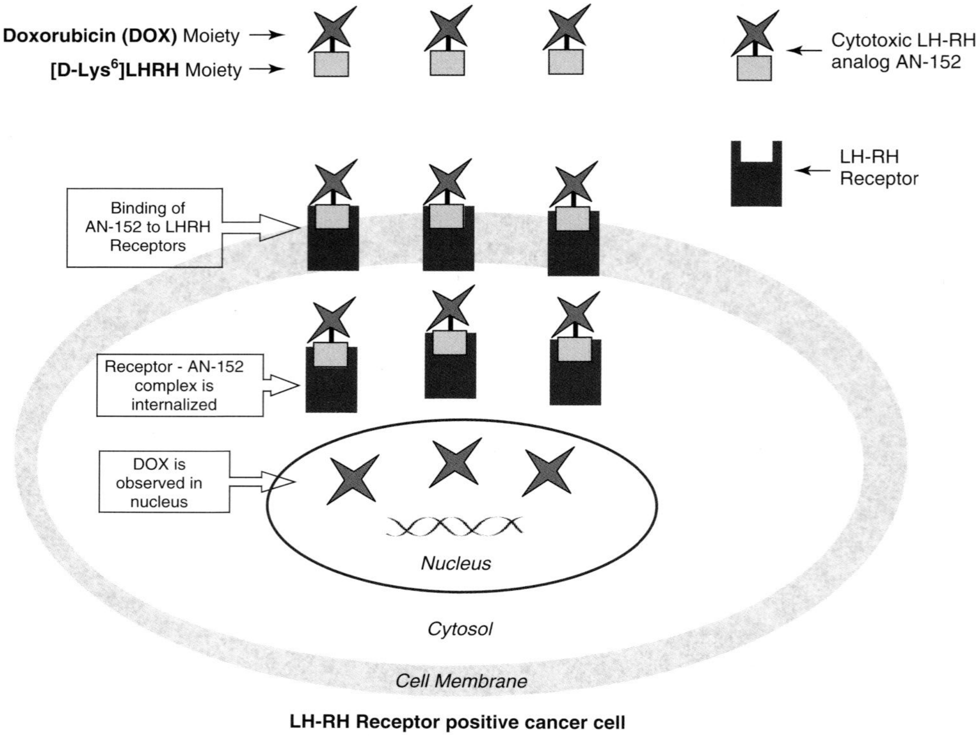

Figure 38.4 Active targeting of cytotoxic LHRH1 analog AN-152 to receptors for LHRH1 on tumors. A schematic representation of binding of LHRH1 analog AN-152 to LHRH1 receptors on human ovarian, endometrial, and breast cancer cells. The binding is followed by internalization of the ligand–receptor complex. This representation is based on the findings obtained by two-photon laser scanning microscopy of fluorophore-labeled AN-152 and confocal laser scanning microscopy using the autofluorescence of the DOX moiety in AN-152 [7, 41–44] at an excitation wavelength of 488 nm. An aggregation of the fluorescent signal of AN-152 on the cell membrane could be observed within a few minutes, indicating binding of the ligand to the receptors. This was followed by the appearance of signals in cytoplasmic granules, demonstrating internalization of AN-152. Within 15–60 min after exposure, the fluorescent signal of free DOX was found in the nucleus. AN-152 entered only LHRH1 receptor-positive cells as demonstrated in the MCF-7 human breast cancer cell line, the Ishikawa human ovarian cancer cell line, and the Hec-1A human endometrial cancer cell line, but not in the LHRH1 receptor-negative human ovarian cancer lines UCI-107 and SKOV-3. The receptor-mediated entry and antiproliferative activity of AN-152 could be diminished by a pretreatment of the cells with LHRH1 agonist [D-Trp^6]LHRH1. In contrast, DOX entered all cell types tested, regardless of their LHRH1 receptor status, and accumulated in the nucleus within a few minutes after exposure. The effects of DOX could not be inhibited by a preincubation with [D-Trp6]LHRH1 [7, 41–44]. (Modified from [7].)

into pituitary cells was shown to be much faster than that of the antagonists, we studied the mechanism of internalization of cytotoxic LHRH1 agonists on tumors.

The interaction with the LHRH1 receptors and the entry into cell cytoplasm of cytotoxic LHRH1 agonist AN-152 containing DOX was investigated in LHRH1 receptor-positive and LHRH1 receptor-negative human ovarian and endometrial cancer cell lines, and in the MCF-7 breast cancer line (Figure 38.4) [7, 41–44]. These processes were revealed by two-photon laser scanning microscopy of fluorophore-labeled AN-152 and confocal laser scanning microscopy using the autofluorescence of the DOX moiety in AN-152 in human ovarian and endometrial cancer cell lines (Figures 38.5 and 38.6). AN-152 entered only into LHRH1 receptor-positive cells while unconjugated DOX entered all cell types independently of their receptor status. A significantly higher fluorescence signal could be detected

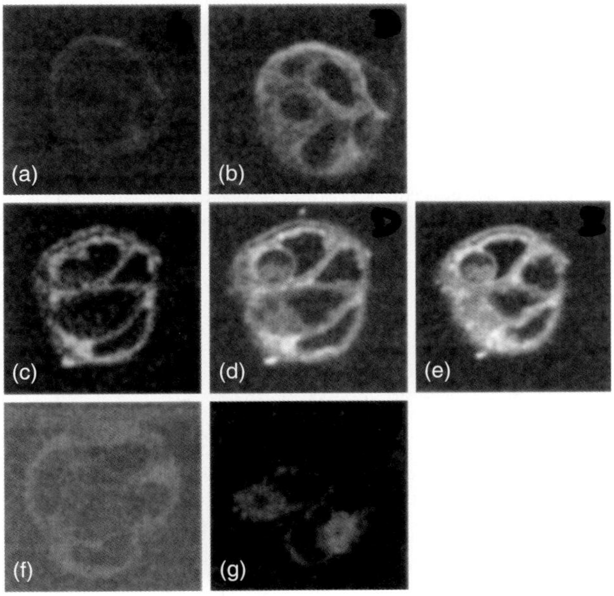

Figure 38.5 Regulation of entry of chromophore-labeled AN-152 (AN-152:C625) into LHRH1 receptor-positive cells (MCF-7) by hormones and comparison of entry into LHRH1 receptor-negative cells (UCI-107): MCF-7 cells were imaged by two-photon laser scanning microscopy after exposure to AN-152:C625. Cells receiving no pretreatment (control) displayed labeling of membranes after 30 min (a), and entry into the cytoplasm and nucleus after 60 min (b). Drug uptake into cells was enhanced by EGF pretreatment, such that labeling of membranes was clear after 10 min (c), uptake into the cytoplasm and nucleus was detected within 30 min (d), and increasing aggregation was seen in the nucleus at 60 min (e). Drug entry into cells is diminished by pretreatment with the somatostatin analog RC-160, such that only faint labeling of membranes and a low entry of the drug was observed at 60 min (f). Entry of AN-152:C625 into UCI-107 (receptor-negative control) is negligible after 90 min (g). (Reproduced from [43].)

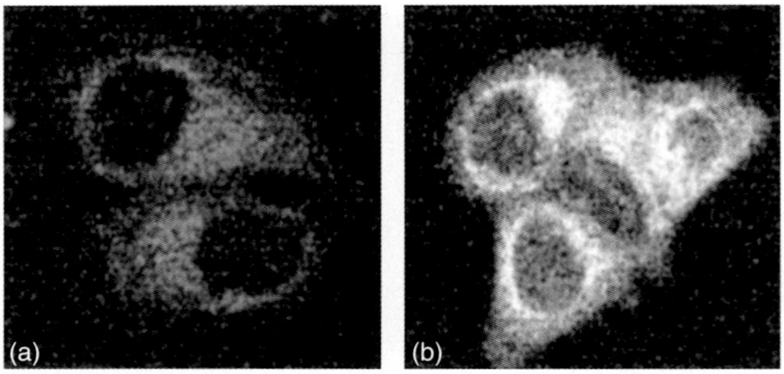

Figure 38.6 Competition assay. [D-Trp^6]LHRH1 competes with AN-152:C625 for binding sites. MCF-7 cells were pretreated with EGF, exposed to AN-152:C625 (0.6 μM), and imaged by two-photon laser scanning microscopy. Image in the presence of [D-Trp^6]LHRH1 (1 μM) after 50 min (a) or after 20 min (without a competitor present; (b) incubation with AN-152:C625. Note that even with 2.5 times as long exposure, the cells exposed to LHRH1 analog showed significantly less uptake of the labeled drug. (Reproduced from [43].)

in the nuclei of LHRH1 receptor-positive cells after treatment with AN-152 than was the case with DOX. Accordingly, AN-152 was significantly more cytotoxic than DOX in these cells [41].

Similar results were obtained in human estrogen-dependent MCF-7 breast cancer cells *in vitro*. Two-photon emission fluorophores were linked to the free amino group of the daunosamine moiety of AN-152 or to the ε-amino group of the carrier [D-Lys^6]LHRH1. The energy required for the excitation of these fluorophore tags allowed "real-time" optical tracking of the conjugate and the carrier in the different compartments of living MCF-7 cells [7, 42, 43]. The labeled carrier peptide was localized mainly in the cytosols of MCF-7 cells and not in the nucleus, but the fluorescent label linked to AN-152 and coupled to the daunosamine nitrogen of DOX was found only in the nuclei. No entry of labeled AN-152 could be observed in LHRH1 receptor-negative UCI-107 human ovarian cancer cells [43]. AN-152 is sensitive to carboxylesterase-catalyzed deconjugation into DOX and probably [D-Lys^6]LHRH1-glutarate in blood and aqueous solutions. Since after the internalization of AN-152, DOX is cleaved from LHRH1 and accumulates in the nucleus, carboxylase-like enzymes are likely responsible for this cleavage of the ester bonds in endosomes or lysosomes. However the intact peptide conjugates AN-152 and AN-207 could also exert antitumor activity.

In mammalian COS-7 cells, stably transfected with recombinant human LHRH1 receptors, AN-207 was found to selectively induce apoptosis in receptor-positive cells as measured by DNA fragmentation and the expression of proapoptotic (BAX) and antiapoptotic (BCL-2) proteins [45].

38.3.1.4 **Responses of Human Experimental Cancers Expressing Receptors for LHRH1 to Targeted Cytotoxic Analogs of LHRH1**

The activity of targeted cytotoxic LHRH1 analogs AN-152 and AN-207 was evaluated in various cancer models *in vitro* and *in vivo*. The main *in vivo* tests were based on the use of human cancer cell lines that express receptors for LHRH1 and that are xenografted into nude mice [7].

38.3.1.4.1 Breast Cancer The treatment options available for estrogen-independent breast cancers, including chemotherapy and Herceptin, are not completely satisfactory for all subclasses of patients [15–17, 25, 46]. As more than 50% of breast cancer specimens have receptors for LHRH1 [24], we explored cytotoxic LHRH1 analogs in various human breast cancer models. Analog AN-207 caused a complete regression of DOX-resistant MX-1 tumors [47], and inhibited the growth of MDA-MB-231 and MDA-MB-435 estrogen-independent human breast cancers xenografted into nude mice [48]. AN-152 also powerfully suppressed proliferation of MX-1 hormone-independent DOX-resistant human breast cancers xenografted in nude mice [49] (Figure 38.7). Clinical phase II trials of AN-152, now also designated AEZS-108, in women with metastatic breast cancer are in progress.

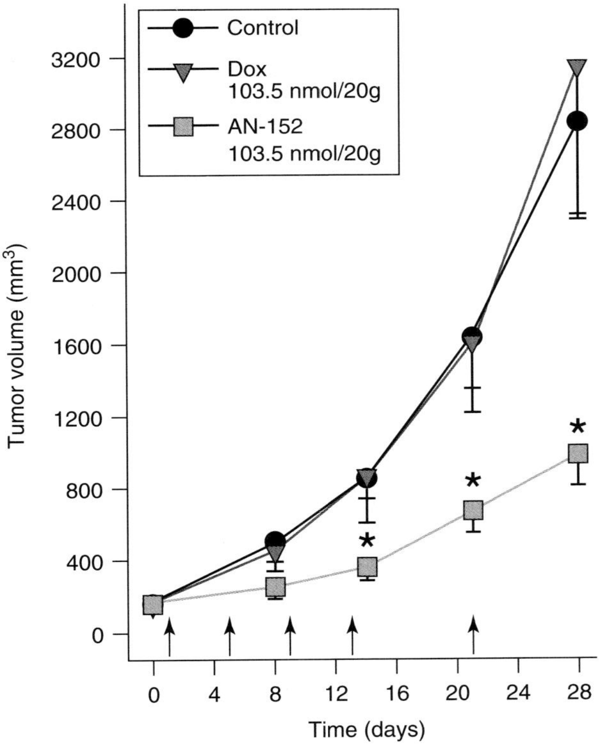

Figure 38.7 Tumor volume in athymic nude mice bearing subcutaneously transplanted xenografts of MX-1 hormone-independent DOX-resistant human breast carcinoma after five intravenous injections of DOX or the cytotoxic LHRH1 analogue AN-152 at doses of 103.5 nmol/20 g, corresponding to 3 mg/kg DOX hydrochloride. Arrows, days of injections. Vertical bars, standard error. $^{*}P < 0.05$ versus control. (Reproduced from [49].)

38.3.1.4.2 Ovarian Cancer Since expression of LHRH1 receptors was found in about 80% of human ovarian cancer specimens and in ovarian cancer cell lines [27], we evaluated targeted cytotoxic LHRH1 analogs in experimental models of human ovarian cancers [7]. Thus, analog AN-152 inhibited the growth of LHRH1 receptor-positive OV-1063 and OVCAR-2 human ovarian cancers in nude mice [50, 51], and was less toxic than DOX [52]. LHRH1 receptor-negative UCI-107 and SK-OV-3 ovarian cancer cell lines did not respond to AN-152 [52]. The proliferation of OV-1063 and ES-2 ovarian cancer (Figure 38.8) *in vivo* was similarly suppressed by cytotoxic LHRH1 analog AN-207 [51, 53]. Cytotoxic LHRH1 analog AN-152 (AEZS-108) is being evaluated for the management of ovarian cancer in phase II clinical trials [54].

38.3.1.4.3 Endometrial Cancer The presence of LHRH1 receptors on more than 80% of endometrial neoplasms [6, 7, 25] provides a rationale of the development of targeted cytotoxic LHRH1 analogs for the treatment of recurrent endometrial cancers. In experimental studies, AN-152 was more effective and less toxic than DOX in tests on HEC-1A, HEC-1B, and RL-95-2 human endometrial cancer cell lines xenografted into nude mice [52, 55] (Figure 38.9). AN-207 also inhibited growth of HEC-1A and RL-95-2 human endometrial cancers, and was more effective than AN-201 [55]. On the basis of these results we started clinical trials, which are now in phase II, with AN-152 (AEZS-108) in women with advanced endometrial cancers [54] (see Section 38.3.2).

38.3.1.4.4 Prostate Cancer Response rates to chemotherapy of patients with androgen-independent castration-resistant prostate cancer are very low [46]. Local

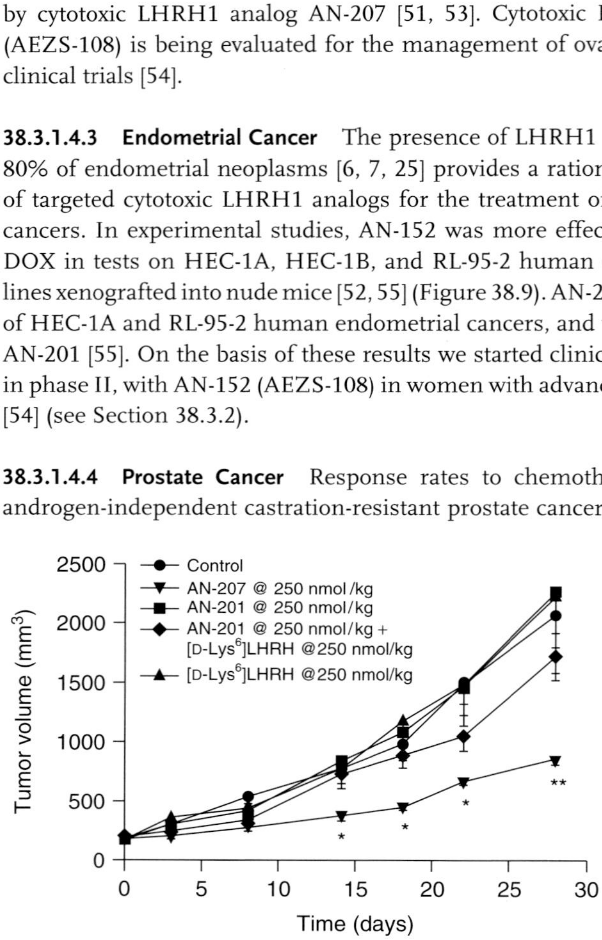

Figure 38.8 Effect of treatment with the cytotoxic LHRH1 analog AN-207 and its components on the growth of ES-2 human ovarian cancers in nude mice. Changes in tumor volume after a single intravenous injection on day 0 at a dose of 250 nmol/kg of AN-207, the cytotoxic radical AN-201, an unconjugated mixture of [D-Lys^6]LHRH1 and AN-201, and the carrier [D-Lys^6]LHRH1. Controls received intravenous injections of the vehicle solution (5% mannitol) $^*p < 0.05$ $^{**}p < 0.01$ versus control. (Reproduced from [53].)

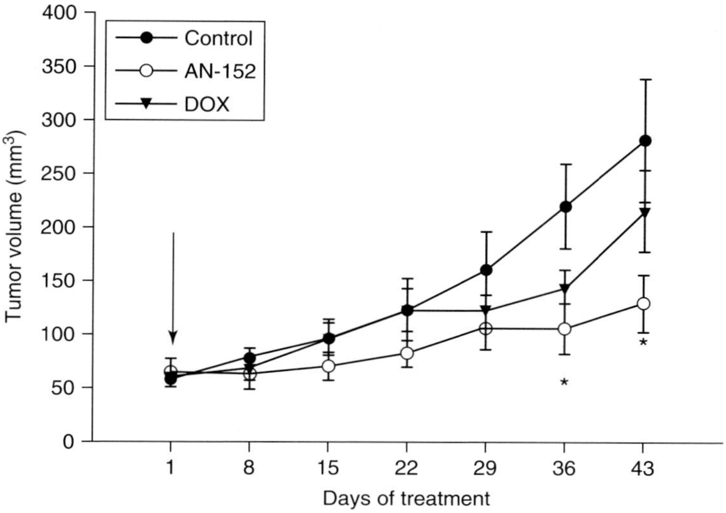

Figure 38.9 Effects of the targeted cytotoxic LHRH1 analog AN-152 at doses equivalent to 10 mg/kg DOX and the radical DOX at equimolar doses on the growth of HEC-1A human endometrial carcinoma xenografts. Mean ± standard error. $^*P < 0.05$. (Reproduced from [55].)

delivery of chemotherapeutic agents would improve their efficacy. Receptors for LHRH1 are expressed by 86% of human prostate cancers as measured by ligand competition assays, RT-PCR analysis [26], or immunohistochemistry [56].

Targeted cytotoxic LHRH1 analogs have been extensively studied in various models of prostate cancer [7, 57–59]. Analog AN-207 strongly inhibited growth of the androgen-independent DU-145 human prostate tumor line (Figure 38.10a) and MDA-PCa-2b human prostate cancers in nude mice, and also lowered prostate-specific antigen (PSA) levels [57, 58]. Analog AN-152 similarly suppressed growth of androgen-sensitive MDA-PCa-2b and LNCaP prostate cancers, and was more effective than DOX [59]. In nude mice bearing androgen-independent intraosseous C4-2 prostate cancers, AN-152 decreased serum PSA levels (Figure 38.10b) and increased apoptosis [59]. The growth of androgen-independent DU-145 human prostate cancer can be also suppressed by AN-152 (Rick and Schally, unpublished). Clinical trials with AN-152 in patients with castration-resistant prostate cancer are pending.

38.3.1.4.5 Urinary Bladder Cancers New therapeutic methods are needed for the treatment of metastatic bladder cancer. Immunohistochemical studies indicate that human bladder cancers express receptors for LHRH1 ([60], and Keller and Schally, unpublished). The growth of human bladder cancer lines xenografted into nude mice is strongly inhibited by cytotoxic LHRH1 analog, AN-152 (Szepeshazi and

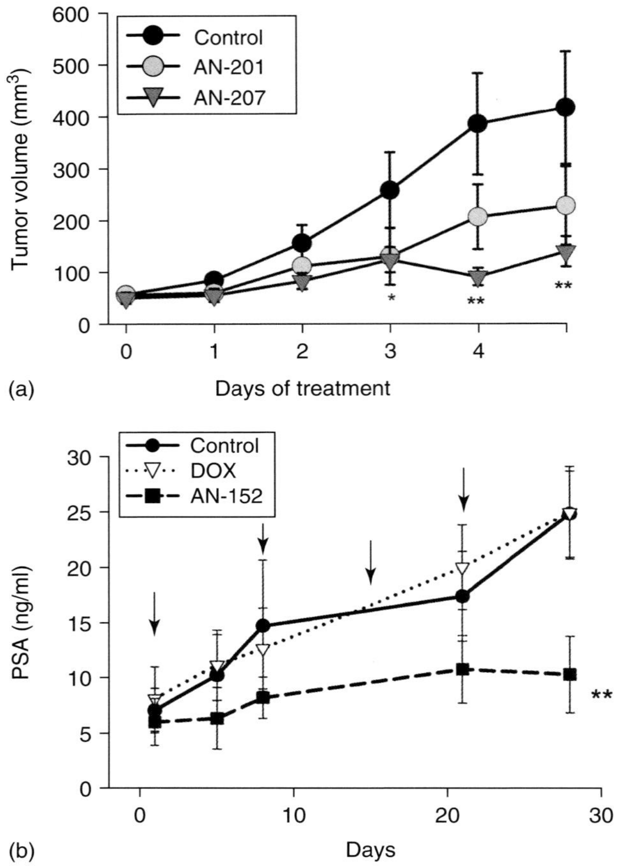

Figure 38.10 Effects of targeted cytotoxic LHRH1 analogs on prostate cancers. (a) Effects of targeted cytotoxic LHRH1 analog AN-207 and cytotoxic radical AN-201 on the growth of DU-145 human androgen-independent prostate cancers xenografted subcutaneously into nude mice. Compounds were injected at 200 nmol/kg body weight on day 0 and day 26. Mean ± standard error. $^{*}P < 0.05$ versus control, $^{**}P < 0.01$ versus control. (Reproduced from [57].) (b) The effect of four intravenous injections of AN-152 or DOX at 138 nmol/kg body weight on days 1, 7, 14, and 21 on serum PSA levels of C4-2 human androgen-independent prostate cancers implanted into the tibiae of nude mice. Vertical bars, standard error. $^{**}P < 0.01$ versus control. Arrows indicate days of injection. (Reproduced from [59].)

Schally, in press). A phase I/II clinical trial with AN-152 (AEZS-108) in patients with metastatic urothelial carcinoma, resistant to platinum chemotherapy, is pending.

38.3.1.4.6 RCCs The expression of LHRH1 receptors was demonstrated by immunohistochemistry in surgically removed specimens of RCC [30]. LHRH1 binding sites, mRNA for LHRH1 receptor, and LHRH1 receptor protein were also detected in three RCC cell lines (A-498, ACHN, and 786-0); analog AN-207 suppressed growth of xenografts of these tumors [30]. Thus, LHRH1 receptors, expressed in human RCC specimens, could be used for targeted chemotherapy with cytotoxic LHRH1 analogs [7].

38.3.1.4.7 NHL The presence of LHRH1 receptors in surgical biopsy specimens of human NHL was detected by immunohistochemistry [29]. The expression of LHRH1 receptors in two human NHL cell lines, RL and HT, was also shown by RT-PCR, Western blot, and radioligand-binding studies [29]. Analog AN-207 significantly inhibited the growth of RL and HT tumors (Figure 38.11) [29]. Our findings indicate that LHRH1 receptors on human NHL could be considered for targeted therapy with the cytotoxic LHRH1 analogs [7].

38.3.1.4.8 Malignant Melanomas Surgical specimens of human malignant melanoma and MRI-H255 and MRI-H187 human melanoma cancer cell lines were found to express LHRH1 receptors by immunohistochemistry, binding assays, Western immunoblotting, and RT-PCR analyses [28]. Analog AN-207 significantly inhibited the growth of MRI-H255 (Figure 38.12) and MRI-H187 xenografts *in vivo* [28]. These results indicate that LHRH1 receptors found in a high percentage of human malignant melanoma specimens could be used for targeting cytotoxic LHRH1 analogs [7].

38.3.1.4.9 Hepatic Cancers The presence of receptors for LHRH1 in SK-Hep-1 human hepatic carcinoma cell line [61] was ascertained by radioreceptor assays and immunohistochemistry. Cytotoxic LHRH1 analog AN-207 inhibited growth of SK-Hep-1 tumors in nude mice [61]. However, more extensive studies with cytotoxic

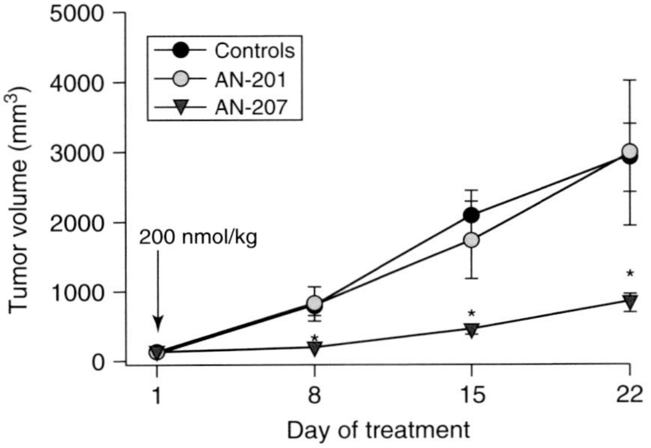

Figure 38.11 Effects of targeted cytotoxic LHRH1 analog AN-207 and its radical AN-201 on the growth of xenografts of RL human NHL. Arrows indicate treatment. $^*P < 0.01$ versus controls and AN-201. (Reproduced from [29].)

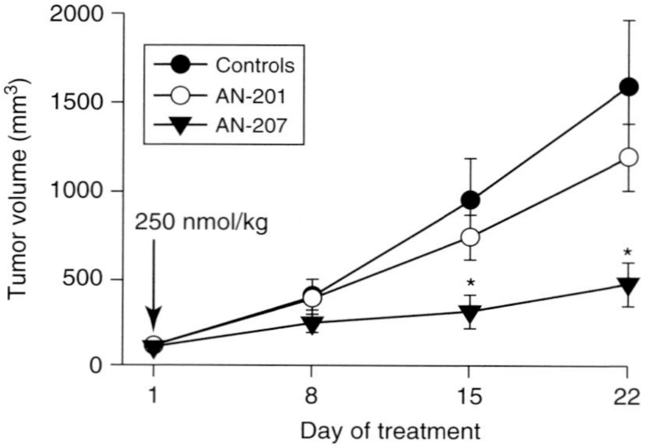

Figure 38.12 Effects of targeted cytotoxic LHRH1 analog AN-207 and its radical AN-201 on the growth of MRI-H255 human malignant melanoma xenografted into nude mice. $^*P < 0.05$ versus controls. (Reproduced from [28].)

LHRH1 analogs in models of human hepatocellular carcinoma are necessary before any clinical trials are considered [61].

38.3.1.4.10 Colorectal Cancer Advanced cases of colorectal cancers can be treated with chemotherapy [11, 46]. Five colon cancer lines investigated, HT-29, HCT-116, HCT-15, LoVo, and Colo-320DM, showed high-affinity binding sites for LHRH1 and expressed mRNA for the LHRH1 receptor [62]. Cytotoxic LHRH1 analogs AN-207 and AN-152 strongly inhibited growth of all five colon cancer cell lines [62]. Thus, targeted therapy with cytotoxic LHRH1 analogs could be also considered for the treatment of metastatic colorectal cancer [7, 17].

38.3.1.4.11 Pancreatic Cancers The prognosis for patients with ductal pancreatic cancers is extremely poor and it is essential to develop new therapeutic approaches [7, 11, 17, 46]. Human pancreatic cancers express LHRH1 receptors [63] localized mostly in the cell nuclei [64]. Treatment with cytotoxic LHRH1 analog AN-152 inhibits growth of human pancreatic cancer lines xenografted into nude mice (Szepeshazi and Schally, in preparation). phase I/II clinical trials with cytotoxic LHRH1 analog AN-152 (AEZS-108) in patients with advanced pancreatic cancers are pending.

38.3.1.5 **Side-Effects of Cytotoxic LHRH1 Analogs**

Targeted cancer therapy should improve the efficacy of treatment and reduce side-effects as compared with standard systemic chemotherapy [6, 7, 46]. During targeted chemotherapy to LHRH1 receptors, the gonadotroph cells of the anterior pituitary could also be affected by cytotoxic LHRH1 analogs [7]. However, damage to the gonadotroph cells might not be harmful to patients afflicted by sex-hormone-dependent tumors such as breast and prostate cancers and hormone replacement therapy could, in any case, restore normal hormonal balance [6, 7, 46].

When rats were treated with a high dose of AN-207, there was a transient selective damage to pituitary gonadotroph cells, but not to growth hormone (GH)-producing somatotroph or prolactin-producing cells and the pituitary function recovered within 1 week [65]. The absence of permanent damage can be explained by the fact that the cytotoxic radicals, DOX and AN-201, primarily kill rapidly proliferating cells, such as tumor and bone marrow cells, but not those of the pituitary, which are known to proliferate slowly [7, 54, 65]. The main side-effect of cytotoxic LHRH1 analogs appears to be myelosuppression caused by the respective cleaved cytotoxic radicals DOX or AN-201 [6, 7, 46, 54, 65]. On the other hand, the development of chemoresistance, mediated by MDR, may be decreased or delayed in some types of tumors treated by targeted chemotherapy [11–14, 44].

38.3.2 Clinical Development

38.3.2.1 Clinical Phase I and Phase II Trials of Cytotoxic LHRH1 Analog AN-152 (AEZS-108) in Women with Ovarian and Endometrial Cancers

In preclinical studies in dogs, AN-152 had no effect on cardiovascular, electrocardiographic, and respiratory variables. In rats and dogs, elimination half-life ($t_{1/2} < 1$ h) and time of peak concentration ($t_{max} = 0.08$ h) of AEZS-108 and DOX were similar. Dose linearity for AN-152 was demonstrated when based on maximum plasma concentration (C_{max}) and area under the curve (AUC). The AUCs of AN-152 were higher (3–9 times in rats and 7–12 times in dogs) than those of DOX after single or multiple doses and no clear accumulation of AN-152 was observed following infusions every other week.

DLTs, maximum tolerated dose (MTD), and pharmacokinetics of AN-152 (now AEZS-108, formerly also ZEN-008) were assessed in recent phase I clinical trials in patients with ovarian, fallopian tube, endometrial, or breast cancers [54, 66]. The most important exclusion criteria were history of diagnosed angina pectoris, or myocardial infarction within the last 6 months, serious arrhythmia or congestive heart failure, radiotherapy to pericardial area, or prior use of anthracyclines corresponding to greater than 70% of the recommended lifetime cumulative dose for DOX. Based on pharmacokinetic studies the half-lives of AN-152 in mouse, rat, and human serum were found to be about 20, 60, and 120 min, respectively [54]. DLT was not observed at 160 mg/m^2. Consequently the dose administered to patients could be increased to reach the MTD of AEZS-108 of 267 mg/m^2. Seventeen patients, with tumors proven immunohistochemically to be LHRH1 receptor-positive, entered the study. LHRH1 receptor expression was centrally assessed by immunohistochemistry. Doses of AN-152 (AEZS-108) were doubled starting at 10 mg/m^2 until grade II side-effects occurred [54, 66]. The patients received AN-152 by intravenous infusion over 2 h at dosages of 10, 20, 40, 80, 160, and 267 mg/m^2 once every 3 weeks. As these patients had previously received several other cytotoxic regimens, the study limited them to 70% of the recommended maximum lifetime dose for DOX. AN-152 (AEZS-108) was well tolerated [54, 66], but dose-limiting leukopenia and neutropenia were observed at the highest dose. Following 160 and 267 mg/m^2 AN-152, maximum plasma concentrations (C_{max}) ranged from 728 to 6661 ng/ml. Only a weak dose dependency was found in C_{max} and AUC. The calculated $t_{1/2}$ and the clearance of AEZS-108 were approximately 2 h and 1 l/min·m^2, respectively. Average C_{max} values of DOX ranged from 600 to 700 ng/ml. Owing to the known cardiotoxic effect of DOX, cardiac safety was monitored by repeated evaluation of left ventricular ejection fraction (LVEF) and the electrocardiogram (ECG). ECG results suggested a small average increase in QTc, but the data for LVEF were not altered. In all, our data suggest that cardiotoxicity would not be relevant for AN-152 up to 267 mg/m^2. A small reduction in LH and FSH was also found. An objective response was achieved in three of 13 patients treated with 160 or 267 mg/m^2 of AN-152, equivalent to 46 and 77 mg/m^2 of DOX. This response consisted of complete normalization of pathological CA125 levels, partial remission of liver metastasis, and complete disappearance of lymph node metastasis. Three other patients experienced disease stabilization (stable hepatic metastasis, minor response in spleen metastasis, and stable spleen metastasis) [54, 66].

A phase II clinical trial in patients with heavily pretreated taxane- and platinum-resistant ovarian cancer or with disseminated endometrial cancer is currently in progress. The dose of 267 mg/m^2 AN-152 (AEZS 108), which was well tolerated and therapeutically active in the phase I trial, is used every 3 weeks, for up to six cycles. This ongoing open-label, noncomparative multicenter trial will involve up to 82 women in 15 centers in Europe [67]. About 38% of patients have a partial response or stabilization of disease. AN-152 was well tolerated. The favorable safety profile confirms the recommended dose of 267 mg/m^2 every 3 weeks. Hematological toxicity was rapidly reversible. Overall survival is encouraging as all patients treated with AN-152 were platinum resistant. Cytotoxic analogs of LHRH1 would be an important addition to the clinical armamentarium for cancer [7, 46].

38.4 Example 2: Targeted Cytotoxic Somatostatin Analogs

38.4.1 Preclinical Considerations and Development

38.4.1.1 Somatostatin and its Receptors

The hypothalamic neuropeptide somatostatin exists in the form of a 14-amino-acid peptide (somatostatin-14) and an extended version consisting of 28 amino acids (somatostatin-28) [17, 46, 68]. Both forms of somatostatin are also present in the gastrointestinal tract and inhibit the secretion therein of many hormones, including GH, insulin and glucagon, gastrin, secretin, and cholecystokinin (CCK). Somatostatin is also present in the gastric mucosa, pancreas, and duodenum where it suppresses exocrine secretions, including gastric acid, pancreatic enzymes, and bicarbonate respectively [17, 46, 68]. Owing to the short half-life of somatostatin-14, more stable and more potent synthetic somatostatin analogs have been developed, including octreotide (Sandostatin®) [69], vapreotide (RC-160, Octastatin®) [70], and lanreotide (Somatulin®) [17, 46]. Somatostatin and its octapeptide analogs exert their effects through specific GPCRs that are widely distributed in normal and cancerous cells [17, 68].

At least five distinct somatostatin receptor subtypes, designated sst_{1-5}, have been cloned and characterized [71, 72]. These five subtypes of somatostatin receptors are encoded by five genes that were mapped to chromosomes 14, 17, 22, 20, and 16, respectively [73]. The sst_2 gene generates two splice variants, sst_{2A} and sst_{2B}, which have a shorter cytoplasmic domain. While native somatostatin shows similar high affinity to sst_{1-5}, the synthetic octapeptides, such as octreotide, RC-160, and RC-121, bind preferentially to sst_2 and sst_5, display moderate affinity to sst_3, and a low affinity to sst_1 and sst_4 [17, 71, 72].

In recent years, the molecular basis of the antitumor activity of somatostatin has been extensively investigated. These actions of somatostatin and its analogs appear to be exerted through both direct and indirect mechanisms [73]. Direct antitumor effects, mediated through somatostatin receptors expressed on tumor cells include blockage of autocrine/paracrine GH and growth factor production, inhibition of growth factor-mediated mitogenic signals, mainly through the regulation of phosphotyrosine phosphatase and MAPK activities, and induction of cell cycle arrest or apoptosis [73]. Indirect antitumor effects include suppression of secretion of GH, prolactin, and growth factors, and inhibition of tumor angiogenesis [73, 74]. Thus, by inhibition of angiogenesis, somatostatin and its analogs can also indirectly control tumor development and metastasis [74]. Tumor angiogenesis is essential for tumor growth, invasion, and metastasis. Somatostatin octapeptide RC-160 also stimulates tyrosine phosphatase [75], which appears to be a transducer of the growth inhibition signal in sst_2-expressing cells. However, in sst_5-expressing cells, the phosphatase pathway is not involved in the inhibitory effect of RC-160 on cell growth; inositol phospholipid/calcium is the implicated pathway [76, 77].

Ligand binding to sst_1 can activate the MAPK cascades and limit the proliferative signals generated by growth factor receptors [78]. After ligand binding, somatostatin receptors undergo internalization. Various sst subtypes differentially internalize somatostatin or its analogs [79]. Somatostatin analogs, including RC-160, are powerful tumor growth suppressors in experimental models of various cancers, including pancreatic, colorectal, and gastric cancers [17, 46]. Consequently, attempts have been made to use modern somatostatin analogs for the therapy of various human cancers, but relevant clinical benefits have been obtained only in hepatocellular carcinoma [80]. To improve therapeutic efficacy, new analogs have been synthesized, including the cyclohexapeptide, designated SOM230 (oasireotide), which binds with high affinity to $sst_{1?-3}$ and sst_5 [81]. The presence of somatostatin receptors, mainly sst_2 on tumors, permits the localization of some primary tumors and their metastases using scintigraphic techniques [82–85]. Radiolabeled analogs of somatostatin, such as [^{111}In-DTPA-D-Phe^1]octreotide (OctreoScan®) are used clinically for the localization of tumors expressing receptors for somatostatin

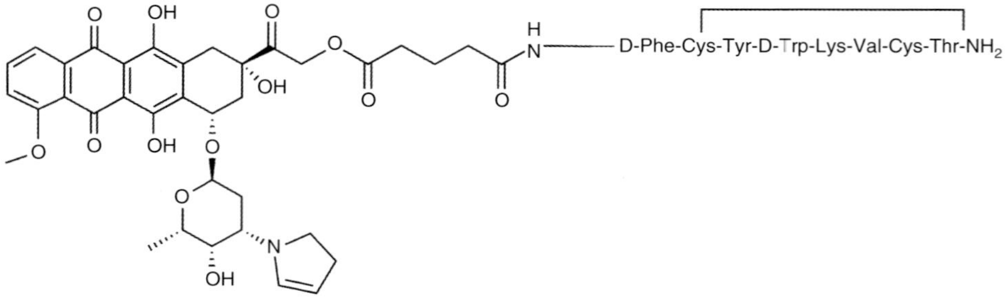

Figure 38.13 Structure of targeted cytotoxic somatostatin analog AN-238 containing 2-pyrrolino-DOX.

[83, 84]. Targeted radiotherapy, in which somatostatin analogs are linked to various radionuclides such as ^{68}Ga or ^{90}Y, is also being developed [46, 82, 84]. These applications are described in other chapters of this volume.

38.4.1.2 **Synthesis of Cytotoxic Analogs of Somatostatin**

In an endeavor to develop chemotherapy targeted to somatostatin receptors, we have synthesized cytotoxic hybrids of somatostatin containing DOX or AN-201 and conjugated to octapeptide analogs RC-121 or RC-160 [6, 7, 46, 86]. This synthesis involved the use of [Lys(Fmoc)^5]RC-121 or RC-160 as an intermediate. The most active cytotoxic analog was AN-238 (Figure 38.13), in which RC-121 is conjugated at its N-terminal D-Phe moiety through a glutaric acid spacer to the 14-OH group of 2-pyrrolino-DOX (AN-201) yielding 2-pyrrolino-DOX-14-*O*-glt-D-Phe-Cys-Tyr-D-Trp-Lys-Val-Cys-Thr-NH_2 [7, 86]. AN-258 (2-pyrrolino-DOX-14-*O*-glt-RC-160) was prepared in a similar way by using [Lys(Fmoc)^5]RC-160 as an intermediate. Analogs AN-162 and AN-163, containing DOX, were also synthesized in a similar manner by using N-Fmoc-DOX-14-*O*-hemiglutarate [7, 86]. Cytotoxic analog AN-162 (Figure 38.14) consists of somatostatin analog RC-121 linked through an α-amino group of its N-terminal D-Phe-moiety and a glutaric acid spacer to the 14-OH group of DOX, giving the following structure: DOX-14-*O*-glt-D-Phe-Cys-Tyr-D-Trp-Lys-Val-Cys-Thr-NH_2 [6, 7, 86]. Somatostatin analogs thus act as carriers and provide the homing mechanism to tumors expressing these somatostatin receptors.

Although many normal tissues express receptors for somatostatin, no receptor-specific toxicity was observed in our studies with cytotoxic analogs AN-162 or AN-238 [6, 7, 46, 86]. The cytotoxic radicals, DOX and AN-201, affect mostly cells with high mitotic activity, therefore damage to cells with a slow turnover is smaller. AN-162 and AN-238 have been evaluated in various tumor models.

38.4.1.2.1 Breast Cancer It is well established that somatostatin receptor subtypes are expressed in human breast cancer [87, 88]. The effects of targeted somatostatin analogs AN-238 and AN-162 were investigated in various human breast cancer cell lines xenografted into nude mice [88]. In the MCF-7-MIII

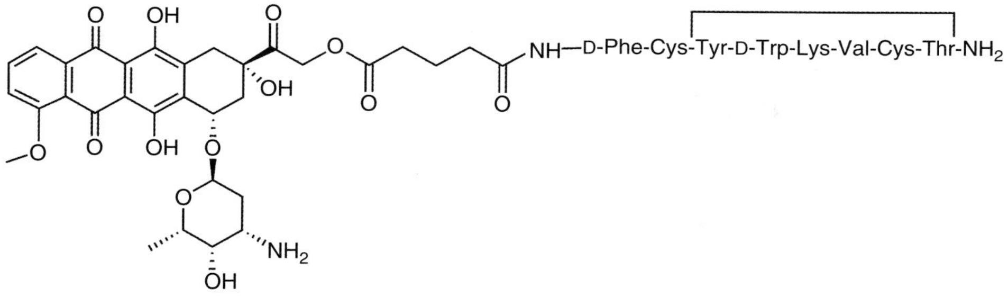

Figure 38.14 Structure of targeted cytotoxic somatostatin analog AN-162 containing DOX.

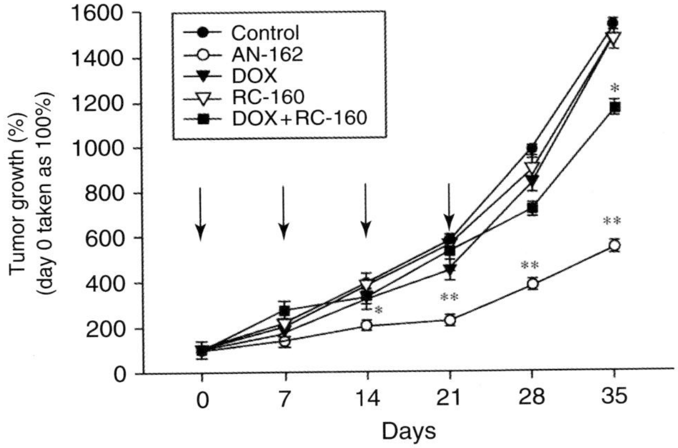

Figure 38.15 Effect of treatment with cytotoxic somatostatin analog AN-162 on the growth of MDA-MB-231 estrogen-independent human breast carcinoma cell line xenografted into nude mice (mean ± standard error). AN-162, DOX, somatostatin analog RC-160, and the unconjugated mixture of DOX plus RC-160 were administered at 2.5 μmol/kg. Arrows mark intravenous injections into the jugular vein. $^{*}P < 0.05$ $^{**}P < 0.01$ (AN-162 versus all other groups), analysis of variance tests. (Three animals died in the RC-160 + DOX group, but this group still contained seven tumors in four animals.) (Reproduced from [89].)

model, several tumors regressed after administration of AN-238. The growth of estrogen-independent human breast cancers, MDA-MB-231 and DOX-resistant MX-1 tumors, expressing sst_2 and sst_3 receptor subtypes, was strongly inhibited by treatment with AN-238 [88]. The radical AN-201 alone was more toxic and less effective than AN-238. AN-162 (AEZS-124) also significantly inhibited growth of the MDA-MB-231 estrogen-independent human breast cancer cell line xenografted into nude mice [89] (Figure 38.15). AN-162 was stable in human serum [89], and appeared to be a safe and effective compound for the treatment of estrogen-independent metastatic breast cancer; however, more extensive experimental studies are first required.

38.4.1.2.2 Ovarian Cancer Human ovarian cancers express receptors for somatostatin and mRNA subtypes for sst_2, sst_3, and sst_5 [90]. Cytotoxic analog AN-238 inhibited growth of somatostatin receptor-positive and LHRH1 receptor-negative UCI-107 human ovarian cancers xenografted into nude mice [91]. Analog AN-162 suppressed growth of ES-2 human platinum-resistant ovarian cancers. Thus, AN-162 or AN-238 might provide a new therapeutic modality for patients with advanced ovarian carcinoma.

38.4.1.2.3 Endometrial Cancer Endometrial cancers also express subtype 2 of somatostatin receptors [92]. Cytotoxic analog AN-238 was shown to inhibit the growth of estrogen receptor-negative HEC-1A and RL-95-2 human endometrial cancers [92]. Additional studies are required to evaluate the effects of AN-162 in endometrial cancers.

38.4.1.2.4 Prostate Cancer Binding sites for somatostatin and expression of sst_2 and sst_5 subtypes were demonstrated in 65% of prostate cancer specimens, and in human prostatic cancer lines as well as in metastases [93]. In nude mice bearing subcutaneous xenografts of androgen-independent PC-3 (Figure 38.16) and DU-145 human prostate cancers, AN-238 strongly inhibited growth and increased apoptosis [94]. In an orthotopic model of PC-3, AN-238 reduced the size of tumors and prevented the development of metastases [94]. AN-238 also

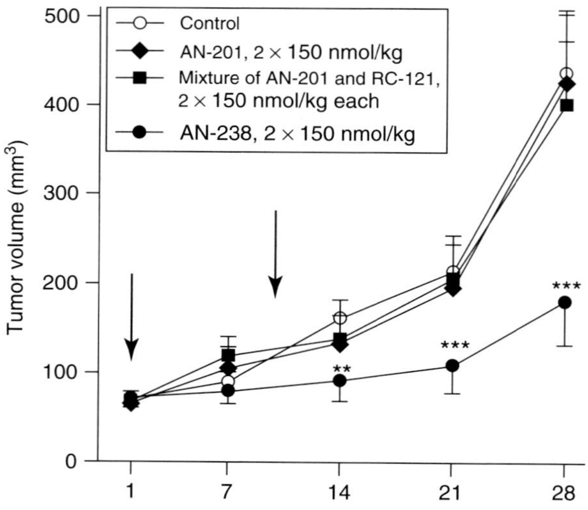

Figure 38.16 Effect of cytotoxic analog of somatostatin AN-238 or its components on the growth of subcutaneous xenografts of PC-3 human hormone-independent prostate cancer in nude mice. Two injections of 150 nmol/kg AN-201, AN-238, or the mixture of AN-201 and the carrier were given 10 days apart when the initial tumor volume had reached 65–70 mm^3. No deaths related to toxicity occurred. Arrows, day of injection; bars, standard error. $^{**}P < 0.01$ versus control, $^{***}P < 0.001$ versus control, $P < 0.05$ versus AN-201. (Reproduced from [94].)

arrested the growth of subcutaneous MDA-PCa-2b as well as intraosseously implanted C4-2 human prostate cancers; serum PSA levels were also reduced [95]. Cytotoxic somatostatin analog AN-162 also inhibited the growth of PC-3 human androgen-independent prostate cancers better than DOX alone. Based on these results, targeted chemotherapy with cytotoxic analogs AN-162 and AN-238 could be considered for the management of patients with castration-resistant prostate cancer and/or metastatic disease.

38.4.1.2.5 RCC and Bladder Cancer Most human RCCs express receptors for somatostatin [87]. AN-238 inhibited *in vivo* growth of human SW-839 and 786-0 RCC lines, which express receptors for somatostatin; the incidence of metastases was greatly reduced [96]. In somatostatin receptor-negative CAKI-1 xenografts AN-238 had no effect [96]. Analog AN-162 was shown to inhibit growth of the HT-1376 human urinary bladder cancer cell line, which expresses somatostatin receptors (Szepeshazi and Schally, in preparation). Targeted cytotoxic somatostatin analogs could provide an effective therapy for RCC and bladder cancers.

38.4.1.2.6 SCLC and NSCLC Improved therapeutic methods are needed for both small-cell lung carcinoma (SCLC) and NSCLC [17, 46]. Most SCLC and their metastases express somatostatin receptors [17, 46, 87, 97, 98]. Somatostatin receptors also are present in the peritumoral vasculature of NSCLC [87, 98, 99]. Treatment of nude mice bearing H-69 SCLC xenografts with analogs AN-238 or AN-162 inhibited tumor growth [99]. Therapy with AN-238 similarly strongly suppressed growth of H-157 and H-838 NSCLC tumors [7, 99]. AN-162 also significantly inhibited the growth of H460 and H1299 NSCLC tumors [97] (Figure 38.17a and b). Therapy, based on targeting of cytotoxic analogs to somatostatin receptors on SCLC and NSCLC tumors or their vasculature, should be superior to systemic chemotherapy.

38.4.1.2.7 Brain Tumors Glioblastomas are the most common brain tumors and also express somatostatin receptors, especially the sst_2 subtype [7, 46, 84, 87]. AN-238 strongly inhibited growth of U-87 MG and U118MG human glioblastomas, which express receptors for somatostatin, xenografted into nude mice [7, 46, 100]. Blocking somatostatin receptors with an excess of somatostatin analog RC-121 nullified the inhibitory effects of AN-238. In mice with orthotopic U-87 MG tumors, AN-238 prolonged the survival time. Recently, analog AN-162 was shown to inhibit the growth *in vivo* of the DBTRG-05 human glioblastomas which express sst_2 and sst_3 subtypes. Thus, cytotoxic somatostatin analogs could be considered for targeted therapy of malignant brain tumors.

38.4.1.2.8 Pancreatic Cancer In view of the dismal prognosis for patients with carcinoma of the pancreas, the development of new treatment methods would be extremely welcome [17, 46]. Gene expression for sst_2 appears to be lost in human pancreatic and colorectal cancers [101], but mRNA for sst_5 and sst_3 is present, and these subtypes can be used for targeting. The growth of SW-1990 pancreatic cancers and other pancreatic tumors containing sst_3 and sst_5 was significantly inhibited by

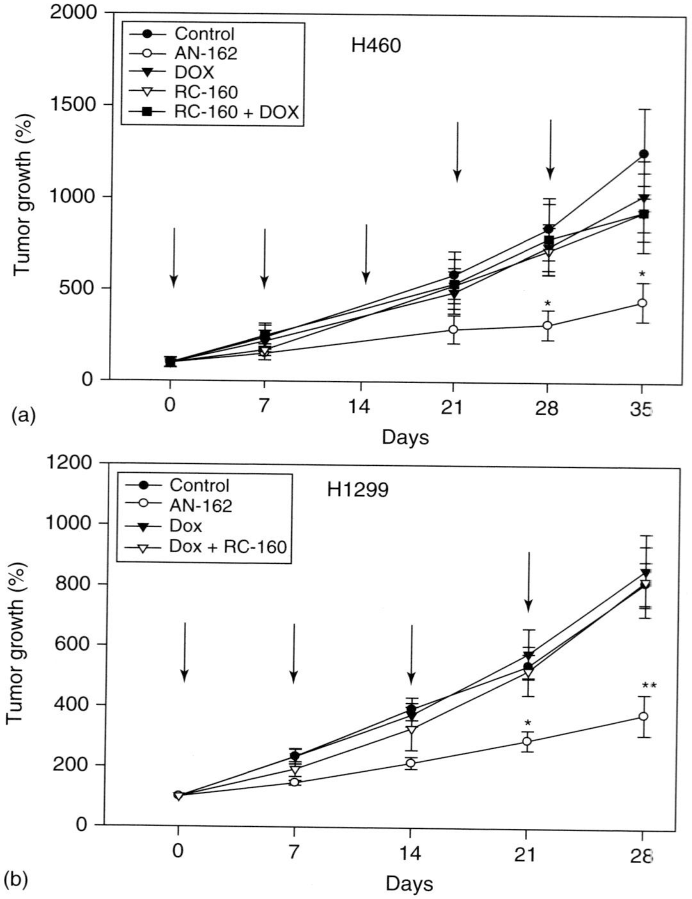

Figure 38.17 Effect of treatment with cytotoxic somatostatin analog AN-162, DOX, somatostatin analog RC-160, and combination of DOX and RC-160 on the growth of (a) H460 and (b) H1299 human NSCLC xenografted into nude mice. Arrows mark days of intravenous injections of the cytotoxic compounds. Animals received all substances in equimolar doses of 2.5 μmol/kg. Day 0 was set at 100%. $^{*}P < 0.05$ for animals treated with AN-162 versus all groups, $^{**}P < 0.05$ for animals treated with AN-162 versus all groups. Vertical bars, standard error of the mean. (Reproduced from [97].)

AN-238 [102]. Analog AN-162 also strongly suppressed growth of Panc-1 tumors in nude mice (Szepeshazi and Schally, unpublished). Thus, patients with pancreatic cancers, expressing sst_3 and/or sst_5, could benefit from treatment with cytotoxic somatostatin analogs.

38.4.1.2.9 Colorectal Cancers Owing to the presence of sst_5 and other subtypes of somatostatin receptors in colorectal carcinomas, we evaluated the effects of cytotoxic somatostatin analogs in these tumors [103]. AN-238 inhibited the growth of HCT-15 and HT-29 colorectal cancer cell lines. Targeted cytotoxic somatostatin analog AN-162 effectively reduced the volume of HCT-15, HT-29, and HCT-116 human colorectal cancer cell lines xenografted into nude mice [104]. Thus, analogs AN-162 and AN-238 could be considered for the therapy of colon cancers [104].

38.4.1.2.10 Gastric Cancers Gastric cancer is a major health problem in Asia and in some European countries, and new therapies for advanced disease are sorely needed. The effects of analog AN-238 were investigated on AGS, Hs746T, and NCI-N87 human gastric cancer cell lines, which express sst_2 and sst_5 receptors [105]. A strong suppression of the growth of NCI-N87 and Hs746T tumors xenografted into nude mice was demonstrated [105]. The results support the merit of continued investigation of AN-162 and AN-238 for the therapy of advanced gastric cancers that express somatostatin receptors [105].

38.4.1.2.11 Hepatocellular Carcinoma Somatostatin receptors are expressed in Hep-3B, Hep-G2, and SK-Hep-1 human hepatocellular carcinoma cell lines, and analog AN-238 was found to inhibit the growth of SK-Hep-1 tumors in nude mice [106]. In addition, in HepG2 and Hep3B human hepatoma cell lines, AN-238 induced apoptosis through its interaction with somatostatin receptor subtypes [107].

38.4.1.2.12 Melanomas Malignant melanomas are generally characterized by a high intrinsic resistance to chemotherapy, which is mediated by transport proteins such as MDR-1 [13]. AN-238 inhibited growth of the melanoma cell lines MRI-H255 and MRI-H187, and did not induce mRNA of MDR-1; AN-201 was ineffective [13]. Thus, targeted chemotherapy with cytotoxic somatostatin analog could be considered for treatment of malignant melanomas.

38.4.1.2.13 NHL Somatostatin receptors are found in a high percentage of human NHL [108]. When AN-238 was tested in nude mice bearing xenografts of RL and HT human NHL, it was found to strongly inhibit the growth of both lines [108]. After additional studies and clinical trials, AN-162 and AN-238 could be considered for the treatment of patients with NHLs.

38.4.1.3 Side-Effects of Cytotoxic Somatostatin Analogs

Since the pituitary, kidneys, and many other normal tissues, such as those of the gastroenteropancreatic system, express high-affinity receptors for somatostatin, side-effects of cytotoxic analog AN-238 in animal models were expected. However, in our studies, no receptor-specific toxicity was observed after treatment with AN-238, possibly because it was used in relatively low doses [7, 17]. For example, no significant changes were found in the basal or GHRH-stimulated GH release from the pituitaries of mice after treatment with AN-238 [7, 17]. The lack of permanent damage to the pituitary caused by AN-238 could be explained by the fact that AN-201, AN-238, and DOX affect mainly cells with high mitotic activity such as neoplastic cells, and the damage to well-differentiated cells with slow turnover ratios is probably smaller than that inflicted on neoplastic tissues. In addition, the resting cells of the gastrointestinal tract can eventually replace the damaged cells, restoring normal organ function [7]. In conclusion, our findings on the toxicity of AN-238 in animal models are in agreement with the clinical observation. Using radionuclide-labeled analogs, only low-grade toxicities to the kidneys and the pituitary were demonstrated after therapy with analogs of somatostatin. Analog AN-162 was also found to be relatively free of side-effects at a MTD of 2.5 μmol/kg in preliminary studies in rodents [89].

38.4.2 Clinical Development

Cytotoxic analogs of somatostatin have not yet been tested clinically. In view of problems in large-scale synthesis of AN-238, analog AN-162 is also being developed.

38.5 Example 3: Cytotoxic Analogs of Bombesin/Gastrin-Releasing Peptide

38.5.1 Preclinical Considerations and Development

38.5.1.1 Bombesin/Gastrin-Releasing Peptide and their Receptors

Bombesin-like peptides are found in amphibians and mammals, including humans [17, 109, 110]. The tetradecapeptide, bombesin, was purified from toad skin; subsequently gastrin-releasing peptide (GRP) – a 27-amino-acid peptide with the C-terminal decapeptide similar to that of bombesin [109] – was isolated from porcine stomach. Neuromedin B, which is also related to bombesin, was purified from spinal cord. Bombesin-like peptides are not hypothalamic hormones, but are present in mammalian brain, including the hypothalamus, as well as in lung and gastrointestinal tract, and may function as gastrointestinal hormones, neurotransmitters, and growth factors [17, 46]. The most important oncological action of bombesin/GRP is to modulate the proliferation or differentiation of various tumors including not only SCLC [111], but others, such as breast, prostatic, and pancreatic cancer [17, 46]. GRP and its receptors are expressed in several types of tumors [87, 111, 112].

Four receptor subtypes for the bombesin-like peptides have been characterized. Subtypes 1–3 are found in mammals [17, 46, 87, 113]. Receptor subtype 1 (termed *GRP-R*) binds bombesin and GRP with high affinity and subtype 2 (NMB-R) is more selective for neuromedin B [17, 46]. The natural ligand for bombesin receptor subtype 3 (BRS-3) has not yet been identified. The genes for GRP-R and BRS-3 have been mapped on human chromosome X, and the gene for NMB-R is located on human chromosome 6 [17, 113]. These receptors share about 50% amino acid sequence homology and any of them may contribute to regulation of mitogenesis *in vivo* [17]. The bombesin/GRP receptor subtype 1 is overexpressed on various human malignancies including SCLC, breast, ovarian, prostate, pancreatic, gastric, and colon cancer as well as brain tumors [17, 46, 87, 113]. In contrast, neuroendocrine tumors express mostly subtype 2 or 3 of bombesin receptors [113]. NMB-R and BRS-3 also seem to be expressed in various human cancers [113]. A fourth subtype has a higher affinity for the amphibian peptide bombesin than for GRP [114].

These receptors are coupled to G-protein via their intracellular domain and thus, belong to the GPCR superfamily [114]. Several signaling mechanisms are activated through the binding of GRP receptors, including phospholipase A_2, β_1, β_3, and D, as well as cAMP, PKC, and cyclooxygenase (COX) [17, 87, 113, 114]. Protein kinase cascades including Raf/MEK (MAPK kinase)/ERK (extracellular signal-regulated kinase) kinase cascade, protein kinase D, and $p70^{s6k}$ are also involved, resulting in an increased expression of c-Myc, c-Jun, c-Fos, and Akt [114]. Both GRP-R and NMB-R subtypes lead to the activation of PLC, generation of IP_3, release of intracellular calcium, and activation of PKC [114]. Stimulation of GRP-R induces activation of tyrosine kinases, tyrosine phosphorylation of p125 focal adhesion kinase, ERK kinase, and Src kinase family members, and leads to a transactivation of the EGFR [17, 114].

The finding that bombesin and GRP can function as autocrine growth factors for SCLC and other tumors [17, 111] stimulated several groups to develop bombesin/GRP antagonists [17, 46, 115, 116]. Various bombesin/GRP antagonists were also synthesized in our laboratory including RC-3095 [D-Tpi^6, Leu^{13} $\psi(CH_2NH)Leu^{14}$]bombesin(6–14) and RC-3940-II [Hca^6, Leu^{13} $(CH_2N)Tac^{14}$]bombesin(6–14) with even stronger antitumor activity [17, 46, 115]. Bombesin/GRP antagonists affect intracellular second messengers causing changes in calcium concentrations [116]. In addition to intracellular calcium mobilization and PKC activation, bombesin/GRP antagonists also affect ERK and JNK (c-Jun N-terminal kinase) MAPK pathways [114]. In this way antagonists can interfere with growth promoting signals originating from other receptors. The main mechanisms of inhibitory action of bombesin/GRP antagonists on tumors involve the decrease in levels of members of the HER family of receptors including EGFR, HER2, and HER3 [17, 116, 117], reduction of oncogene expression including c-*fos*, c-*jun*, pAkt, K-RAS, COX-2, protein kinases including MAPK and PKC isoforms, modulation of the tumor suppressor gene p53, an alteration in BCL-2/BAX ratio, and an effect on growth factors such as VEGF, resulting in inhibition of neovascularization [114]. After administration, bombesin/GRP antagonists are rapidly eliminated from the bloodstream, but EGFRs remain down-regulated for many hours [17]. No side-effects of treatment with bombesin/GRP antagonist RC-3095 have been detected in clinical phase I/II trials.

38.5.1.2 **Radiolabeled and Cytotoxic Bombesin Analogs**

The application of radiolabeled bombesin/GRP analogs for tumor detection has been proposed [17, 46]. Various radiolabeled GRP analogs have been developed [114]. The use of radiolabeled bombesin/GRP analogs for tumor imaging has been reviewed by Reubi [87]. Clinical studies with ^{99m}Tc- and ^{68}Ga-labeled bombesin-based peptides have been reported for imaging metastasized prostate, breast, and gastrointestinal tumors [87, 114]. A potent, radiolabeled analog ^{177}Lu-AMBA has been proposed for both imaging and treatment [118]. This topic is covered elsewhere in this volume.

Safay *et al.* constructed a cytotoxic peptide consisting of bombesin(7–13) and the anticancer drug paclitaxel [119] for targeted therapy. The cytotoxicity of this targeted taxane conjugate against H1299 human NSCLC was enhanced compared with that of the unconjugated taxane. Moody *et al.* synthesized a camptothecin–bombesin conjugate that binds to all three bombesin receptor classes with high affinity [120]. This conjugate inhibited the growth of NSCLC *in vitro* [120].

We have synthesized targeted cytotoxic bombesin analogs using as carriers, bombesin antagonists, which have high binding affinity to bombesin/GRP receptor subtype 1 [121] and using DOX or AN-201 as cytotoxic agents. The cytotoxic bombesin analog AN-215 (Figure 38.18) was made by linking the N-terminal of des-D-Tpi-RC-3095 through a glutaric acid spacer to the 14-OH group of 2-pyrrolino-DOX (AN-201) giving the following structure: 2-pyrrolino-DOX-14-*O*-glt-Gln-Trp-Ala-Val-Gly-His-Leu-Ψ(CH_2-NH)-Leu-NH_2 [121]. This compound is targeted to bombesin/GRP receptor subtype 1. Thus the proliferation of xenografts of human tumors such as SCLC (Figure 38.19) as well as prostatic, renal, mammary, ovarian, endometrial, pancreatic and gastric cancers, and brain tumors was strongly inhibited in nude mice by AN-215 [14, 17, 46, 122–124]. The use of bombesin/GRP analogs as homing carriers for cytotoxic and radioactive compounds might offer new options for diagnosis and treatment of diverse malignancies overexpressing these bombesin/GRP receptors.

38.5.2 Clinical Development

It remains for cytotoxic analogs of bombesin/GRP to be tested clinically.

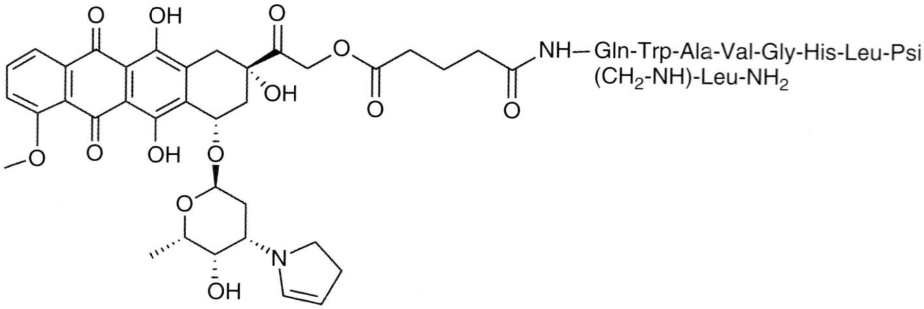

Figure 38.18 Structure of targeted cytotoxic bombesin/GRP analog AN-215 containing 2-pyrrolino-DOX. (Modified from [121].)

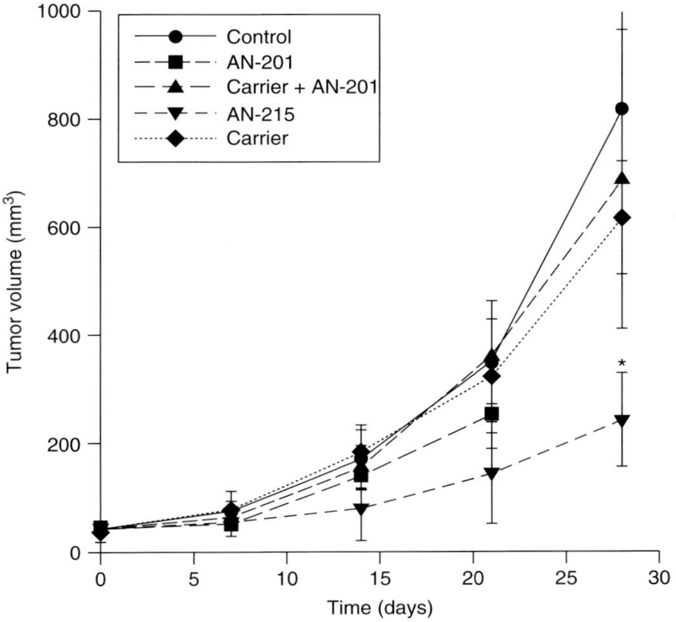

Figure 38.19 Changes in tumor volume in athymic nude mice bearing subcutaneous xenografts of H-69 SCLC after treatment with 200 nmol/kg of cytotoxic bombesin analog AN-215, cytotoxic radical AN-201, unconjugated mixture of AN-201, and the carrier peptide RC-3094 or the carrier peptide RC-3094. Vertical bars, standard error of the mean. $^{*}P < 0.05$ versus control. Three mice in the AN-201-treated group died during the fourth week of treatment and the volume of tumors recorded on day 21 is shown. (Reproduced from [124].)

38.6 Example 4: Antagonists of GHRH

38.6.1 Preclinical Considerations and Development

38.6.1.1 GHRH and GHRH Receptors in Tumors

GHRH is secreted by the hypothalamus, and stimulates the synthesis and release of GH in the pituitary. GHRH is also present in diverse extrahypothalamic tissues, including the gastrointestinal tract and many tumors [9, 17, 46]. The 44- and 40- amino-acid forms of GHRH were first isolated and identified from human pancreatic tumors, and only subsequently purified from hypothalamic tissue [9, 17, 46]. The full biological activity is contained in the N-terminal 29-amino-acid sequence [GHRH(1–29)NH_2] [9, 17, 46] (Table 38.1). The expression of mRNA for GHRH and the presence of biologically or immunologically active GHRH has been demonstrated in various human tumors, including those of the breast, endometrium, ovary, prostate, lung, pancreas, stomach, and colon [9, 17, 46].

Table 38.1 Structures of GHRH and some of its antagonists. (Modified from [9].)

Peptide	Structure
hGHRH(1–29)NH_2	Tyr^1-Ala^2-Asp-Ala-Ile-Phe^6-Thr-Asn^8-Ser^9-Tyr^{10}-Arg^{11}-Lys^{12}-Val-Leu-Gly^{15}-Gln-Leu-Ser-Ala-Arg^{20}-Lys^{21}-Leu-Leu-Gln-Asp-Ile-Met^{27}-Ser^{28}-Arg^{29}-NH_2
D-Arg^2 antagonist	[Ac-Tyr^1, D-Arg^2]hGHRH(1–29)NH_2
MZ-4-71	[Ibu-Tyr^1, D-Arg^2, Phe(4-Cl)^6, Abu^{15}, Nle^{27}]hGHRH(1–28)Agm
MZ-5-156	[PhAc-Tyr^1, D-Arg^2, Phe(4-Cl)^6, Abu^{15}, Nle^{27}]hGHRH(1–28)Agm
JV-1-36	[PhAc-Tyr^1, D-Arg^2, Phe(4-Cl)^6, Arg^9, Abu^{15}, Nle^{27}, D-Arg^{28}, Har^{29}]hGHRH(1–29)NH_2
JV-1-38	[PhAc0-Tyr^1, D-Arg^2, Phe(4-Cl)^6, Har^9, Tyr(Me)^{10}, Abu^{15}, Nle^{27}, D-Arg^{28}, Har^{29}]hGHRH(1–29)NH_2
MZ-J-7-132	[$PhAc^0$-Tyr^1, D-Arg^2, Phe(4-Cl)^6, Har^9, Tyr(Me)^{10}, His^{11}, Abu^{15}, His^{20}, Nle^{27}, D-Arg^{28}, Har^{29}]hGHRH(1–29)NH_2
MIA-602	[(PhAc-Ada)^0-Tyr^1, D-Arg^2, Phe(F)$_5$^{6}, Ala^8, Har^9, Tyr(Me)^{10}, His^{11}, Orn^{12}, Abu^{15}, His^{20}, Orn^{21}, Nle^{27}, D-Arg^{28}, Har^{29}]hGHRH(1–29)NH_2

Abu, α-aminobutyric acid; Ac, acetyl; Ada, (12-aminododecanoyl); Agm, agmatine; Amp, *p*-amidino-phenylalanine; Har, homoarginine; Ibu, isobutyryl; Nle, norleucine; Oct, octyl; Orn, ornithine; PhAc, phenylacetyl; Tyr(Et), *O*-ethyltyrosine; Tyr(Me), *O*-methyltyrosine.

In studies *in vitro* with pancreatic, colonic, gastric, lung, and other human cancer lines, exogenously added GHRH(1–29)NH_2 increased the rate of cell proliferation [9, 125]. Conversely the "knocking down" (silencing) of GHRH gene expression suppressed the proliferation of breast cancer, prostate cancer, and NSCLC cell lines *in vitro* [125]. Replacement of the "knocked down" GHRH expression by exogenous GHRH(1–29)NH_2 re-established the proliferation of these cancer cell lines with silenced genes [125]. These results support the role of GHRH as a tumor growth factor.

Our group has also identified peptide receptors on tumors that appear to mediate the effects of GHRH and its antagonists [126, 127]. The sequencing of cDNAs encoding tumoral GHRH receptors revealed that they are splice variants (SVs) of the pituitary GHRH receptors (pGHRH-R) [126]. The major part of the cDNA sequence for SV_1 is identical with the corresponding cDNA sequence of the pituitary GHRH receptor, but the first 334 nucleotides of SV_1 and SV_2 genes are different from those of the pituitary GHRH receptor gene [7, 126]. SV_1 appears to be the major isoform of GHRH receptors [7, 126]. The deduced protein sequence of SV_1 differs from the pGHRH-R only in the N-terminal extracellular domain – the first 89 amino acids of the pGHRH-R being replaced by a different 25-amino-acid sequence [7, 126]. Thus, SV_1 encodes a functional GPCR with seven transmembrane domains, with the third intracellular loop critical for interaction with G-protein. SV_2 may encode a GHRH-R isoform truncated after the second transmembrane domain [126]. Using antisera generated against the N-terminal

25-amino-acid sequence, which is present in SV_1 [128], we detected by Western blots the approximately 40-kDa SV_1 protein in cell lines of human endometrial, lung and pancreatic cancers, lymphomas, and glioblastomas, as well as in surgical specimens of endometrial, breast, and lung cancers [9, 129]. Using RT-PCR and Western blots with antibodies specific for the pGHRH-R, we showed that the pituitary-type receptor is also detectable in human lymphoma, glioblastomas, and SCLC cell lines, and in surgical specimens of human lung cancers [9, 129]. Consequently, many tumors have been shown to express splice variants as well as pGHRH-R. All in all, the expression of GHRH receptors has been found in primary human prostatic, lung, endometrial, breast, and adrenal carcinomas [129–132], and in cell lines of virtually all major types of malignancies, including prostatic, lung (SCLC and NSCLC), breast, ovarian, endometrial, gastric, pancreatic, colorectal, and renal cancers, glioblastomas, osteogenic and Ewing's sarcomas, and lymphomas [9, 17]. Collectively, these findings suggest that in various tumors, GHRH and its tumoral receptors may form an autocrine/paracrine mitogenic loop involved in the control of malignant growth [9, 17]. The inhibitory effects of GHRH antagonists on cancers appear to be based in part on the interference with this local stimulatory GHRH system. Thus, GHRH antagonists can directly block the tumoral receptors for GHRH and prevent the activation of the tumoral autocrine/paracrine GHRH. In addition, GHRH antagonists may directly inhibit the production of tumoral insulin-like growth factor (IGF)-I and -II. The antitumor action of GHRH antagonists can be also indirect and exerted through the inhibition of GH secretion from the pituitary with the resultant suppression of the pituitary GH/hepatic IGF-I axis. The mechanisms of tumor inhibition by GHRH antagonists could also vary among different tumors [9, 17].

38.6.1.2 **Antagonistic Analogs of GHRH**

The development of GHRH antagonists was started after it was established that somatostatin analogs do not adequately suppress GH and IGF-I levels in patients with tumors dependent on IGF-I. It was found that replacement of Ala^2 by D-Arg^2 in GHRH(1–29)NH_2 resulting in [Ac-Tyr^1, D-Arg^2]hGHRH(1–29)NH_2 generates GHRH antagonism [133] (Table 38.1). Systematic efforts to develop better GHRH antagonists led to antagonists MZ-4-71 and MZ-5-156 [9, 17, 134] (Table 38.1). Other substitutions were then incorporated into GHRH analogs yielding antagonists such as JV-1-36, JV-1-38, and JV-1-65, which all manifested increased inhibitory activity [9, 50, 135]. During the past 4 years we have synthesized, in Miami, several hundred new antagonists of GHRH, incorporating various substitutions with less common noncoded amino acids. Some of these antagonists contained ω-amino fatty acids, such as Ada (12-aminododecanoyl), at the N- or C-terminus and exerted very potent inhibitory effects at small doses on various tumors (Table 38.1). We are now engaged in an active selection of the antagonist candidate best suited for clinical development.

Antagonists of GHRH bind with a high affinity to receptors for GHRH, and inhibit the proliferation of various cancer cell lines *in vitro* and the growth of many human cancer cell lines xenografted into nude mice [9, 17]. These include

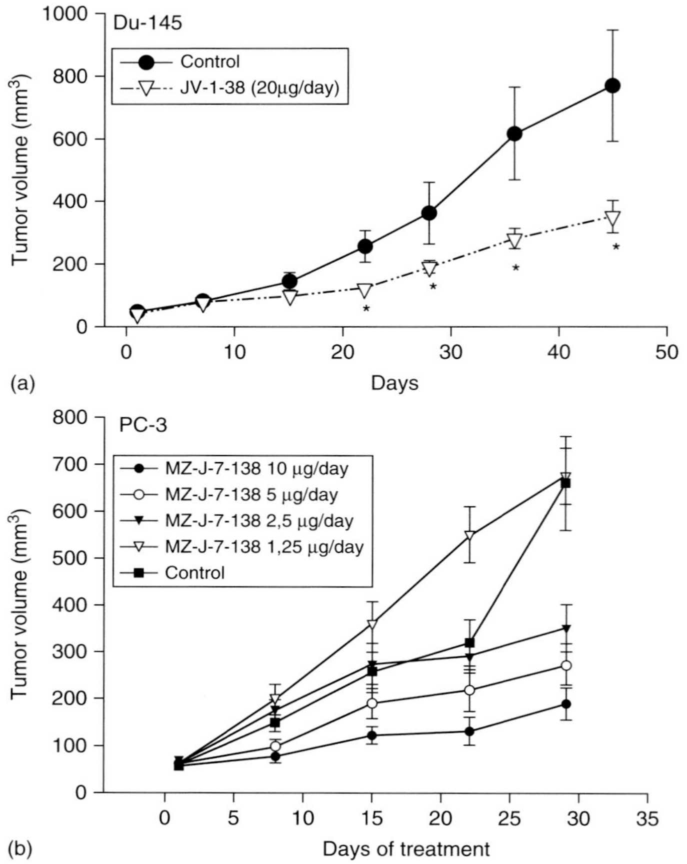

Figure 38.20 (a) Effect of GHRH antagonist JV-1-38 (20 μg/day subcutaneous) on the growth of subcutaneous xenografted DU-145 human prostate carcinomas in nude mice. The treatment lasted for 45 days. Vertical bars, standard error. $^*P < 0.05$ versus control. (Reproduced from [136].) (b) Growth of PC-3 tumors treated with different doses of the GHRH antagonist MZ-J-7-138. Significant differences from the control are marked by asterisks ($P < 0.001$). (Reproduced from [137].)

mammary, ovarian, endometrial, and prostate cancers (Figure 38.20), SCLCs and NSCLCs (Figure 38.21), renal, esophageal, pancreatic, gastric, colorectal and hepatocellular carcinomas, malignant gliomas, osteosarcomas, and NHLs [9, 17, 136–139]. GHRH antagonists also appear to reduce the invasive and metastatic potentials of human cancer cell lines [140]. Although GHRH antagonists do not deliver a cytotoxic radical, it is considered that they are actively targeted (homed) to the specific GHRH receptors on tumors. This view is based on their interaction with the receptors represented by the binding process. GHRH antagonists may offer important advantages over chemotherapy. As GHRH antagonists also inhibit

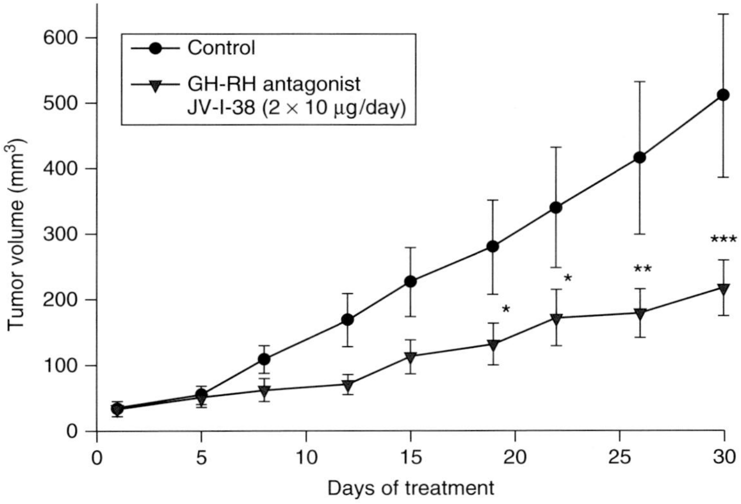

Figure 38.21 Changes in tumor volume in athymic nude mice bearing subcutaneously transplanted H838 NSCLC during treatment with GHRH antagonist JV-1-38 administered by subcutaneous injections at a dose of 10 µg/animal twice a day. Bars, standard error. $^*P < 0.05$, $^{**}P < 0.01$, $^{***}P < 0.001$. (Reproduced from [139].)

IGF-II-dependent tumors, they should be superior to GH antagonists, as the synthesis of IGF-II is not controlled by GH [9, 17].

38.6.2 Clinical Developments

No clinical trials have been carried out so far with our advanced GHRH antagonists. The administration of an early GHRH antagonist was reported to reduce GH hypersecretion in a patient with metastatic GHRH-secreting carcinoid tumor, but the effect of large intravenous doses lasted only 3–4 h [141].

38.7 Conclusions and Perspectives

The presence of specific receptors for LHRH1, somatostatin, and bombesin/GRP on various cancers provided a rationale for the conceptualization and synthesis of cytotoxic hybrids, consisting of chemotherapeutic agents conjugated to the analogs of these peptides, which can be targeted to the respective tumoral receptors. Receptors for GHRH were also found on a variety of tumors and antagonistic analogs of GHRH have been developed. GHRH antagonists inhibit the growth of a variety of tumors and may be devoid of side-effects. Therapeutic peptides, targeting to tumors, were tested on many human cancer lines xenografted into nude mice. Thus, cytotoxic analogs of LHRH1 AN-152 and AN-207, containing DOX or 2-pyrrolino-DOX (AN-201), targeting LHRH1 receptors, inhibited growth of prostatic, bladder, breast, ovarian, and endometrial cancers, NHLs, melanomas, and RCCs. DOX and AN-201 were also linked to analogs of somatostatin, which are targeted to the receptors on prostatic, mammary, ovarian, gastric, renal, colorectal and pancreatic cancers, NHLs, as well as glioblastomas and lung cancer, thus suppressing the growth of experimental models of these tumors. A cytotoxic analog of bombesin/GRP containing AN-201 was shown to inhibit growth of human cancer lines expressing these receptors. Antagonists of GHRH were also shown to strongly inhibit growth of the many cancers mentioned previously. The clinical profile of the cytotoxic LHRH1 analog AN-152 was assessed in a phase I trial in women with gynecologic cancers and this analog is now in phase II trials. Other clinical trials are pending. Continued development of targeted cytotoxic peptide analogs and GHRH antagonists could lead to a more efficacious and less toxic therapy for many human cancers.

Acknowledgments

Experimental studies cited in this chapter were supported by the Medical Research Service of the Veterans Affairs Department and Departments of Pathology and Medicine, Division of Hematology/Oncology of the Miller Medical School, University of Miami and AEterna/Zentaris GmbH through the South Florida Veterans Affairs Foundation for Research and Education (all to A.V.S.) and the Hungarian Scientific Research Fund (OTKA) K81596 and TAMOP 4.2.1/B-09/1/KONV-2010-007 Project (G.H.). We are grateful to Dr. Norman Block for valuable suggestions, and to Peter Goldstein for expert editorial assistance and help in the preparation of the manuscript.

References

1. FitzGerald, D. and Pastan, I. (1989) Targeted toxin therapy for the treatment of cancer. *J. Natl. Cancer Inst.*, **81**, 1455–1463.
2. Pastan, I., Hassan, R., FitzGerald, D., and Kritman, R. (2006) Immunotoxin therapy of cancer. *Nat. Rev. Cancer*, **6**, 559–565.
3. Mendelsohn, J. and Baselga, J. (2003) Status of epidermal growth factor receptor antagonists in the biology and treatment of cancer. *J. Clin. Oncol.*, **21**, 2787–2799.
4. Slamon, D.J., Leyland-Jones, B., Shak, S., Fuchs, H., Paton, V., Bajamonde, A. *et al.* (2001) Use of chemotherapy plus a monoclonal antibody against HER2 for metastatic breast cancer that overexpresses HER2. *N. Engl. J. Med.*, **344**, 783–792.
5. Hurwitz, H., Fehrenbacher, L., Novotny, W., Cartwright, T., Hainsworth, J., Heim, W. *et al.* (2004) Bevacizumab plus irinotecan, fluorouracil, and leucovorin for metastatic colorectal cancer. *N. Eng. J. Med.*, **350**, 2335–2342.
6. Schally, A.V. and Nagy, A. (1999) Cancer chemotherapy based on targeting of cytotoxic peptide conjugates to their receptors on tumors. *Eur. J. Endocrinol.*, **141**, 1–14.
7. Schally, A.V. and Nagy, A. (2004) Chemotherapy targeted to cancers

through tumoral hormone receptors. *Trends Endocrinol. Metab.*, **15**, 300–310.
8. Ehrlich, P. (1956) The relationship existing between chemical constitution, distribution, and pharmacological action in *The Collected Papers of Paul Ehrlich*, vol. **1** (eds F. Himmelweite, M. Marguardt, and H.D. Elmsford), Pergamon, London, pp. 596–618.
9. Schally, A.V., Varga, J.L., and Engel, J.B. (2008) Antagonists of growth hormone-releasing hormone: an emerging new therapy for cancer. *Nat. Clin. Pract. Endocrinol. Metab.*, **4**, 33–43.
10. Aina, O.H., Sroka, T.C., Chen, M.L., and Lam, K.S. (2002) Therapeutic cancer targeting peptides. *Biopolymers*, **66**, 184–199.
11. Kufe, D.W., Pollock, R.E., Weichselbaum, R.R., Bast, R.C. Jr., Gansler, T.S., Holland, J.F., and Frei, E. III (eds) (2006) *Cancer Medicine*, 7th edn, Decker, Hamilton.
12. Goda, K., Bacso, Z., and Szabo, G. (2009) Multidrug resistance through the spectacle of P-glycoprotein. *Curr. Cancer Drug Targets*, **9**, 281–297.
13. Keller, G., Schally, A.V., Nagy, A., Baker, B., Halmos, G., and Engel, J.B. (2006) Effective therapy of experimental human malignant melanomas with a targeted cytotoxic somatostatin analogue without induction of multi-drug resistance proteins. *Int. J. Oncol.*, **28**, 1507–1513.
14. Keller, G., Schally, A.V., Nagy, A., Halmos, G., Baker, B., and Engel, J.B. (2005) Targeted chemotherapy with cytotoxic bombesin analogue AN-215 can overcome chemoresistance in experimental renal cell carcinomas. *Cancer*, **104**, 2266–2274.
15. Schally, A.V., Halmos, G., Rekasi, A., and Arencibia, J.M. (2001) The actions of luteinizing hormone-releasing hormone agonists, antagonists, and cytotoxic analogues on the luteinizing hormone-releasing hormone receptors on the pituitary and tumors in *Infertility and Reproductive Medicine Clinics of North America: GnRH Analogs* (ed. P. Devroey), Saunders, Philadelphia, PA, pp. 17–44.
16. Engel, J.B. and Schally, A.V. (2007) Drug insight: clinical use of agonists and antagonists of luteinizing-hormone-releasing hormone. *Nat. Clin. Pract. Endocrinol. Metab.*, **3**, 157–167.
17. Schally, A.V., Comaru-Schally, A.M., Nagy, A., Kovacs, M., Szepeshazi, K., Plonowski, A. *et al.* (2001) Hypothalamic hormones and cancer. *Front. Neuroendocrinol.*, **22**, 248–291.
18. Mamputha, S., Lu, Z., Roeske, R., Millar, R., Katz, A., and Flanagan, C. (2007) Conserved amino acid residues that are important for ligand binding in the Type I gonadotropin-releasing hormone (GnRH) receptor are required for high potency of GnRH II at the type II GnRH receptor. *Mol. Endocrinol.*, **21**, 281–292.
19. Pawson, A., Faccenda, E., Maudsley, S., Lu, Z., Noar, Z., and Millar, R. (2008) Mammalian type I gonadotropin-releasing hormone receptors undergo slow, constitutive, agonist-independent internalization. *Endocrinology*, **149**, 1415–1422.
20. Franklin, J., Hislop, J., Flynn, A., and McArdle, C.A. (2003) Signaling and anti-proliferative effects mediated by gonadotropin-releasing hormone receptors after expression in prostate cancer cells using recombinant adenovirus. *J. Endocrinol.*, **176**, 275–284.
21. Grundker, C., Volker, P., Cunthert, A.R., and Emons, G. (2001) Antiproliferative signaling of LHRH1 in human endometrial and ovarian cancer cells through G-protein αi-mediated activation of phosphotyrosine phosphatase. *Endocrinology*, **142**, 2369–2380.
22. Emons, G., Grundker, C., Gunthert, A.R., Westphalen, S., Kavanagh, J., and Verschraegen, C. (2003) GnRH antagonists in the treatment of gynecological and breast cancers. *Endocr. Relat. Cancer*, **10**, 291–299.
23. Eidne, K.A., Flanagan, C.A., and Millar, R.P. (1985) Gonadotropin-releasing hormone binding sites in human breast carcinoma. *Science*, **229**, 989–991.
24. Fekete, M., Wittliff, J.L., and Schally, A.V. (1989) Characteristics and distribution of receptors for

[D-Trp[6]]-luteinizing hormone-releasing hormone, somatostatin, epidermal growth factor and sex steroids in 500 biopsy samples of human breast cancer. *J. Clin. Lab. Anal.*, **3**, 137–147.

25. Emons, G. and Schally, A.V. (1994) The use of luteinizing hormone releasing hormone agonists and antagonists in gynecological cancers. *Reproduction*, **9**, 1364–1379.
26. Halmos, G., Arencibia, J.M., Schally, A.V., Davis, R., and Bostwick, D.G. (2000) High incidence of receptors for luteinizing hormone-releasing hormone (LH-RH) and LH-RH receptor gene expression in human prostate cancers. *J. Urol.*, **163**, 623–629.
27. Srkalovic, G., Schally, A.V., Wittliff, J.L., Day, T.G. Jr., and Jenison, E.L. (1998) Presence and characteristics of receptors for [D-Trp[6]]-luteinizing hormone-releasing hormone and epidermal growth factor in human ovarian cancer. *Int. J. Oncol.*, **12**, 489–498.
28. Keller, G., Schally, A.V., Gaiser, T., Nagy, A., Baker, B., Westphal, G. *et al.* (2005) Human malignant melanomas express receptors for luteinizing hormone releasing hormone allowing targeted therapy with cytotoxic luteinizing hormone releasing hormone analogue. *Cancer Res.*, **65**, 5857–5863.
29. Keller, G., Schally, A.V., Gaiser, T., Nagy, A., Baker, B., Halmos, G. *et al.* (2005) Receptors for luteinizing hormone releasing hormone (LH-RH) expressed in human non-Hodgkin's lymphomas can be targeted for therapy with the cytotoxic LH-RH analogue AN-207. *Eur. J. Cancer*, **41**, 2196–2202.
30. Keller, G., Schally, A.V., Gaiser, T., Nagy, A., Baker, B., Halmos, G. *et al.* (2005) Receptors for luteinizing hormone releasing hormone expressed on human renal cell carcinomas can be used for targeted chemotherapy with cytotoxic luteinizing hormone releasing hormone analogues. *Clin. Cancer Res.*, **11**, 5549–5557.
31. Emons, G., Ortmann, O., Schulz, K.D., and Schally, A.V. (1997) Growth-inhibitory actions of analogs of luteinizing hormone releasing hormone on tumor cells. *Trends Endocrinol. Metab.*, **8**, 355–362.
32. Ben-Yehuda, A. and Lorberboum-Galski, H. (2004) Targeted cancer therapy with gonadotropin-releasing hormone chimeric proteins. *Expert Rev. Anticancer Ther.*, **4**, 151–161.
33. Leuschner, C., Enright, F.M., Gawronska-Kozak, B., and Hansel, W. (2003) Human prostate cancer cells and xenografts are targeted and destroyed through luteinizing hormone-releasing hormone receptors. *Prostate*, **56**, 239–249.
34. Qi, L., Nett, T.M., Allen, M.C., Sha, X., Harrison, G.S., Frederick, B.A. *et al.* (2004) Binding and cytotoxicity for conjugated and recombinant fusion proteins targeted to the gonadotropin-releasing hormone receptors. *Cancer Res.*, **64**, 2090–2095.
35. Gho, Y.S. and Chae, C.B. (1999) Luteinizing hormone releasing hormone–RNase A conjugates specifically inhibit the proliferation of LH-RH-receptor-positive human prostate and breast tumor cells. *Mol. Cells*, **9**, 31–36.
36. Jacobs, E., Watson, S.A., Michaeli, D., Ellis, I.O., and Robertson, J.F. (1999) Anti-gonadotrophin releasing hormone antibodies inhibit the growth of MCF7 human breast cancer xenografts. *Br. J. Cancer*, **80**, 352–359.
37. Ben-Yehuda, A., Yarkoni, S., Nechushtan, A., Belostotskyu, R., and Lorberboum-Galski, H. (1999) Linker-based GnRH–PE chimeric proteins inhibit cancer growth in nude mice. *Med. Oncol.*, **16**, 38–45.
38. Ben-Yehudah, A., Prus, D., and Lorberboum-Galski, H.I.V. (2001) Administration of L-GnRH–PE66 efficiently inhibits growth of colon adenocarcinoma xenografts in nude mice. *Int. J. Cancer*, **92**, 263–268.
39. Schlick, J., Dulieu, P., Desvoyes, B., Adami, P., Radom, J., and Jouvenot, M. (2000) Cytotoxic activity of a recombinant GnRH–PAP fusion toxin on human tumor cell lines. *FEBS Lett.*, **472**, 241–246.

40. Nagy, A., Schally, A.V., Armatis, P., Szepeshazi, K., Halmos, G., Kovacs, M. *et al.* (1996) Cytotoxic analogs of luteinizing hormone-releasing hormone containing doxorubicin or 2-pyrrolinodoxorubicin, a derivative 500–1000 times more potent. *Proc. Natl. Acad. Sci. USA*, **93**, 7269–7273.
41. Westphalen, S., Kotulla, G., Kaiser, F., Krauss, W., Werning, G., Elsasser, H.P. *et al.* (2000) Receptor mediated antiproliferative effects of the cytotoxic LH-RH agonist AN-152 in human ovarian and endometrial cancer cell lines. *Int. J. Oncol.*, **17**, 1063–1069.
42. Wang, X., Krebs, L.H., Al-Nuri, M., Pudavar, H.E., Ghosal, S., Liebo, C. *et al.* (1999) A chemically labeled cytotoxic agent: two-photon fluorophore for optical tracking of cellular pathway in chemotherapy. *Proc. Natl. Acad. Sci. USA*, **96**, 11081–11084.
43. Krebs, L., Wang, X., Pudavar, H.E., Bergey, E.J., Schally, A.V., Nagy, A. *et al.* (2000) Regulation of targeted chemotherapy with cytotoxic luteinizing hormone-releasing hormone analogue by epidermal growth factor. *Cancer Res.*, **60**, 4294–4299.
44. Günthert, A.R., Grundker, C., Bongertz, T., Schlott, T., Nagy, A., Schally, A.V. *et al.* (2004) Internalization of cytotoxic analog AN-152 of luteinizing hormone-releasing hormone induces apoptosis in human endometrial and ovarian cancer cell lines independent of multidrug resistance-1 (MDR-1) system. *Am. J. Obstet. Gynecol.*, **191**, 1164–1172.
45. Danila, D.C., Schally, A.V., Nagy, A., and Alexander, J.M. (1999) Selective induction of apoptosis by the cytotoxic analog AN-207 in cells expressing recombinant receptor for luteinizing hormone releasing hormone. *Proc. Natl. Acad. Sci. USA*, **96**, 669–673.
46. Schally, A.V. and Comaru-Schally, A.M. (2006) Hypothalamic and other peptide hormones in *Cancer Medicine*, 7th edn (eds D.W. Kufe, R.E. Pollock, R.R. Weichselbaum Jr., R.C. Bast, T.S. Gansler, J.F. Holland, and E.B.C Frei III), Decker, Hamilton, pp. 802–816.
47. Kahán, Z., Nagy, A., Schally, A.V., Halmos, G., and Arencibia, J.M. (1999) Complete regression of MX-1 human breast carcinoma xenografts after targeted chemotherapy with a cytotoxic analog of luteinizing hormone-releasing hormone, AN-207. *Cancer*, **85**, 2608–2615.
48. Kahán, Z., Nagy, A., Schally, A.V., Halmos, G., Arencibia, J.M., and Groot, K. (2000) Administration of a targeted cytotoxic analog of luteinizing hormone-releasing hormone inhibits growth of estrogen-independent MDA-MB-231 human breast cancers in nude mice. *Breast Cancer Res. Treat.*, **59**, 255–262.
49. Bajo, A.M., Schally, A.V., Halmos, G., and Nagy, A. (2003) Targeted doxorubicin-containing luteinizing hormone-releasing hormone analogue AN-152 inhibits the growth of doxorubicin-resistant MX-1 human breast cancers. *Clin. Cancer Res.*, **9**, 3742–3748.
50. Miyazaki, M., Nagy, A., Schally, A.V., Lamharzi, N., Halmos, G., Szepeshazi, K. *et al.* (1997) Growth inhibition of human ovarian cancers by cytotoxic analogues of luteinizing hormone-releasing hormone. *J. Natl. Cancer Inst.*, **89**, 1803–1809.
51. Miyazaki, M., Schally, A.V., Nagy, A., Lamharzi, N., Halmos, G., Szepeshazi, K. *et al.* (1999) Targeted cytotoxic analog of luteinizing hormone-releasing hormone AN-207 inhibits growth of OV-1063 human epithelial ovarian cancers in nude mice. *Am. J. Obstet. Gynecol.*, **180**, 1095–1103.
52. Grundker, C., Volker, P., Griesinger, F., Ramaswamy, A., Nagy, A., Schally, A.V. *et al.* (2002) Antitumor effects of the cytotoxic LH-RH analog AN-152 on human endometrial and ovarian cancers xenografted into nude mice. *Am. J. Obstet. Gynecol.*, **187**, 528–537.
53. Arencibia, J.M., Bajo, A.M., Schally, A.V., Krupa, M., Chatzistamou, I., and Nagy, A. (2002) Effective treatment of experimental ES-2 human ovarian cancers with cytotoxic analog of luteinizing hormone-releasing hormone AN-207. *Anti-Cancer Drugs*, **13**, 949–956.

54. Emons, G., Kaufmann, M., Gorchev, G., Tsekova, V., Grunker, C., Gunthert, A. *et al.* (2010) Dose escalation and pharmacokinetic study of AEZS-108 (AN-152) an LHRH1 agonist linked to doxorubicin, in women with LHRH1 receptor positive tumors. *Gynecol. Oncol.*, **119**, 457–461.
55. Engel, J.B., Keller, G., Schally, A.V., Nagy, A., Chism, D.D., and Halmos, G. (2005) Effective treatment of experimental human endometrial cancers with targeted cytotoxic LH-RH analogs AN-152 and AN-207. *Fertil. Steril.*, **83** (Suppl.), 1125–1133.
56. Szabo, J., Vegh, A., Racz, G., and Szende, B. (2005) Immunohistochemical demonstration of gonadotropin-releasing hormone receptors in prostate carcinoma. *Urol. Oncol.*, **23**, 399–401.
57. Stangelberger, A., Schally, A.V., Nagy, A., Szepeshazi, K., Kanashiro, C.A., and Halmos, G. (2006) Inhibition of human experimental prostate cancers by a targeted cytotoxic luteinizing hormone-releasing hormone analog AN-207. *Prostate*, **66**, 200–210.
58. Plonowski, A., Schally, A.V., Nagy, A., Groot, K., Krupa, M., Navone, N.M., *et al.* (2002) Inhibition of *in vivo* proliferation of MDA-PCa-2b human prostate cancer by a targeted cytotoxic analog of luteinizing hormone-releasing hormone AN-207. *Cancer Lett.*, **176**, 57–63.
59. Letsch, M., Schally, A.V., Szepeshazi, K., Halmos, G., and Nagy, A. (2003) Preclinical evaluation of targeted cytotoxic luteinizing hormone-releasing hormone analog AN-152 in androgen sensitive and insensitive prostate cancers. *Clin. Cancer Res.*, **9**, 4505–4513.
60. Bahk, J.Y., Kim, M.O., Park, M.S., Lee, H.Y., Lee, J.H., Chung, B.C. *et al.* (2008) Gonadotropin-releasing hormone (GnRH) and GnRH receptor in bladder cancer epithelia and GnRH effect on bladder cancer cell proliferation. *Urol. Int.*, **80**, 431–438.
61. Szepeshazi, K., Schally, A.V., Treszl, A.V., Seitz, S., and Halmos, G. (2008) Therapy of experimental hepatic cancers with cytotoxic peptide analogs targeted to receptors for luteinizing hormone-releasing hormone, somatostatin or bombesin. *Anti-Cancer Drugs*, **19**, 349–358.
62. Szepeshazi, K., Schally, A.V., and Halmos, G. (2007) LH-RH receptors in human colorectal cancers: unexpected molecular targets for experimental therapy. *Int. J. Oncol.*, **30**, 1485–1492.
63. Fekete, M., Zalatnai, A., Comaru-Schally, A.M., and Schally, A.V. (1989) Membrane receptors for peptides in experimental and human pancreatic cells. *Pancreas*, **4**, 521–528.
64. Szende, B., Srkalovic, G., Timar, J., Mulchahey, J., Niell, J., Lapis, K. *et al.* (1991) Localization of receptors for luteinizing hormone-releasing hormone in pancreatic and mammary cancer cells. *Proc. Natl. Acad. Sci. USA*, **88**, 4153–4156.
65. Kovacs, M., Schally, A.V., Nagy, A., Koppan, M., and Groot, K. (1997) Recovery of pituitary function after treatment with a targeted cytotoxic analog of luteinizing hormone-releasing hormone. *Proc. Natl. Acad. Sci. USA*, **94**, 1420–1425.
66. Emons, G., Sinermann, H., Engel, J., Schally, A.V., and Grundker, C. (2009) Luteinizing hormone-releasing hormone receptor-targeted chemotherapy using AN-152. *Neuroendocrinology*, **90**, 15–18.
67. Emons, G., Tomov, S., Hartner, P., Sehouli, J., Wimberger, E.P., Staehle, A. *et al.* (2010) Phase II study of AEZS-108 (AN-152), a targeted cytotoxic LHRH1 analog, in patients with LHRH1 receptor positive platinum resistant ovarian cancer, American Society of Clinical Oncology Annual Meeting, Chicago, IL, abstract 5035.
68. Schally, A.V., Szepeshazi, K.A., Nagy, A.M., and Comaru-Schally, Halmos, G. (2004) Biomedicine and disease: new approaches to therapy of cancers of the stomach, colon and exocrine pancreas based on peptide analogs. *Cell. Mol. Life Sci.*, **61**, 1042–1068.
69. Bauer, W., Briner, U., Doepfner, W., Haller, R., Huguenin, R., Marbach, P. *et al.* (1982) SMS 201-995: a very potent and selective octapeptide analogue of

somatostatin with prolonged action. *Life Sci.*, **31**, 1133–1140.
70. Cai, R.-Z., Szoke, B., Lu, R., Fu, D., Redding, T.W., and Schally, A.V. (1986) Synthesis and biological activity of highly potent octapeptide analogs of somatostatin. *Proc. Natl. Acad. Sci. USA*, **83**, 1896–1900.
71. Patel, Y.C. (1999) Somatostatin and its receptor family. *Front. Neuroendocrinol.*, **20**, 157–198.
72. Reisine, T. and Bell, G.I. (1995) Molecular biology of somatostatin receptors. *Endocr. Rev.*, **16**, 427–442.
73. Guillermet-Guibert, J., Lahlou, H., Cordelier, P., Bousquet, C., Pyronnet, S., and Susini, C. (2005) Physiology of somatostatin receptors. *J. Endocrinol. Invest.*, **28**, 5–9.
74. Pyronnet, S., Bousquet, C., Najib, S., Azar, R., Laklai, H., and Susini, C. (2008) Antitumor effects of somatostatin. *Mol. Cell. Endocrinol.*, **286**, 230–237.
75. Liebow, C., Reilly, C., Serrano, M., and Schally, A.V. (1989) Somatostatin analogues inhibit growth of pancreatic cancer by stimulating tyrosine phosphatase. *Proc. Natl. Acad. Sci. USA*, **86**, 2003–2007.
76. Buscail, L., Esteve, J.P., Saint-Laurent, N., Bertrand, V., Reisine, T., O'Carroll, A.M. *et al.* (1995) Inhibition of cell proliferation by the somatostatin analogue RC-160 is mediated by SSTR2 and SSTR5 somatostatin receptor subtypes through different mechanisms. *Proc. Natl. Acad. Sci. USA*, **92**, 1580–1584.
77. Bousquet, C., Puente, E., Buscail, L., Vaysse, N., and Susini, C. (2001) Antiproliferative effect of somatostatin and analogs. *Chemotherapy*, **47**, 30–39.
78. Florio, T., Yao, H., Carey, K.D., Dillon, T.J., and Stork, P.J.S. (1999) Somatostatin activation of mitogen-activated protein kinase via somatostatin receptor 1 (SSTR1). *Mol. Endocrinol.*, **13**, 24–37.
79. Hofland, L.J. and Lamberts, S.W. (2003) The pathophysiological consequences of somatostatin receptor internalization and resistance. *Endocrinol. Rev.*, **24**, 28–47.
80. Kouroumalis, E., Skordilis, P., Thermos, K., Vasilaki, A., Moschandrea, J., and Manousos, O.N. (1998) Treatment of hepatocellular carcinoma with octreotide: a randomized controlled study. *Gut*, **42**, 442–447.
81. Bruns, C., Lewis, I., Briner, U., Meno-Tetang, G., and Weckbecker, G. (2002) SOM230: a novel somatostatin peptidomimetic with broad somatotropin release inhibiting factor (SRIF) receptor binding and a unique antisecretory profile. *Eur. J. Endocrinol.*, **146**, 707–716.
82. Reubi, J.-C. and Laissue, J.A. (1995) Multiple actions of somatostatin in neoplastic disease. *Trends Pharmacol. Sci.*, **16**, 110–115.
83. Krenning, E.P., Kwekkeboom, D.J., Bakker, W.H., Breeman, W.A., Kooij, P.P., Oei, H.Y. *et al.* (1993) Somatostatin receptor scintigraphy with [^{111}In-DTPA-D -Phe^{1}]- and [^{123}I-Tyr^{3}]octreotide: the Rotterdam experience with more than 1,000 patients. *Eur. J. Nucl. Med.*, **20**, 716–731.
84. Lamberts, S.W., de Herder, W.W., and Hofland, L.J. (2002) Somatostatin analogs in the diagnosis and treatment of cancer. *Trends Endocrinol. Metab.*, **13**, 451–457.
85. Kwekkeboom, D.J., Krenning, E.P., Bakker, W.H., Oei, H.Y., Kooij, P.P.M., and Lamberts, S.W.J. (1993) Somatostatin analogue scintigraphy in carcinoid tumors. *Eur. J. Nucl. Med.*, **20**, 283–292.
86. Nagy, A., Schally, A.V., Halmos, G., Armatis, P., Cai, R.Z., Csernus, V. *et al.* (1998) Synthesis and biological evaluation of cytotoxic analogs of somatostatin containing doxorubicin or its intensely potent derivative 2-pyrrolinodoxonubicin. *Proc. Natl. Acad. Sci. USA*, **95**, 1794–1799.
87. Reubi, J.C. (2003) Peptide receptors as molecular targets for cancer diagnosis and therapy. *Endocrinol. Rev.*, **24**, 389–427.
88. Kahán, Z., Nagy, A., Schally, A.V., Hebert, F., Sun, B., Groot, K. *et al.* (1999) Inhibition of growth of MX-1, MCF-7-MIII and MDA-MB-231 human

breast cancer xenografts after administration of a targeted cytotoxic analog of somatostatin, AN-238. *Int. J. Cancer*, **82**, 592–598.

89. Seitz, S., Schally, A.V., Treszl, A., Papadia, A., Rick, F., Szalontay, L. *et al.* (2009) Preclinical evaluation of properties of a new targeted cytotoxic somatostatin analog, AN-162 (AEZS-124), and its effects on tumor growth inhibition. *Anti-Cancer Drugs*, **20**, 553–558.
90. Halmos, G., Sun, B., Schally, A.V., Hebert, F., and Nagy, A. (2000) Human ovarian cancers express somatostatin receptors. *J. Clin. Endocrinol. Metab.*, **85**, 3509–3512.
91. Plonowski, A., Schally, A.V., Koppan, M., Nagy, A., Arencibia, J.M., Csernus, B. *et al.* (2001) Inhibition of the UCI-107 human ovarian carcinoma cell line by a targeted cytotoxic analog of somatostatin, AN-238. *Cancer*, **92**, 1168–1176.
92. Engel, J.B., Schally, A.V., Halmos, G., Baker, B., Nagy, A., and Keller, G. (2005) Targeted therapy with a cytotoxic somatostatin analog, AN-238, inhibits growth of human experimental endometrial carcinomas expressing multidrug resistance protein MDR-1. *Cancer*, **104**, 1312–1321.
93. Halmos, G., Schally, A.V., Sun, B., Davis, R., Bostwick, D.G., and Plonowski, A. (2000) High expression of somatostatin receptors and ribonucleic acid for its receptor subtypes in organ-confined and locally advanced human prostate cancers. *J. Clin. Endocrinol. Metab.*, **85**, 2564–2571.
94. Plonowski, A., Schally, A.V., Nagy, A., Sun, B., and Szepeshazi, K. (1999) Inhibition of PC-3 human androgen-independent prostate cancer and its metastases by cytotoxic somatostatin analogue AN-238. *Cancer Res.*, **59**, 1947–1953.
95. Letsch, M., Schally, A.V., Szepeshazi, K., Halmos, G., and Nagy, A. (2004) Effective treatment of experimental models of androgen-sensitive and androgen-independent prostate cancer metastatic to the bone with targeted cytotoxic somatostatin analog AN-238. *J. Urol.*, **171**, 911–915.
96. Plonowski, A., Schally, A.V., Nagy, A., Kiaris, H., Hebert, F., and Halmos, G. (2000) Inhibition of metastatic renal cell carcinomas expressing somatostatin receptors by a targeted cytotoxic analog of somatostatin AN-238. *Cancer Res.*, **60**, 2996–3001.
97. Treszl, A., Schally, A.V., Seitz, S., Szalontay, L., Rick, F., Szepeshazi, K. *et al.* (2009) Inhibition of human non-small cell lung cancers with a targeted cytotoxic somatostatin analog, AN-162. *Peptides*, **30**, 1643–1650.
98. O'Byrne, K.J., Schally, A.V., Thomas, A., Carney, D.N., and Steward, W.P. (2001) Somatostatin, its receptors and analogs, in lung cancer. *Chemotherapy*, **47** (Suppl. 2), 78–108.
99. Kiaris, H., Schally, A.V., Nagy, A., Szepeshazi, K., Hebert, F., and Halmos, G. (2001) A targeted cytotoxic somatostatin (SST) analogue AN-238 inhibits the growth of H-69 small cell lung carcinoma (SCLC) and H-157 non-SCLC in nude mice. *Eur. J. Cancer*, **37**, 620–628.
100. Kiaris, H., Schally, A.V., Nagy, A., Sun, B., Szepeshazi, K., and Halmos, G. (2000) Regression of U-87MG human glioblastomas in nude mice after treatment with a cytotoxic somatostatin analog AN-238. *Clin. Cancer Res.*, **6**, 709–717.
101. Buscail, L., Saint-Laurent, N., Chastre, E., Vaillant, J.C., Gespach, C., Capella, G. *et al.* (1996) Loss of sst_2 somatostatin receptor gene expression in human pancreatic and colorectal cancer. *Cancer Res.*, **56**, 1823–1827.
102. Szepeshazi, K., Schally, A.V., Halmos, G., Sun, B., Hebert, F., Csernus, B. *et al.* (2001) Targeting of cytotoxic somatostatin analog AN-238 to somatostatin receptor subtypes 5 and/or 3 in experimental pancreatic cancer. *Clin. Cancer Res.*, **7**, 2854–2861.
103. Szepeshazi, K., Schally, A.V., Halmos, G., Armatis, P., Hebert, F., Sun, B. *et al.* (2002) Targeted cytotoxic somatostatin analogue AN-238 inhibits somatostatin receptor-positive experimental colon cancers independently

of their p53 status. *Cancer Res.*, **62**, 781–788.

104. Hohla, F., Buchholz, S., Schally, AV., Krishan, A., Rick, F., Szalontay, L. *et al.* (2010) Targeted cytotoxic somatostatin analog AN-162 inhibits growth of human colon carcinomas and overcomes resistance to doxorubicin in murine leukemia cells. *Cancer Lett.*, **294**, 35–42.

105. Szepeshazi, K., Schally, A.V., Nagy, A., Wagner, B.W., Bajo, A.M., and Halmos, G. (2003) Preclinical evaluation of therapeutic effects of targeted cytotoxic analogs of somatostatin and bombesin on human gastric carcinomas. *Cancer*, **98**, 1401–1410.

106. Szepeshazi, K., Schally, A.V., Treszl, A., Seitz, S., and Halmos, G. (2008) Therapy of experimental hepatic cancers with cytotoxic peptide analogs targeted to receptors for luteinizing hormone-releasing hormone, somatostatin or bombesin. *Anti-Cancer Drugs*, **19**, 349–358.

107. Lasfer, M., Vadrot, N., Schally, A.V., Nagy, A., Halmos, G., Pessayre, D. *et al.* (2005) Potent induction of apoptosis in human hepatoma cell lines by targeted cytotoxic somatostatin analogue AN-238. *J. Hepatol.*, **42**, 230–237.

108. Keller, G., Engel, J.B., Schally, A.V., Nagy, A., Hammann, B., and Halmos, G. (2005) Growth inhibition of experimental non-Hodgkins's lymphomas with the targeted cytotoxic somatostatin analogue AN-238. *Int. J. Cancer*, **115**, 831–835.

109. Spindel, E.R., Giladi, E., Segerson, T.P., and Nagalla, S. (1993) Bombesin-like peptides: of ligands and receptors. *Recent Prog. Horm. Res.*, **48**, 365–391.

110. Sunday, M.E., Kaplan, L.M., Motoyama, E., Chin, W.W., and Spindel, E.R. (1988) Gastrin-releasing peptide (mammalian bombesin) gene expression in health and disease. *Lab. Invest.*, **59**, 5–24.

111. Cuttitta, F., Carney, D.N., Mulshine, J., Moody, T.W., Fedorko, J., Fischler, A. *et al.* (1985) Bombesin-like peptides can function as autocrine growth factors in human small cell lung cancer. *Nature*, **316**, 823–826.

112. Jensen, J.A., Carroll, R.E., and Benya, R.V. (2001) The case for gastrin-releasing peptide acting as a morphogen when it and its receptor are aberrantly expressed in cancer. *Peptides*, **22**, 689–699.

113. Reubi, J.C., Wenger, S., Schmuckli-Maurer, J., Schaer, J.C., and Gugger, M. (2002) Bombesin receptor subtypes in human cancers: detection with the universal radioligand ^{125}I-[D -TYR6, beta-ALA11, PHE13, NLE14] bombesin(6–14). *Clin. Cancer Res.*, **8**, 1139–1146.

114. Hohla, F. and Schally, A.V. (2010) Targeting gastrin releasing peptide receptors. New options for the therapy and diagnosis of cancer. *Cell Cycle*, **9**, 1–4.

115. Cai, R.-Z., Reile, H., Armatis, P., and Schally, A.V. (1994) Potent bombesin antagonists with C-terminal Leu $\psi(CH_2N)$-Tac-NH_2 or its derivatives. *Proc. Natl. Acad. Sci. USA*, **91**, 12664–12668.

116. Moody, T.W. and Jensen, R.T. (1998) Bombesin receptor antagonists. *Drugs Future*, **23**, 1305–1315.

117. Bajo, M., Schally, A.V., Krupa, M., Hebert, F., Groot, K., and Szepeshazi, K. (2001) Bombesin antagonists inhibit growth of (MDA-MB-435) estrogen-independent breast cancers and decrease the expression of the ErbB-2/HER-2 oncoprotein and c-*jun* and c-*fos* oncogenes. *Proc. Natl. Acad. Sci. USA*, **99**, 3836–3841.

118. Waser, B., Eltschinger, V., Linder, K., Nunn, A., and Reubi, J.C. (2007) Selective *in vitro* targeting of GRP and NMB receptors in human tumours with the new bombesin tracer ^{177}Lu-AMBA. *Eur. J. Nucl. Med. Mol. Imaging*, **34**, 95–100.

119. Safavy, A., Raisch, K.P., Khazaeli, M.B., Buchsbaum, D.J., and Bonner, J.A. (1999) Paclitaxel derivatives for targeted therapy of cancer: toward the development of smart taxanes. *J. Med. Chem.*, **42**, 4919–4924.

120. Moody, T.W., Mantey, S.A., Pradhan, T.K., Schumann, M.,

Nakagawa, T., Martinez, A. *et al.* (2004) Development of high affinity camptothecin–bombesin conjugates that have targeted cytotoxicity for bombesin receptor-containing tumor cells. *J. Biol. Chem.*, **279**, 23580–23589.

121. Nagy, A., Armatis, P., Cai, R.Z., Szepeshazi, K., Halmos, G., and Schally, A.V. (1997) Design, synthesis and *in vitro* evaluation of cytotoxic analogs of bombesin-like peptides containing doxorubicin or its intensely potent derivative, 2-pyrrolinodoxorubicin. *Proc. Natl. Acad. Sci. USA*, **94**, 652–656.

122. Engel, J.B., Schally, A.V., Halmos, G., Baker, B., Nagy, A., and Keller, G. (2005) Experimental therapy of human endometrial cancers with a targeted cytotoxic bombesin analog AN-215: low induction of multidrug resistance proteins. *Eur. J. Cancer*, **41**, 1824–1830.

123. Engel, J.B., Schally, A.V., Halmos, G., Baker, B., Nagy, A., and Keller, G. (2005) Targeted cytotoxic bombesin analog AN-215 effectively inhibits experimental human breast cancers with a low induction of multi-drug resistance proteins. *Endocr. Relat. Cancer*, **12**, 999–1009.

124. Kiaris, H., Schally, A.V., Nagy, A., Sun, B., Armatis, P., and Szepeshazi, K. (1999) Targeted cytotoxic analog of bombesin/gastrin-releasing peptide inhibits the growth of H-69 human small-cell lung carcinoma in nude mice. *Br. J. Cancer*, **81**, 966–971.

125. Barabutis, N. and Schally, A.V. (2008) Knocking down gene expression for growth hormone-releasing hormone inhibits proliferation of human cancer cell lines. *Br. J. Cancer*, **98**, 1790–1796.

126. Rekasi, Z., Czompoly, T., Schally, A.V., and Halmos, G. (2000) Isolation and sequencing of cDNAs for splice variants of growth hormone-releasing hormone receptors from human cancers. *Proc. Natl. Acad. Sci. USA*, **97**, 10561–10566.

127. Halmos, G., Schally, A.V., Varga, J.L., Plonowski, A., Rekasi, Z., and Czompoly, T. (2000) Human renal cell carcinoma expresses distinct binding sites for growth hormone-releasing hormone. *Proc. Natl. Acad. Sci. USA*, **97**, 10555–10560.

128. Toller, G.L., Horvath, J.E., Schally, A.V., Halmos, G., Varga, J.L., Groot, K. *et al.* (2004) Development of a polyclonal antiserum for the detection of the isoforms of the receptors for human growth hormone-releasing hormone on tumors. *Proc. Natl. Acad. Sci. USA*, **101**, 15160–15165.

129. Havt, A., Schally, A.V., Halmos, G., Varga, J.L., Toller, G.L., Horvath, J.E. *et al.* (2005) The expression of the pituitary GHRH receptor and its splice variants in normal and neoplastic human tissues. *Proc. Natl. Acad. Sci. USA*, **102**, 17424–17429.

130. Halmos, G., Schally, A.V., Czompoly, T., Krupa, M., Varga, J.L., and Rekasi, Z. (2002) Expression of growth hormone-releasing hormone and its receptor splice variants in human prostate cancer. *J. Clin. Endocrinol. Metab.*, **87**, 4707–4714.

131. Freddi, S., Arnaldi, G., Fazioli, F., Scarpelli, M., Appolloni, G., Mancini, T. *et al.* (2005) Expression of growth hormone-releasing hormone receptor splicing variants in human primary adrenocortical tumours. *Clin. Endocrinol.*, **62**, 533–538.

132. Chatzistamou, I., Schally, A.V., Kiaris, H., Politi, E., Varga, J., Kanellis, G. *et al.* (2004) Immunohistochemical detection of growth hormone-releasing hormone and its receptor splice variant 1 in primary human breast cancers. *Eur. J. Endocrinol.*, **151**, 391–396.

133. Robberecht, P., Coy, D.H., Waelbroeck, M., Heiman, M.L., de Neef, P., Camus, J.C. *et al.* (1985) Structural requirements for the activation of rat anterior pituitary adenylate cyclase by growth hormone-releasing factor (GRF): discovery of (N-Ac-Tyr1, D-Arg2)-GRF(1–29)-NH_2 as a GRF antagonist on membranes. *Endocrinology*, **117**, 1759–1764.

134. Zarandi, M., Horvath, J.E., Halmos, G., Pinski, J., Nagy, A., Groot, K. *et al.*

(1994) Synthesis and biological activities of highly potent antagonists of growth hormone-releasing hormone. *Proc. Natl. Acad. Sci. USA*, **91**, 12298–12302.

135. Varga, J.L., Schally, A.V., Horvath, J.E., Kovacs, M., Halmos, G., Groot, K. *et al.* (2004) Increased activity of antagonists of growth hormone-releasing hormone substituted at positions 8, 9 and 10. *Proc. Natl. Acad. Sci. USA*, **101**, 1708–1713.

136. Letsch, M., Schally, A.V., Busto, R., Bajo, A.M., and Varga, J.L. (2003) Growth hormone-releasing hormone (GH-RH) antagonists inhibit the proliferation of androgen-dependent and -independent prostate cancers. *Proc. Natl. Acad. Sci. USA*, **100**, 1250–1255.

137. Heinrich, E., Schally, A., Buchholz, S., Rick, F., Halmos, G., Mile, M. *et al.* (2008) Dose-dependent growth inhibition *in vivo* of PC-3 prostate cancer with a reduction in tumoral growth factors after therapy with GHRH antagonist MZ-J-7-138. *Prostate*, **68**, 1763–1772.

138. Pozsgai, E., Schally, A.V., Zarandi, M., Varga, J.L., Vidaurre, I., and Bellyei, S. (2010) The effect of GHRH antagonists on human glioblastomas and their mechanism of action. *Int. J. Cancer*, **127**, 2313–2322.

139. Szereday, Z., Schally, A.V., Varga, J.L., Kanashiro, C., Hebert, F., Armatis, P. *et al.* (2003) Antagonists of growth hormone-releasing hormone inhibit the proliferation of experimental non-small cell lung carcinoma. *Cancer Res.*, **63**, 7913–7919.

140. Bellyei, S., Schally, A.V., Zarandi, M., Varga, J., Vidaurre, I., and Pozsgai, E. (2010) GHRH antagonists appear to reduce the invasive and metastatic potential of human cancer cell lines *in vitro*. *Cancer Lett.*, **293**, 31–40.

141. Jaffe, C.A., DeMott-Friberg, R., Frohman, L.A., and Barkan, A.L. (1997) Suppression of growth hormone (GH) hypersecretion due to ectopic GH-releasing hormone (GHRH) by a selective GHRH antagonist. *J. Clin. Endocrinol. Metab.*, **82**, 634–637.

39
Aptamer Conjugates: Emerging Delivery Platforms for Targeted Cancer Therapy

Zeyu Xiao, Jillian Frieder, Benjamin A. Teply, and Omid C. Farokhzad

39.1
Introduction

Targeted therapeutic platforms that have the ability to deliver drugs in a cell- or tissue-specific manner provide enhanced therapeutic efficacy and reduced cytotoxicity [1–3]. Targeted delivery is an area of vigorous research and a variety of delivery platforms have been described by using different recognition ligands, which include antibodies [4–6] and their fragments [7, 8], small molecules (peptides, vitamins, and carbohydrates) [9], and nucleic acids (aptamers) [10–12].

An optimal targeted delivery platform would possess the following features: (i) differential accumulation or internalization into a particular organ or cell, (ii) straightforward assembly processes that facilitate scale-up and manufacturing, and (iii) biostability and biocompatibility for *in vivo* applications [12–17].

However, many approaches are limited by the paucity of available targeting ligands against the cell or tissue of interest, technical complexity that provides a barrier to translation, and toxicity or immunogenicity profile that prevent repetitive treatment cycles [18]. Since aptamers may provide solutions to these limitations, they represent a promising new class of targeting ligands. Aptamers are nucleic acid or peptide molecules that bind to a specific target molecule (Figure 39.1). Aptamers are usually created by selecting them from a large random sequence pool, but natural aptamers also exist in riboswitches. Specifically, aptamers can be classified as peptide aptamers or nucleic acid (DNA or RNA) aptamers. Peptide aptamers are artificial recognition molecules that consist of a variable peptide sequence inserted into a constant scaffold protein [19, 20]. Compared with other classes of constrained combinatorial proteins (such as antibodies, antibody fragments, and other nonantibody scaffold-based molecules), peptide aptamers have distinguishing features that include their small size, their simple design, and their disulfide-independent folding; the latter enables them to function inside living cells [21, 22] (Figure 39.1b). Nucleic acid (DNA or RNA) aptamers are single-stranded,

Drug Delivery in Oncology: From Basic Research to Cancer Therapy, First Edition.
Edited by Felix Kratz, Peter Senter, and Henning Steinhagen.

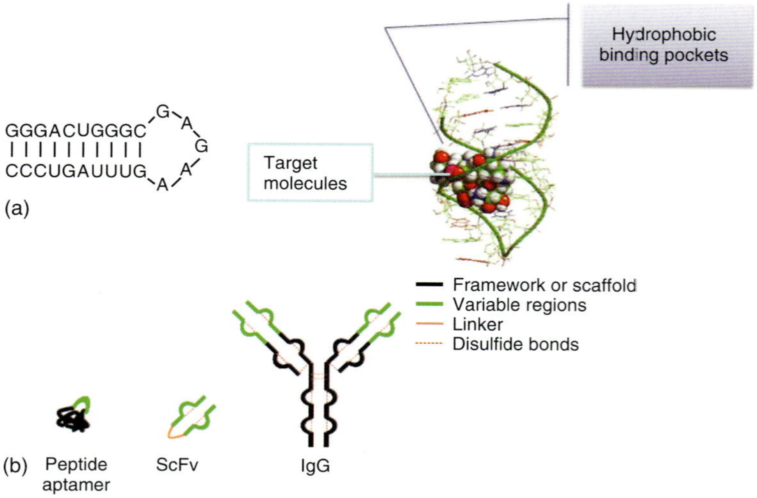

Figure 39.1 (a) Schematic secondary structure of an aptamer. Aptamers fold through intramolecular interactions to create tertiary conformations with hydrophobic binding pockets, which bind to their target molecules with high specificity and affinity. (b) Comparison between different constrained combinatorial recognition proteins, showing their approximate size and complexity (not to scale). IgG, immunoglobulin G; scFv, single-chain Fv antibody fragment.

natural or modified, oligonucleotides that are isolated from an iterative process called *in vitro* selection [23] or systematic evolution of ligands by exponential enrichment (SELEX) [24]. With high affinity and specificity for their targets and a chemical synthesis production process, nucleic acid aptamers satisfy most of the desirable characteristics for targeted therapeutic applications. Compared with antibodies, these kinds of aptamers have lower immunogenicity because of their nucleic acid composition. They also have a smaller size (5–15 kDa) than antibodies (around 155 kDa), allowing for more efficient penetration into biological compartments [25]. Unlike antibodies, which are produced via a biological process, nucleic acid aptamers can be manipulated by a chemical synthesis process, which is less prone to batch-to-batch variability [18]. Compared with peptides and small molecules, nucleic acid aptamers provide higher specificity and affinity, mainly due to the stability of the folded three-dimensional structure with specific binding pockets (Figure 39.1a) [26]. Moreover, nucleic acid aptamers can be internalized into cells by binding to certain types of receptors that participate in the receptor-mediated endocytosis [11]. Despite the relative infancy of the field, recent studies have demonstrated an emerging interest in the development of nucleic acid aptamer conjugates as drug delivery platforms [10, 27–32]. Herein, we summarize the recent progress of using nucleic acid aptamers as delivery platforms for targeted cancer therapy. The isolation process of these aptamers, their applications, and considerations for *in vivo* applications are the primary focus of this chapter.

39.2
Isolating Aptamers for Targeted Delivery

39.2.1
SELEX Against Purified Proteins

Many cell surface antigens or receptors are internalized by receptor-mediated endocytosis [33]. Aptamers that bind to these types of antigens or receptors could potentially be internalized into cells and unload their conjugated cargos inside the cells. Most of the aptamers that are currently available for targeted delivery were isolated by utilizing recombinant proteins. For example, prostate-specific membrane antigen (PSMA) is a well-characterized transmembrane protein that is strongly expressed in human prostate cancer and the vascular endothelium [34, 35]. Importantly, PSMA is continually recycled from the plasma membrane and is constitutively endocytosed in PSMA-positive cells, making it an attractive portal to deliver cargos intracellularly [11]. Using a purified target protein containing a modified extracellular form of PSMA, Lupold *et al.* selected two 2′-fluoro-modified RNase-resistant RNA aptamers with high binding affinity [36]. Since these anti-PSMA aptamers can be internalized, they have recently been engineered for cell-type-specific delivery of various cargos [37–39], such as chemotherapeutic agents, drug-encapsulated nanoparticles, toxins, enzymes, and small interfering RNAs (siRNAs). Similarly, several other aptamers against purified cell surface biomarkers or receptors have been successfully selected for targeted delivery, including anti-CD4 aptamers [40], anti-HIV glycoprotein 120 aptamers [41–43], anti-tenascin-C protein (TN-C) aptamers [44], anti-mouse transferrin receptor (TfR) aptamers [29], anti-nucleolin (NCL) aptamers [45], and anti-mucin 1 (MUC1) aptamers [46]. A brief summary of these aptamers and their various cargos and methods of conjugation are detailed in Table 39.1.

39.2.2
SELEX Against Living Cells

Despite the successful isolation of aptamers against purified proteins, efficient development of new cell-type-specific aptamers for targeted delivery is challenged by the limited number of purified receptors that can be used for aptamer selection when the protein targets are insoluble or the targets are functionally part of multiprotein complexes [54]. In these situations, traditional selections against purified proteins are not feasible. Therefore, selection protocols based on living cells present an alternative method for identifying aptamers against either cell surface or internal proteins [55]. In contrast to the selection processes against purified proteins, cell-based SELEX [56] can be performed without prior knowledge of targets or multiprotein complexes expressed on the cell surface. Moreover, intact living cells with many native receptor proteins are used as targets during the selection procedure. This allows for panels of aptamers targeting several proteins on the same cells to be isolated from such screenings [57]. As this strategy relies on the

Table 39.1 Aptamers utilized for targeted delivery.

Aptamers	Nucleic acid	Isolation targets	Cargos	Strategy for conjugation	Literature
Anti-PSMA	RNA	purified proteins	nanoparticles encapsulated with chemotherapeutic agents (such as dextran, DTX, Pt(IV), and DOX)	chemically covalently conjugate via amino and carboxylic acid chemistry	[10, 11, 47]
			toxin	chemically covalently conjugate toxin with aptamer via SPDP reagent	[30]
			drug (DOX)	physical conjugates via intercalation interaction	[27]
			siRNA	noncovalently conjugate siRNA with aptamer via a streptavidin connector	[31]
				aptamer–siRNA chimeras	[32, 48]
				bivalent aptamer–siRNA conjugates	[49]
Anti-CD4	RNA	purified proteins	siRNA	noncovalently assemble pRNA–siRNA chimera with pRNA–aptamer into dimer or trimer	[50]
Anti- HIV gp120	RNA	purified proteins	siRNA	aptamer–siRNA chimeras	[51]
				noncovalently conjugate siRNA with aptamer via a "sticky bridge"	[41]
Anti- TN-C	RNA	purified proteins	radionuclide and fluorescent agents	chemically covalently conjugate ^{99m}Tc or fluorescent agents with aptamers	[44]

Anti-PTK7	DNA	living cells	drug (DOX)	chemically covalently conjugate DOX with aptamer via an acid-labile linkage	[52]
			viral capsid	chemically covalently conjugate MS2 viral capsid with aptamer via an oxidative coupling reaction	[53]
Anti-TfR	DNA	purified proteins	enzyme	chemically covalently conjugate α-L-iduronidase with aptamer via an oxidative coupling reaction	[29]
Anti-NCL	DNA	purified proteins	liposomes and chemotherapeutic agents	cisplatin was encapsulated into liposomes that was noncovalently coated with aptamers	[45]
Anti-MUC1	DNA	purified proteins	photodynamic therapy agents	chemically covalently conjugate chlorin e6 with aptamer via EDC (1-(3-(dimethylamino)propyl)-3-ethylcarbodiimide hydrochloride) chemistry	[46]

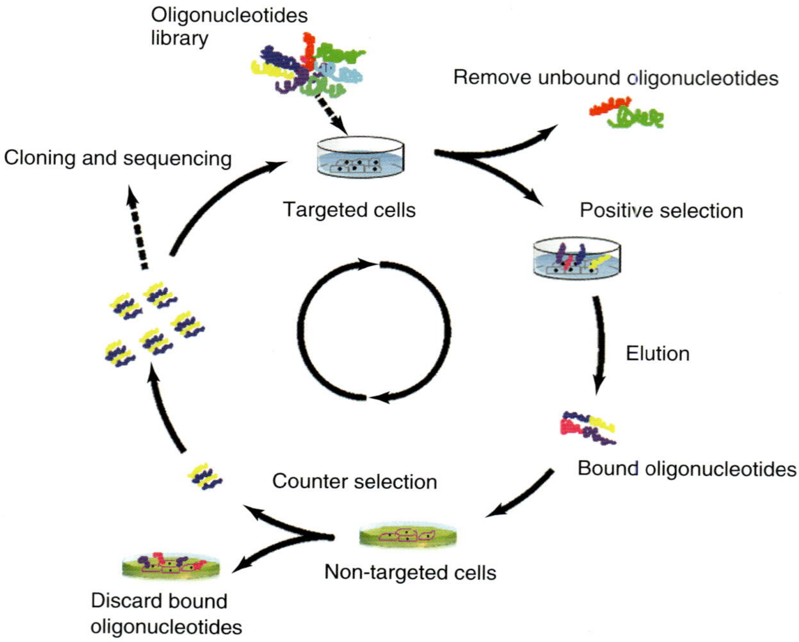

Figure 39.2 Schematic representation of cell-based aptamer selection. Briefly, the initial oligonucleotide library was incubated with target cells. After washing, the bound DNAs were eluted by heating to 95 °C. The eluted oligonucleotides were then incubated with nontargeted cells for counterselection. After centrifugation, the supernatant was collected and the selected oligonucleotides was amplified by polymerase chain reaction. The polymerase chain reaction products were separated for next-round selection or cloned and sequenced for aptamer identification in the last-round selection.

differences between the target cell population and the control cell population used for counterselection (e.g., defined phenotype, protein expression levels, different protein conformations), multiple aptamers that recognize only the target cells and not the control cells can be identified (Figure 39.2). For example, Shangguan *et al.* isolated a panel of aptamers that can distinguish leukemia T-cells from B-cells using cell-based SELEX [58]. Subsequently, an internalizing aptamer that binds to PTK7 receptor (anti-PTK7 aptamer) was identified from the isolated panel [53, 59]. Despite these advantages, one disadvantage of this approach is that it does not discriminate between dead cells with reduced cell membrane integrity and living cells [26]. Dead cells can yield a sequence-independent binding of nucleic acids [60]. During the process of exposing the cells to the SELEX libraries, any damage to fragile cells may result in selection failure. Compared with the traditional SELEX methods using a single target protein [61], cell-based SELEX typically requires more selection cycles (more than 20) and longer processing periods for efficient enrichment of the aptamer candidates. Furthermore, increasing the number of selection cycles could favor the enrichment of nonspecific or unwanted species, which preferentially adapt to the enzymatic amplification reactions rather than to the target binding. These limitations demonstrate that aptamer selection based on living cells is a difficult task and is still in its infancy. Although successful in individual cases [57], further optimization of selection schemes is required to increase the general applicability of cell-based selection. For example, living and dead cells within a cultured cell mixture could be discriminated and separated on the basis of their different light-scattering characteristics [60].

39.3
Applications of Aptamer Conjugates for Targeted Cancer Therapy

Aptamers can bind to the cell surface and become internalized into cells by receptor-mediated endocytosis. In addition, because of their accessibility for backbone or end-chain modifications [26], they can be adapted for delivery of various therapeutic cargos (small-molecule drugs, nanoparticles, or siRNAs) in a cell- or tissue-specific manner (Figure 39.3). Approaches in which aptamers have been linked to cargos to yield targeted therapeutics have recently been described [62, 63]. For small-molecule delivery, aptamers can be conjugated by either physical interaction or chemical linkage. For nanoparticle delivery, aptamers are mainly incorporated by covalent chemical bonds. For siRNA delivery, aptamers have been conjugated by different designs, including streptavidin–biotin association, covalent chemical linkage, and stick-bridge strategies. The detailed strategies of aptamer–cargo conjugation and their applications will be described in this section.

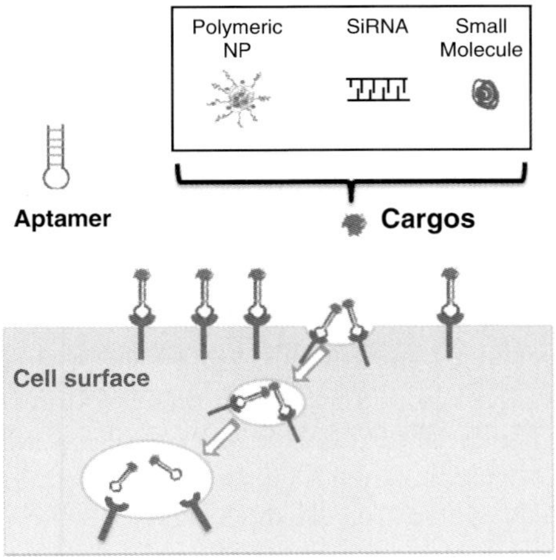

Figure 39.3 Aptamers with their conjugated cargos are taken up into the cells by receptor-mediated endocytosis.

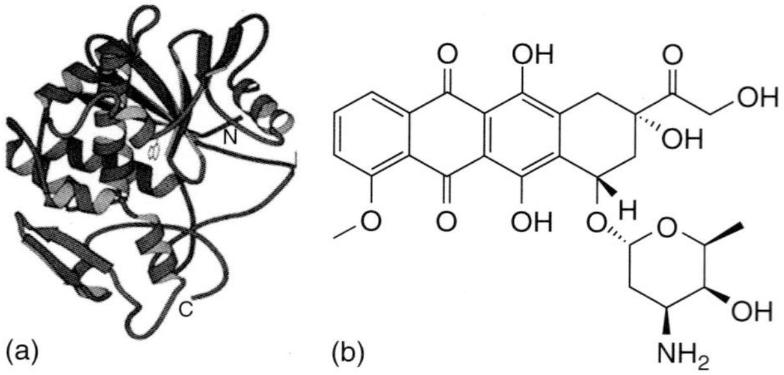

Figure 39.4 (a) Mimic structure of gelonin. Gelonin is a 28-kDa protein toxin found in the seeds of the Himalayan plant *Gelonium multiflorum*. Gelonin is a 60S ribosome-inactivating glycoprotein that inhibits protein synthesis. (b) Molecular structure of DOX. DOX is a cytotoxic anthracycline antibiotic used as a drug for cancer chemotherapy. The molecule contains acidic functions in the ring phenolic groups and a basic function in the sugar amino group, making it amphoteric.

39.3.1
Small-Molecule Delivery via Aptamer Conjugates

Conventional small-molecule therapeutics have been delivered via aptamers. For example, gelonin (Figure 39.4a) is a 28-kDa glycoprotein that inhibits protein synthesis [64]. However, gelonin has very little inherent cytotoxicity due to the lack of a translocation domain; therefore, it cannot be efficiently internalized into the cells at significant concentrations [65]. By conjugating anti-PSMA aptamers, these aptamer–toxin conjugates greatly increase the cytotoxicity of gelonin. They have an IC_{50} value of 27 nM and have an increased potency of at least 600-fold in PSMA-expressing cells relative to cells that do not express PSMA [30]. Similarly, doxorubicin (DOX) (Figure 39.4b), an anthracycline drug, is widely used for anticancer treatment and is well known to interact with the double helix of DNA. It was recently reported that the anti-PSMA aptamer physically interacts with DOX and that the aptamer could be directly used for drug delivery (Figure 39.5a) [27]. The aptamer–DOX conjugates were specifically taken up by LNCaP, but not PC-3 cells. The aptamer–DOX conjugates were in the cytosol and nuclei, unlike free DOX, which exclusively appears in nuclei. This observation demonstrated that the aptamer–DOX conjugates were being delivered by receptor-mediated endocytosis following binding of aptamer–DOX conjugates to PSMA on the cell surface. Interestingly, both this study and the previous study with gelonin showed that aptamer–drug conjugates have even lower background cytotoxicity than free drugs. Conjugating drugs to aptamers may be beneficial not only because of cell-specific delivery, but also because aptamers reduce the spontaneous uptake of free drug into nontarget cells. In another aptamer-based targeted drug delivery system, DOX was covalently linked to the anti-PTK7 aptamer that specifically targets T-cell acute lymphoblastic leukemia cells [52]. In this design format, an acid-labile linkage was used to facilitate the release of DOX when the aptamer–DOX complex was internalized

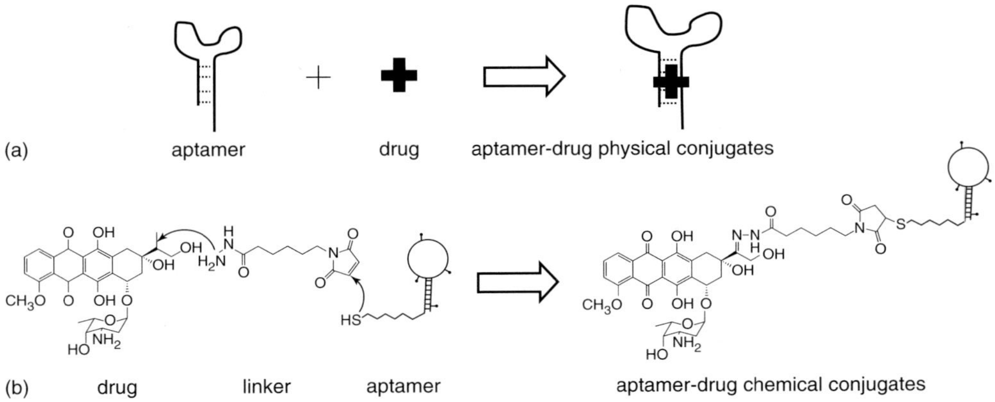

Figure 39.5 Aptamer-based drug (DOX) delivery by physical conjugation (a) or chemical conjugation (b).

into the endosomal compartment (Figure 39.5b). Consequently, the aptamer–DOX conjugates show a 6.7-fold increase in toxicity to their target CCRF-CEM cells compared to that of nontarget NB-4 cells [52]. Similarly, another study showed that anti-MUC1 aptamers selected against unique short *O*-glycan-peptide signatures on the surface of breast, colon, lung, ovarian, and pancreatic cancer cells can be used for targeted delivery of a phototoxic cancer therapy agent [46]. When modified at their 5′-end with the photodynamic therapy agent chlorin e6 and delivered to epithelial cancer cells, these phototoxic aptamers exhibited a remarkable enhancement (above 500-fold increase) in toxicity upon light activation compared with the drug alone. In addition, they were not cytotoxic toward normal cell types, which lack *O*-glycan-peptide markers. Taken together, these results show that aptamer-based targeted delivery of anticancer agents is a promising drug delivery technology that can increase the efficacy of chemotherapeutics, while at the same time mitigate the overall side-effect toxicity.

39.3.2
Nanoparticle Delivery via Aptamer Conjugate

Aptamers can also be used to direct the delivery of nanoparticles. Farokhzad *et al.* [11] pioneered the development of aptamer-targeted polymeric systems. The first such system consisted of poly(lactide)-*b*-poly(ethylene glycol) (PEG) block copolymers self-assembled via a double-emulsion method. Anti-PSMA aptamers were NH_2 modified at the 3′-terminus and coupled to the carboxyl-terminated PEG block (Figure 39.6a). The resulting nanoparticle–aptamer (NP-Apt) bioconjugates were incubated with PSMA-overexpressed LNCaP cells [11]. A 77-fold increase of binding and uptake in LNCaP cells was observed in the NP-Apt groups compared to the NP groups with Apt conjugation [11]. After loading with docetaxel (DTX), a chemotherapy drug, these DTX-encapsulated nanoparticle–aptamer (DTX-NP-Apt) bioconjugates bound and were subsequently taken up by LNCaP cells, resulting

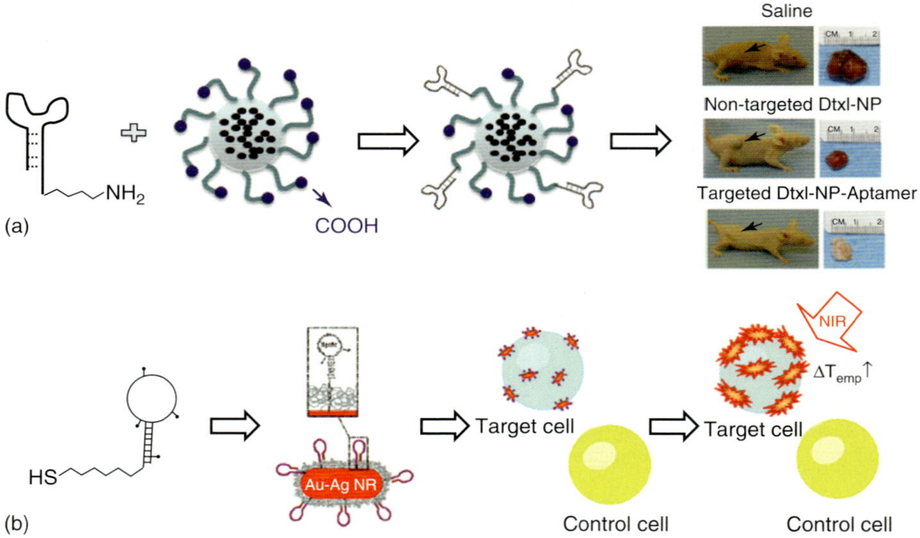

Figure 39.6 (a) Aptamer and organic nanoparticle conjugation for targeted chemotherapy. (b) Aptamer and inorganic nanoparticle conjugation for targeted thermotherapy.

in significantly enhanced *in vitro* cellular toxicity as compared with nontargeted nanoparticles that lack the PSMA aptamer (DTX-NP) [10]. The DTX-NP-Apt bioconjugates also exhibited remarkable *in vivo* efficacy and reduced toxicity as measured by tumor reduction, nearly 60% less mean body weight loss, and 100% survival compared with 57% survival for DTX-NP and 14% for DTX alone in the 109-day study in LNCaP xenograft nude mice [10]. Using the same anti-PSMA aptamer, efficacy was also demonstrated with the chemotherapeutic drug cisplatin delivered to tumor cells via aptamer functionalized poly(D,L-lactic-*co*-glycolic acid)–PEG nanoparticle conjugates [47]. Similarly, an anti-NCL aptamer was conjugated to a liposome in order to deliver encapsulated chemotherapeutic cisplatin to tumors [45]. In that study, the controlled release of the conjugates to tumors was achieved by using an antisense oligonucleotide. These targeted encapsulation strategies may decrease the systemic toxicity normally associated with chemotherapy.

Besides organic nanoparticles, inorganic nanoparticles of Au–Ag nanorods have also been conjugated with multiple anti-PTK7 aptamers for targeted cancer photothermal therapy (Figure 39.6b) [66, 67]. Some aptamers have moderate binding affinities that prevent themselves from efficient targeting to the desirable cell lines. By using Au–Ag nanorods that can be conjugated to around 80 aptamers, 26 times higher binding affinity was obtained compared to individual aptamer strands [66]. Subsequently, selective photothermal therapeutic effects for mixed cancer cells were achieved by using this anti-PTK7 aptamer–nanorod conjugate [67]. In this study, the aptamer–nanorod conjugates were incubated with the cell mixtures of aptamer-targeted CEM cells and nontarget NB-4 cells. Under a specific laser intensity and duration of laser exposure, about 50% of CEM cells were severely damaged, while more than 87% of NB-4 cells remained intact [67]. These results showed a great potential of utilizing aptamer–nanoparticles conjugates for targeted cancer therapy.

39.3.3
siRNA Delivery via Aptamer Conjugates

Beyond nanoparticle and small-molecule delivery, aptamers could also be useful for delivering siRNAs, which have potential clinical applications as antisense therapeutics [68]. One of the major difficulties for the development of siRNA therapeutics is effective delivery [69, 70]. To address this limitation, several independent groups have successfully employed the anti-PSMA, anti-CD4 [50], and anti-gp120 [51] RNA aptamers to specifically deliver different siRNAs into targeted cells. In a proof-of-concept study [31], Chu *et al.* reported noncovalent conjugation of biotinylated anti-PSMA aptamer with biotinylated 27mer lamin A/C or GAPDH siRNAs via a modular streptavidin connector (Figure 39.7a). By using such a streptavidin

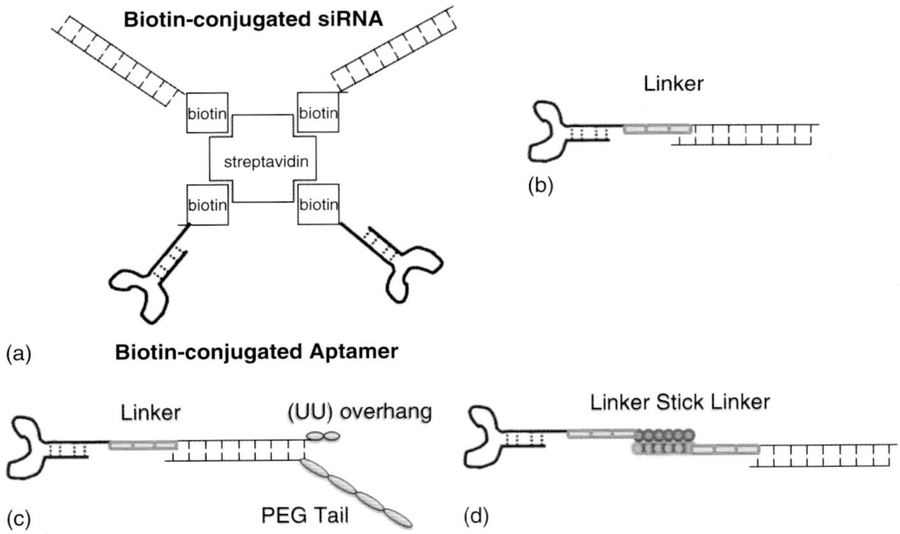

Figure 39.7 Aptamer-based siRNA delivery. (a) Aptamer–streptavidin–siRNA conjugates. (b) First-generation aptamer–siRNA chimeras. The 2′-fluoro-modified aptamer and siRNA sense strand were cotranscribed, followed by annealing of the complementary siRNA antisense strand to complete the chimeric molecule. (c) Optimized second-generation chimeras. Compared with the first-generation chimeras, the aptamer portion of the chimera was truncated, and the sense and antisense strands of the siRNA portion were swapped. A two-nucleotide (UU) overhang and a PEG tail were added to the 3′-end of the guide strand and the 5′-end of the passenger strand, respectively. (d) Aptamer–"sticky bridge"–siRNA conjugates. Either the antisense or the sense strand of the 27mer Dicer substrate RNA duplex and the aptamer were attached with to complementary "sticky" sequences.

connector, two aptamers and two siRNAs were elegantly assembled into a multivalent construct, displaying effective PSMA receptor-mediated internalization of aptamer–siRNAs and specific silencing of the targeted transcripts in tumor cells. In another approach developed by Giangrande *et al.* [32], the anti-PSMA aptamer (A10) was covalently conjugated to the sense strand of a 21mer siRNA, which in turn was hybridized to the 21mer antisense strand (Figure 39.7b). The resulting aptamer–chimeric RNA was shown to be selectively internalized into cells expressing PSMA and to effectively knockdown expression of the targeted tumor survival genes (PLK1 and BCL2) both in cell culture and *in vivo* via intratumoral administration [32]. More recently, the same group extended their investigations of delivering aptamer–siRNA chimeras *in vivo* via systematic administration. To achieve this goal, the PSMA A10–Plk1 chimera was truncated from 71 to 39 nucleotides, while still maintaining high binding affinity. Furthermore, a two-nucleotide (UU) overhang was added at the 3′-end of the siRNA duplex, which favors Dicer recognition and loading of the guide strand (containing the two-base 3′ overhang) into an RNA-induced silencing complex, hence increasing the silencing activity and specificity. Finally, a PEG moiety with a molecular weight of 20 kDa was conjugated with the siRNA passenger, substantially increasing the circulating half-life of the chimeric molecule (Figure 39.7c). As a result, the optimized second-generation aptamer–siRNA chimeras lead to obvious regression of PSMA-expressing tumors after systemic administration in athymic mice.

Other efforts to further refine aptamer-conjugated siRNA delivery and targeting efficiency are being attempted through multimerization of the aptamer portion. Previous studies with aptamers have revealed that multivalent aptamers can increase the potency and antitumor response, and promote receptor activation [71–74]. The multivalent aptamer–siRNA construct has also been recently exploited for facilitating receptor internalization, further improving the therapeutic potential. Wullner *et al.* generated two different bivalent anti-PSMA aptamer–siRNA chimeras in which the siRNAs targeted eukaryotic elongation factor-2 [49]. Their modifications included using the siRNA itself as a linker to join the two aptamers or appending the siRNAs onto the 3′-ends of each aptamer. Compared with the monovalent aptamer–siRNA chimeras (55% target knockdown), these bivalent aptamer–siRNA constructs resulted in an almost complete loss of PSMA-positive cell viability, suggesting that bivalent aptamers promote internalization of chimeras. These efforts have encouraged new design of multiple aptamer–siRNA conjugates. In a study by Zhou *et al.* [41], a "sticky bridge" strategy was developed to noncovalently conjugate the anti-gp120 aptamer with various siRNAs (Figure 39.7d). In this design format, one pair of complementary GC-rich sticky bridge sequences was chemically attached to the 3′-end of the aptamer. The complement to this sequence was attached to one of the two siRNA strands, and the aptamer and siRNA were joined by Watson–Crick base pairing. A flexible three-carbon atom hinge (C3) was added as a spacer between the adhesive (sticky) sequence and the aptamer to allow spatial and structural flexibility. Most importantly, this sticky bridge-based strategy can be used to facilitate the effective interchange of different siRNAs with a single aptamer, which is required to avert viral resistance to the siRNA component. These results demonstrated the potential use of aptamer–siRNA conjugates as a systemic, cell type-specific, siRNA cocktail delivery system for a myriad of diseases.

39.4
Considerations of Aptamer Characteristics for *In Vivo* Applications

Although great progress has been made in isolating and applying aptamers for targeted delivery and cancer therapy *in vitro*, the translation of these aptamers for clinical applications has faced considerable challenges. Herein, we summarize some major considerations for utilizing those aptamers *in vivo*, which may facilitate the translation of selected aptamers for further development.

39.4.1
Nuclease Resistance

The half-lives of RNA aptamers composed of unmodified nucleotides in the blood can be as short as 2 min [75], mainly due to the degradation by serum endo- or exonucleases [26]. During the endonuclease cleavage, the ribose 2′-OH engages in nucleophilic attack on the neighboring 3′-phosphodiester bond. Therefore, 2′ RNA modifications, by replacing the 2′-position with either a fluoro, amino, or *O*-methyl group, can be performed. This results in at least 1000-fold more resistance to degradation in plasma than their unmodified RNA counterparts [76]. These modified nucleotides can be introduced either chemically or enzymatically. Apart from degradation by endonucleases, aptamers are also subject to degradation by exonucleases. To overcome this limitation, inverted end caps that involve reversing the polarity of the chain can be incorporated at the 3′-terminus [18], as 3′-exonuclease activity in serum is much higher than 5′-exonuclease activity. Linkers are commonly modified at the 5′-terminus to provide handles for conjugation or to alter pharmacokinetic properties.

39.4.2
Optimal Circulating Half-Life

The molecular mass cutoff for renal glomerulus is around 50 kDa [77]. Aptamers have a molecular mass range of 5–15 kDa [25] and thus they are susceptible to renal filtration regardless of how well they resist nuclease-mediated degradation. To reduce the renal filtration rate and increase the circulating half-life, one strategy is to conjugate polymers with the size range larger than the filter cutoff of the renal glomerulus. For example, unconjugated aptamers were cleared from the mouse circulatory system with a half-life of 5–10 min, whereas conjugation of a 40-kDa PEG to a 2′-fluoro/2′-*O*-methyl-modified aptamer increased its circulating half-life to 12 h when administered to Sprague-Dawley rats [78]. Moreover, a 40-kDa PEG conjugated to a fully 2′-*O*-methyl aptamer persisted in circulation with a half-life of 23 h in mice [79]. Cholesterol conjugation has also been reported as an alternative strategy to reduce renal filtration rates, although the extent of this effect is less than for PEG conjugation [80]. Rusconi *et al.* reported the conjugation of cholesterol to a Factor IXa-specific aptamer that resulted in an increase in half-life from 5–10 min to 1–1.5 h in swine [81]. Notably, protein modification is generally performed stochastically through lysine side-chains, which often results in a mixture of products and a loss of activity [18]. By contrast, aptamers are chemically synthesized and lack many of the functional groups commonly present in proteins, hence a single functional group (such as an alkyl amine) can be site-specifically introduced and conjugated to the aptamer without disrupting structure or function [26].

39.4.3
Rapid Penetration and Longer Retention Time in Target Tissue

Aptamers have shown rapid uptake in the target tissue. An investigation comparing tumor imaging by an aptamer and an antibody binding to the same protein shows that the antibody requires days to achieve an appreciable signal/noise ratio, whereas the aptamer rapidly develops a far higher signal/noise ratio that results in high-quality tumor images [82]. After intravenous injection of two different ^{99m}Tc-radiolabeled aptamers, maximal levels were observed in either clots or tumors within 10–30 min. The slower uptake and clearance of antibodies is due in part to their larger size [83]. The desirable uptake kinetics of aptamers fit well with the anticipated clinical needs.

Another feature of aptamers is their durable retention in the preferred tissue, with a half-life of more than 12 h for a tumor-targeting aptamer in the mouse [82]. Although the reason for long retention has not been addressed, it has been found that tumor- and clot-associated aptamers remain mostly intact for hours, with some variation depending on the aptamer and the animal species [84]. In contrast to target-bound aptamers, nuclease degradation of blood-bound aptamers occurs rapidly, with greater than 95% destruction within 30 min in blood. The possible reason might be that the degradation occurs at sites (perhaps the liver and kidney) that are anatomically separate from the target tissue [84]. Consistent with this model, it has been noted that aptamer clearance from the blood is dramatically slower in hepatectomized rats [60]. Therefore, the observed protection of target-bound aptamers from nucleases has implications for the development of function-blocking nucleic acids, including aptamers, antisense, and ribozymes, which operate in extravascular tissue.

39.4.4
Toxicology

Another consideration of *in vivo* applications of aptamers is their toxicity. Using aptamer-based drug delivery platforms is a relatively young field and still in preclinical investigations, and thus there is only limited published information concerning the toxicology of aptamers. Many studies have been performed concerning the toxicology of antisense therapeutics [85], specifically with regard to complement activation and innate immune stimulation. Aptamer and oligonucleotide antisense therapeutics differ in several respects, including chemical substitution, size, and secondary structure; however, some parallels can be drawn.

Complement activation has been attributed to the interaction of oligonucleotides with complement Factor H [86], which is a control protein for the alternative complement pathway. Complement activation has been observed in studies conducted in nonhuman primates in which effects are predominantly acute and seemed to manifest themselves only after a high oligonucleotide concentration had been reached. Observations included hypotension, elevated heart rate, and can include cardiovascular collapse when severe [87].

Innate immune activation occurs as a consequence of the activation of Toll-like receptor (TLR)-3, -7, -8, or -9. TLR-3 responds to double-stranded RNA, TLR-7 and -8 respond to single-stranded RNA, and TLR-9 responds to unmethylated CG motifs in DNA (CpG motifs) [88]. Since unmodified RNA is highly sensitive to endogenous nucleases and since 2′-modification abrogates the TLR response [89], TLR-9 is probably the most relevant to the study of potential adverse effects of therapeutic aptamers, although other TLRs may be relevant to the interpretation of *in vivo* responses to siRNA. Innate immune responses mediated by TLR-9 include secretion of cytokines interleukin-6 and interferon [90]. Nevertheless, TLR-9-mediated immune responses to oligonucleotides are being considered for therapeutic applications in which immune stimulation is desirable, such as in oncology [91].

39.5 Conclusions and Perspectives

Aptamers have many favorable characteristics, including high binding affinity and specificity, relatively small size, and a chemical synthesis process, making them attractive for a variety of applications in targeted delivery. In this regard, nucleic acid aptamers targeting cell surface proteins are emerging in several promising delivery platforms to target a particular cell population or tissue, thus providing enhanced therapeutic efficacy and reduced cellular toxicity.

To date, significant advances have been made to develop aptamer conjugates as platforms to deliver therapeutic cargos into diseased cells or tissues in a cell-type-specific manner. Some examples of applying aptamer conjugates for targeted therapy have been discussed in this chapter. Despite substantial progress in aptamer-mediated targeted delivery, three major efforts are still required for clinical translation: (i) the development of more efficient selection methods to generate new cell-internalizing aptamers with high affinity and specificity; (ii) the development of straightforward strategies for conjugating aptamers with their therapeutic cargos; and (iii) efforts to increase the yield of synthesis and to improve pharmacokinetic properties. By addressing these challenges, the promise of aptamer-based drug delivery platform may appear in the clinical trials in the near future.

Acknowledgments

This work was supported by National Institutes of Health grants CA119349 and EB003647, and Koch-Prostate Cancer Foundation Award in Nanotherapeutics.

References

1. Langer, R. (1998) Drug delivery and targeting. *Nature*, **392** (Suppl. 6679), 5–10.
2. Ferrari, M. (2005) Cancer nanotechnology: opportunities and challenges. *Nat. Rev. Cancer*, **5**, 161–171.
3. Davis, M.E., Chen, Z.G., and Shin, D.M. (2008) Nanoparticle therapeutics: an emerging treatment modality for cancer. *Nat. Rev. Drug Discov.*, **7**, 771–782.
4. Boerman, O.C. *et al.* (1999) Pretargeting of renal cell carcinoma: improved tumor targeting with a bivalent chelate. *Cancer Res.*, **59**, 4400–4405.
5. Paganelli, G. *et al.* (1999) Antibody-guided three-step therapy for high grade glioma with yttrium-90 biotin. *Eur. J. Nucl. Med.*, **26**, 348–357.
6. Axworthy, D.B. *et al.* (2000) Cure of human carcinoma xenografts by a single dose of pretargeted yttrium-90 with negligible toxicity. *Proc. Natl. Acad. Sci. USA*, **97**, 1802–1807.
7. Adams, G.P. and Schier, R. (1999) Generating improved single-chain Fv molecules for tumor targeting. *J. Immunol. Methods*, **231**, 249–260.
8. Wu, A.M. *et al.* (1996) Tumor localization of anti-CEA single-chain Fvs: improved targeting by non-covalent dimers. *Immunotechnology*, **2**, 21–36.
9. Alexis, F. *et al.* (2008) HER-2-targeted nanoparticle-affibody bioconjugates for cancer therapy. *ChemMedChem*, **3**, 1839–1843.
10. Farokhzad, O.C. *et al.* (2006) Targeted nanoparticle–aptamer bioconjugates for cancer chemotherapy *in vivo*. *Proc. Natl. Acad. Sci. USA*, **103**, 6315–6320.
11. Farokhzad, O.C. *et al.* (2004) Nanoparticle–aptamer bioconjugates: a new approach for targeting prostate cancer cells. *Cancer Res.*, **64**, 7668–7672.
12. Farokhzad, O.C., Karp, J.M., and Langer, R. (2006) Nanoparticle–aptamer bioconjugates for cancer targeting. *Expert Opin. Drug Deliv.*, **3**, 311–324.
13. Peer, D. *et al.* (2007) Nanocarriers as an emerging platform for cancer therapy. *Nat. Nanotechnol.*, **2**, 751–760.
14. Farokhzad, O.C. (2008) Nanotechnology for drug delivery: the perfect partnership. *Expert Opin. Drug Deliv.*, **5**, 927–929.
15. Farokhzad, O.C. *et al.* (2006) Drug delivery systems in urology – getting "smarter". *Urology*, **68**, 463–469.
16. Farokhzad, O.C. and Langer, R. (2006) Nanomedicine: developing smarter therapeutic and diagnostic modalities. *Adv. Drug Deliv. Rev.*, **58**, 1456–1459.
17. Farokhzad, O.C. and Langer, R. (2009) Impact of nanotechnology on drug delivery. *ACS Nano*, **3**, 16–20.
18. Keefe, A.D., Pai, S., and Ellington, A. (2010) Aptamers as therapeutics. *Nat. Rev. Drug Discov.*, **9**, 537–550.
19. Colas, P. *et al.* (1996) Genetic selection of peptide aptamers that recognize and inhibit cyclin-dependent kinase 2. *Nature*, **380**, 548–550.
20. Bickle, M.B., Dusserre, E., Moncorge, O., Bottin, H., and Colas, P. (2006) Selection and characterization of large collections of peptide aptamers through optimized yeast two-hybrid procedures. *Nat. Protoc.*, **1**, 1066–1091.
21. Colas, P. (2008) The eleven-year switch of peptide aptamers. *J. Biol.*, **7**, 2.
22. Baines, I.C. and Colas, P. (2006) Peptide aptamers as guides for small-molecule drug discovery. *Drug Discov. Today*, **11**, 334–341.
23. Ellington, A.D. and Szostak, J.W. (1990) *In vitro* selection of RNA molecules that bind specific ligands. *Nature*, **346**, 818–822.

24. Tuerk, C. and Gold, L. (1990) Systematic evolution of ligands by exponential enrichment: RNA ligands to bacteriophage T4 DNA polymerase. *Science*, **249**, 505–510.
25. Bouchard, P.R., Hutabarat, R.M., and Thompson, K.M. (2010) Discovery and development of therapeutic aptamers. *Annu. Rev. Pharmacol. Toxicol.*, **50**, 237–257.
26. Mayer, G. (2009) The chemical biology of aptamers. *Angew. Chem. Int. Ed. Engl.*, **48**, 2672–2689.
27. Bagalkot, V., Farokhzad, O.C., Langer, R., and Jon, S. (2006) An aptamer–doxorubicin physical conjugate as a novel targeted drug-delivery platform. *Angew. Chem. Int. Ed.*, **45**, 8149–8152.
28. Bagalkot, V. *et al.* (2007) Quantum dot-aptamer conjugates for synchronous cancer imaging, therapy, and sensing of drug delivery based on bi-fluorescence resonance energy transfer. *Nano Lett.*, **7**, 3065–3070.
29. Chen, C.H. *et al.* (2008) Aptamer-based endocytosis of a lysosomal enzyme. *Proc. Natl. Acad. Sci. USA*, **105**, 15908–15913.
30. Chu, T.C. *et al.* (2006) Aptamer:toxin conjugates that specifically target prostate tumor cells. *Cancer Res.*, **66**, 5989–5992.
31. Chu, T.C., Twu, K.Y., Ellington, A.D., and Levy, M. (2006) Aptamer mediated siRNA delivery. *Nucleic Acids Res.*, **34**, e73.
32. McNamara, J.O. II *et al.* (2006) Cell type-specific delivery of siRNAs with aptamer–siRNA chimeras. *Nat. Biotechnol.*, **24**, 1005–1015.
33. Tsui, P., Rubenstein, M., and Guinan, P. (2005) Correlation between PSMA and VEGF expression as markers for LNCaP tumor angiogenesis. *J. Biomed. Biotechnol.*, **2005**, 287–290.
34. Tasch, J., Gong, M., Sadelain, M., and Heston, W.D. (2001) A unique folate hydrolase, prostate-specific membrane antigen (PSMA): a target for immunotherapy? *Crit. Rev. Immunol.*, **21**, 249–261.
35. Liu, H. *et al.* (1998) Constitutive and antibody-induced internalization of prostate-specific membrane antigen. *Cancer Res.*, **58**, 4055–4060.
36. Lupold, S.E., Hicke, B.J., Lin, Y., and Coffey, D.S. (2002) Identification and characterization of nuclease-stabilized RNA molecules that bind human prostate cancer cells via the prostate-specific membrane antigen. *Cancer Res.*, **62**, 4029–4033.
37. Levy-Nissenbaum, E., Radovic-Moreno, A.F., Wang, A.Z., Langer, R., and Farokhzad, O.C. (2008) Nanotechnology and aptamers: applications in drug delivery. *Trends Biotechnol.*, **26**, 442–449.
38. Yan, A.C. and Levy, M. (2009) Aptamers and aptamer targeted delivery. *RNA Biol.*, **6**, 316–320.
39. Thiel, K.W. and Giangrande, P.H. (2009) Therapeutic applications of DNA and RNA aptamers. *Oligonucleotides*, **19**, 209–222.
40. Kraus, E., James, W., and Barclay, A.N. (1998) Cutting edge: novel RNA ligands able to bind CD4 antigen and inhibit $CD4^+$ T lymphocyte function. *J. Immunol.*, **160**, 5209–5212.
41. Zhou, J. *et al.* (2009) Selection, characterization and application of new RNA HIV gp 120 aptamers for facile delivery of Dicer substrate siRNAs into HIV infected cells. *Nucleic Acids Res.*, **37**, 3094–3109.
42. Dey, A.K., Griffiths, C., Lea, S.M., and James, W. (2005) Structural characterization of an anti-gp120 RNA aptamer that neutralizes R5 strains of HIV-1. *RNA*, **11**, 873–884.
43. Dey, A.K. *et al.* (2005) An aptamer that neutralizes R5 strains of human immunodeficiency virus type 1 blocks gp120–CCR5 interaction. *J. Virol.*, **79**, 13806–13810.
44. Hicke, B.J. *et al.* (2001) Tenascin-C aptamers are generated using tumor cells and purified protein. *J. Biol. Chem.*, **276**, 48644–48654.
45. Cao, Z. *et al.* (2009) Reversible cell-specific drug delivery with aptamer-functionalized liposomes. *Angew. Chem. Int. Ed.*, **48**, 6494–6498.
46. Ferreira, C.S., Cheung, M.C., Missailidis, S., Bisland, S., and Gariepy, J. (2009) Phototoxic aptamers selectively

enter and kill epithelial cancer cells. *Nucleic Acids Res.*, **37**, 866–876.

47. Dhar, S., Gu, F.X., Langer, R., Farokhzad, O.C., and Lippard, S.J. (2008) Targeted delivery of cisplatin to prostate cancer cells by aptamer functionalized Pt(IV) prodrug–PLGA–PEG nanoparticles. *Proc. Natl. Acad. Sci. USA*, **105**, 17356–17361.
48. Dassie, J.P. *et al.* (2009) Systemic administration of optimized aptamer–siRNA chimeras promotes regression of PSMA-expressing tumors. *Nat. Biotechnol.*, **27**, 839–849.
49. Wullner, U. *et al.* (2008) Cell-specific induction of apoptosis by rationally designed bivalent aptamer–siRNA transcripts silencing eukaryotic elongation factor 2. *Curr. Cancer Drug Targets*, **8**, 554–565.
50. Hu-Lieskovan, S., Heidel, J.D., Bartlett, D.W., Davis, M.E., and Triche, T.J. (2005) Sequence-specific knockdown of EWS-FLI1 by targeted, nonviral delivery of small interfering RNA inhibits tumor growth in a murine model of metastatic Ewing's sarcoma. *Cancer Res.*, **65**, 8984–8992.
51. Zhou, J., Li, H., Li, S., Zaia, J., and Rossi, J.J. (2008) Novel dual inhibitory function aptamer–siRNA delivery system for HIV-1 therapy. *Mol. Ther.*, **16**, 1481–1489.
52. Huang, Y.F. *et al.* (2009) Molecular assembly of an aptamer–drug conjugate for targeted drug delivery to tumor cells. *ChemBioChem*, **10**, 862–868.
53. Tong, G.J., Hsiao, S.C., Carrico, Z.M., and Francis, M.B. (2009) Viral capsid DNA aptamer conjugates as multivalent cell-targeting vehicles. *J. Am. Chem. Soc.*, **131**, 11174–11178.
54. Sawyers, C.L. (2008) The cancer biomarker problem. *Nature*, **452**, 548–552.
55. Daniels, D.A., Chen, H., Hicke, B.J., Swiderek, K.M., and Gold, L. (2003) A tenascin-C aptamer identified by tumor cell SELEX: systematic evolution of ligands by exponential enrichment. *Proc. Natl. Acad. Sci. USA*, **100**, 15416–15421.
56. Guo, K.T., Ziemer, G., Paul, A., and Wendel, H.P. (2008) CELL-SELEX: Novel perspectives of aptamer-based therapeutics. *Int. J. Mol. Sci.*, **9**, 668–678.
57. Fang, X. and Tan, W. (2009) Aptamers generated from cell-SELEX for molecular medicine: a chemical biology approach. *Acc. Chem. Res.*, **43**, 48–57.
58. Shangguan, D., Cao, Z.C., Li, Y., and Tan, W. (2007) Aptamers evolved from cultured cancer cells reveal molecular differences of cancer cells in patient samples. *Clin. Chem.*, **53**, 1153–1155.
59. Xiao, Z., Shangguan, D., Cao, Z., Fang, X., and Tan, W. (2008) Cell-specific internalization study of an aptamer from whole cell selection. *Chemistry*, **14**, 1769–1775.
60. Raddatz, M.S. *et al.* (2008) Enrichment of cell-targeting and population-specific aptamers by fluorescence-activated cell sorting. *Angew. Chem. Int. Ed. Engl.*, **47**, 5190–5193.
61. Kulbachinskiy, A.V. (2007) Methods for selection of aptamers to protein targets. *Biochemistry.*, **72**, 1505–1518.
62. Zhou, J. and Rossi, J.J. (2010) Aptamer-targeted cell-specific RNA interference. *Silence*, **1**, 4.
63. Chu, T., Ebright, J., and Ellington, A.D. (2007) Using aptamers to identify and enter cells. *Curr. Opin. Mol. Ther.*, **9**, 137–144.
64. Stirpe, F., Olsnes, S., and Pihl, A. (1980) Gelonin, a new inhibitor of protein synthesis, nontoxic to intact cells. Isolation, characterization, and preparation of cytotoxic complexes with concanavalin A. *J. Biol. Chem.*, **255**, 6947–6953.
65. Better, M. *et al.* (1994) Gelonin analogs with engineered cysteine residues form antibody immunoconjugates with unique properties. *J. Biol. Chem.*, **269**, 9644–9650.
66. Huang, Y.F., Chang, H.T., and Tan, W. (2008) Cancer cell targeting using multiple aptamers conjugated on nanorods. *Anal. Chem.*, **80**, 567–572.
67. Huang, Y.F., Sefah, K., Bamrungsap, S., Chang, H.T., and Tan, W. (2008) Selective photothermal therapy for mixed cancer cells using aptamer-conjugated nanorods. *Langmuir*, **24**, 11860–11865.
68. Cullen, B.R. (2002) RNA interference: antiviral defense and genetic tool. *Nat. Immunol.*, **3**, 597–599.

69. Sioud, M. (2005) On the delivery of small interfering RNAs into mammalian cells. *Expert Opin. Drug Deliv.*, **2**, 639–651.
70. Xie, F.Y., Woodle, M.C., and Lu, P.Y. (2006) Harnessing *in vivo* siRNA delivery for drug discovery and therapeutic development. *Drug Discov. Today*, **11**, 67–73.
71. Shi, H., Hoffman, B.E., and Lis, J.T. (1999) RNA aptamers as effective protein antagonists in a multicellular organism. *Proc. Natl. Acad. Sci. USA*, **96**, 10033–10038.
72. Santulli-Marotto, S., Nair, S.K., Rusconi, C., Sullenger, B., and Gilboa, E. (2003) Multivalent RNA aptamers that inhibit CTLA-4 and enhance tumor immunity. *Cancer Res.*, **63**, 7483–7489.
73. McNamara, J.O. *et al.* (2008) Multivalent 4-1BB binding aptamers costimulate $CD8^+$ T cells and inhibit tumor growth in mice. *J. Clin. Invest.*, **118**, 376–386.
74. Dollins, C.M. *et al.* (2008) Assembling OX40 aptamers on a molecular scaffold to create a receptor-activating aptamer. *Chem. Biol.*, **15**, 675–682.
75. Griffin, L.C., Tidmarsh, G.F., Bock, L.C., Toole, J.J., and Leung, L.L. (1993) *In vivo* anticoagulant properties of a novel nucleotide-based thrombin inhibitor and demonstration of regional anticoagulation in extracorporeal circuits. *Blood*, **81**, 3271–3276.
76. Pieken, W.A., Olsen, D.B., Benseler, F., Aurup, H., and Eckstein, F. (1991) Kinetic characterization of ribonuclease-resistant 2′-modified hammerhead ribozymes. *Science*, **253**, 314–317.
77. Chow, W.H., Dong, L.M., and Devesa, S.S. (2010) Epidemiology and risk factors for kidney cancer. *Nat. Rev. Urol.*, **7**, 245–257.
78. Ng, E.W. *et al.* (2006) Pegaptanib, a targeted anti-VEGF aptamer for ocular vascular disease. *Nat. Rev. Drug Discov.*, **5**, 123–132.
79. Burmeister, P.E. *et al.* (2005) Direct *in vitro* selection of a 2′-*O*-methyl aptamer to VEGF. *Chem. Biol.*, **12**, 25–33.
80. Soutschek, J. *et al.* (2004) Therapeutic silencing of an endogenous gene by systemic administration of modified siRNAs. *Nature*, **432**, 173–178.
81. Rusconi, C.P. *et al.* (2004) Antidote-mediated control of an anticoagulant aptamer *in vivo*. *Nat. Biotechnol.*, **22**, 1423–1428.
82. Hicke, B.J. and Stephens, A.W. (2000) Escort aptamers: a delivery service for diagnosis and therapy. *J. Clin. Invest.*, **106**, 923–928.
83. Lister-James, J., Moyer, B.R., and Dean, T. (1996) Small peptides radiolabeled with ^{99m}Tc. *Q. J. Nucl. Med.*, **40**, 221–233.
84. Hicke, B.J. *et al.* (2006) Tumor targeting by an aptamer. *J. Nucl. Med.*, **47**, 668–678.
85. Jason, T.L., Koropatnick, J., and Berg, R.W. (2004) Toxicology of antisense therapeutics. *Toxicol. Appl. Pharmacol.*, **201**, 66–83.
86. Levin, A.A. (1999) A review of the issues in the pharmacokinetics and toxicology of phosphorothioate antisense oligonucleotides. *Biochim. Biophys. Acta*, **1489**, 69–84.
87. Henry, S.P. *et al.* (2002) Complement activation is responsible for acute toxicities in rhesus monkeys treated with a phosphorothioate oligodeoxynucleotide. *Int. Immunopharmacol.*, **2**, 1657–1666.
88. Lenert, P.S. (2010) Classification, mechanisms of action, and therapeutic applications of inhibitory oligonucleotides for Toll-like receptors (TLR) 7 and 9. *Mediators Inflamm.*, **2010**, 986596.
89. Yu, D. *et al.* (2009) Modifications incorporated in CpG motifs of oligodeoxynucleotides lead to antagonist activity of toll-like receptors 7 and 9. *J. Med. Chem.*, **52**, 5108–5114.
90. Cooper, C.L. *et al.* (2008) Immunostimulatory effects of three classes of CpG oligodeoxynucleotides on PBMC from HCV chronic carriers. *J. Immune Based Ther. Vaccines*, **6**, 3.
91. Krieg, A.M. (2008) Toll-like receptor 9 (TLR9) agonists in the treatment of cancer. *Oncogene*, **27**, 161–167.

40
Design and Synthesis of Drug Conjugates of Vitamins and Growth Factors

Iontcho R. Vlahov, Paul J. Kleindl, and Fei You

> If we picture an organism as infected by a certain species of bacterium, it will ... be easy to effect a cure if substances have been discovered which have a specific affinity for these bacteria and act ... on these alone ... while they possess no affinity for the normal constituents of the body ... such substances would then be ... magic bullets.
>
> *Paul Ehrlich, 1908 Nobel Prize in Medicine*

40.1
Introduction

It is only a matter of time before most medicines will discriminate between pathologic and healthy cells. Paul Ehrlich envisaged a "magic bullet" – a chemical substance directed toward pathogens and toxins with high affinity for the causative agent. After more than 25 years of determined pursuit, he was triumphant with the discovery of preparation 606 [1]. In November 1910, his "magic bullet," Salvarsan, was brought to market. Today, one elegant approach to implement Ehlrich's vision in oncology is to link drugs possessing nonspecific toxicities to ligands that recognize and bind selectively to receptors overexpressed on the surface of pathologic cells.

Several vitamins and growth factors exhibit high affinity toward their selective receptors, thus becoming increasingly popular ligands for targeting cytotoxic agents to malignant cells. For flawless delivery to tumors, a perfectly constructed conjugate should serve as an "inactive" prodrug, and only upon binding and internalization should action on a specific chemical motif trigger the release of the payload. The purpose of this chapter is: (i) to gain insight into the rational chemical design of ligand–drug conjugates, (ii) to provide an overview of synthetic methodologies for preparing such complex molecules, and (iii) to exemplify efficient mechanisms for releasing intact parent cytotoxic molecules. This chapter begins with vitamin conjugates of folic acid (FA), cobalamin, and biotin, and touches briefly on conjugates of vitamins E and B_6. Conjugates of growth factors are then discussed,

Drug Delivery in Oncology: From Basic Research to Cancer Therapy, First Edition.
Edited by Felix Kratz, Peter Senter, and Henning Steinhagen.

including: epidermal growth factor (EGF), insulin-like growth factor (IGF), and fibroblast growth factor (FGF). The chapter concludes with a brief examination of synthetic peptides that target growth factor receptors.

40.2 Chemical Aspects of FA–Drug Conjugate Design

40.2.1 Folate Receptor-Mediated Endocytosis for Targeted Drug Delivery

FA (synonyms: folate, vitamin B_9; Figure 40.1), pteroyl-L-glutamic acid, is itself not biologically active, rather tetrahydrofolate and other derivatives perform biological functions after metabolism by dihydrofolate reductase in the liver [2]. Inside the cell, FA is needed to carry one carbon for methylation reactions and *de novo* synthesis of nucleotide bases (most notably thymine, but also purine bases). Therefore, it is essential to the viability of proliferating cells.

In the body two independent and mechanistically different systems mediate the cellular uptake of FA. (i) Reduced folate carrier (RFC) is a low-affinity ($K_d \sim 10^{-5}$ M), high-capacity membrane-spanning anion transport protein that delivers reduced FAs across the plasma membrane in a bidirectional fashion [3]. RFC is ubiquitously present in tissues, and is responsible for the majority of FA transport in and out of all cells of the body. (ii) *Folate receptor* (FR) is a high-affinity ($K_d \sim 10^{-10}$ M), single-chain FA-binding protein, which internalizes FA through active receptor-mediated endocytosis (also known as potocytosis) [4–7]. To date, three isoforms of FR have been identified and cloned: FR-α, FR-β, and FR-γ and its truncated cogener, FR-γ′ [8–13]. In normal tissues, the distribution of measurable levels of FR-α is limited only to the apical membrane surface of certain polarized epithelial cells, in placental trophoblasts, and on the apical side of kidney proximal tubule cells, the latter serving as a salvaging route for FAs prior to urinary excretion [14–21]. In contrast, in many human malignant cells FR-α is highly overexpressed, especially in aggressively growing cancers [22–26]. Conjugation of molecules to FA at its γ-carboxy moiety influences its affinity for the FR; however, in many cases this effect is not biologically significant. Therefore, FA can be exploited as a molecular "Trojan horse" for the targeted delivery of covalently attached,

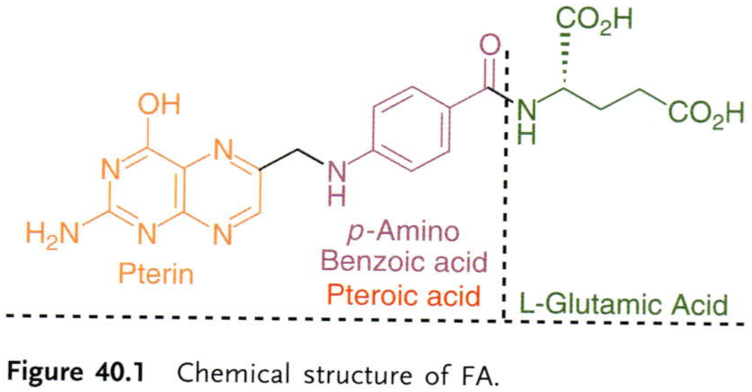

Figure 40.1 Chemical structure of FA.

biologically active molecules via the FR [27–29]. The effectiveness of FA targeting can be demonstrated by examining the biodistribution of ^{111}In-diethylene triamine pentaacetic acid (DTPA)-FA, an imaging agent, in patients that are tumor-free and those that possess FR-positive tumors (Figure 40.2) (*www.endocyte.com*). In the healthy patient, accumulation of ^{111}In-DTPA-FA is only seen in the kidneys. In the ovarian cancer patient, FR-positive tumors are evident throughout the body.

FR-mediated endocytosis (Figure 40.3) follows the same pathway for FA or for FA–drug conjugates [30]. In brief, after binding, the cellular membrane invaginates to form an early endosome, which entraps the FA or FA–drug moiety. Next, proton pumps lower the pH of the vesicle lumen to between 5 and 6, thus causing a conformational change in the FR that subsequently enables the FA (FA–drug)

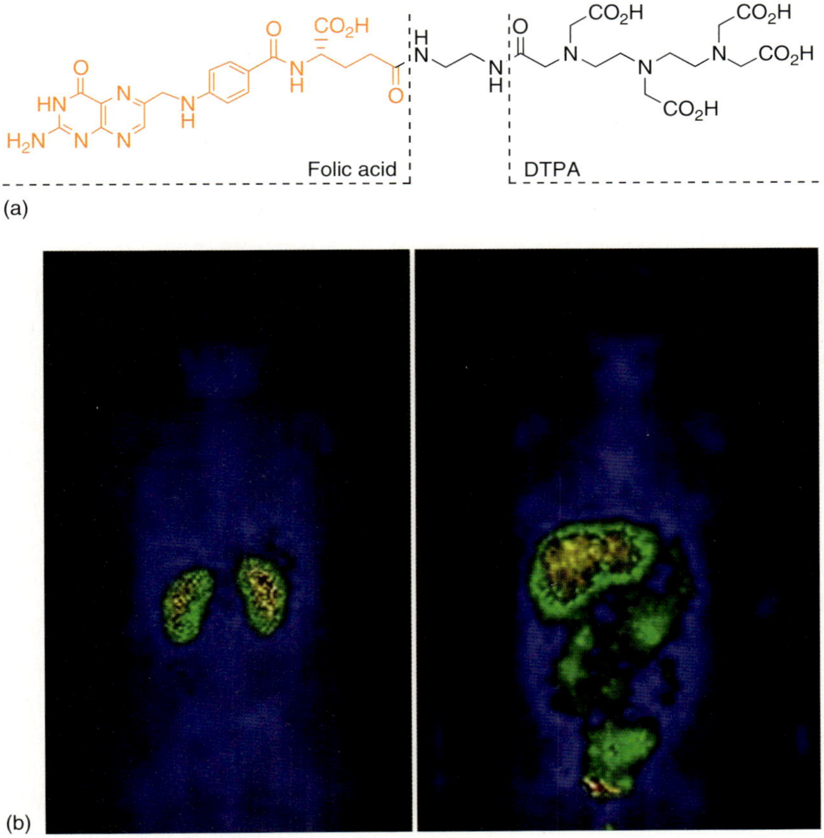

Figure 40.2 (a) Structure of DTPA–FA (b) Images of ^{111}In-DTPA–FA in a healthy patient (on left) and a patient with advanced ovarian cancer (on right).

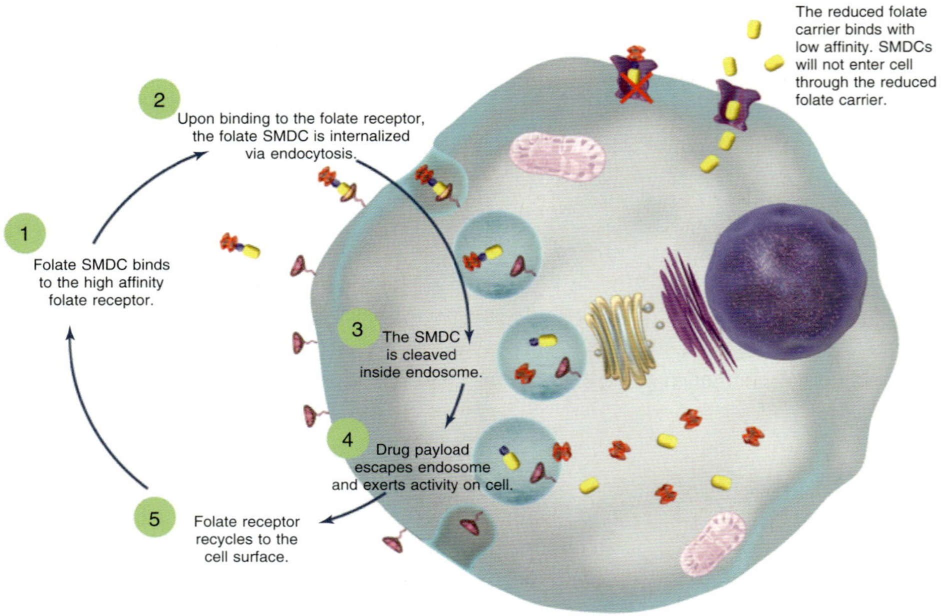
The reduced folate carrier binds with low affinity. SMDCs will not enter cell through the reduced folate carrier.
2
Upon binding to the folate receptor, the folate SMDC is internalized via endocytosis.
1
Folate SMDC binds to the high affinity folate receptor.
3
The SMDC is cleaved inside endosome.
4
Drug payload escapes endosome and exerts activity on cell.
5
Folate receptor recycles to the cell surface.

Figure 40.3 Schematic presentation of cellular uptake of FA–drug conjugates by FR-mediated endocytosis (SMDC, small-molecule drug conjugate, consisting of FA (shown in yellow) and the drug payload (shown in red)).

moiety to be detached from its receptor [31]. The FR protein recycles back to the cellular membrane where it can participate in another round of internalization/drug delivery, whereas the released ligand (i.e., FA or FA–drug) remains inside the cell. On the other hand, the anion transporter RFC can shuttle FA molecules inside the cell; however, FA–drug conjugates are not substrates for the RFC, consequently, acquisition of FA–drug molecules in normal cells is avoided.

40.2.2
General Criteria for the Design of FA–Drug Conjugates and their Intracellular Release Mechanisms

In early studies, researchers focused mainly on the ability of the FR to deliver FA conjugates inside tumor cells, thus ignoring structure–activity relationships, and were met with limited success [32]. Initial examples of chemotherapeutic agents covalently attached to FA or pteroic acid included bis(haloethyl) phosphoramidites [33], poly(ethylene glycol) (PEG)–carboplatin [34], a 10mer conjugate of a thymidylate synthase inhibitor 5-fluoro-2′-deoxyuridine-5′-*O*-monophosphate [35], Taxol® [36], and maytansine [37]. After years of intensive effort in this area of research, successful FA–drug conjugates have been found to share several common characteristics:

- *Highly potent drugs* with IC_{50} values for intrinsic cytotoxicity in the low nanomolar range are a prerequisite for producing activity since the number of FRs on the surface of the cell is restricted and the FR recycling rate is of the order of 8–12 h [38].
- The *low molecular weight* of most cytotoxic drugs is important for drug delivery applications, and is the basis for better penetration into solid tumors and rapid systemic clearance of the conjugates from which they are derived.
- The lipophilicity of the vast majority of small-molecule chemotherapeutic compounds allows for their passive diffusion through cell membrane bilayers at random. FA–drug conjugates with *enhanced hydrophilicity* (e.g., introducing a discrete number of charged residues) will enable the molecule to enter only FR-positive cells via FR-mediated endocytosis.
- *Highly stable* conjugates prevent exposure of normal cells to "leaking" free drug during systemic circulation, emphasizing the FR-specific mode of action of the conjugate.

Importantly, the activity of a highly potent FA–drug molecule is closely dependent on an efficient cleavable linker system that is capable of releasing the parent drug from its targeting ligand at a predictable and reliable rate. Two different trigger systems have been utilized to promote the programmed collapse of the linker system within the endosome. The most successful approach – a disulfide-bond-based linker system – takes advantage of the reductive environment in the endosome [39]. The second approach – a pH-sensitive linker system – releases the active parent drug from its FA conjugate as the result of the drop in the pH in the endosome [31]. Studies have shown pH values in endosomal compartments populated by monovalent FA conjugates to be around 6, whereas endosomes encapsulating multivalent FA conjugates have been found to have pH values as low as 5.0 [40, 41]. After release occurs by either of these two methods, highly lipophilic drugs cross the endosomal membrane and find their pharmacological target within the cytosol.

To meet the demand for expedient and efficient regioselective synthesis of releasable FA–drug conjugates and considering the requirements detailed above, we designed a modular approach (Figure 40.4) for facile assembly of these complex molecules.

The ligand FA serves as Module 1, while the active drug is represented as Module 4. The role of the spacer unit (Module 2) is (i) to properly position ligand and cargo, thereby optimizing FR binding, and (ii) to provide the desired

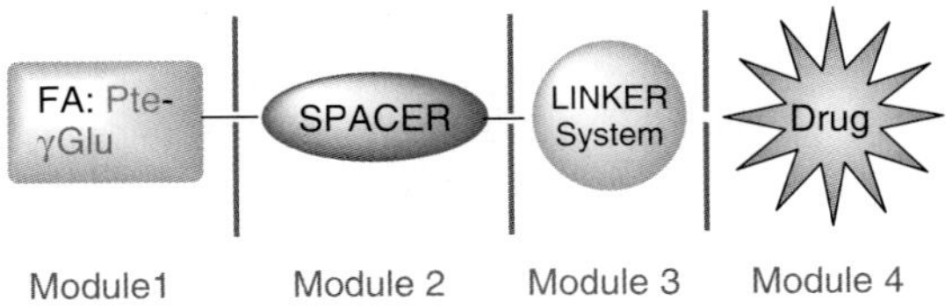

Figure 40.4 Modular design of releasable FA–drug conjugates (Pte, pteroic acid; Glu, glutamic acid).

hydrophilicity to the construct. Juxtaposed between the spacer and the drug is a cleavable linker system represented as Module 3.

40.2.3 Synthesis of FA–Cancer Drug Conjugates Containing Disulfide-Based Linker Systems

The *retro*-synthetic analysis presented in Scheme 40.1 was the roadmap for expedient assembly of FA–drug conjugates containing cleavable disulfide-based, self-immolative linker systems. As indicated by the double-lined arrows, strategic disconnection reveals two key synthons: a FA–spacer terminated by a thiol group and a thiophilic linker–drug derivative.

40.2.3.1 Exploiting Peptide-Based Spacers

The FA–spacer unit **1** (Figure 40.5) was synthesized using standard fluorenylmethyloxycarbonyl (Fmoc)-based solid-phase peptide synthesis (SPPS) techniques on a cysteine-loaded polymeric support [42]. Aspartic acid and arginine were added to the peptide to improve the water solubility of the final drug conjugate. The thiol group of cysteine served as the attachment site for the cleavable linker system.

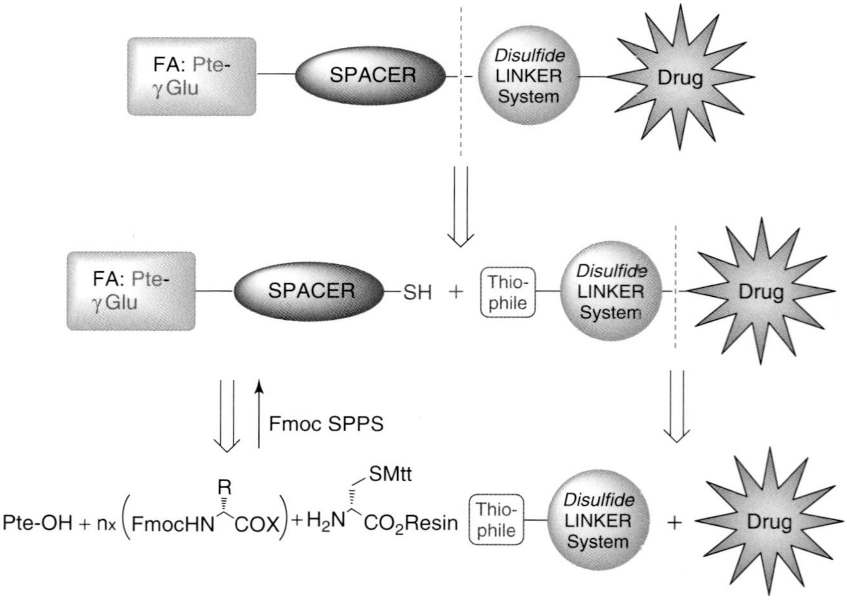

Scheme 40.1 *Retro*-synthetic analysis of disulfide-based FA–drug conjugates containing self-immolative linker systems (strategic disconnections depicted with dotted lines).

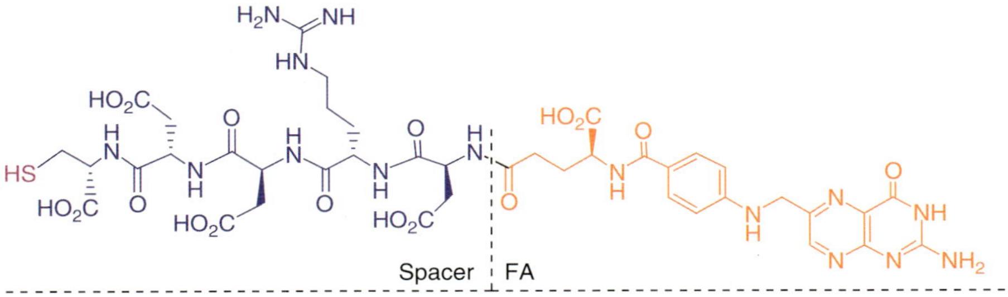

1

Figure 40.5 Peptidic FA–spacer unit **1**.

We developed novel thiophilic heterobifunctional cross-linker **2** to incorporate disulfide linker systems into our conjugates (Scheme 40.2) [42]. Activated carbonate **2** has been found to react under mild conditions with many *N*- and *O*-nucleophiles, and as a result can be applied in the synthesis of a wide variety of drug conjugates. Activated carbonate **2** was utilized to link FA to highly potent drugs such as the microtubule-destabilizing agent desacetyl vinblastine hydrazide (DAVLBH) **3** – a semisynthetic derivative of the *Vinca* alkaloid vinblastine (Scheme 40.2).

Hydrazide **3** was treated with **2** and diisopropylethylamine (DIPEA) to yield 2-(vinblastinyl)hydrazinecarboxylic acid 2-pyridyldisulfanylethyl ester **4**. To a solution of **1** in aqueous solution (pH 6.5), under argon, was added a solution of **4** in tetrahydrofuran, providing conjugate EC145, in 15 min.

Release of parent drug **3** from the conjugate was examined by treating a 1 mM solution of EC145 in phosphate-buffered saline (PBS; pH 7.4) with 20 mM of the reducing agent L-glutathione (GSH) at 37 °C. Complete cleavage of the disulfide bond with concomitant release of the FA–spacer **1** occurred within 6 h ($t_{1/2} = 1$ h, Scheme 40.3). Formation of **3** was also confirmed by liquid chromatography/mass spectrometry.

Following similar synthetic protocols, several representative conjugates utilizing spacer **1** have been prepared by our group [43], in our collaboration with scientists from Bristol-Myers Squibb [44] or ImmunoGen [45], as well as P. Low's group [46] (Figure 40.6). FA–paclitaxel and FA–daunomycin conjugates lacking a spacer region (therefore of limited hydrophilicity) were also synthesized [47]. In addition, Suzuki *et al.* synthesized a FA conjugate of the histone deacetylase inhibitor NCH-31 [48].

The preclinical pharmacology for most of these FA conjugates revealed persistent antitumor effects against FR-positive tumors in multiple animal models [45, 49–51]. Applying well-tolerated treatment regimens typically resulted in cures with the added benefit of little to no weight loss. For example, EC145 was found to have an IC_{50} of 9 nM in a FR-positive KB cell line. Competition was observed, The addition of excess FA displaced EC145 from the FRs, resulting in a loss of activity, thus proving the observed toxicity is the result of FR targeting,

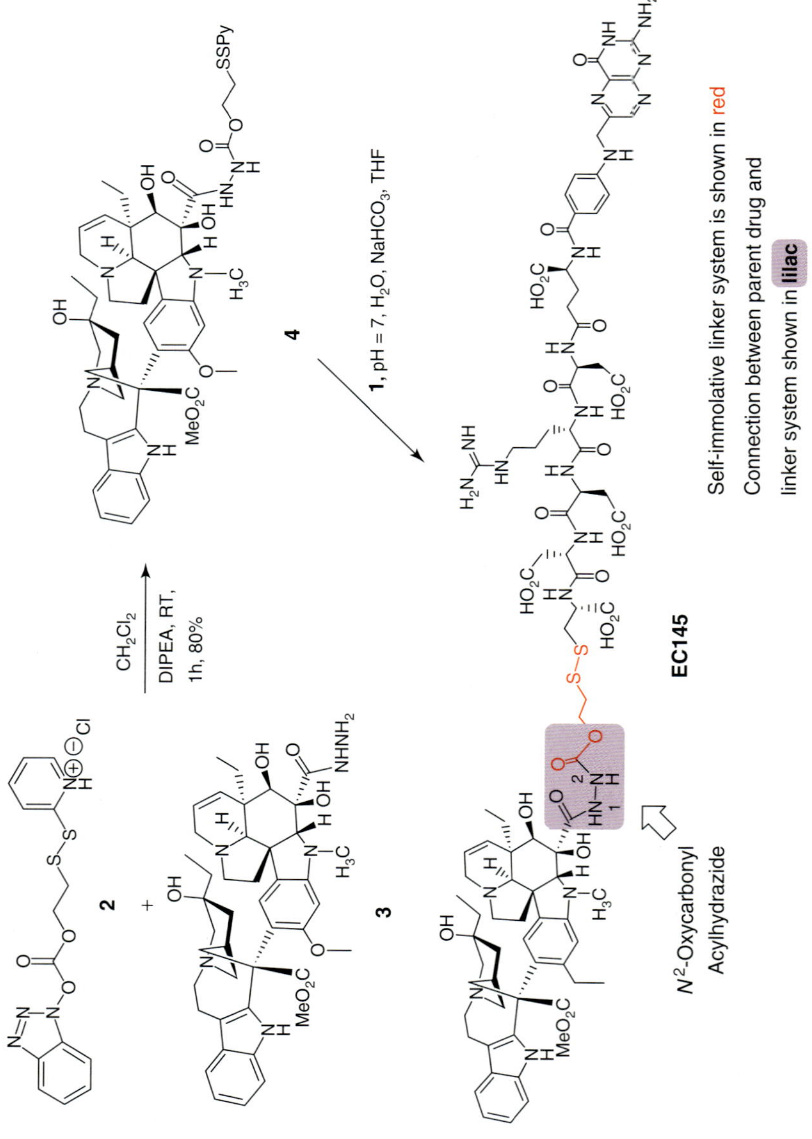

Scheme 40.2 Expedient synthesis of EC145 – a FA conjugate possessing a disulfide-based self-immolative linker system.

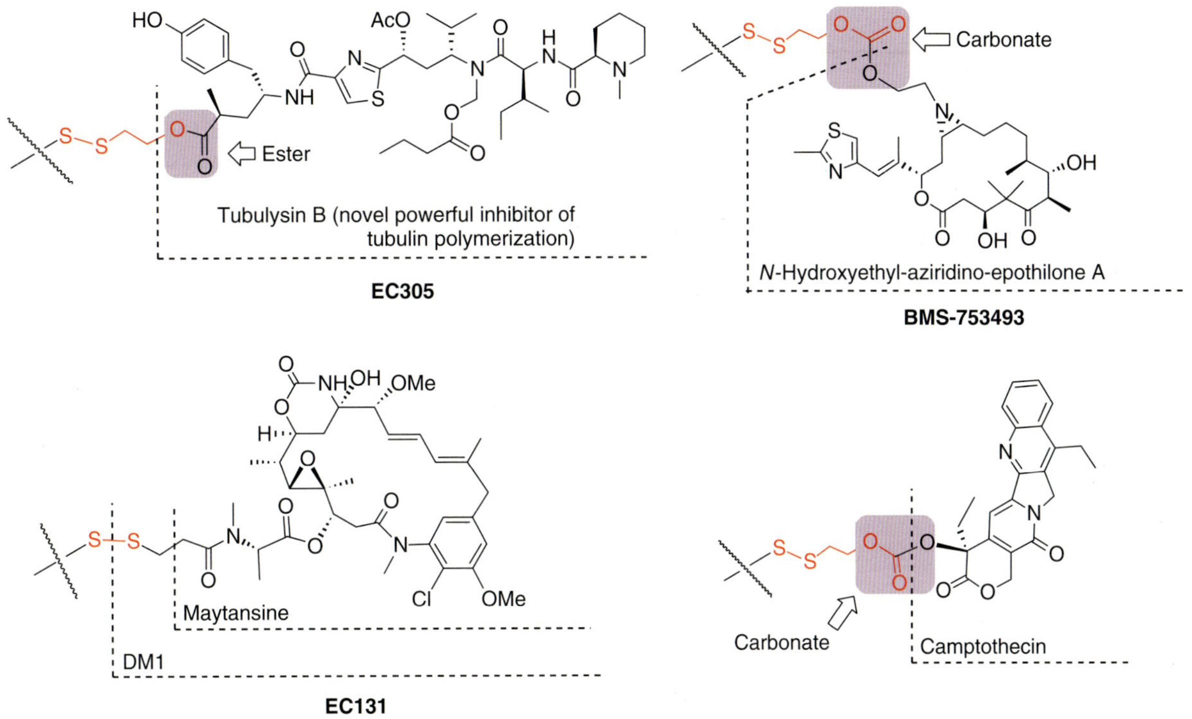

Figure 40.6 Chemical structures of representative FA–drug conjugates utilizing FA–spacer **1** and possessing a disulfide-based linker system.

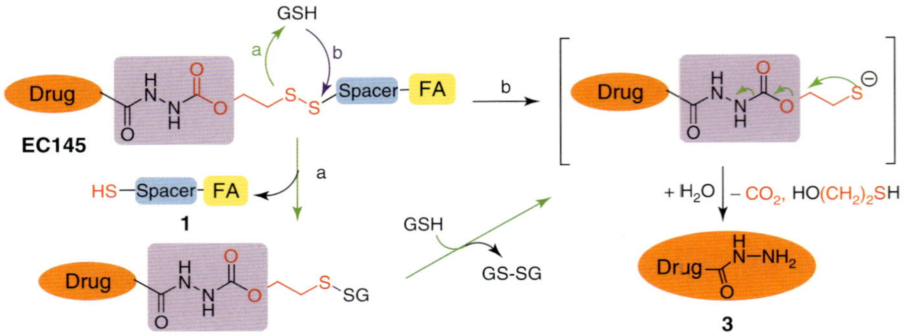

Scheme 40.3 Release study of the self-immolative disulfide-based linker system in the FA–drug conjugate in a reductive environment.

rather than some other mode of delivery (Figure 40.7a). Treatment of nude mice implanted with FR-positive KB tumors with EC145 at a dosage of 5 μmol/kg, 3 times a week, resulted in all five animals in the study exhibiting a complete response. Little weight loss was observed (Figure 40.7b and c) [52]. EC145 represents the first FR-targeted drug to enter clinical trials and two phase II trials have been completed (*http://www.clinicaltrials.gov/ct2/show/NCT00507741, http://clinicaltrials.gov/ct2/show/NCT00722592 and http://clinicaltrials.gov/ct2/show/NCT01002924*). In the first phase II clinical trial, patients with advanced non-small-cell lung cancer were treated with EC145 and also the FA–^{99}Tc imaging agent EC20 to identify tumors that were FR-positive [53]. Of the patients with FR-positive tumors, 45% completed 4 months of therapy without disease progression. Little toxicity was observed. Mild-to-moderate constipation was the most common side-effect of treatment. The second phase II study (known as PRECEDENT), which is a comparison of EC145 plus Doxil® verses Doxil alone for the treatment of women with platinum-resistant ovarian cancer, showed a 2.3 month (85%) improvement in progression free survival (PFS) in patients who received the combination therapy. In the subset of patients whose tumors were 100% FR-positive, a 4.0 month (260%) increase in PFS was observed [54]. EC145 in combination with Doxil® showed limited additional toxicity compared to standard therapy with Doxil® alone. The most commonly occurring adverse events were neutropenia, small intestine obstruction, and palmar-plantar erythrodysesthesia. BMS-753493 is also being evaluated in two phase I/II clinical trials in patients with advanced solid cancers (*http://clinicaltrials.gov/ct2/show/NCT00546247 and http://clinicaltrials.gov/ct2/show/NCT00550017*). Each of these studies attempts to determine the maximum tolerated dose (MTD) following an open-label dose-escalation scheme. The studies differ only in the frequency of dosing, with one study dosing on days 1–4 of a 21-day cycle, and the other study dosing on days 1, 4, 8, and 11 [55, 56]. Preliminary data has shown that more frequent dosing results in a MTD of 17 mg, whereas spreading the dosing over 11 days results in

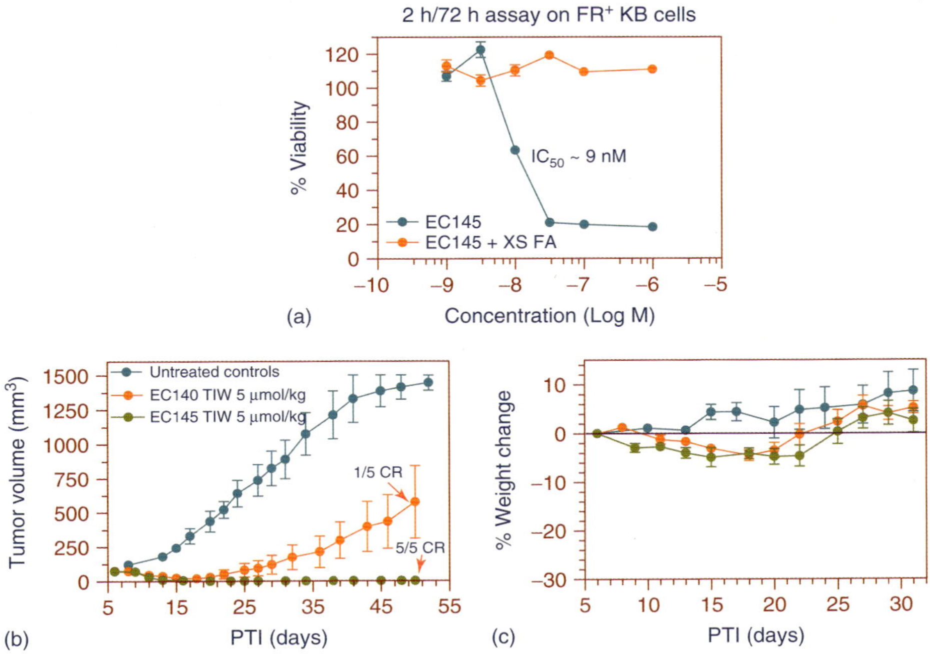

Figure 40.7 *In vitro* and *in vivo* testing of EC145 on FR-positive KB tumor cells. (a) *In vitro* test of FR-positive KB cells treated with EC145 alone and EC145 plus FA. Cells were treated with the analytes for 2 h and viability was assessed by ^{3}H-thymidine uptake at 72 h. (b) Treatment of subcutaneous FR-positive KB tumors in *nu/nu* mice with EC145 and EC140 (discussed later in this chapter). Dosing continued for 2 weeks (PTI, post-tumor implantation; CR, complete response). (c) Percent weight change of mice treated with EC145 and EC140.

an MTD of 33 mg. Neither of these studies has reported any complete or partial responses; however, tumor shrinkage of up to 23% has been observed with the accelerated dosing schedule. Similar toxicities were observed in both studies, with fatigue, diarrhea, nausea, vomiting, anorexia, and elevated liver enzymes the most commonly observed adverse events.

40.2.3.2 **Exploiting Carbohydrate-Based Spacers**

The dose-limiting toxicity for EC145 in the phase I clinical trial was found to be related to ileus, albeit in heavily pretreated patients [57]. Owing to the low-to-undetectable levels of the FR expressed in hepatic tissue [58], it was suspected that non-FR-related liver clearance, with subsequent metabolic release of free DAVLBH, may have been (in part) responsible for producing the observed gastrointestinal toxicity. A novel, chemistry-based approach was developed to substantially decrease the hepatobiliary route of clearance of free DAVLBH without affecting the conjugate's targeted antitumor activity [59]. Thus, selective placement of structurally optimized carbohydrate segments in the spacer region resulted in conjugates that were equipotent, but less toxic than EC145. Our carbohydrate-containing FA–spacer unit **6** was designed to be bifunctional, containing alternately repeating acidic (glutamic acid) and novel saccharo-amino acids, thus providing the high water solubility of the final drug conjugate under physiological conditions. This unit was assembled using standard Fmoc SPPS techniques. The structural design of the protected saccharo-amino acid **5** was of crucial importance to the successful execution of a simple and high-yielding SPPS protocol. The selected approach relied on a ring-opened carbohydrate chain rather than on cyclic pyranoside or furanoside units. Pyranosides and furanosides are of limited usefulness for a simplified SPPS-based protocol because they require inherently tedious protecting/deprotecting strategies, utilize sensitive glycosyl donors, and generate diastereomeric glycosidic linkages. Therefore, we designed and synthesized the uniformly protected **5** by connecting via amide bonds two easily accessible molecular constructs – glutamic acid and glucamine (Scheme 40.4). Treatment of FA–spacer **6** with **4** under the same conditions as described for the synthesis of EC145 resulted

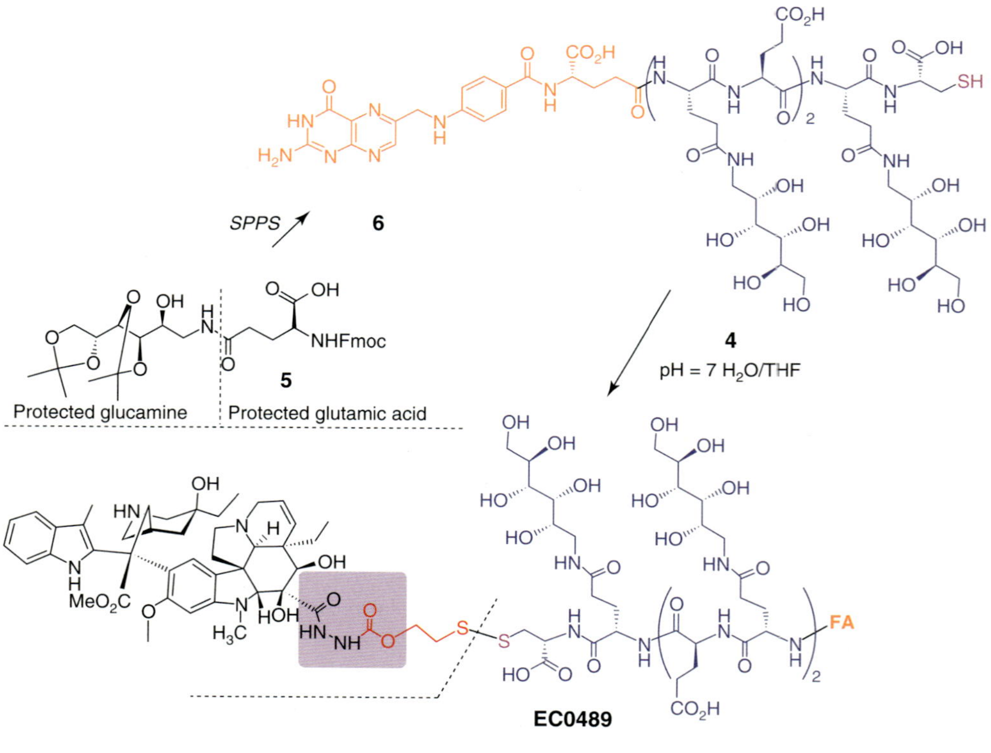

Scheme 40.4 Synthesis of the novel carbohydrate-based FA–spacer unit **6** and the conjugate EC0489.

in the novel conjugate EC0489. EC0489 was found to be equally efficacious as EC145 for the treatment of KB tumor xenographs in nude mice. Also, EC0489 showed a 70% decrease in bile clearance compared to EC145 in rats, resulting in a doubling of the MTD and therapeutic index [60]. EC0489 is currently in phase I trials for the treatment of refractory or metastatic cancers for patients who have exhausted standard therapeutic options (*http://www.clinicaltrials.gov/ct2/show/NCT00852189*). Early results have shown that patients can receive doses of EC0489 equivalent to twice the amount of DAVLBH that would be able to be safely dosed with EC145 [61].

40.2.3.3 **Introduction of a Second Unsymmetrical Disulfide Bond: Synthesis of Releasable Dual-Drug Conjugates**

A logical expansion in the design of FA–drug conjugates involved a novel synthetic strategy, which allows for the introduction of a second reductively labile disulfide linker system (or simply a disulfide bond) into a molecular framework with a pre-existing disulfide linker system. Such methodology ensures the delivery and release of multiple cargos (parent drugs, reporter molecules, etc.) in targeted cells. Synthetic efforts have resulted in the synthesis of EC0225 (Figure 40.8), the first FR targeting conjugate possessing two different biologically active agents: DAVLBH (Drug 1) and the highly chemically sensitive alkylating agent mitomycin C (MMC, Drug 2) [62]. Both cargos are covalently attached to a FA–spacer unit via two disulfide-based release systems.

As indicated in the *retro*-synthetic analysis (Scheme 40.5), the key precursor to the final construct **I** (simplified representation of dual-drug conjugate EC0225) is the thiol-containing disulfide conjugate **II**. Molecules such as **II**, which possess a disulfide bond as well as a free thiol functionality, are highly reactive and unstable, and are prone to rearrangement and intramolecular cyclization (Scheme 40.5a and b). An elegant solution to this challenging stability-related problem involves a synthetic route in which **II** is generated *in situ* from the stable *S*-protected monoconjugate **III**. Trapping the thiol group of **II** with a Drug 2-containing, disulfide-forming synthon **IV** results in the desired dual-drug conjugate **I**. Monoconjugate **III** was synthesized using the same conjugation techniques as described for EC145.

The activity of EC0225 [63] was superior to that of its monodrug–FA counterparts (FA–MMC and FA–DAVLBH) at equimolar concentrations and when the monodrug–FA conjugates are used in combination. The conjugate retained high affinity for FR-positive cells, and exhibited potent *in vitro* and curative *in vivo* activities. For example, animals with well-established human tumor xenografts responded to EC0225 therapy completely. KB tumors as large as 750 mm^3 have been effectively treated with EC0225 (Figure 40.9) [64]. The extensive *in vivo* evaluation has led to the advancement of EC0225 to a phase I clinical trial in patients with refractory or metastatic cancer [65]. The phase I trial has established a MTD of 2.3 mg/m^2 (six doses in the first 2 weeks of a 28-day cycle). Patients with colorectal, breast, and prostate cancer, as well as patients with leiomyosarcoma and mesothelioma were found to have disease stabilization for 4 months or more. The most common treatment-related adverse events were anemia, constipation, leukopenia, and fatigue.

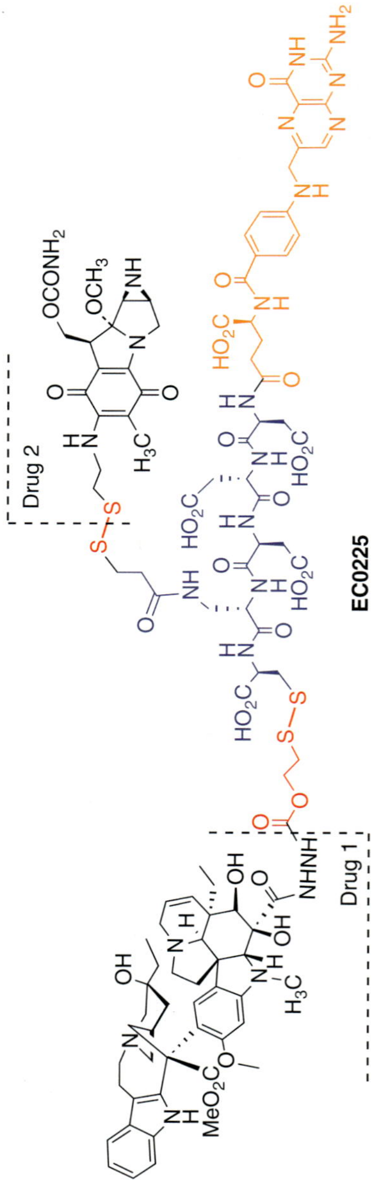

EC0225

Figure 40.8 DAVLBH- and MMC-containing FA conjugate.

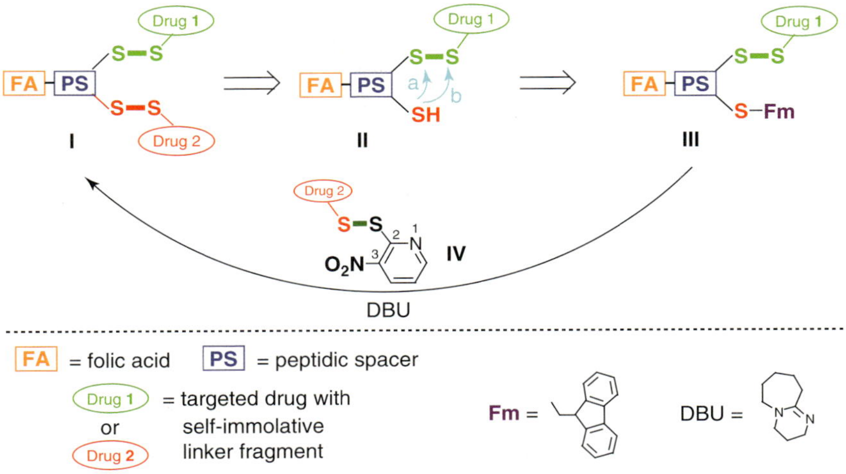

Scheme 40.5 Assembly concept for the consecutive introduction of unsymmetrical disulfide bonds.

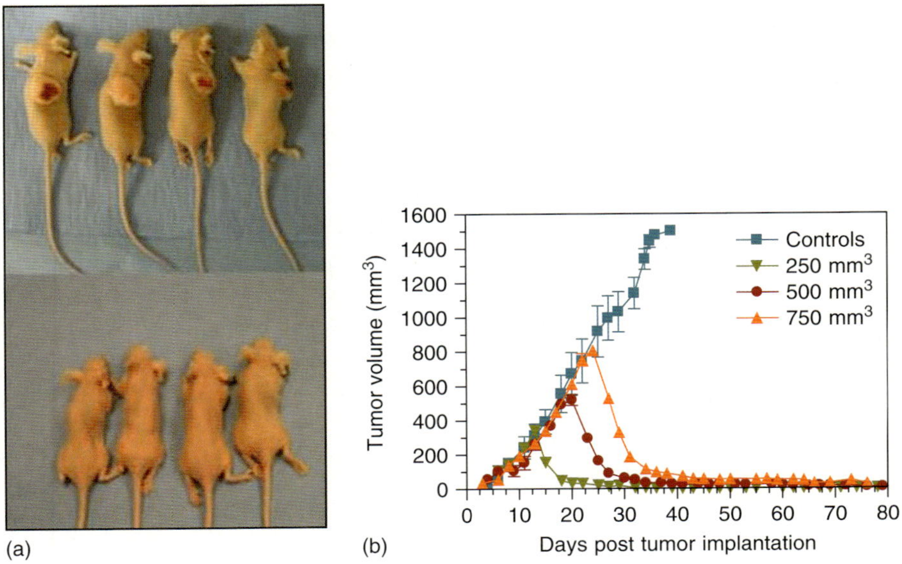

Figure 40.9 Treatment of *nu/nu* mice with subcutaneous KB tumors of varying size with EC0225 (intravenous), 2 mmol/kg, TIW, for 2 weeks. (a) Mice with large KB tumors prior to treatment (top) and mice after treatment (bottom). (b) Tumor volume versus post-tumor implantation for KB tumors of 250, 500, and 750 mm^3.

40.2.4 Application of pH-Responsive Linker Systems for the Synthesis of FA–Drug Conjugates

A second approach to release a parent drug from its FA conjugate exploits the lowered pH within the endosome. The concept of using a pH-sensitive linker system in FR-targeted drug delivery was first demonstrated with the design and synthesis of EC140 – a FA–DAVLBH conjugate containing the acyl hydrazone functionality.

In general, based on the delocalization of their π-electrons, hydrazones are hydrolytically much more stable than imines. Therefore, an electron-withdrawing group (e.g., an acyl) has to be placed into hydrazone systems in order to curb electron delocalization and moderate their overall hydrolytic stability. As a result, these molecular constructs can find application in the design of releasable drug conjugates. Acyl hydrazones are easily accessible from aldehydes or ketones and acyl hydrazides under mild conditions.

The synthesis of acyl hydrazone conjugate EC140 [66] was pursued in two steps and is presented in Scheme 40.6. Treatment of **3** with an equimolar amount of 4-maleimido benzophenone **7** resulted in the desired vinblastenyl acyl hydrazide **8**. Subsequently, the thiol moiety of the FA–spacer unit **1** was reacted with the maleimide moiety of **8**, thus providing the N^1-acyl hydrazone-linked conjugate. Drug release studies were performed in pH 5.0 and 7.4 buffers at 37 °C. It was shown that at the lower pH, the hydrazone bond in EC140 was cleaved with a hydrolysis rate of $t_{1/2} \sim 5.5$ h. In contrast, at pH 7.4 the rate was found to be $t_{1/2} \sim 22$ h.

This water-soluble conjugate was found to retain high affinity for FR-positive cells and it produced specific, dose-responsive activity *in vitro*. Initial *in vivo* tests confirmed EC140's activity in both syngeneic and xenograft models. Hence, enduring complete responses were observed in animals bearing established, subcutaneous tumors using regimens that produced minor toxicity (Figure 40.7).

The design and synthesis of FA-targeted liposomes, nanoparticles for delivery of chemotherapeutic cargo, as well as radiopharmaceuticals, will not be discussed in this chapter due to space restrictions. The interested reader is referred to other relevant chapters in this volume as well as invited to explore the novel approaches published in the specialized scientific literature [67–72].

40.2.5 FR-Targeted Immunotherapy

An alternative strategy for the treatment of FR-positive tumors exploits FA for the delivery of highly immunogenic haptens to the cell surface [73]. In this approach, patients are first immunized against the hapten (e.g., against fluorescein, used by Endocyte in a clinical trial known as FolateImmune) and then treated with the FA–hapten (FA–fluorescein) conjugate (EC17, Figure 40.10). After such targeted decoration, the cancer cells are seen as "foreign" by the immune system. Subsequently, antihapten (antifluorescein) antibodies bind to the marked tumor cells,

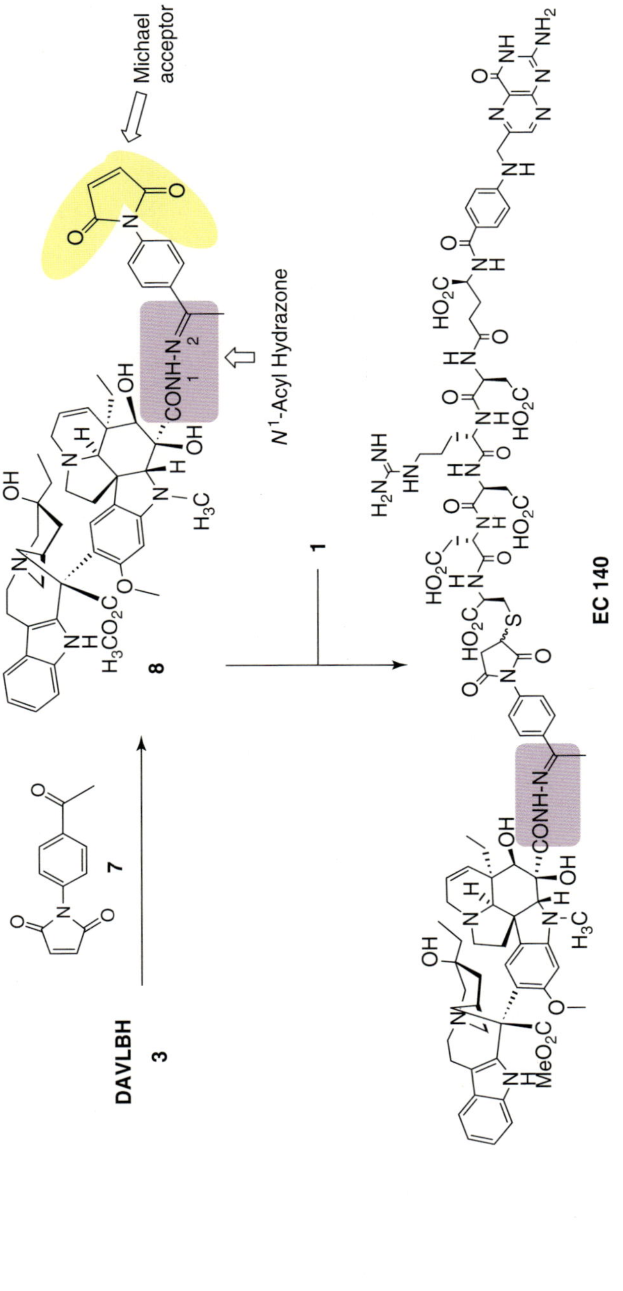

Scheme 40.6 Synthesis of the pH-sensitive acyl hydrazone-based conjugate EC140.

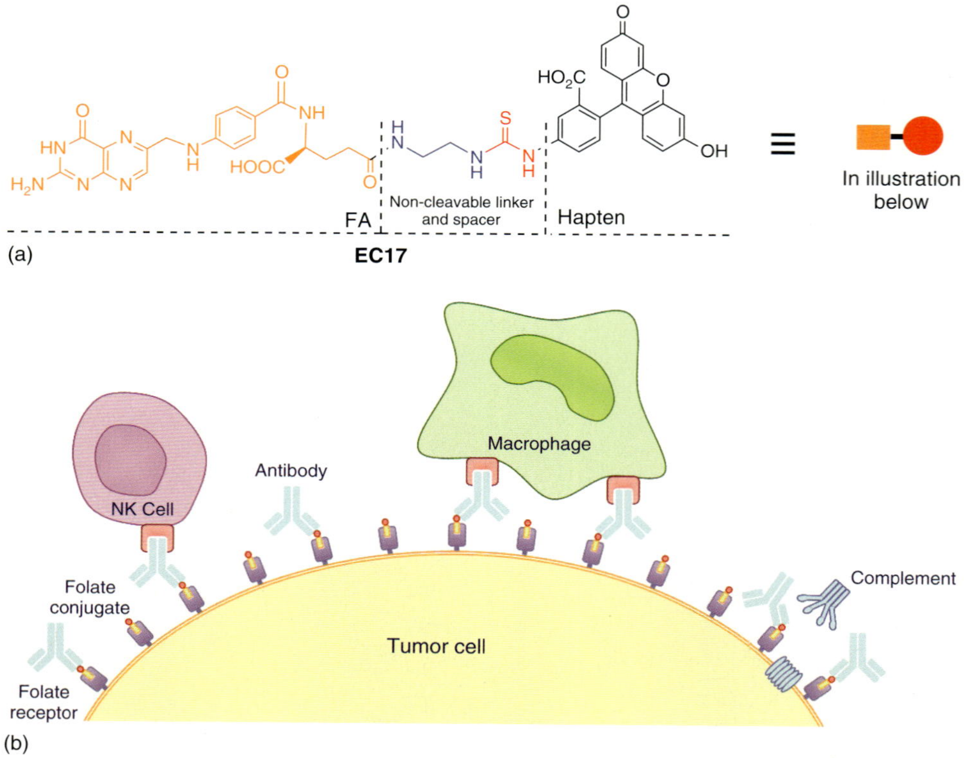

Figure 40.10 FA–fluorescein conjugate, EC17 (a), and an illustration of FA-hapten-mediated immunotherapy (b). ((b) Reprinted with permission from [74]. © 2008 American Chemical Society.)

and trigger their destruction by macrophages, natural killer cells, and complement. No drug release is required for therapeutic efficacy.

40.3 Chemical Aspects of Vitamin B_{12}–Drug Conjugate Design

40.3.1 Vitamin B_{12}-Binding Proteins and Cellular Transport

Vitamin B_{12} (cobalamin) is a natural nutrient cofactor that plays a role in the synthesis of methionine and thymidine in cells [75]. Rapidly dividing cancer cells have an increased need for vitamin B_{12} and, as a result, researchers have focused on this vitamin as a potential targeting moiety. Three binding proteins are involved in the transport of vitamin B_{12} throughout the body [76]. These proteins are known as:

haptocorrin (HC, also known as transcobalamin I (TCI)), intrinsic factor (IF), and transcobalamin II (TCII). During digestion, each of these proteins plays a role in the transport of cobalamin from the digestive tract into the cells of the body. Binding with HC allows for the passage of cobalamin through the acidic environment of the stomach into the intestine. The cobalamin then is released from HC and binds with IF. This complex is then transported via endocytosis by the IF-B_{12} receptor known as cubulin into the bloodstream. In the bloodstream, vitamin B_{12} then binds with TCII and is internalized via endocytosis into cells by the TCII-B_{12} receptor. Based on this mechanism of vitamin B_{12} internalization, substantial work has been focused on identifying cancer cell lines that overexpress the TCII-B_{12} receptor. Human breast cells [77, 78], ovarian cells [77], glioma cells [79], and leukemia cell lines [80] have all been found to be TCII receptor-positive. Unfortunately, the TCII receptor is also found in high concentrations in the kidneys, placenta, intestines, and liver [81]. Transport via TCII binding also slows clearance of vitamin B_{12} conjugates, which limits its usefulness for targeting radiopharmaceutical drugs [82]. As a result, several research groups have focused their research on identifying cell lines that express the IF receptor or the TCI receptor. Work by several groups has been successful in making modifications so as to favor uptake by one of these two receptors over the TCII pathway [83, 84].

40.3.2 Structural Considerations in Vitamin B_{12} Conjugate Design

Several excellent reviews discussing the use of vitamin B_{12} for targeting and oral delivery of active species have been published in the past few years [76, 85, 86]. Herein, we will focus on the chemistries of recent vitamin B_{12}–cancer drug conjugates, with a particular emphasis on small-molecule conjugates with releasable linkers and established biological efficacies. The structure of vitamin B_{12} is shown in Figure 40.11. The most common sites of conjugation have been the *e*-propionamide, the 5′-hydroxyl group of the ribose unit, the phosphate moiety, and the β-ligand site directly attached to the cobalt atom [76]. These sites have the least impact on receptor binding and the chemistries are relatively straightforward. Spacers are also employed in some vitamin B_{12} conjugates. As we have seen for other vitamin conjugates, these spacers are used to improve or modify properties such as solubility, cell permeability, or receptor binding, or to allow for the release of the drug payload from the conjugate. Russell-Jones provides an overview of a number of the spacers used for the oral delivery of proteins via vitamin B_{12} conjugation [85].

40.3.3 Synthesis of Vitamin B_{12}–Drug Conjugates

40.3.3.1 Releasable β-Ligand Conjugates

Grissom *et al.* have synthesized a number of vitamin B_{12} conjugates utilizing the β-ligand site for attachment of chemotherapeutically active drugs, including

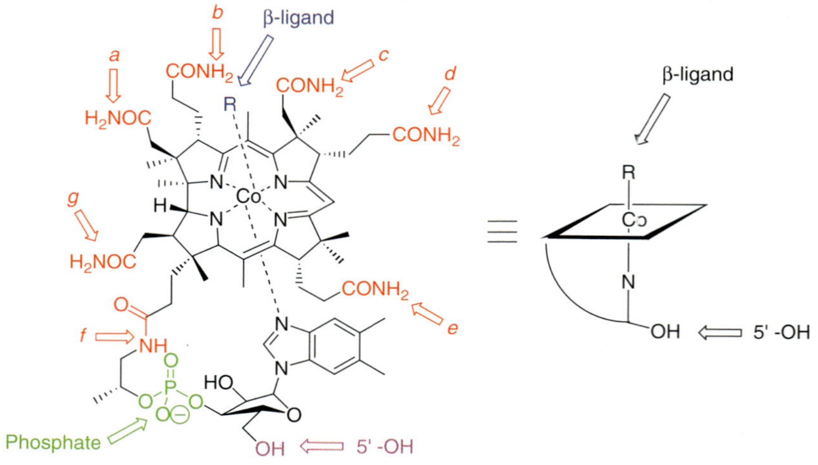

Figure 40.11 Structure of vitamin B_{12}. R = OH, hydroxocobalamin; CN, cyanocobalamin; Ado, 5′-deoxyadenosylcobalamin.

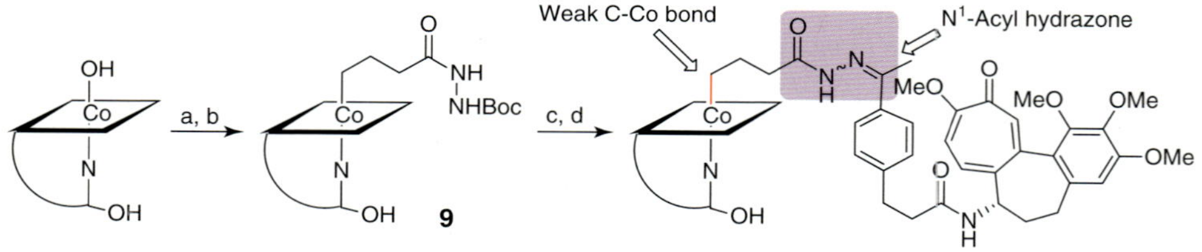

Scheme 40.7 Synthesis of colbalamin–cochicine conjugate. (a) Zn, HN_4Cl, H_2O. (b) $ClCH_2CH_2CH_2CONHNH$-Boc, MeOH. (c) Trifluoroacetic acid. (d) Colchicine-acetylphenoxyacetic acid adduct, MeOH.

chlorambucil and doxorubicin (DOX). More recently, his group has synthesized a conjugate of colchicine that employs an acid-labile hydrazone linker as well as the inherently weak carbon–cobalt bond to effect release (Scheme 40.7) [87]. Hydroxocobalamin was reacted with *t*-butoxycarbonyl (Boc)-protected chloropropyl carbazide under reducing conditions to yield adduct **9**. After deprotection, the modified B_{12} was reacted with a colchicine–acetylphenoxyacetic acid adduct. Grissom *et al.* report that this conjugate undergoes rapid and complete hydrolysis under acidic conditions, and exhibits only a minimal loss of toxicity compared to authentic colchicine.

Bauer *et al.* have described the synthesis of nitrosylcobalamin (NO-Cbl) from hydroxocobalamin acetate upon treatment with NO gas at 150 psi [78, 88]. The release of nitric oxide from this conjugate as well as its toxicity to a number of human cancer cell lines has been reported. Also reported is a possible synergy between NO-Cbl and interferon (IFN)-β against the OVCAR-3 cell line. IFN-β is believed to enhance TCII receptor expression, thereby enhancing NO-Cbl binding.

40.3.3.2 Other Vitamin B_{12}–Drug Conjugates

Several authors have detailed the use of radiolabeled vitamin B_{12} conjugates for imaging. Of the many strategies employed, several modify vitamin B_{12} with a chelating moiety such as DTPA. For example, Collins *et al.* synthesized a DTPA-polylysine modified CN-Cbl [89]. DTPA has also been used to coordinate radioisotopes for the treatment of disease. Siega *et al.* detail the use of this chelating moiety along with triethylenetetraamine-*N,N,N′,N″,N″,N‴,N‴*-hexaacetic acid (TTHA) to coordinate Gd^{3+} to vitamin B_{12} to treat K562 leukemia cells (Figure 40.12) [90]. The Gd^{3+} coordinate of **11** was found to have a half-life of 33 h in PBS and little Gd^{3+} was internalized into K562 cells. The Gd^{3+} coordinate of **10**, on the other hand, was reported to have a half-life of only 2.5 h and showed increasing uptake of Gd^{3+} with increasing concentrations of **10**. The open coordination shell in DTPA results in the involvement of the ester oxygen atoms in Gd^{3+} coordination, making the ester more susceptible to hydrolysis. The weaker coordination of DTPA also allows for hydrogen-bonding interactions on the cell surface resulting in the release of Gd^{3+} in close proximity to the targeted cells. Previous reports have shown that Gd^{3+} can be easily internalized through the cellular membrane [91]. K562 cells treated with the Gd^{3+} coordinate of compound **10** show a marked decrease in cell viability at 1 mM concentrations.

The selective inhibition of gene expression by small interfering RNA (siRNA) has shown promise as a novel form of chemotherapy and, as a result, has received considerable attention in recent years. Plenat *et al.* describe the synthesis of vitamin B_{12}–oligonucleotide conjugates following the most common strategy used for coupling active agents to the propionamide moieties of vitamin B_{12} [92]. CN-Cbl was hydrolyzed under acidic conditions and the typically formed monocarboxylic acid isomers the *b*-, *d*-, and *e*-acids, were then separated. The Cbl *d*-acid was then

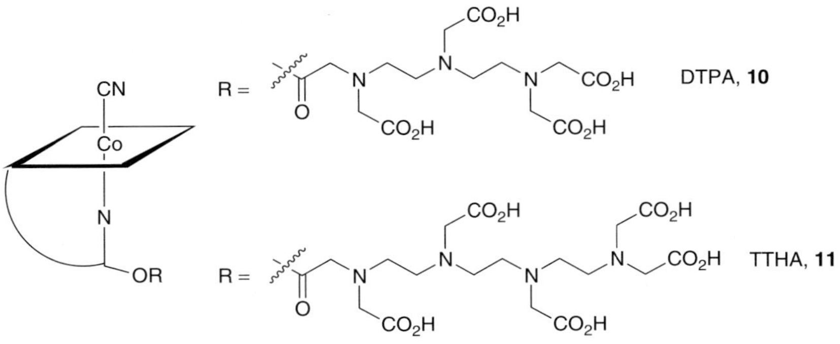

Figure 40.12 Vitamin B_{12}–DTPA/TTHA adducts.

dissolved in a pH 6 buffer and 1-ethyl-3-(3-dimethylaminopropyl)carbodiimide hydrochloride, and a 3′-amino-modified antisense oligonucleotide was added according to the method described by Russell-Jones *et al.*

40.4
Chemical Aspects of Biotin–Drug Conjugate Design

40.4.1
Biotin and Biotin Conjugate Targeting in Cancer Therapy

Biotin (vitamin B_7, Figure 40.13) is a cofactor responsible for carbon dioxide transfer in several carboxylase enzymes, and, as a result, is important in fatty acid synthesis, branched-chain catabolism, and gluconeogenesis, and an essential micronutrient for normal cellular function, growth, and development [93]. In the area of targeted cancer therapy, biotin is involved in two distinct ways. (i) As has been seen with FA and vitamin B_{12}, for a number of rapidly dividing cancer cell lines, biotin uptake is greater than that seen with normal tissues [94]. In fact, biotin receptors are overexpressed more than FA and/or vitamin B_{12} receptors on several cancer cell lines, including leukemia (L1210FR), lung (M109), renal (RENCA, RD0995), and breast (4T1, JC, MMT06056) [95, 96]. The structure(s) of the biotin receptor(s) are not known [95, 97]; however, the sodium-dependent multivitamin transporter is believed to be involved in biotin uptake [98, 99]. Biotin conjugates have been shown to target cells that overexpress biotin receptors. After binding, these conjugates are internalized via endocytosis [100]. (ii) Biotin has been found to bind with the proteins avidin and streptavidin with a dissociation constant of the order of 10^{-15}. This is one of the strongest known protein–ligand interactions [101]. The affinity for these two proteins has been exploited in what is referred to generically as biotin–avidin systems (BASs) or biotin–avidin technology [102–104]. In these systems, avidin–biotin binding acts as a bridge between some cell targeting moiety and a payload. Several recent examples of the use of biotin–avidin technology in cancer research can be found in the literature [102–108]. A ^{90}Y -tetra-azacyclodocecanetetra acetic acid–biotin conjugate and a NR-LU-10 antibody–streptavidin conjugate entered a phase II trial for the treatment of metastatic colon cancer [109]. Sixteen percent of the patients achieved a stable disease state for a period of 10–20 weeks and considerable toxicities were observed that had not been anticipated based on the results of the phase I trial. As BASs depend upon not only the affinity of biotin for avidin, but also upon the affinity of the targeting moiety and subsequent delivery based on that targeting moiety's specific receptor, further discussion of this methodology will not

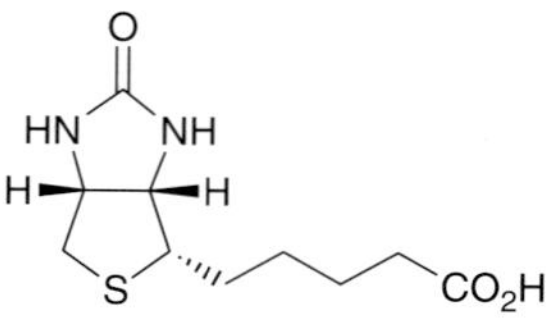

Figure 40.13 Structure of biotin.

take place in this chapter. Rather, we will focus on the targeting of active species by conjugation to biotin via the biotin receptors.

40.4.2
Synthesis of Biotin–Drug Conjugates

Camptothecin (CPT) is an anticancer agent that causes DNA damage by targeting topoisomerase I. Unfortunately, CPT has low water solubility and poor *in vivo* stability. To address these issues, Sinko *et al.* synthesized biotinylated and nonbiotinylated PEG–CPT conjugates (Scheme 40.8), and evaluated them on A2780 human ovarian cancer cells [99]. CPT was first treated with Boc-protected glycine in the presence of 1,3-diisoproplycarbodiimide (DIPC) and 4-dimethylaminopyridine (DMAP) to yield the CPT-glycinate. The gylcinate was then reacted with PEG-*N*-hydroxysuccinimide (NHS) (MW 5000) or biotin-PEG-NHS (MW 3400) to yield the target conjugates. Tests on sensitive and multidrug-resistant A2780 cells showed a 12-fold increase in toxicity for the PEGylated CPT, and a further 5.2 and 2.1 times increase in toxicity for the biotin-NHS-CPT in the sensitive and drug-resistant cell lines, respectively.

Ojima *et al.* describe the synthesis of biotin–taxoid conjugates that feature a reductively labile disulfide linker [110]. The linker was constructed and incorporated into the biotin–SB-T-1214 conjugate **13** as shown (Scheme 40.9). Reduction of the disulfide bond in **13** with GSH or other endosomal reducing agents begins a cascade whereby free SB-T-1214 is released upon the formation of thiolactone **14**. The effectiveness of this reductively labile disulfide linker system was demonstrated on L1210FR cells that were treated with a similarly linked biotin–coumarin conjugate followed by GSH-OEt. Compound **13** was found to have an IC_{50} of 8.8 nM against L1210FR cells, whereas on the L1210 and WI38 cell lines where biotin receptors are not expressed, the IC_{50} values were 522 and 570 nM, respectively. The IC_{50} of the SB-T-1214 base drug on all three of these cell lines has been reported to be around 10 nM.

In addition to **13**, Ojima has also reported the synthesis of a dual drug–biotin conjugate comprised of a taxoid and topotecan, as well as a taxoid conjugate with both biotin- and FA-targeting ligands [111]. Each of these conjugates use the reductively labile disulfide linkage previously described.

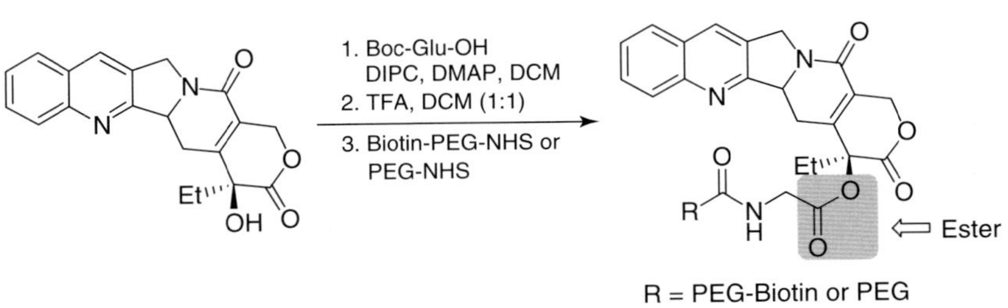

Scheme 40.8 Synthesis of biotin-PEG–CPT conjugate.

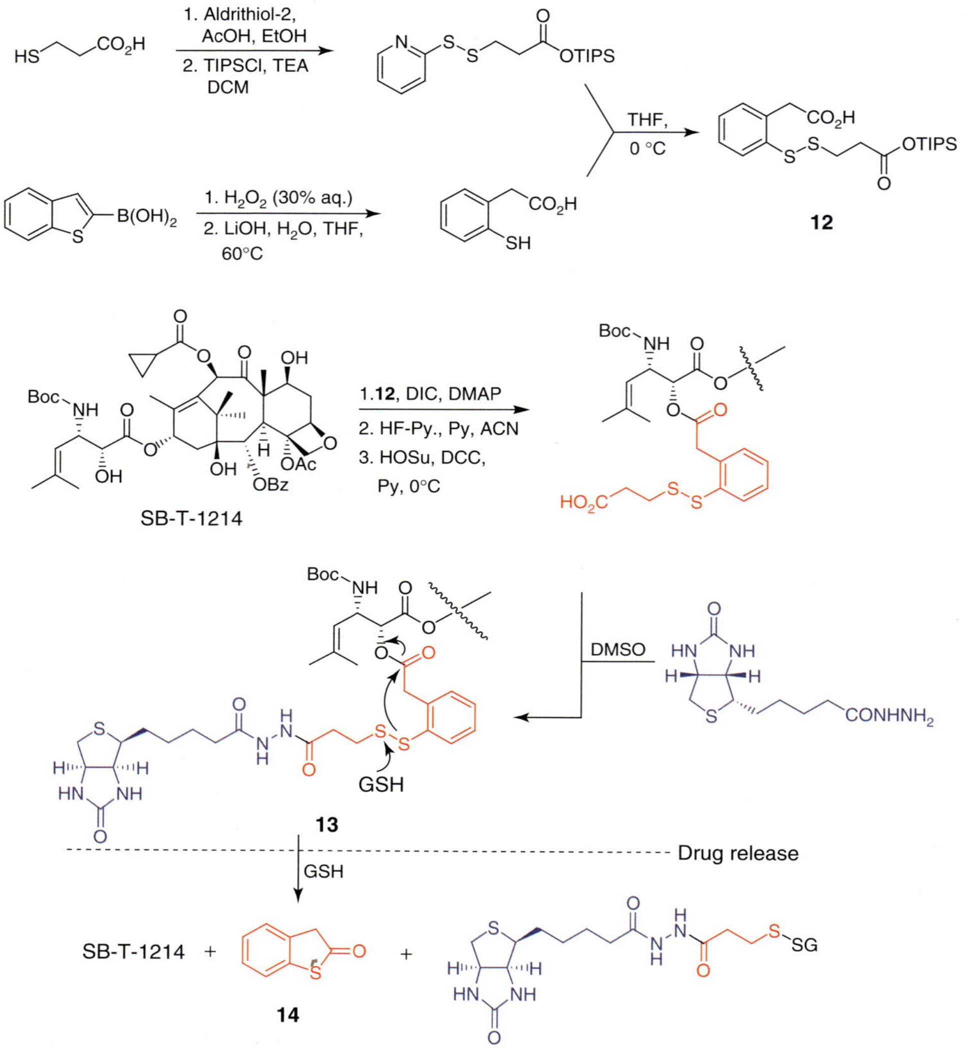

Scheme 40.9 Synthesis and reductive release of SB-T-1214–biotin conjugate **13**.

Russell-Jones and McEwan describe the synthesis of a number of macromolecular biotin–cytotoxin conjugates that incorporate polymers, dendrimers, and nanoparticles [96]. The most developed example is a conjugate of biotin and DOX. The drug and targeting moiety are linked through a *N*-(2-hydroxypropyl)methacrylamide (HPMA), *N*-methacryloylglycylphenyllecinylglycine copolymer. This conjugate was compared to analogous B_{12} and FA conjugates for the treatment of Colo-26 colorectal cancer in nude mice.

40.5 Other Vitamin–Drug Conjugates

40.5.1 Conjugates of Vitamin E

Yokota *et al.* describe a α-tocopherol (vitamin E)–siRNA conjugate. α-Tocopherol binds to apolipoproteins in chylomicrons. Conjugation allows for the delivery of the siRNA conjugate to liver cells via lipoprotein receptors on the cell surface of liver cells [112].

40.5.2 Conjugates of Vitamin B_6

Vitamin B_6 (pyridoxine, Figure 40.14) is a series of compounds containing the pyridinyl structure, such as pyridoxol (PN), pyridoxamine (PM), pyridoxal (PL), and their derivatives [113]. Pyridoxal 5′-phosphate (PLP), the metabolically active form of vitamin B_6, serves as a coenzyme for many reactions, and can help facilitate decarboxylation, transamination, racemization, elimination, replacement, and β-group interconversion reactions. The vitamin B_6 structure is recognized by specific pyridoxine transporters on cells within the liver. As a result, vitamin B_6 has been used to target magnetic resonance imaging (MRI) contrast agents and anticancer agents [113]. Yan *et al.* describe the synthesis of polymeric pyridoxine–5-fluorouracil (5-FU) conjugates for the treatment of hepatic cancer (Scheme 40.10) [114]. 5-FU, a thymidylate synthesis inhibitor, and PM were each treated with phosgene to form their respective isocyanates. The activated drug and targeting ligand were then reacted with four polyaspartamides with differing side-chain modifications: poly-α, β-(*N*-(2-hydroxyethyl)-L-aspartamide) (PHEA), poly-α, β-(*N*-(2-aminoethyl)-L-aspartamide) (PAEA), poly-α, β-((*N*-(3-hydroxypropyl)-L-aspartamide) (PHPA), and poly-α, β-(*N*-(6-aminohexyl)-L-aspartamide) (PAHA). The polyaspartamides were chosen because they are water soluble, biologically well tolerated synthetic polymers with a protein-like structure that is nontoxic, nonantigenic, and degradable in living systems. 5-FU–PAEA–PM's biodistribution and ability to induce apoptosis on Bel-7204 human hepatic tumor cells was examined. The addition of PM to the 5-FU–PAEA conjugate greatly increases the uptake of the

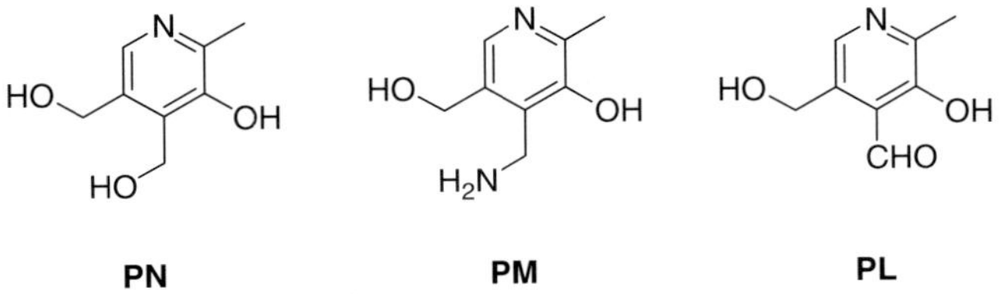

Figure 40.14 Three forms of vitamin B_6.

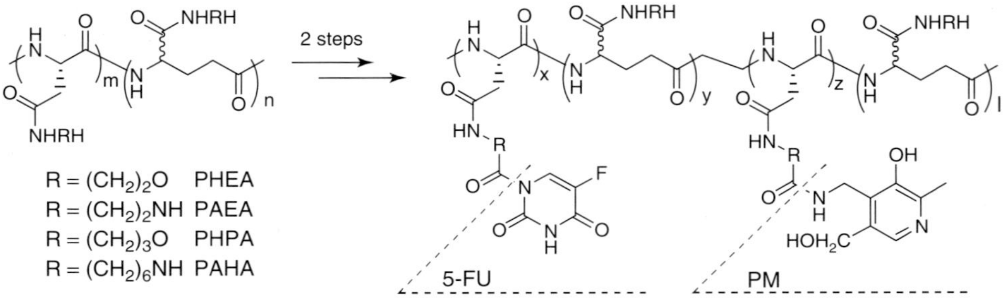

Scheme 40.10 Synthesis of vitamin B_6–5-FU conjugates.

targeted conjugate in the liver of mice at early timepoints. 5-FU–PAEA–PM was able to induce apoptosis in 62% of Bel-7204 cells at a concentration of 135 μg/ml.

40.6
Concluding Remarks on Vitamin Targeting

The synthesis and evaluation of therapies based on vitamin receptor-targeting, including conjugates of chemotherapeutics, diagnostic imaging agents, and immunogenic haptens, has emerged as an area of research that has seen exponential growth in the last two decades. There are still challenges, such as developing drug conjugates of sufficient toxicity and stability to exploit the finite delivery capacity of the various receptors, developing reliable release mechanisms tailored to the functionality of each particular drug, enhancing the ability of complex molecules to escape the endosome for optimal intracellular delivery, and improving the oral bioavailability of drug conjugates. Nevertheless, the promise of vitamin targeting, avoiding the toxicities that have compromised traditional therapies while maintaining high efficacy, will keep researchers searching for creative strategies to overcome the challenges that currently exist. Results from current and future clinical trials will expose the benefits and full potential of these targeted delivery strategies.

40.7
Growth Factor Conjugates for Tumor Targeting

40.7.1
Growth Factors and Growth Factor Receptors

Growth factors are natural substances, usually proteins or steroid hormones, capable of stimulating cellular growth, proliferation, and differentiation. There are many families of growth factors, including nerve growth factor (NGF), epidermal growth factor (EGF) [115], Fibroblast growth factor (FGF), vascular endothelial growth factor (VEGF), transforming growth factor (TGF-α), and granulocyte macrophage colony-stimulating factor. Growth factors bind to their receptors specifically and efficiently (e.g., EGF binds to high binding affinity EGF receptor (EGFR) with $K_d = 70$ pM [116]). Human EGF is a single-chain polypeptide consisting of 53 amino acid residues with three internal disulfide bridges [117]. Human EGFR (HER1; ErbB-1) is a 1186-amino-acid transmembrane (TM) glycoprotein, with extracellular domains (domain I–IV), a single spanning TM domain, an intracellular juxtamembrane (JM) region, a tyrosine kinase domain, and a C-terminal regulatory region, as shown (Figure 40.15) [118, 119]. The binding of the growth factor to the extracellular domain of the receptor leads to the activation of the intracellular domain, resulting in signal transduction that increases cellular growth or differentiation. Following ligand binding, growth factor receptors are rapidly internalized from the cell surface via several pathways that attenuate the receptor signals and diminish the level of cell activation. The endosomes containing internalized receptors mature into late endosomes and multivesicular bodies, and growth factor receptors are either recycled back to the plasma membrane or destroyed in the lysosome [120].

Cancer cells are known to overexpress or activate growth factor receptors by mutation (e.g., EGFR is overexpressed in many cancer cells, including non-small-cell

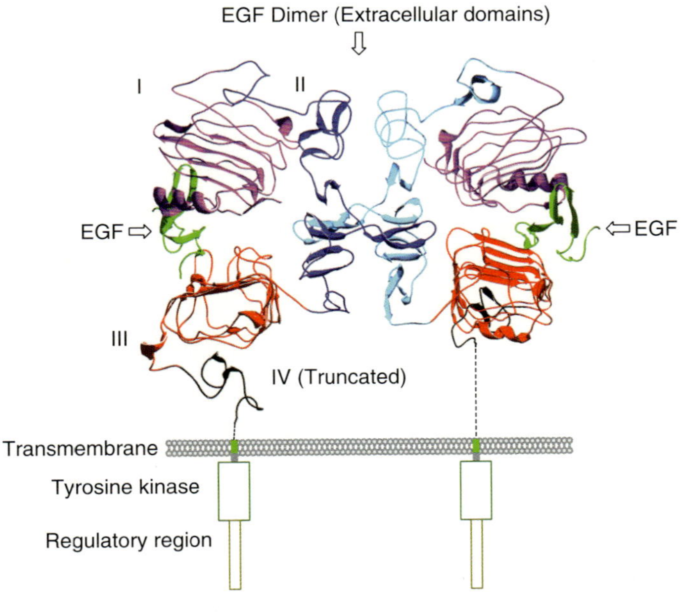

Figure 40.15 Pictorial representation of the EGF–EGFR complex. The crystal structure portion shows the complex of EGF and EGFR extracellular domains (domain I–IV). After EGF binds to EGFR binding domains (domain I and III), EGFR forms an activated homodimer with another EGFR or an activated heterodimer with another member of the ErbB family. The crystal structure was generated using Swiss PDB Viewer 4.0 (*http://www.expasy.org/spdbv* [121]) and POV Ray 3.62 (Persistence of Vision, Williamstown, Victoria, Australia; *www.povray.org*).

lung cancer, breast, head and neck, gastric, colorectal, esophageal, prostate, bladder, renal, pancreatic, and ovarian cancers [122]). As growth factors bind to their receptors with high affinity and specificity, growth factors can be used to target therapeutics to cancer cells overexpressing growth factor receptors. Researchers also use antibodies [123, 124] or antibody fragments [125] as ligands instead of growth factors to maintain high binding affinity and specificity, while achieving kinase inhibition at the same time. Alternatively, peptides derived from the growth factor [126, 127] are utilized to avoid the immunogenicity and proliferation effects common with growth factor targeting. This section focuses on targeted delivery with growth factors as ligands.

40.7.2
Growth Factor Targeted Delivery of Protein Toxin

Early studies of growth factor targeted delivery focused on growth factor–protein toxin conjugates. EGF was linked to protein toxins like the ricin A chain and diphtheria A chain by reaction with *N*-succinimidyl-3-(2-pyridyldithio)-propionate (SPDP) on the N-terminus of EGF (Figure 40.16). The diphtheria A chain was also linked to the C-terminus of EGF by cystamine. Conjugates linked to the N- or C-terminus of EGF were able to compete against EGF for binding to EGFR [128–131]. Using SPDP, basic FGF (bFGF) and saporin-6 (SAP, ribosome-inactivating protein) were also conjugated. FGF–SAP showed bFGF receptor-specific cytotoxicity (IC_{50} = 25 pM) on baby hamster kidney fibroblast cells. Animal models showed excellent tumor inhibition with minimal toxicity in mice treated with FGF–SAP [132, 133]. The conjugates of cytotoxic proteins with growth factors were also obtained by recombinant DNA methods [134, 135]. There were several clinical trials on fusion toxins of growth factors (e.g., DT388MCSF for acute myelogenous leukemia and chronic myelomonocytic leukemia (*http://www.clinicaltrials.*

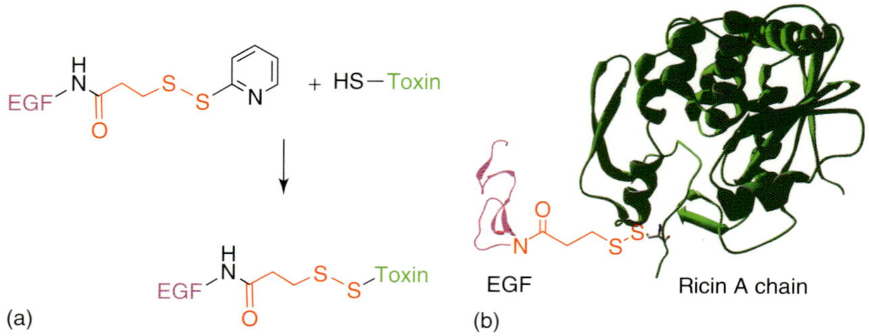

Figure 40.16 (a) Synthesis of EGF–ricin A chain conjugate. (b) Ribbon diagram of the conjugate of EGF and ricin A chain. The ribbon structure of EGF was generated from 1IVO [119] and the structure of ricin A chain was generated from 3HIO [136].

gov/ct2/show/NCT00074750), and PE-38 (TGF-α–*Pseudomonas* exotoxin conjugate) for malignant brain tumors (*http://www.clinicaltrials.gov/ct2/show/NCT00104091 and http://clinicaltrials.gov/ct2/show/NCT00074334*)) (see Chapter 45).

40.7.3
Growth Factor Targeted Delivery of Chemotherapeutics

Growth factors are used to target drug-loaded nanoparticles or polymers to tumors cells. EGF-modified nanoparticles have been used to enhance cisplatin accumulation in lung tumors via inhalation [137]. An EGF-modified single-wall carbon nanotube (SWNT) was used to deliver cisplatin to head and neck squamous cell carcinoma, achieving rapid regression of tumor growth relative to nontargeted SWNT–cisplatin [138]. EGFR-targeted immunoliposomes significantly enhance the efficacy of drugs *in vivo*, including DOX, epirubicin, and vinorelbine [139, 140]. An EGFR-targeted human recombinant EGF_L–poly-L-ornithine–β-amanitin conjugate (Figure 40.17) was 80 times more cytotoxic than β-amanitin and 20 times more cytotoxic than poly-L-ornithine–β-amanitin on A431 cells [141].

Apart from delivering macromolecules to tumor cells, growth factors can be linked to small molecules directly. EGF was cross-linked to DOX by glutaldehyde in a one-pot reaction. EGF–DOX showed higher activities *in vitro* and *in vivo* than free DOX [125]. Methotrexate (MTX) was linked to Insulin-like growth factor (IGF) by amide bond formation as well (Figure 40.18). Against MCF-7 xenografts, IGF–MTX was more effective than free MTX, even with a 4-fold lower dosage [142].

40.7.4
Growth Factor Targeted Delivery in Radiotherapy and Photodynamic Therapy

In addition to the targeted delivery of toxins, growth factors are also used to deliver radioactive compounds and photosensitizers. EGF–Dex–^{131}I–tyrosine showed a

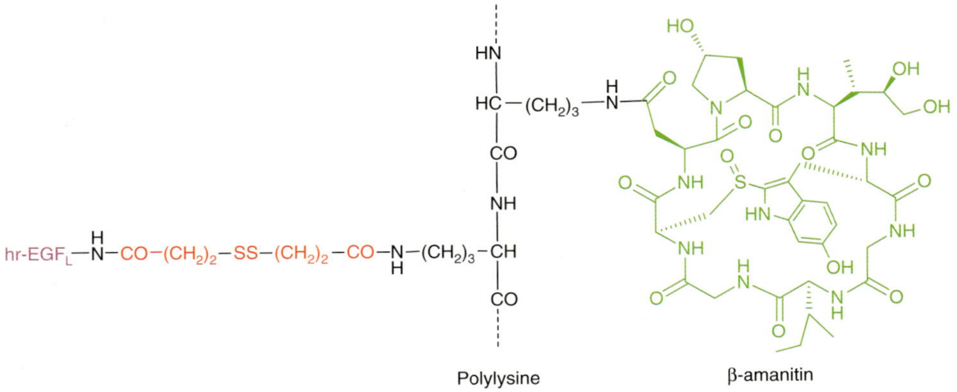

Figure 40.17 EGF–polylysine-β-amanitin.

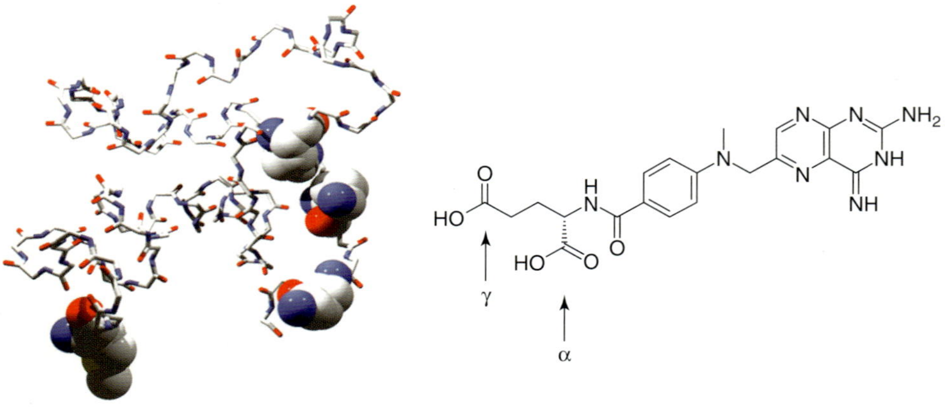

Figure 40.18 Protein structure of long-R^3-IGF-I (a potent analog of IGF-I that has been modified by a Glu(3) to Arg mutation and a 13-amino-acid extension appended to the N-terminus) [143] indicates that the three lysine residues plus the N-terminal methionine amino group could react with the activated carboxy groups of MTX. MTX has two potential reaction sites – the less sterically hindered γ-carboxyl group and the α-carboxyl group. Most likely, conjugation will result in a mixture of regioisomers.

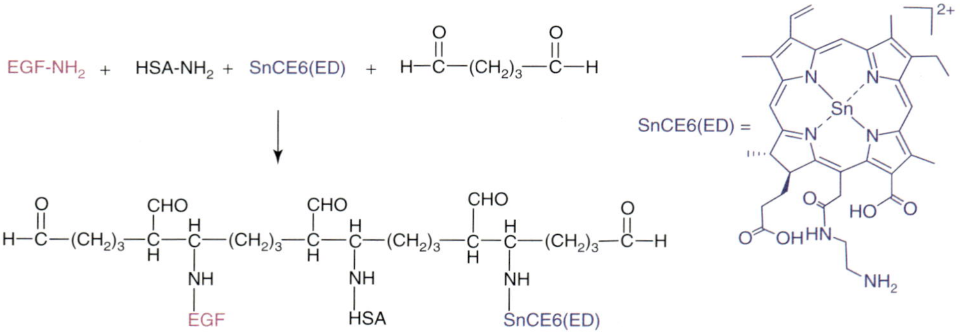

Figure 40.19 Representative structure of EGF–HSA–SnCE6(ED).

good therapeutic effect on glioma cells [144]. Photosensitizers can be targeted to tumor cells by growth factors to enhance photocytotoxicity in photodynamic therapy. EGF was linked to human serum albumin (HSA) and Sn(IV) chlorin e6 ethylenediamine (SnCE6(ED)) by glutaraldehyde (Figure 40.19). EGF–HSA–SnCE6(ED) conjugates showed EGFR-specific photocytotoxicities (IC_{50}, 63 nM) on MDA-MB-468 cells at a light dose of 27 kJ/m^2 [145].

40.7.5
Peptides Targeting Growth Factor Receptor

To avoid the immunogenicity or proliferation effects of growth factors, small peptides have been designed to have high binding affinity to growth factor receptors. By screening phage-display libraries, peptide GE11 (YHWYGYTPQNVI) with a K_d of 22.28 nM to EGFR was identified. GE11–polyethylenimine conjugates can effectively transfect genes into cancer cells overexpressing EGFR via a receptor-mediated mechanism [126]. By virtual screening, EGFR-targeted peptide ligand D4 (Leu-Ala-Arg-Leu-Leu-Thr) was identified. Peptide D4 directed liposomes toward cancer cells overexpressing EGFR [127]. The peptide with the sequence KRTGQYKL (bFGFp) was found to inhibit binding of bFGF to FGF receptor and bFGF-induced proliferation of vascular endothelial cells [146]. Uptake of conjugates of bFGFp–bovine serum albumin and bFGFp–liposomes by FGF receptor-overexpressing NIH 3T3 cells was significantly enhanced [147].

40.7.6
Concluding Remarks on Growth Factor Targeting

Targeted delivery of therapeutics to tumors holds great promise. Growth factors have been used as ligands for targeted delivery to tumors overexpressing growth factor receptors with high specificity. Several growth factor conjugates of protein toxin are in clinical trials for cancer therapy. One of the concerns with using growth factors as targeting ligands is that growth factors can cause cancer cells to proliferate. However, growth factor targeting may help to eradicate otherwise dormant cancer cells, enhancing the activity of drugs that would normally be more effective on actively dividing cells. The outcome of these clinical trials will help to further our understanding of the mechanism of targeted delivery by growth factors and the criteria for the choice of cytotoxic agents. In addition, to avoid the potential proliferation effect and the immunogenicity of growth factor conjugates, small peptides with good binding affinities for growth factor receptors have been developed. With the small peptides as ligands, selective and flexible synthetic methods can be applied, thereby generating a variety of conjugates with different release mechanisms. Hopefully, small peptide ligands will broaden the application of growth factor receptor targeted delivery in oncology.

Acknowledgments

The authors wish to recognize the talent and scientific contributions of every single member of the Discovery Department at Endocyte Inc., and especially Drs. Christopher Leamon and Philip Low for their pioneering work, dedication, and creativity in the field of FA targeting.

References

1. Ehrlich, P. (1910) Diskussionsbemerkungen zum Vortrag von Wechselmann (Chemotherapie der Syphilis). *Ber. Tagung Freien Ver Mikrobiol.*, **47**, 223–224.
2. Bailey, S.W.A.J. (2009) The extremely slow and variable activity of dihydrofolate reductase in human liver and its implications for high folic acid intake. *Proc.*

Natl. Acad. Sci. USA, **106**, 15424–15429.

3. Antony, A.C. (1992) The biological chemistry of folate receptors. *Blood*, **79**, 2807–2820.
4. Kamen, B.A., Wang, M.T., Streckfuss, A.J., Peryea, X., and Anderson, R.G.W. (1988) Delivery of folates to the cytoplasm of ma104 cells is mediated by a surface-membrane receptor that recycles. *J. Biol. Chem.*, **263**, 13602–13609.
5. Anderson, R.G.W., Kamen, B.A., Rothberg, K.G., and Lacey, S.W. (1992) Potocytosis – sequestration and transport of small molecules by caveolae. *Science*, **255**, 410–411.
6. Antony, A.C. (1996) Folate receptors. *Annu. Rev. Nutr.*, **16**, 501–521.
7. Kamen, B.A. and Capdevila, A. (1986) Receptor-mediated folate accumulation is regulated by the cellular folate content. *Proc. Natl. Acad. Sci. USA*, **83**, 5983–5987.
8. Sadasivan, E. and Rothenberg, S.P. (1989) The complete amino-acid sequence of a human folate-binding protein from KB cells determined from the cDNA. *J. Biol. Chem.*, **264**, 5806–5811.
9. Lacey, S.W., Sanders, J.M., Rothberg, K.G., Anderson, R.G.W., and Kamen, B.A. (1989) Complementary DNA for the folate binding-protein correctly predicts anchoring to the membrane by glycosyl-phosphatidylinositol. *J. Clin. Invest.*, **84**, 715–720.
10. Elwood, P.C. (1989) Molecular cloning and characterization of the human folate-binding protein cDNA from placenta and malignant-tissue culture (KB) cells. *J. Biol. Chem.*, **264**, 14893–14901.
11. Ratnam, M., Marquardt, H., Duhring, J.L., and Freisheim, J.H. (1989) Homologous membrane folate-binding proteins in human placenta – cloning and sequence of a cDNA. *Biochemistry*, **28**, 8249–8254.
12. Shen, F., Ross, J.F., Wang, X., and Ratnam, M. (1994) Identification of a novel folate receptor, a truncated receptor, and receptor-type-beta in hematopoietic-cells – cDNA cloning, expression, immunoreactivity, and tissue-specificity. *Biochemistry*, **33**, 1209–1215.
13. Shen, F., Wu, M., Ross, J.F., Miller, D., and Ratnam, M. (1995) Folate receptor-type-gamma is primarily a secretory protein due to lack of an efficient signal for glycosylphosphatidylinositol modification – protein characterization and cell-type specificity. *Biochemistry*, **34**, 5660–5665.
14. Weitman, S.D., Lark, R.H., Coney, L.R., Fort, D.W., Frasca, V., Zurawski, V.R., and Kamen, B.A. (1992) Distribution of the folate receptor gp38 in normal and malignant-cell lines and tissues. *Cancer Res.*, **52**, 3396–3401.
15. Weitman, S.D., Weinberg, A.G., Coney, L.R., Zurawski, V.R., Jennings, D.S., and Kamen, B.A. (1992) Cellular localization of the folate receptor: potential role in drug toxicity and folate homeostasis. *Cancer Res.*, **52**, 6708–6711.
16. Birn, H., Nielsen, S., and Christensen, E.I. (1997) Internalization and apical-to-basolateral transport of folate in rat kidney proximal tubule. *Am. J. Physiol.*, **272**, F70–F78.
17. Birn, H., Selhub, J., and Christensen, E.I. (1993) Internalization and intracellular transport of folate-binding protein in rat kidney proximal tubule. *Am. J. Physiol.*, **264**, C302–C310.
18. Garin-Chesa, P., Campbell, I., Saigo, P.E., Lewis, J.L., Old, L.J., and Rettig, W.J. (1993) Trophoblast and ovarian cancer antigen LK26. Sensitivity and specificity in immunopathology and molecular identification as a folate-binding protein. *Am. J. Pathol.*, **142**, 557–567.
19. Holm, J., Hansen, S.I., Hoiermadsen, M., and Bostad, L. (1992) A high-affinity folate binding-protein in proximal tubule cells of human kidney. *Kidney Int.*, **41**, 50–55.
20. Prasad, P.D., Ramamoorthy, S., Moe, A.J., Smith, C.H., Leibach, F.H., and Ganapathy, V. (1994) Selective expression of the high-affinity isoform of the folate receptor (FR-α) in the human placental syncytiotrophoblast and choriocarcinoma cells. *Biochim. Biophys. Acta*, **1223**, 71–75.

21. Rettig, W.J., Cordoncardo, C., Koulos, J.P., Lewis, J.L., Oettgen, H.F., and Old, L.J. (1985) Cell-surface antigens of human trophoblast and choriocarcinoma defined by monoclonal-antibodies. *Int. J. Cancer*, **35**, 469–475.
22. Campbell, I.G., Jones, T.A., Foulkes, W.D., and Trowsdale, J. (1991) Folate-binding protein is a marker for ovarian cancer. *Cancer Res.*, **51**, 5329–5338.
23. Hartmann, L.C., Keeney, G.L., Lingle, W.L., Christianson, T.J.H., Varghese, B., Hillman, D., Oberg, A.L., and Low, P.S. (2007) Folate receptor overexpression is associated with poor outcome in breast cancer. *Int. J. Cancer*, **121**, 938–942.
24. Ross, J.F., Chaudhuri, P.K., and Ratnam, M. (1994) Differential regulation of folate receptor isoforms in normal and malignant-tissues in-vivo and in established cell-lines – physiological and clinical implications. *Cancer*, **73**, 2432–2443.
25. Toffoli, G., Cernigoi, C., Russo, A., Gallo, A., Bagnoli, M., and Boiocchi, M. (1997) Overexpression of folate binding protein in ovarian cancers. *Int. J. Cancer*, **74**, 193–198.
26. Toffoli, G., Russo, A., Gallo, A., Cernigoi, C., Miotti, S., Sorio, R., Tumolo, S., and Boiocchi, M. (1998) Expression of folate binding protein as a prognostic factor for response to platinum-containing chemotherapy and survival in human ovarian cancer. *Int. J. Cancer*, **79**, 121–126.
27. Leamon, C.P. (2008) Folate-targeted drug strategies for the treatment of cancer. *Curr. Opin. Invest. Drugs*, **9**, 1277–1286.
28. Leamon, C.P. and Low, P.S. (1991) Delivery of macromolecules into living cells – a method that exploits folate receptor endocytosis. *Proc. Natl. Acad. Sci. USA*, **88**, 5572–5576.
29. Reddy, J.A., Allagadda, V.M., and Leamon, C.P. (2005) Targeting therapeutic and imaging agents to folate receptor positive tumors. *Curr. Pharm. Biotechnol.*, **6**, 131–150.
30. Leamon, C.P. and Low, P.S. (1993) Membrane folate-binding proteins are responsible for folate protein conjugate endocytosis into cultured cells. *Biochem. J.*, **291**, 855–860.
31. Lee, R.J., Wang, S., and Low, P.S. (1996) Measurement of endosome pH following folate receptor-mediated endocytosis. *Biochim. Biophys. Acta*, **1312**, 237–242.
32. Leamon, C.P. and Reddy, J.A. (2004) Folate-targeted chemotherapy. *Adv. Drug Deliv. Rev.*, **56**, 1127–1141.
33. Steinberg, G. and Borch, R.F. (2001) Synthesis and evaluation of pteroic acid-conjugated nitroheterocyclic phosphoramidates as folate receptor-targeted alkylating agents. *J. Med. Chem.*, **44**, 69–73.
34. Aronov, O., Horowitz, A.T., Gabizon, A., and Gibson, D. (2003) Folate-targeted PEG as a potential carrier for carboplatin analogs. Synthesis and *in vitro* studies. *Bioconjug. Chem.*, **14**, 563–574.
35. Liu, J.Q., Kolar, C., Lawson, T.A., and Gmeiner, W.H. (2001) Targeted drug delivery to chemoresistant cells: folic acid derivatization of FdUMP[10] enhances cytotoxicity toward 5-FU-resistant human colorectal tumor cells. *J. Org. Chem.*, **66**, 5655–5663.
36. Lee, J.W., Lu, J.Y., Low, P.S., and Fuchs, P.L. (2002) Synthesis and evaluation of taxol–folic acid conjugates as targeted antineoplastics. *Bioorg. Med. Chem.*, **10**, 2397–2414.
37. Ladino, C.A., Chari, R.V.J., Bourret, L.A., Kedersha, N.L., and Goldmacher, V.S. (1997) Folate-maytansinoids: target-selective drugs of low molecular weight. *Int. J. Cancer*, **73**, 859–864.
38. Paulos, C.M., Reddy, J.A., Leamon, C.P., Turk, M.J., and Low, P.S. (2004) Ligand binding and kinetics of folate receptor recycling *in vivo*: impact on receptor-mediated drug delivery. *Mol. Pharm.*, **66**, 1406–1414.
39. Yang, J., Chen, H., Vlahov, I.R., Cheng, J.X., and Low, P.S. (2006) Evaluation of disulfide reduction during receptor-mediated endocytosis by using

FRET imaging. *Proc. Natl. Acad. Sci. USA*, **103**, 13872–13877.

40. Yang, J., Chen, H.T., Vlahov, I.R., Cheng, J.X., and Low, P.S. (2007) Characterization of the pH of folate receptor-containing endosomes and the rate of hydrolysis of internalized acid-labile folate–drug conjugates. *J. Pharm. Exp. Ther.*, **321**, 462–468.
41. Lee, R.J., Wang, S., Turk, M.J., and Low, P.S. (1998) The effects of pH and intraliposomal buffer strength on the rate of liposome content release and intracellular drug delivery. *Biosci. Rep.*, **18**, 69–78.
42. Vlahov, I.R., Santhapuram, H.K.R., Kleindl, P.J., Howard, S.J., Stanford, K.M., and Leamon, C.P. (2006) Design and regioselective synthesis of a new generation of targeted chemotherapeutics. Part 1: EC145, a folic acid conjugate of desacetylvinblastine monohydrazide. *Bioorg. Med. Chem. Lett.*, **16**, 5093–5096.
43. Vlahov, I.R., Wang, Y., Kleindl, P.J., and Leamon, C.P. (2008) Design and regioselective synthesis of a new generation of targeted chemotherapeutics. Part II: folic acid conjugates of tubulysins and their hydrazides. *Bioorg. Med. Chem. Lett.*, **18**, 4558–4561.
44. Vlahov, I., Vite, G., Kleindl, P., Wang, Y., Santhapuram, H., You, F., Howard, S., Kim, S., Lee, F., and Leamon, C. (2010) Regioselective synthesis of folate receptor-targeted agents derived from epothilone analogs and folic acid. *Bioorg. Med. Chem. Lett.*, **20**, 4578–4581.
45. Reddy, J.A., Westrick, E., Santhapuram, H.K.R., Howard, S.J., Miller, M.L., Vetzel, M., Vlahov, I., Chari, R.V.J., Goldmacher, V.S., and Leamon, C.P. (2007) Folate receptor-specific antitumor activity of EC131, a folate-maytansinoid conjugate. *Cancer Res.*, **67**, 6376–6382.
46. Henne, W.A., Doorneweerd, D.D., Hilgenbrink, A.R., Kularatne, S.A., and Low, P.S. (2006) Synthesis and activity of a folate peptide camptothecin prodrug. *Bioorg. Med. Chem. Lett.*, **16**, 5350–5355.
47. Satyam, A. (2008) Design and synthesis of releasable folate–drug conjugates using a novel heterobifunctional disulfide-containing linker. *Bioorg. Med. Chem. Lett.*, **18**, 3196–3199.
48. Suzuki, T., Hisakawa, S., Itoh, Y., Suzuki, N., Takahashi, K., Kawahata, M., Yamaguchi, K., Nakagawa, H., and Miyata, N. (2007) Design, synthesis, and biological activity of folate receptor-targeted prodrugs of thiolate histone deacetylase inhibitors. *Bioorg. Med. Chem. Lett.*, **17**, 4208–4212.
49. Leamon, C.P., Reddy, J.A., Vetzel, M., Dorton, R., Westrick, E., Parker, N., Wang, Y., and Vlahov, I. (2008) Folate targeting enables durable and specific antitumor responses from a therapeutically null tubulysin B analogue. *Cancer Res.*, **68**, 9839–9844.
50. Reddy, J.A., Dorton, R., Westrick, E., Dawson, A., Smith, T., Xu, L.C., Vetzel, M., Kleindl, P., Vlahov, I.R., and Leamon, C.P. (2007) Preclinical evaluation of EC145, a folate–vinca alkaloid conjugate. *Cancer Res.*, **67**, 4434–4442.
51. Covello, K., Flefleh, C., Menard, K., Wiebesiek, A., McGlinchey, K., Wen, M., Westhaus, R., Reddy, J., Vlahov, I., Hunt, J., Rose, W., Leamon, C., Vite, G., and Lee, F. (2008) Preclinical pharmacology of epothilone-folate conjugate BMS-753493, a tumor targeting agent selected for clinical development. American Association of Cancer Researchers Annual Meeting, San Diego, CA, abstract 2326.
52. Vlahov, I.R., Santhapuram, H.R., Kleindl, P.J., Howard, S.J., Stanford, K.M., and Leamon, C.P. (2006) Design and synthesis of a folate receptor-targeted chemotherapeutics: folic acid conjugate of desacetylvinblastine hydrazide (EC145). 232nd ACS National Meeting, San Francisco, CA, MEDI-054.
53. Symanowski, J.T., Maurer, A.H., Naumann, R.W., Shah, N.P., Morgenstern, D., and Messmann, R.A. (2010) Use of 99mTc-EC20 (a folate-targeted imaging agent) to predict response to therapy with EC145

(folate-targeted therapy) in advanced ovarian cancer. American Society of Clinical Oncology Annual Meeting, Chicago, IL, abstract 5034.

54. Naumann, R.W., Coleman, R.L., Burger, R.A., Herzog, T.J., Morris, R., Sausville, E.A., Kutarska, E., Ghamande, S.A., Gabrail, N.Y., De Pasquale, S., Nowara, E., Gilbert, L., Caton, J.R., Gersh, R.H., Teneriello, M.G., Harb, W.A., Konstantinopoulos, P., Symanowski, J.T., Lovejoy, C., and Messmann, R.A. (2010) Precedent: a randomized phase II trial comparing EC145 and pegylated liposomal doxorubicin (PLD) in combination, versus PLD alone, in subjects with platinum-resistant ovarian cancer. American Society of Clinical Oncology Annual Meeting, Chicago, IL, abstract 5045.

55. Peethambaram, P.P., Hartmann, L.C., Goss, G.D., Jonker, D.J., and Plummer, R. (2010) A phase I pharmacokinetic and safety analysis of epothilone folate (BMS-753493): a first-in-human clinical experience of a folate receptor-targeted chemotherapeutic agent dosed once daily on days 1, 2, 3, and 4 of a 21-day cycle. American Society of Clinical Oncology Annual Meeting, Chicago, IL, abstract e13005.

56. De Jonge, M.J., Sleijfer, S., Martin, L.P., Marshall, J., Deeken, J.F., Konner, L.A., and Aghajanian, C. (2010) Phase I pharmacokinetic and safety analysis of epothilone folate (BMS-753493): first-in-human clinical experience of a folate receptor-targeted chemotherapeutic agent administered on days 1, 4, 8, and 11 of a 21-day cycle. American Society of Clinical Oncology Annual Meeting, Chicago, IL, abstract 2607.

57. Li, J., Sausville, E.A., Klein, P.J., Morgenstern, D., Leamon, C.P., Messmann, R.A., and LoRusso, P. (2009) Clinical pharmacokinetics and exposure-toxicity relationship of a folate–vinca alkaloid conjugate EC145 in cancer patients. *J. Clin. Pharm.*, **49**, 1467–1476.

58. Parker, N., Turk, M.J., Westrick, E., Lewis, J.D., Low, P.S., and Leamon, C.P. (2005) Folate receptor expression in carcinomas and normal tissues determined by a quantitative radioligand binding assay. *Anal. Biochem.*, **338**, 284–293.

59. Vlahov, I.R., Santhapuram, H.K.R., You, F., Wang, Y., Kleindl, P.J., Hahn, S.J., Vaughn, J.F., Reno, D.S., and Leamon, C.P. (2010) Carbohydrate-based synthetic approach to control toxicity profiles of folate–drug conjugates. *J. Org. Chem.*, **75**, 3685–3691.

60. Leamon, C.P., Reddy, J.A., Vlahov, I.R., Klein, P.J., Dorton, R., Bloomfield, A., Westrick, E., Emsweller, K., Vetzel, M., Wang, Y., Santhapuram, H.K., Kleindl, P., and You F. (2009) Preclinical evaluation of a spacer-optimized folate-targeted Vinca alkaloid conjugate with increased therapeutic index. American Society of Cancer Researchers Annual Meeting, Denver, CO, abstract 1681.

61. Harb, W.A., Conley, B.A., LoRusso, P., Sausville, E.A., Heath, E.I., Chandana, S.R., Hamm, M., Carter, J., Perez, W.J., and Messmann, R.A. (2010) A phase I study of the folate-targeted conjugate EC0489 in patients with refractory or advanced metastatic cancer. American Society of Clinical Oncology Annual Meeting, Chicago, IL, abstract 3088.

62. Vlahov, I.R., Santhapuram, H.K.R., Wang, Y., Kleindl, P.J., You, F., Howard, S.J., Westrick, E., Reddy, J.A., and Leamon, C.P. (2007) An assembly concept for the consecutive introduction of unsymmetrical disulfide bonds: synthesis of a releasable multidrug conjugate of folic acid. *J. Org. Chem.*, **72**, 5968–5972.

63. Leamon, C.P., Reddy, J.A., Vlahov, I.R., Westrick, E., Dawson, A., Dorton, R., Vetzel, M., Santhapuram, H.K., and Wang, V. (2007) Preclinical antitumor activity of a novel folate-targeted dual drug conjugate. *Mol. Pharm.*, **4**, 659–667.

64. Vlahov, I.R., Santhapuram, H.R., Wang, Y., Kleindl, P.J., You, F., Howard, S.J., Westrick, E., Reddy, J.A., and Leamon, C.P. (2007) Releasable dual-drug conjugates of folic

acid (EC0225): an assembly concept for the consecutive introduction of unsymmetrical disulfide bonds. 234th ACS National Meeting, Boston, MA, MEDI-406.

65. Sharma, S., Sausville, E.A., LoRusso, P., Vogelzang, N.J., Samlowski, W.E., Carter, J., Forman, K., Bever, S., and Messmann, R.A. (2010) A phase I study of EC0225 administered weeks 1 and 2 of a 4-week cycle. American Society of Clinical Oncology Annual Meeting, Chicago, IL, abstract 3082.
66. Leamon, C.P., Reddy, J.A., Vlahov, I.R., Kleindl, P.J., Vetzel, M., and Westrick, E. (2006) Synthesis and biological evaluation of EC140: a novel folate-targeted vinca alkaloid conjugate. *Bioconjug. Chem.*, **17**, 1226–1232.
67. Gabizon, A., Shmeeda, H., Horowitz, A.T., and Zalipsky, S. (2004) Tumor cell targeting of liposome-entrapped drugs with phospholipid-anchored folic acid–PEG conjugates. *Adv. Drug Deliv.Rev.*, **56**, 1177–1192.
68. Hilgenbrink, A.R. and Low, P.S. (2005) Folate receptor-mediated drug targeting: from therapeutics to diagnostics. *J. Pharm. Sci.*, **94**, 2135–2146.
69. Low, P.S. and Kularatne, S.A. (2009) Folate-targeted therapeutic and imaging agents for cancer. *Curr. Opin. Chem. Biol.*, **13**, 256–262.
70. Salazar, M.D.R.M. (2007) The folate receptor: what does it promise in tissue-targeted therapeutics. *Cancer Metastasis Rev.*, **26**, 141–152.
71. Stephenson, S.M., Low, P.S., and Lee, R.J. (2004) Folate receptor-mediated targeting of liposomal drugs to cancer cells. in *Methods in Enzymology: Liposomes D* (ed. N. Duzgunes), Elsevier Academic Press, San Diego, CA, pp. 33–50.
72. Zhao, X.B., Li, H., and Lee, R.J. (2008) Targeted drug delivery via folate receptors. *Exp. Opin. Drug Deliv.*, **5**, 309–319.
73. Lu, Y.J., Sega, E., Leamon, C.P., and Low, P.S. (2004) Folate receptor-targeted immunotherapy of cancer: mechanism and therapeutic potential. *Adv. Drug Deliv. Rev.*, **56**, 1161–1176.
74. Low, P.S., Henne, W.E., and Doorneweerd, D.D. (2007) Discovery and development of folic-acid-based receptor targeting for imaging and therapy of cancer and inflammatory diseases. *Acc. Chem. Res.*, **41**, 120–129.
75. Higashi, K., Clavo, A.C., and Wahl, R.L. (1993) Invitro assessment of 2-fluoro-2-deoxy-D -glucose, L-methionine and thymidine as agent to monitor the early response of a human adenocarcinoma cell-line to radiotherapy. *J. Nucl. Med.*, **34**, 773–779.
76. Petrus, A.K., Fairchild, T.J., and Doyle, R.P. (2009) Traveling the vitamin B-12 pathway: oral delivery of protein and peptide drugs. *Angew. Chem. Int. Ed.*, **48**, 1022–1028.
77. Rachmilewitz, B., Sulkes, A., Rachmilewitz, M., and Fuks, Z. (1981) Serum transcobalamin-II levels in breast-carcinoma patients. *Isr. J. Med. Sci.*, **17**, 874–878.
78. Bauer, J.A., Morrison, B.H., Grane, R.W., Jacobs, B.S., Dabney, S., Gamero, A.M., Carnevale, K.A., Smith, D.J., Drazba, J., Seetharam, B., and Lindner, D.J. (2002) Effects of interferon beta on transcobalamin II-receptor expression and antitumor activity of nitrosylcobalamin. *J. Natl. Cancer Inst.*, **94**, 1010–1019.
79. Fiskerstrand, T., Riedel, B., Ueland, P.M., Seetharam, B., Pezacka, E.H., Gulati, S., Bose, S., Banerjee, R., Berge, R.K., and Refsum, H. (1998) Disruption of a regulatory system involving cobalamin distribution and function in a methionine-dependent human glioma cell line. *J. Biol. Chem.*, **273**, 20180–20184.
80. Amagasaki, T., Green, R., and Jacobsen, D.W. (1990) Expression a transcobalamin-II receptors by human leukemia L562 and HL-60 cells. *Blood*, **76**, 1380–1386.
81. Bose, S., Seetharam, S., and Seetharam, B. (1995) Membrane expression and interactions of human transcobalamin-II receptor. *J. Biol. Chem.*, **270**, 8152–8157.

82. Seetharam, B., Bose, S., and Li, N. (1999) Cellular import of cobalamin (vitamin B-12). *J. Nutr.*, **129**, 1761–1764.

83. Viola-Villegas, N., Rabideau, A.E., Bartholoma, M., Zubieta, J., and Doyle, R.P. (2009) Targeting the cubilin receptor through the vitamin B-12 uptake pathway: cytotoxicity and mechanistic insight through fluorescent Re(I) delivery. *J. Med. Chem.*, **52**, 5253–5261.

84. Waibel, R., Treichler, H., Schaefer, N.G., van Staveren, D.R., Mundwiler, S., Kunze, S., Kuenzi, M., Alberto, R., Nuesch, J., Knuth, A., Moch, H., Schibli, R., and Schubiger, P.A. (2008) New derivatives of vitamin B12 show preferential targeting of tumors. *Cancer Res.*, **68**, 2904–2911.

85. Russell-Jones, G. (1998) Use of vitamin B12 conjugates to deliver protein drugs by the oral route. *Crit. Rev. Ther. Drug Carrier Syst.*, **15**, 557–586.

86. Gupta, Y., Kohli, D.V., and Jain, S.K. (2008) Vitamin B-12-mediated transport: a potential tool for tumor targeting of antineoplastic drugs and imaging agents. *Crit. Rev. Ther. Drug Carrier Syst.*, **25**, 347–379.

87. Bagnato, J.D., Eilers, A.L., Horton, R.A., and Grissom, C.B. (2004) Synthesis and characterization of a cobalamin–colchicine conjugate as a novel tumor-targeted cytotoxin. *J. Org. Chem.*, **69**, 8987–8996.

88. Bauer, J.A. (1998) Synthesis, characterization and nitric oxide release profile of nitrosylcobalamin: a potential chemotherapeutic agent. *Anti-Cancer Drugs*, **9**, 239–244.

89. Collins D.H.H. (2007) Cobaltamin conjugates useful as imaging and therapeutic agents. US Patent Application 7175449 B2.

90. Siega, P., Wuerges, J., Arena, F., Gianolio, E., Fedosov, S.N., Dreos, R., Geremia, S., Aime, S., and Randaccio, L. (2009) Release of toxic Gd^{3+} ions to tumour cells by vitamin B-12 bioconjugates. *Chem. Eur. J.*, **15**, 7980–7989.

91. Cabella, C., Crich, S.G., Corpillo, D., Barge, A., Ghirelli, C., Bruno, E., Lorusso, V., Uggeri, F., and Aime, S. (2006) Cellular labeling with Gd(III) chelates: only high thermodynamic stabilities prevent the cells acting as "sponges" of Gd^{3+} ions. *Contrast Media Mol. Imaging*, **1**, 23–29.

92. Guy, M., Olszewski, A., Monhoven, N., Namour, F., Gueant, J.L., and Plenat, F. (1998) Evaluation of coupling of cobalamin to antisense oligonucleotides by thin-layer and reversed-phase liquid chromatography. *J. Chromatogr. B*, **706**, 149–156.

93. Zempleni, J.W.S. and Hassan, Y.I. (2009) Biotin. *Biofactors*, **35**, 36–46.

94. Yang, W.J., Cheng, Y.Y., Xu, T.W., Wang, X.Y., and Wen, L.P. (2009) Targeting cancer cells with biotin–dendrimer conjugates. *Eur. J. Med. Chem.*, **44**, 862–868.

95. Russell-Jones, G., McTavish, K., McEwan, J., Rice, J., and Nowotnik, D. (2004) Vitamin-mediated targeting as a potential mechanism to increase drug uptake by tumours. *J. Inorg. Biochem.*, **98**, 1625–1633.

96. Russell-Jones, G. and McEwan, J. (2004) Amplification of biotin-mediated targeting. PCT WO2004/045647.

97. Na, K., Lee, T.B., Park, K.H., Shin, E.K., Lee, Y.B., and Cho, H.K. (2003) Self-assembled nanoparticles of hydrophobically-modified polysaccharide bearing vitamin H as a targeted anti-cancer drug delivery system. *Eur. J. Pharm. Sci.*, **18**, 165–173.

98. Yellepeddi, V.K., Kumar, A., and Palakurthi, S. (2009) Biotinylated poly(amido)amine (PAMAM) dendrimers as carriers for drug delivery to ovarian cancer cells *In vitro*. *Anti-Cancer Res.*, **29**, 2933–2943.

99. Minko, T., Paranjpe, P.V., Qiu, B., Lalloo, A., Won, R., Stein, S., and Sinko, P.J. (2002) Enhancing the anticancer efficacy of camptothecin using biotinylated poly(ethyleneglycol) conjugates in sensitive and multidrug-resistant human ovarian carcinoma cells. *Cancer Chemother. Pharm.*, **50**, 143–150.

100. Horn, M.A., Heinstein, P.F., and Low, P.S. (1990) Biotin-mediated delivery of exogenous macromolecules

into soybean cells. *Plant Physiol.*, **93**, 1492–1496.

101. Green, N.M. (1990) Avidin and streptavidin. *Methods Enzymol.*, **184**, 51–67.
102. Cheng, C., Wei, H., Zhu, J.L., Chang, C., Cheng, H., Li, C., Cheng, S.X., Zhang, X.Z., and Zhuo, R.X. (2008) Functionalized thermoresponsive micelles self-assembled from biotin-PEG-*b*-P(NIPAAm-*co*-HMAAm)-*b*-PMMA for tumor cell target. *Bioconjug. Chem.*, **19**, 1194–1201.
103. Laitinen, O.H., Airenne, K.J., Raty, J.K., Wirth, T., and Yla-Herttuala, S.Y. (2005) Avidin fusion protein strategies in targeted drug and gene delivery. *Lett. Drug Des. Discov.*, **2**, 124–132.
104. Ouchi, T., Yamabe, E., Hara, K., Hirai, M., and Ohya, Y. (2004) Design of attachment type of drug delivery system by complex formation of avidin with biotinyl drug model and biotinyl saccharide. *J. Control. Release*, **94**, 281–291.
105. Pulkkinen, M., Pikkarainen, J., Wirth, T., Tarvainen, T., Haapa-Acho, V., Korhonen, H., Seppala, J., and Jarvinen, K. (2008) Three-step tumor targeting of paclitaxel using biotinylated PLA–PEG nanoparticles and avidin–biotin technology: formulation development and *in vitro* anticancer activity. *Eur. J. Pharm. Biopharm.*, **70**, 66–74.
106. Su, F.M., Beaumier, P., Axworthy, D., Atcher, R., and Fritzberg, A. (2005) Pretargeted radioimmunotherapy in tumored mice using an *in vivo* Pb-212/Bi-212 generator. *Nucl. Med. Biol.*, **32**, 741–747.
107. Xiao, Z., McQuarrie, S.A., Suresh, M.R., Mercer, J.R., Gupta, S., and Miller, G.G. (2002) A three-step strategy for targeting drug carriers to human ovarian carcinoma cells *in vitro*. *J. Biotechnol.*, **94**, 171–184.
108. Tseng, C.L., Wang, T.W., Dong, C.C., Wu, S.Y.H., Young, T.H., Shieh, M.J., Lou, P.J., and Lin, F.H. (2007) Development of gelatin nanoparticles with biotinylated EGF conjugation for lung cancer targeting. *Biomaterials*, **28**, 3996–4005.
109. Knox, S.J., Goris, M.L., Tempero, M., Weiden, P.L., Gentner, L., Breitz, H., Adams, G.P., Axworthy, D., Gaffigan, S., Bryan, K., Fisher, D.R., Colcher, D., Horak, I.D., and Weiner, L.M. (2000) Phase II trial of yttrium-90-DOTA-biotin pretargeted by NR-LU-10 antibody/streptavidin in patients with metastatic colon cancer. *Clin. Cancer Res.*, **6**, 406–414.
110. Chen, S.Y., Zhao, X.R., Chen, J.Y., Chen, J., Kuznetsova, L., Wong, S.S., and Ojima, I. (2010) Mechanism-based tumor-targeting drug delivery system. Validation of efficient vitamin receptor-mediated endocytosis and drug release. *Bioconjug. Chem.*, **21**, 979–987.
111. Zuniga, E.S., Shah, P., Reimer, A., and Ojima, I. (2010) Towards novel tumor-targeting anticancer drug conjugates, MEDI 381. 239th ACS National Meeting General Poster Session, San Francisco, CA, abstract 344916.
112. Yokota, T., Nishina, K., Mizusawa, H., and Unno, T. (2009) System for delivering nucleic acids for suppressing target gene expression bu utilizing endogenous chylormicron. WIPO WO2009069313.
113. Yan, G., Wang, X., and Mei, L. (2008) Vitamin B6 as liver-targeting group in drug delivery, in *Vitamin B* (ed. C. Elliot), Nova Science, Hauppauge, NY, pp. 153–174.
114. Yan, G.P., Zhuo, R.X., and Zheng, C.Y. (2001) Study on the anticancer drug 5-fluorouracil-conjugated polyaspartamide containing hepatocyte-targeting group. *J. Bioact. Compat. Polym.*, **16**, 277–293.
115. Carpenter, G. and Cohen, S. (1990) Epidermal growth factor. *J. Biol. Chem.*, **265**, 7709–7712.
116. King, A.C. and Cuatrecasas, P. (1982) Resolution of high and low affinity epidermal growth factor receptors. Inhibition of high affinity component by low temperature, cycloheximide, and phorbol esters. *J. Biol. Chem.*, **257**, 3053–3060.
117. Gregory, H. (1975) Isolation and structure of urogastrone and its relationship to epidermal growth factor. *Nature*, **257**, 325–327.

s

118. Ullrich, A., Coussens, L., Hayflick, J.S., Dull, T.J., Gray, A., Tam, A.W., Lee, J., Yarden, Y., Libermann, T.A., Schlessinger, J., Downward, J., Mayes, E.L.V., Whittle, N., Waterfield, M.D., and Seeburg, P.H. (1984) Human epidermal growth factor receptor cDNA sequence and aberrant expression of the amplified gene in A431 epidermoid carcinoma cells. *Nature*, **309**, 418–425.
119. Ogiso, H., Ishitani, R., Nureki, O., Fukai, S., Yamanaka, M., Kim, J.H., Saito, K., Sakamoto, A., Inoue, M., Shirouzu, M., and Yokoyama, S. (2002) Crystal structure of the complex of human epidermal growth factor and receptor extracellular domains. *Cell*, **110**, 775–787.
120. Waterman, H. and Yarden, Y. (2001) Molecular mechanisms underlying endocytosis and sorting of ErbB receptor tyrosine kinases. *FEBS Lett.*, **490**, 142–152.
121. Guex, N. and Peitsch, M.C. (1997) SWISS-MODEL and the Swiss-PdbViewer: an environment for comparative protein modeling. *Electrophoresis*, **18**, 2714–2723.
122. Salomon, D.S., Brandt, R., Ciardiello, F., and Normanno, N. (1995) Epidermal growth factor-related peptides and their receptors in human malignancies. *Crit. Rev. Oncol. Hematol.*, **19**, 183–232.
123. Phillips, G.D.L., Li, G.M., Dugger, D.L., Crocker, L.M., Parsons, K.L., Mai, E., Blattler, W.A., Lambert, J.M., Chari, R.V.J., Lutz, R.J., Wong, W.L.T., Jacobson, F.S., Koeppen, H., Schwall, R.H., Kenkare-Mitra, S.R., Spencer, S.D., and Sliwkowski, M.X. (2008) Targeting HER2-positive breast cancer with Trastuzumab-DM1, an antibody-cytotoxic drug conjugate. *Cancer Res.*, **68**, 9280–9290.
124. Ojima, I. (2008) Guided molecular missiles for tumor-targeting chemotherapy – case studies using the second-generation taxolds as warheads. *Acc. Chem. Res.*, **41**, 108–119.
125. Lutsenko, S.V., Feldman, N.B., and Severin, S.E. (2002) Cytotoxic and antitumor activities of doxorubicin conjugates with the epidermal growth factor and its receptor-binding fragment. *J. Drug Target.*, **10**, 567–571.
126. Li, Z.H., Zhao, R.J., Wu, X.H., Sun, Y., Yao, M., Li, J.J., Xu, Y.H., and Gu, J.R. (2005) Identification and characterization of a novel peptide ligand of epidermal growth factor receptor for targeted delivery of therapeutics. *FASEB J.*, **19**, 1978–1985.
127. Song, S., Liu, D., Peng, J., Deng, H., Guo, Y., Xu, L.X., Miller, A.D., and Xu, Y. (2009) Novel peptide ligand directs liposomes toward EGF-R high-expressing cancer cells *in vitro* and *in vivo*. *FASEB J.*, **23**, 1396–1404.
128. Cawley, D.B., Herschman, H.R., Gilliland, D.G., and Collier, R.J. (1980) Epidermal growth factor–toxin A chain conjugates – EGF–ricin-A is a potent toxin while EGF–diphtheria fragment-A is nontoxic. *Cell*, **22**, 563–570.
129. Simpson, D.L., Cawley, D.B., and Herschman, H.R. (1982) Killing of cultured-hepatocytes by conjugates of asialofetuin and EGF linked to the A-chains of ricin or diphtheria-toxin. *Cell*, **29**, 469–473.
130. Shimizu, N., Miskimins, W.K., and Shimizu, Y. (1980) A cytotoxic epidermal growth-factor cross-linked to diphtheria toxin-A-fragment. *FEBS Lett.*, **118**, 274–278.
131. Yoon, J.M., Han, S.H., Kown, O.B., Kim, S.H., Park, M.H., and Kim, B.K. (1999) Cloning and cytotoxicity of fusion proteins of EGF and angiogenin. *Life Sci.*, **64**, 1435–1445.
132. Lappi, D.A., Martineau, D., and Baird, A. (1989) Biological and chemical characterization of basic FGF–saporin mitotoxin. *Biochem. Biophys. Res. Commun.*, **160**, 917–923.
133. Beitz, J.G., Davol, P., Clark, J.W., Kato, J., Medina, M., Frackelton, A.R., Lappi, D.A., Baird, A., and Calabresi, P. (1992) Antitumor-activity of basic fibroblast growth factor–saporin mitotoxin *in vitro* and *in vivo*. *Cancer Res.*, **52**, 227–230.
134. Veenendaal, L.M., Jin, H., Ran, S., Cheung, L., Navone, N., Marks, J.W., Waltenberger, J., Thorpe, P., and

Rosenblum, M.G. (2002) *In vitro* and *in vivo* studies of a VEGF121/rGelonin chimeric fusion toxin targeting the neovasculature of solid tumors. *Proc. Natl. Acad. Sci. USA*, **99**, 7866–7871.

135. Liu, T.F., Cohen, K.A., Ramage, J.G., Willingham, M.C., Thorburn, A.M., and Frankel, A.E. (2003) A diphtheria toxin–epidermal growth factor fusion protein is cytotoxic to human glioblastoma multiform cells. *Cancer Res.*, **63**, 1834–1837.

136. Ho, M.-C., Sturm, M.B., Almo, S.C., and Schramm, V.L. (2009) Transition state analogues in structures of ricin and saporin ribosome-inactivating proteins. *Proc. Natl. Acad. Sci. USA*, **106**, 20276–20281.

137. Tseng, C.L., Su, W.Y., Yen, K.C., Yang, K.C., and Lin, F.H. (2009) The use of biotinylated-EGF-modified gelatin nanoparticle carrier to enhance cisplatin accumulation in cancerous lungs via inhalation. *Biomaterials*, **30**, 3476–3485.

138. Bhirde, A.A., Patel, V., Gavard, J., Zhang, G.F., Sousa, A.A., Masedunskas, A., Leapman, R.D., Weigert, R., Gutkind, J.S., and Rusling, J.F. (2009) Targeted killing of cancer cells *in vivo* and *in vitro* with EGF-directed carbon nanotube-based drug delivery. *ACS Nano*, **3**, 307–316.

139. Mamot, C., Drummond, D.C., Greiser, U., Hong, K., Kirpotin, D.B., Marks, J.D., and Park, J.W. (2003) Epidermal growth factor receptor (EGFR)-targeted immunoliposomes mediate specific and efficient drug delivery to EGFR- and EGFRvIII-overexpressing tumor cells. *Cancer Res.*, **63**, 3154–3161.

140. Mamot, C., Drummond, D.C., Noble, C.O., Kallab, V., Guo, Z., Hong, K., Kirpotin, D.B., and Park, J.W. (2005) Epidermal growth factor receptor-targeted immunoliposomes significantly enhance the efficacy of multiple anticancer drugs *in vivo*. *Cancer Res.*, **65**, 11631–11638.

141. Bermbach, U. and Faulstich, H. (1990) Epidermal growth-factor labeled beta-amanitin poly-L-ornithine – preparation and evidence for specific cytotoxicity. *Biochemistry*, **29**, 6839–6845.

142. McTavish, H., Griffin, R.J., Terai, K., and Dudek, A.Z. (2009) Novel insulin-like growth factor–methotrexate covalent conjugate inhibits tumor growth *in vivo* at lower dosage than methotrexate alone. *Trans. Res.*, **153**, 275–282.

143. Laajoki, L.G., Francis, G.L., Wallace, J.C., Carver, J.A., and Keniry, M.A. (2000) Solution structure and backbone dynamics of long-[Arg(3)]insulin-like growth factor-I. *J. Biol. Chem.*, **275**, 10009–10015.

144. Andersson, A., Capala, J., and Carlsson, J. (1992) Effects of EGF–dextran–tyrosine-^{131}I conjugates on the clonogenic survival of cultured glioma cells. *J. Neuro-Oncol.*, **14**, 213–223.

145. Gijsens, A., Missiaen, L., Merlevede, W., and de Witte, P. (2000) Epidermal growth factor-mediated targeting of chlorin e6 selectively potentiates its photodynamic activity. *Cancer Res.*, **60**, 2197–2202.

146. Yayon, A., Aviezer, D., Safran, M., Gross, J.L., Heldman, Y., Cabilly, S., Givol, D., and Katchalski-Katzir, E. (1993) Isolation of peptides that inhibit binding of basic fibroblast growth factor to its receptor from a random phage-epitope library. *Proc. Natl. Acad. Sci. USA*, **90**, 10643–10647.

147. Terada, T., Mizobata, M., Kawakami, S., Yabe, Y., Yamashita, F., and Hashida, M. (2006) Basic fibroblast growth factor-binding peptide as a novel targeting ligand of drug carrier to tumor cells. *J. Drug Target.*, **14**, 536–545.

41
Drug Conjugates with Polyunsaturated Fatty Acids

Joshua Seitz and Iwao Ojima

41.1
Introduction

Polyunsaturated fatty acids (PUFAs) are a major class of biochemicals that are utilized as cellular membrane components, energy sources, and signaling molecules. It has been shown that PUFAs distinctly affect a number of cellular processes involved in human diseases. Based on the fact that PUFA uptake is substantially elevated in malignant tissues, numerous PUFA–drug conjugates have been investigated and are currently in all stages of drug development. Conjugation of PUFAs to cytotoxic drugs has proven to be an effective method for delivering the drugs to tumors, which increases the efficacy *in vivo* and considerably decreases serious side-effects. The role of PUFAs in cancer progression and control, potential benefits of their conjugation to chemotherapeutic agents, and actual efficacy of these PUFA–drug conjugates demonstrated in preclinical and clinical trials will be discussed in this chapter.

41.2
Rationale for the Potential Benefits of PUFA Conjugation to Chemotherapeutic Drugs

Conjugation of cytotoxic drugs to PUFAs has been found to drastically change the pharmacokinetics and distribution of the drugs, resulting in specific accumulation of the drugs in tumor tissues and cells. The PUFA component of a drug conjugate readily binds to human serum albumin (HSA) to form a HSA–drug conjugate complex, which solubilizes the hydrophobic drug conjugate, lowers the rate of clearance, and enhances tumor-specific accumulation of the drug conjugate. It has been shown that glycoprotein 60 (gp60) and "secreted protein acidic and rich in cysteine" (SPARC) play a key role in the tumor-specific transport of HSA-bound nutrients as well as drugs from the tumor blood vessels to the tumor interstitium via caveolae and the containment of the drug in the tumor interstitium (Figure 41.1), as exemplified by Abraxane® (HSA-bound paclitaxel nanoparticles) [1–3]. Based on the findings that certain PUFAs are avidly taken up by tumor cells, it is very

Drug Delivery in Oncology: From Basic Research to Cancer Therapy, First Edition.
Edited by Felix Kratz, Peter Senter, and Henning Steinhagen.

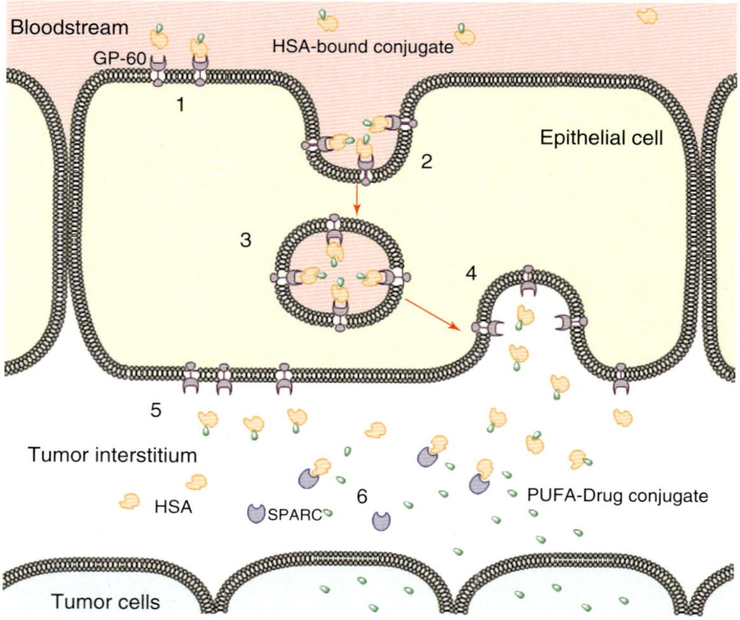

Figure 41.1 gp60-mediated transcytosis. (1) HSA (orange) bound to drug conjugate (green) travels through the bloodstream and binds to gp60 (purple) on the tumor epithelial cell surface. (2) Ligand binding initiates transcytosis. (3) Vesicles containing drug conjugate–protein complex are transported across the cell. (4) Fusion of the vesicle to the interstitial cell wall occurs. (5) Drug conjugate–HSA complex is released into the tumor interstitium. (6) Binding of SPARC (blue) to HSA causes release of free drug conjugate, which permeates into tumor cells.

likely that PUFA–drug conjugates would also be greedily accumulated into the tumor cells, wherein the PUFA–drug linkage is cleaved to release the free drug and PUFA. A substantial body of evidence suggests that once inside the tumor cells, certain PUFAs and their metabolites affect a number of signaling pathways, resulting in synergism with various cytotoxic drugs. Therefore, it is anticipated that conjugation of cytotoxic drugs to PUFAs results in not only tumor-specific accumulation of the drug, but also that of the PUFA and its metabolites, which may further enhance the efficacy of the drug.

41.2.1
PUFAs in Cancer Progression and Control

Pronounced effects of dietary PUFA intake on cancer development and progression have been demonstrated; most notably, the ratio of certain PUFAs present in the diet can lead to either a stimulation or inhibition of cancer growth *in vitro* and *in vivo* [4]. For instance, populations that consume significant amounts of n–3 PUFAs, such as docosahexaenoic acid (DHA) and eicosapentaenoic acid (EPA), have lower cancer incidents than populations with a diet rich in n–6 PUFAs, such as linoleic acid (LA) and arachidonic acid (AA) [5]. Deep-water fish and fish oil are typically high in n–3 PUFAs, whereas n–6 PUFAs are found in terrestrial plants such as corn and olive oil, as well as the animals fed from these plants, such as chicken and cattle. The biochemical and physiological reasons for these trends in cancer incident rates are rapidly emerging as more detailed information has been disclosed for PUFA transport, internalization, metabolism, and their effects on cellular signaling.

41.2.2
Effects of PUFA Internalization on Membrane Composition and Signaling

Although there has been some debate as to the mechanism of PUFA internalization, a more cohesive model is emerging, with an increasing body of evidence that suggests a hybrid of the passive diffusion and enzyme-assisted processes [6] (Figure 41.2). Free PUFAs are transported through the bloodstream primarily by HSA and related binding proteins, where they are carried to the capillaries at the outer extremities of the cardiovascular system. It has been shown that the transcytosis of HSA-bound nutrients as well as drugs from the blood capillaries to the interstitial tissues is mediated by gp60 [1]. Once in the extracellular space, the PUFA is slowly released from albumin (or swiftly by the action of SPARC in tumor tissues) and subsequently desorbed into the external membrane of the cell. Once embedded in the membrane, PUFAs penetrate into the inner leaflet of

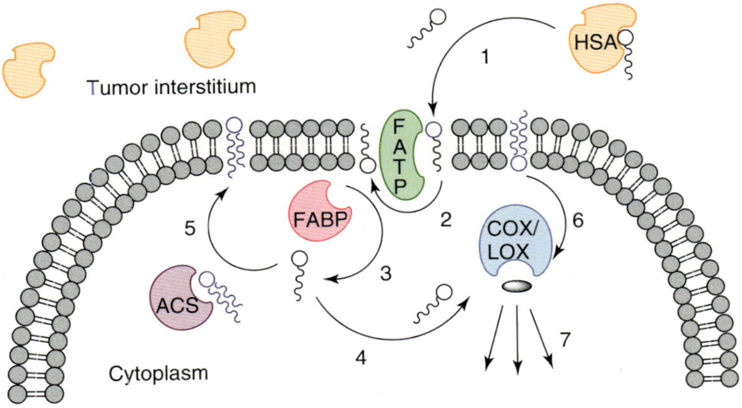

Figure 41.2 Schematic illustration of PUFA internalization. (1) PUFAs (black) are released from HSA (orange) and passively embed into the lipid membrane (gray). (2) "Flip-flop" process is assisted by FATPs (green), resulting in PUFAs on the inner membrane leaflet. (3) PUFAs are excised by FABPs (pink) into the cytoplasm. (4) Free PUFAs are metabolized into a number of signaling molecules. (5) Alternatively, PUFAs are incorporated into phospholipids (dark blue) by ACS (purple) and returned to the membrane. (6) PUFA-containing phospholipids are excised and metabolized. (7) PUFAs and their metabolites serve as signaling mediators causing numerous downstream events.

the membrane by a "flip-flop" process [6]. This process may also occur actively with the help of membrane fatty acid transport proteins (FATPs) – a family of proteins with at least seven members, each with a distinctive tissue distribution pattern [7]. When overexpressed, these proteins increase PUFA internalization in an ATP-dependent manner. Once PUFAs are embedded in the inner leaflet, fatty acid binding proteins (FABPs) remove them from the membrane, allowing metabolism into endogenous signaling molecules or phospholipid components of the membrane [8]. There is no appreciable difference in the internalization rates of different PUFAs through binding to individual members of the FABP family [9]. However, it has been shown that acyl-CoA synthetases (ACSs) that incorporate PUFAs into phospholipids are partially selective in certain tissues. For example, overexpression of ACS2 in neurons is correlated to the enhanced neurite outgrowth and internalization of AA and DHA. This suggests that ACS2 enzyme is responsible for the existence of a relatively large proportion of these PUFAs in the membrane of growing neurites compared to other cell types [10].

When incorporated into the cellular membranes as phospholipids, PUFAs change the physical properties of membranes, such as fluidity and the structural composition of lipid rafts [11]. Lipid rafts are microdomains within the fluid mosaic of the membrane, rich in cholesterol and sphingolipids. There are a number of cell surface receptors that localize in these rafts (caveolae), which allow aggregation and activation or inactivation of the protein in question, wherein the extent of actions depends on the PUFA composition of the raft (caveola) [12]. For example, by altering the composition of these lipid rafts, EPA and DHA were found to lower the proportion of epidermal growth factor receptor (EGFR) in caveolae, leading to subsequent phosphorylation and activation of this receptor [11]. It sounds rather peculiar, but it has been reported that this particular way of EGFR activation leads to apoptosis of human breast cancer cells [11]. Even when acting as structural components, the composition of PUFAs internalized into the cell may lead to major alterations in certain signaling pathways and their downstream effectors. In addition, PUFAs are metabolized into a number of small molecules with profound and diverse consequences on many aspects of cellular development and homeostasis [4, 5, 13, 14].

41.2.3
Suppression of Tumor-Promoting Eicosanoid Biosynthesis by PUFAs

Eicosanoids are 20-carbon short-term signaling molecules metabolically derived from certain PUFAs such as AA, α-linolenic acid (LNA), LA, and EPA. These compounds control and modulate a myriad of biological processes, including cellular growth, differentiation, adhesion, platelet aggregation, inflammation, and angiogenesis [4, 5, 15–18]. The biosynthesis of eicosanoids proceeds as PUFAs are taken up from the membrane bilayer by phospholipases and subsequently modified. Metabolic enzymes that act on PUFAs to produce eicosanoids include cyclooxygenases (COXs) (producing thromboxanes and prostaglandins), lipoxygenases (LOXs) (producing leukotrienes, hydroxy fatty acids, and lipoxins), and cytochrome P450

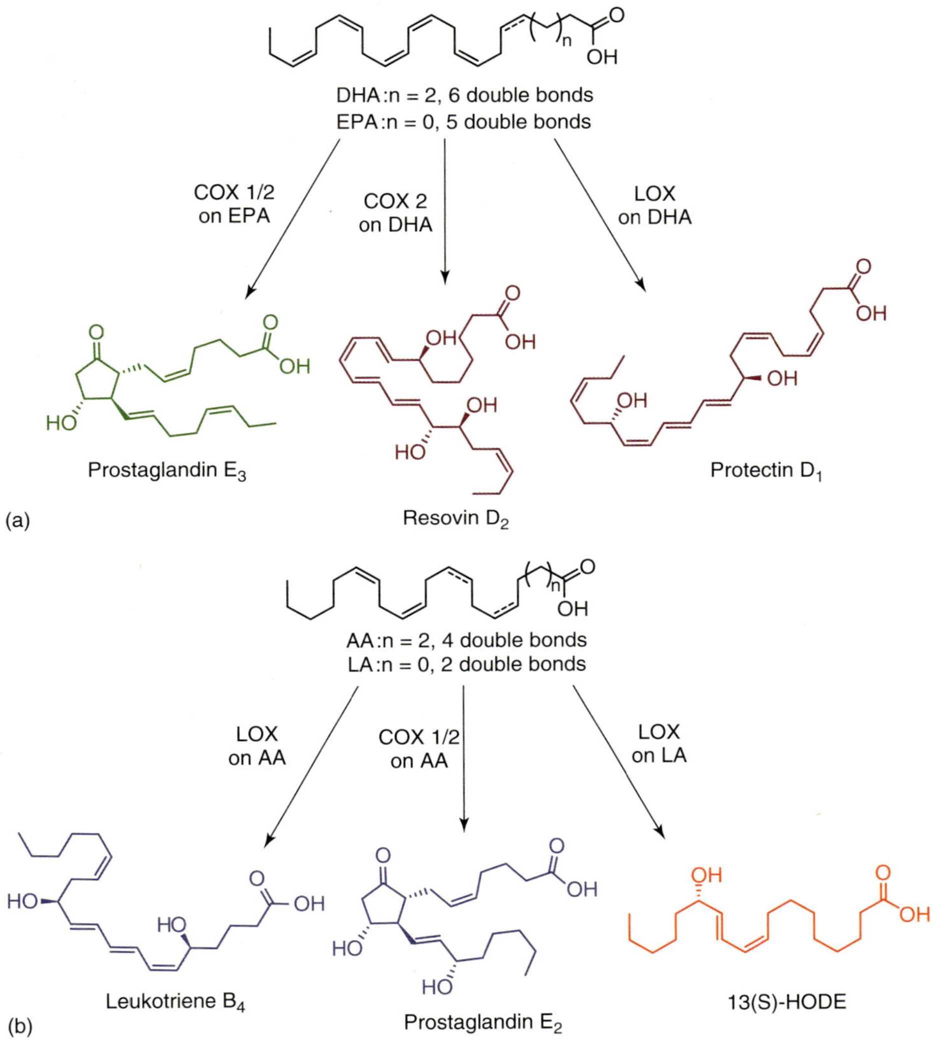

Figure 41.3 Structures of some metabolites relevant to cancer progression derived from: (a) *n*−3 PUFAs DHA (green) and EPA (purple), and (b) *n*−6 PUFAs AA (blue) and LA (red) by the action of LOX and COX 1/2 enzymes.

monooxygenases (producing hydroxy, dihydroxy, and epoxy fatty acids) [5, 19, 20] (Figure 41.3). The regulation of specific eicosanoid production is determined by the type of cells as well as the composition of PUFAs in the membrane that are available for metabolism.

Eicosanoids that are derived from *n*−3 PUFAs generally exhibit an inhibitory effect on inflammation and tumor growth, whereas those from *n*−6 PUFAs produce opposite results [21]. For example, prostaglandin E_2 (PGE_2), derived from AA, a $n-6$ PUFA, through metabolism by COX-1 and COX-2, aids in tumorigenesis through promoting cellular division, angiogenesis, as well as through inhibition of apoptosis [14]. Leukotriene B_4, another AA-derived eicosanoid, is implicated in the generation of reactive oxygen species (ROS) and the modulation of cellular adhesion, which may lead to carcinogenesis and metastasis, respectively [22, 23]. It has been shown that 13-hydroxyoctadecadienoic acid (13-HODE), a metabolite of LA, promotes tumor growth and cell proliferation as indicated by enhanced ^{3}H-thymidine incorporation *in vitro* and *in vivo* [21, 24]. In contrast, the addition of $n-3$ PUFAs was shown to inhibit cellular growth through the competitive inhibition of LOXs involved in 13-HODE synthesis [21, 25]. In addition to eicosanoids, $n-3$ PUFAs are metabolized into resolvins and protectins [26], which exhibit potent anti-inflammatory activity that may impede tumor growth due to the close ties between inflammation and cancer [27].

It has been revealed that $n-3$ PUFAs inhibit the production of carcinogenic eicosanoids derived from $n-6$ PUFAs through various mechanisms [4, 5, 28]. An increased ratio of $n-3/n-6$ PUFAs in the diet usually translates to a greater proportion of $n-3$ PUFAs in cellular membranes. This effectively increases the frequency that $n-3$ PUFAs are removed from the membrane, thus leading to a greater intracellular concentration of free $n-3$ PUFAs and their metabolites [29]. Since both $n-3$ and $n-6$ PUFAs share common enzymes in their metabolic pathways, competitive inhibition occurs between the two groups. The increased intracellular concentration of $n-3$ PUFAs leads to a reduction in $n-6$ PUFA-derived eicosanoids [5, 25, 30]. Eicosanoids derived from $n-6$ and $n-3$ PUFAs have contradictory effects on the expression levels of COX enzymes, and the production of prostaglandins, which indicates that the signals generated by metabolites of $n-3$ PUFAs regulate the biosynthesis of tumorigenic molecules derived from LA and AA at a transcriptional level [31, 32]. Furthermore, $n-3$ PUFAs appear to accelerate the catabolism of $n-6$ PUFA-derived eicosanoids, reducing their intracellular half-life and their ability to propagate growth-promoting signals [33]. These mechanisms of inhibition suggest a complex network wherein PUFA metabolism balances many key biological processes commonly involved in carcinogenesis [33].

41.2.4
Influences of PUFAs on Signal Transduction Pathways and Gene Expression

The signal transduction network in the cell has essential functions as a complex regulatory system that converges in the nucleus, and ultimately shapes the genetic and epigenetic landscape that controls gene transcription. Cancer is inherently a disease wherein this regulatory system fails through a series of malfunctions, leading to uncontrolled cell growth, disconnection from extracellular signals of the host, and invasion into surrounding tissues. A number of transcription factors, which regulate the expression of many genes involved in cellular growth, division, adhesion, and apoptosis, have been implicated in cancer progression by either

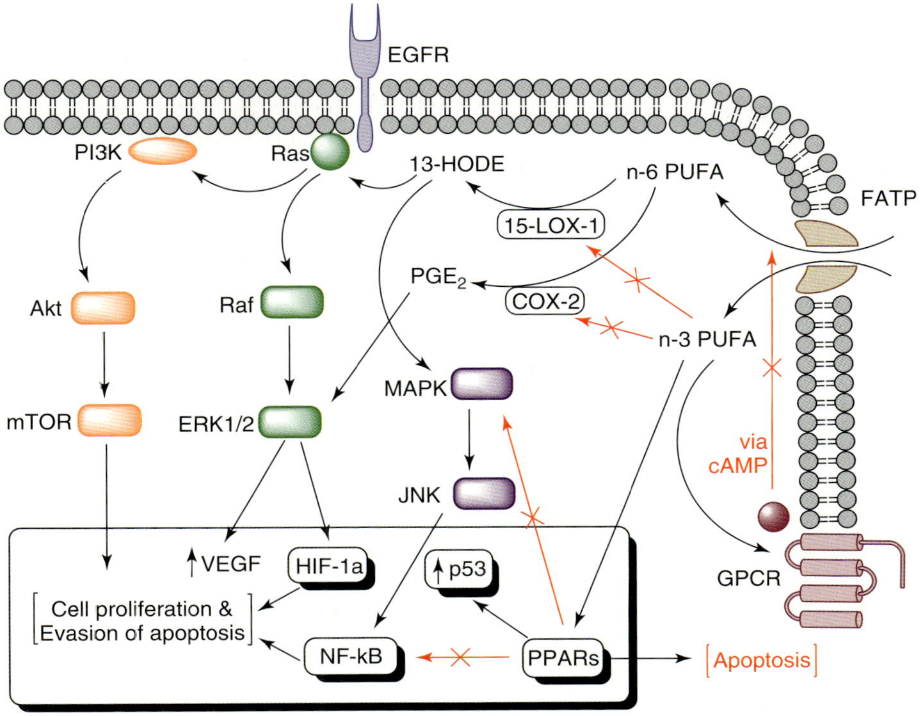

Figure 41.4 Pathways under the influence of PUFAs and their metabolites: *n*–3 PUFAs compete for COX and LOX binding, lowering the intracellular concentrations of 13-HODE and PGE_2, respectively. Reduced levels of these metabolites translate to decreased activation of the Ras–Raf–ERK1/2 pathway (green). 13-HODE levels also affect the phosphoinositide 3-kinase–Akt–mTOR cell survival pathway (orange) as well as MAPK–JNK pathway (purple), which are involved in the evasion of apoptosis. By binding to G-protein-coupled receptors (light purple), *n*–3 PUFAs have been shown to inhibit *n*–6 PUFA uptake in a cAMP-dependent manner, enhancing the previously described effects. PPARs also bind *n*–3 PUFAs, and have been shown to inhibit MAPK and NF-κB transcription. The net effect is the downregulation of proliferative genes and the initiation of apoptosis in the cancer cell.

upregulation or downregulation of their target genes. It has been shown that many of signal transduction pathways and transcription factors that are commonly found in tumor cells are under the influence of PUFAs and their metabolites [4, 5, 34, 35] (Figure 41.4).

Extracellular signal-regulated kinase 1/2 (ERK1/2) function as signaling proteins that are involved in the inhibition of apoptosis, and are highly activated in numerous cancers, including breast and pancreatic cancers, as well as melanoma [36–38]. LA metabolite, 13-HODE, has been implicated in the cAMP-induced phosphorylation and activation of ERK1/2 in the MCF-7 breast cancer cell line, and DHA and EPA have been shown to inhibit this process [24, 25]. ERK1/2 are downstream of the

Ras oncogenic protein family, which is overexpressed in numerous cancers and involved in cellular proliferation [39]. Ras activation, not expression, was found to be differently affected by LA and DHA in colonocytes, and DHA leads to a reduction in Ras membrane localization, GTP binding, and subsequent ERK1/2 phosphorylations [24]. The ERK1/2 pathway has been implicated in drug resistance, which can be inhibited by $n-3$ PUFAs. This may be contributing to the synergy observed between $n-3$ PUFAs and a variety of cytotoxic agents.

The nuclear transcription factor κB (NF−κB) family regulates the expression of numerous genes involved in cell cycle regulation, cellular adhesion, inflammation, apoptosis, and cytokine signaling [40]. Drastic activation of NF−κB has been observed in a variety of cancer cell lines, which occurs through the "Jun N-terminal kinase" (JNK) pathway, leading to the upregulation of the antiapoptotic proteins Bcl-2, Bcl-X_L, and "inhibitor of apoptosis" [41]. Activation of NF−κB in murine macrophages was decreased by the presence of $n-3$ PUFAs [42]. Therefore, the modulation of NF−κB activity is another potential mechanism, through which $n-3$ PUFAs exert their drug-sensitizing and anticancer effects.

Peroxisome proliferator-activated receptors (PPARs) are a family of transcription factors that directly bind various PUFAs, causing ligand-activated gene expression [43]. Each member of the PPAR family binds a specific subset of PUFAs, leading to different gene expression corresponding to a variety of effects, such as lipid transport and metabolism, anti-inflammatory response, cell cycle regulation, and apoptosis [43]. For example, PPARγ binds a number of $n-3$ and $n-6$ PUFAs, as well as selected metabolites that promote apoptosis by binding NF−κB and increasing the expression of p53 [44]. The activation of PPARγ has been implicated in $n-3$ PUFA-induced apoptosis in MCF-7 and Reh cell lines [45, 46]. Another member of this family, PPARα, is activated by DHA in vascular smooth muscle cells, leading to apoptosis via an intrinsic pathway that involves mitogen-activated protein kinase (MAPK), Bax, and cytochrome *c* [47]. It has been indicated that the activation of PPARα is involved in the synergy observed between clioquinol and DHA for the treatment of an ovarian cancer cell line, A2780 [48].

A number of proteins, whose expression profiles are affected by the $n-3$ and $n-6$ PUFA levels, have previously been implicated in the progression and development of cancer [37–40, 45]. It has been shown that the vascular endothelial growth factor (VEGF) receptor, typically involved in angiogenesis for neoplastic growth and a biomarker for poor clinical outcome, is down-regulated via the COX-2/PGE_2 pathway in human colon cancer cell line HT-29 treated with $n-3$ PUFAs [34]. Other relevant proteins whose activities are modulated by PUFA levels include, but are not limited to, the transcription factor c-Myc, cyclins and their dependent kinases, retinoid X receptor, protein kinases C and A, Akt, and mammalian target of rapamycin (mTOR) [49–52]. A comprehensive overview of the current knowledge regarding the various biological pathways affected by PUFAs is beyond the scope of this chapter. Nevertheless, it is evident from these examples that PUFAs and their metabolites have diverse and far-reaching effects on cell-signaling pathways involved in many biological functions.

41.2.5
PUFA Peroxidation and ROS

Although there are enzymes that are responsible for the specific oxidation of PUFAs, it has been suggested that a majority of PUFA peroxidation occurs independently by free radicals within the cytoplasm. The formation of DNA–PUFA adducts and reactive PUFA-derived aldehydes, such as *trans*-4-hydroxy-2-nonenal and malondialdehyde, has been shown to lead to carcinogenesis *in vitro* [53]. The rate of PUFA autooxidation in atmosphere has been shown to correlate with the number of unsaturations in the molecule [54]. However, there is substantial evidence that PUFA peroxidation *in vitro* may not correlate to that *in vivo* [55]. For example, mice that were fed with a diet rich in fish oil were shown to upregulate the expression of certain antioxidant enzymes, including glutathione transferases and manganese superoxide dismutase, which suggests that certain PUFAs may actually protect the organism from oxidative damage [55]. Since PUFAs and their metabolites work to modulate a multitude of biological functions, it is possible that they play a cytoprotective role besides being substrates for direct oxidation and generation of ROS.

The presence of vitamin E, a potent antioxidant, was found to decrease the growth inhibition of cancer cells by PUFA, which suggests that oxidized products of n−3 PUFAs suppress tumor growth [56]. The generation of ROS has been implicated in the initiation of apoptosis, and it is possible that PUFA oxidation products may be involved in the generation and propagation of radical chain reactions that lead to the initiation of the apoptotic cascade. Release of cytochrome *c* from the mitochondrial membrane, a key step in the apoptotic cascade, has been shown to occur during heavy mitochondrial peroxidation of PUFAs [57]. It is likely that these effects occur alongside those previously listed, each at varying degrees, in the PUFA-induced tumor growth inhibition and apoptosis.

41.2.6
Synergy of Cytotoxic Drugs and PUFAs for the Treatment of Cancer Cell Lines

Failures in the regulatory networks of signaling pathways involved in apoptosis and cell cycle progression are common hallmarks of cancer, which are also largely responsible for the ability of many drug-resistant cell lines to survive chemotherapy. Certain PUFAs have been shown to moderate these malfunctions in a dose-dependent manner for many of the signaling pathways implicated in drug resistance [34, 42, 48, 58]. Since some PUFAs modulate diverse processes such as inflammation, cellular adhesion, and metabolism, it has been suggested that treatment with dietary PUFAs during the administration of chemotherapeutic drugs may help protect healthy tissues in addition to increasing the efficacy of the drugs against malignant tumor growth [59]. Therefore, it is not surprising that synergy has been observed when PUFAs are coadministered with cytotoxic drugs against a wide variety of cancer cell lines [48, 60, 61]. For the SGC7901 gastric cancer cell line, DHA was found to exhibit a synergistic effect with 5-fluorouracil

(5-FU, 40 μg/ml of each) and a similar effect was observed with clioquinol (5 μM with 100 μM DHA) against the human ovarian cancer cell line A2780 [48, 60]. Synergism was also observed between EPA and the angiogenesis inhibitor, TNP-470 (EPA, 221 μg/ml: TNP-470, 34.2 μg/ml), as well as the tyrosine kinase inhibitor, genistein (genistein, 93 and 176 μM: EPA, 211 and 609 μM, respectively), against two breast cancer cell lines [61, 62]. A similar synergistic effect has also been reported for coadministration of γ-LNA with vinorelbine or paclitaxel using comparable concentrations of PUFA [63, 64]. Increase in efficacy by coadministration of PUFAs has been demonstrated with a number of other drugs, including, but not limited to, doxorubicin (DOX), mitomycin C, and tamoxifen [65–67]. These unique properties of PUFAs that lead to synergistic cytotoxicity against malignant tissues, combined with their potential as tumor-targeting components, make them highly attractive candidates for drug conjugation and tumor-targeted therapy.

41.3 Drug Conjugates with PUFAs

The conjugation of cytotoxic drugs with PUFAs is an attractive strategy for novel drug development because of the following reasons: (i) PUFAs are US Food and Drug Administration-approved food additives and therefore are nontoxic, (ii) some PUFAs possess cancer-specific toxicity via a myriad of signaling pathways overexpressed in various cancers, (iii) synergism has been observed with a variety of cytotoxic drugs against various cancer cell lines, (iv) PUFAs appear to have protective effects on healthy cells by preventing drug-induced apoptosis, and (v) conjugation may limit systemic toxicity by altering the pharmacokinetic properties of the cytotoxic drugs. For example, as HSA is the primary carrier for PUFAs in the bloodstream, the conjugation of drugs to PUFAs would increase their affinity to HSA, likely leading to enhanced tumor-specific accumulation of the drug conjugates through transcytosis into the tumor interstitium via gp60, followed by drug conjugate release from HSA through interaction with SPARC [3]. Also, tumor cells tend to rapidly divide and thus require an increased level of PUFA uptake for metabolism into signaling molecules or ATP production [21]. Various compounds with proven anticancer activity have recently been conjugated to certain PUFAs, and are currently involved in various stages of preclinical and clinical developments (Figure 41.5).

41.3.1 DHA–Paclitaxel and PUFA–Second-Generation Taxoid Conjugates (1)

Paclitaxel, a member of the taxane family of diterpenoids, was first isolated from the bark of the North American pacific yew tree in the early 1970s, and has since been approved for treatment of a number of malignancies including breast, ovarian, prostate, and non-small-cell lung cancers (NSCLCs) as well as Kaposi's sarcoma (Figure 41.5) [68–70]. Paclitaxel exerts its potent cytotoxicity

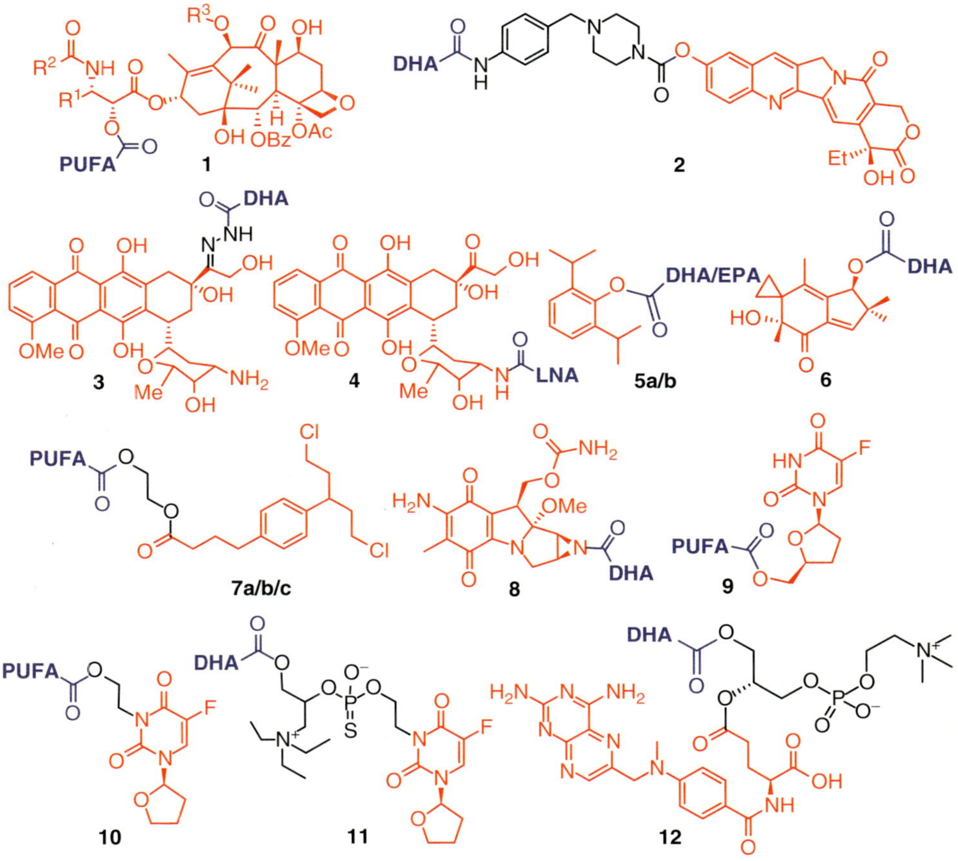

Figure 41.5 Structures of PUFA–drug conjugates: the cytotoxic drug component is depicted in red, the linker (if applicable) in black, and the PUFA component in blue.

through binding to β-tubulin, hyperstabilizing microtubules, and impairing the dynamic instability of the microtubule framework. This causes cell cycle arrest and initiation of apoptosis at the G_2/M stage [71, 72]. In order to manage its poor aqueous solubility, numerous formulations as well as prodrugs of paclitaxel have been developed, including liposome, cyclodextrin, and HSA-bound nanoparticle (Abraxane) formulations [2, 73], as well as paclitaxel conjugates with polyglutamate, amphiphilic triblock copolymers, heparin, and DHA (Taxoprexin® (TXP)) [73–75]. Also, a number of highly potent new-generation taxoids have been developed based on extensive structure–activity relationship studies, which possess dramatically enhanced potency, especially against paclitaxel-resistant cancer cell lines and tumor xenografts [76]. PUFA conjugates of the second-generation taxoids and their *in vivo* efficacy against tumor xenografts, as well as a summary of the clinical results for TXP (**1** : $R^1 = Ph$, $R^2 = Ph$, $R^3 = Ac$) will be described in Sections 41.4 and 41.5

41.3.2
DHA–10-Hydroxycamptothecin (2)

Camptothecin (CPT) is a naturally occurring pentacyclic alkaloid with potent antitumor activity as a topoisomerase I inhibitor through specific binding to the DNA–topoisomerase complex (Figure 41.5). This prevents religation of the DNA, leading to the accretion of single-strand breaks and subsequent apoptosis [77]. Due to its poor solubility, CPT has been largely replaced by pharmacologically better congeners, including 10-hydroxycamptothecin (HCPT), which exhibits less systemic toxicity and more potent topoisomerase I inhibitory activity [78]. Although simple conjugates of HCPT with saturated fatty acids did not exhibit appreciable activity *in vivo*, DHA–HCPT conjugate (**2**) did exhibit improved therapeutic effects over HCPT [79]. Conjugation was made through the carbamate moiety at the 10-position of HCPT with a *p*-aminobenzylpiperazine spacer between HCPT and DHA to improve the stability and solubility of the conjugate.

Although the conjugation of HCPT to DHA caused an 8-fold reduction in potency against the L1210 leukemia cell line, DHA–HCPT substantially outperformed HCPT against a mouse tumor model of the same cell line [79]. The increase in lifespan for DHA–HCPT in this mouse model was 323% at 120 mg/kg dose with three out of six mice surviving for 30 days, while no survivors were observed for HCPT alone at its optimum dose (20 mg/kg) [79]. Similar effects were observed against two other tumor xenografts, including Lewis lung carcinoma and colon 38 adenocarcinoma [79]. In early and more advanced stages of tumor development, DHA–HCPT resulted in tumor growth inhibition of 78 and 80%, respectively, against the colon 38 carcinoma xenografts. The clear improvement in therapeutic effect of HCPT through DHA–conjugation is most likely attributed to prolonged exposure of the tumor to the cytotoxic agent, which is especially important because HCPT has its maximal effect on cells at the S phase of mitosis. Whether this improved therapeutic window *in vivo* is a result of selective delivery to tumor cells or increased half-life through HSA binding has yet to be determined.

41.3.3
DHA/LNA–DOX (3/4)

DOX has been extensively used in the clinic for the treatment of various cancers, including breast, ovarian, leukemia, and lymphoma (Figure 41.5) [80, 81]. DOX is a member of the anthracycline family and inflicts its cytotoxicity through DNA intercalation and topoisomerase II inhibition [82]. Like many other chemotherapeutic agents, its use is limited due to several systemic toxicities, including myelosuppression, cardiotoxicity, and gastrointestinal disorders [81]. To reduce those undesirable side-effects, the conjugation of DOX to DHA via a cleavable hydrazone linker was reported as a method to improve the pharmacokinetic properties of the drug, while lowering its systemic toxicity [83]. The hydrazone linker was chosen based on the fact that the pH is lower in tumors than in healthy tissues and also that the hydrazone bond is stable for long periods of time at pH 7.4 yet rapidly cleaves at pH 4.5 [84]. As expected for the prodrug, the *in vitro* activity of DHA–DOX (**3**) was one order of magnitude weaker than that of free DOX, as exemplified by IC_{50} values of 1.4 and 0.15 μM, respectively, against L1210 leukemia cell lines [83]. The efficacy of DOX and DHA–DOX was then compared *in vivo* using mice injected with L1210 leukemia and B16 melanoma cells. At optimal dosing for the L1210-bearing mice, the conjugation of DOX to DHA improved the increase in lifespan value from 53 to 107%, substantially lowered the weight loss (−19% for free DOX, −4% for DHA–DOX), and had one survivor after 30 days. In the melanoma model, DHA–DOX doubled the tumor growth inhibition from 35 to 70% with significantly less systemic toxicity, as measured by weight loss [83]. However, the exact reasons for the improved preliminary *in vivo* results have yet to be determined.

Another PUFA–DOX conjugate, LNA–DOX (**4**), bearing LNA linkage to the daunosamine moiety of DOX was also evaluated [85]. Interestingly, the *in vitro* cytotoxicity of this conjugate, determined by the standard 3-(4,5-dimethylthiazol-2-yl)-2,5-diphenyltetrazolium bromide (MTT) assay, was significantly increased upon conjugation against MCF-7, MDA-MB-231, and HepG2 cancer cell lines [85]. This increase in toxicity was attributed to rapid internalization of the conjugate compared to free DOX; in fact, the fluorescence microscopy and flow cytometry showed a marked increase in internalization of LNA–DOX [85].

41.3.4
DHA/EPA–Propofol (5a/b)

Propofol is among the most widely used anesthetics, and has recently been shown to aid in the inhibition of tumor growth and metastasis at clinically relevant concentrations (20–50 μM) (Figure 41.5) [86]. To capitalize on the apparently tumor-selective cytotoxicity, propofol was conjugated to DHA and EPA and the effects of the conjugation on MDA-MB-231 breast cancer cells were examined [87]. It is interesting to note that DHA–propofol (**5a**) and LNA–propofol (**5b**) exhibited much greater potency for inhibiting cell growth, slowing migration, increasing cellular adhesion, and initiating apoptosis than either combination of propofol with DHA or LNA [87]. Stability studies showed that the DHA–propofol was stable in blood serum, such that it is unlikely that the ester linkage of this conjugate is cleaved under the experimental conditions employed [88]. Unlike DHA-induced apoptosis in MCF-7, MDA-MB-231, AU565, and MDA-MB-361 breast cancer cell lines, there was no discernable effect on PPARα or PPARγ, suggesting an independent mode of action of DHA–propofol [88]. The inhibition of histone deacetylase (HDAC) by DHA–propofol was observed, which could be responsible for mediating the cytotoxic effects as there is structural similarity to trichostatin A – a known HDAC inhibitor [88]. Most notably, it was reported that at concentrations cytotoxic to cancer cells, the normal cell lines tested were not adversely affected [88].

41.3.5
DHA–Illudin M (6)

The illudins are a class of fungal natural products that are extremely potent alkylators of DNA, RNA, and proteins because of the electrophilic spirocyclopropane and enone moieties in the molecule (Figure 41.5). IC_{50} values in the single-digit nanomolar level were reported against cancer cell lines, such as Panc-1 and HT-29, using MTT assays [89]. Irofulven, a semisynthetic analog, was evaluated in phase II clinical trials for different cancers, with only limited promise in prostate and pancreatic cancers [90, 91]. Due to their highly reactive structure and generally high cytotoxicity, treatment with these compounds resulted in severe side-effects, including thrombocytopenia, which critically narrowed the therapeutic window [91]. In the hope of expanding therapeutic window, Illudin M was conjugated to DHA via an ester linkage, and the *in vitro* activity of DHA–illudin M (**6**) was assessed against Panc-1 and HT-29 cancer cell lines [89]. Although DHA–illudin M was found to be far less cytotoxic than illudin M in the assays, its efficacy against tumor xenografts in mice has yet to be examined.

41.3.6
PUFA–Chlorambucil (7)

Chlorambucil (Chl) – a nitrogen mustard – has been commonly used for the treatment of chronic lymphocytic leukemia and generally inhibits cancer cell growth at the micromolar level IC_{50} values (Figure 41.5) [92]. It has been shown that α-fetoprotein (AFP) is secreted from certain tumor types, binds PUFAs with high affinity, and can be involved in the transport of PUFA into cells [93]. Accordingly, for cancer cells expressing AFP-specific cell surface receptors, significant tumor targeting drug delivery could be attained through PUFA conjugation [93]. Based on this hypothesis, conjugates of Chl with DHA, AA, and oleic acid (**7a–c**) were synthesized to study the effects of PUFA conjugation on tumor-specific uptake and cytotoxicity against human lymphomas and normal human peripheral blood lymphocytes [92]. Synergistic cytotoxicity against CEM and Raji lymphoma cell lines was observed for both AA and DHA conjugates of Chl (**7a** and **b**) (e.g., the IC_{50} value of around 20 μM against Raji cells with DHA–Chl (**7a**) [92]). No significant cytotoxicity was observed for the oleic acid conjugate (**7c**). For cancer cells that express AFP-binding receptors such as B- and T-lymphomas, the DHA and AA conjugates exhibited considerable enhancement in cytotoxicity, compared to quiescent lymphocytes that did not express this receptor [92].

41.3.7
PUFA–Mitomycin C (8)

Another potent DNA alkylator, mitomycin C, has been used to treat gastrointestinal and breast cancers (Figure 41.5) [94, 95]. Alkylation of DNA causes the initiation of either DNA repair mechanisms or, if that fails, apoptosis [96]. In order to develop new inhibitors of protein tyrosine kinases (PTKs), mitomycin C was conjugated to PUFAs [97]. Of all of the conjugates synthesized and examined, only the DHA–mitomycin C conjugate (**10**) showed significant inhibition of PTKs at 3 μg/ml, and it did not appreciably effect protein kinase C or protein kinase A at concentrations up to 100 μg/ml [97]. No PTK inhibition was observed with DHA or mitomycin C alone, or in combination, while DHA completely inhibited protein kinase C at 50 μg/ml [97]. This result provides an example of how conjugation of two compounds with different properties can often produce an entirely novel pharmacological profile, similar to the case of the DHA–propofol conjugate described above.

41.3.8
PUFA–2′-Deoxy-5-fluorouridine (9) and PUFA–Tegafur (10 and 11)

Antimetabolites are an important class of chemotherapeutic agents frequently used for the treatment of cancer, because these compounds are capable of halting necessary anabolic and catabolic processes that are required for cellular growth and division [98]. Of these, 5-FU is especially important in cancer chemotherapy, which inhibits thymidylate synthase that is necessary for DNA replication (Figure 41.5) [98].

PUFA conjugates of 2′-deoxy-5-fluorouridine (d5FU), a prodrug of 5-FU, have been synthesized and their toxicity evaluated *in vitro* against HT-29 cells as well as healthy peripheral blood mononuclear cells (PBMCs). Of the seven PUFA conjugates synthesized, DHA–d5FU (**9**) proved to be the most cytotoxic with IC_{50} value of 10 μM, a comparable value to free d5FU after 48 h of drug exposure [99]. It should be noted that the DHA–5-FU conjugate showed marked improvement in potency in shorter-term incubation times compared to the free drug (2 versus 24 h) [99]. This potency is beyond the synergy observed by coadministration of DHA with d5FU, which may be the result of improved cellular uptake of the conjugate. Phytohemagglutinin (PHA) was used as a mitogen to initiate mitosis in healthy PBMC in order to test the effect of rapid cellular division on the cytotoxicity of DHA–d5FU. In healthy cells, DHA–d5FU was also more cytotoxic than d5FU, albeit there was marked difference in potency against quiescent and PHA-activated PBMCs, with IC_{50} values of around 120 versus around 40 μM, respectively [99]. These findings suggest that increased levels of cell division result in an increased uptake of the PUFA-conjugated drug, leading to higher potency.

Tegafur acts as a prodrug for 5-FU, significantly reducing undesirable side-effects, such as bone marrow depletion, gastrointestinal problems, and damage to the liver and kidney [100]. Although tegafur has been used for the treatment of several adenocarcinomas, its systemic toxicity profile remains a limiting factor. In order to improve the therapeutic window of tegafur, its PUFA conjugates have been synthesized and examined, including PUFA–tegafur (**10**) and PUFA–glycerophospholipid–tegafur (**11**) [100]. Of the five PUFA–tegafur conjugates examined, those bearing oleoyl, linoleoyl, and arachidonoyl groups were reported to show increased potency compared to tegafur alone against Ec9706 and A549 cancer cell lines [100].

41.3.9 DHA–Methotrexate (11)

Methotrexate (MTX) is another commonly used antimetabolite in cancer chemotherapy, as it is a competitive inhibitor of dihydrofolate reductase (DHFR) – an enzyme necessary for the *de novo* synthesis of purines and thymidine during the S phase of the cell cycle (Figure 41.5) [101]. MTX is highly cytotoxic at nanomolar concentrations *in vitro*, and exhibits undesirable side-effects at therapeutic doses, including myelosuppression, anemia, and neutropenia [101]. At physiological pH, MTX exists as a dianion, which must be actively transported into the cell. As a result, drastic decrease in MTX uptake has been observed in various tumors. To overcome this problem, MTX prodrugs, conjugated to lipophilic molecules such as dimyristoylphosphatidylethanolamine (DMPE), were designed and indeed the MTX–DMPE conjugate was shown to inhibit DHFR activity as well as cancer cell proliferation [102].

Accordingly, the phosphatidylcholine conjugate of MTX and DHA was designed by capitalizing on the data suggesting that DHA extended the S phase of mitosis as well as the synergy between MTX with DHA observed upon coadministration [103]. The observed synergy was most pronounced with relatively low levels of MTX and high levels of DHA (i.e., 9.5 nM and 150 μM, respectively) [103]. In the DHA–MTX conjugate (**11**) synthesized, MTX occupies the *sn-2* position of the phosphatidylcholine backbone. Conjugation of MTX to the phosphatidylcholine backbone containing a PUFA in the *sn-1* position allows the DHA–MTX conjugate (**11**) to be incorporated into liposomes to enhance solubility of the compound [103]. The efficacy of DHA–MTX (**11**) was evaluated against leukemia cell line T27A and found to have an IC_{50} of 1.19 μM based on the ^{3}H-thymidine incorporation assay using liposome formulation [103]. An analogous conjugate with stearic acid in the place of DHA was found to be slightly less effective ($IC_{50} = 2.11$ μM), yet significantly less effective at concentrations below 1.5 μM [103]. This data may suggest that there is indeed a level of synergism between DHA and MTX that is not present with stearic acid.

41.4 Case Study in PUFA Conjugation: TXP (DHA–Paclitaxel)

41.4.1 Preclinical Evaluations

Many chemotherapeutic agents target actively dividing cells at either the S or G_2/M phases of mitosis, including paclitaxel, which targets the latter. This makes paclitaxel an excellent choice for the treatment of rapidly dividing tumors [104].

However, many cancers, as well as certain subpopulations of cells within solid tumors, divide much more slowly. Therefore, it would be advantageous to maintain constant levels of anticancer drugs in the tumor interstitium for longer periods of time, so that they may permeate throughout the tumor and affect even the slowly dividing cancer cells. Based on this concept as well as the observation that PUFAs are rapidly taken up by tumors from the bloodstream, TXP was developed by conjugating paclitaxel to DHA [105]. In TXP, DHA was covalently linked to paclitaxel at its 2′-position through an ester linkage. It has been shown that the modification of the 2′-hydroxyl group costs substantial decrease in cytotoxicity of the drug [105]. The resulting prodrug drastically changed the pharmacokinetic profile of paclitaxel, which was suited for the treatment of various solid tumors [105]. Conjugation to DHA also allowed clinical formulation containing 80% saline/10% ethanol/10% Cremophor EL®, which uses 80% less Cremophor EL on a molar basis than the standard formulation of paclitaxel which is administered in Cremophor EL and 49.7% (v/v) anhydrous ethanol [105].

TXP was initially screened against 56 human cancer cell lines from tumors of various organs and showed a marked decrease in potency from an average IC_{50} of around 10^{-9} M for free paclitaxel to that of around 10^{-6} M for TXP [105]. These assays were run with a 72-h drug incubation period. The observed marked decrease in potency is likely due to the stability of the ester bond *in vitro*, which must be hydrolyzed before the compound can display maximal potency [105]. Microtubule polymerization, flow cytometry, and immunofluorescence studies indicated that the mechanism of action for the conjugate was similar to free paclitaxel – providing strong support for the prodrug model [105]. Preliminary *in vivo* studies against syngeneic and xenogeneic M109 and HT-29 tumors in mice showed increased efficacy and reduced systemic toxicity compared to paclitaxel at the optimum dose [105]. In the M109 mouse lung tumor model, TXP eliminated all measurable tumor bulk for 60 days in 10/10 mice after five consecutive daily administrations at the total optimum dose of 120 mg/kg (Figure 41.6). In contrast, free paclitaxel delayed tumor growth only for 10 days before tumor growth comparable to the control was observed in all mice [105]. In a similar study using the HT-29 human colon cancer xenograft, TXP caused complete responses in two and partial responses in three out of five mice tested, while paclitaxel showed only temporary tumor growth delay and no remission [105]. In addition, the hind-limb paralysis observed in paclitaxel-treated mice was not observed in those treated with TXP – implying tumor specificity with decreased systemic toxicity [105].

41.4.2
Pharmacokinetics

In order to obtain a more detailed picture of the factors responsible for the improved efficacy of TXP, detailed pharmacokinetics profiling of the conjugate was performed [105]. Two doses of the TXP were examined (equimolar to paclitaxel and the optimum dose) and compared to the optimum dose of paclitaxel (Figure 41.7). Three major parameters investigated were maximal concentration (C_{max}), time of

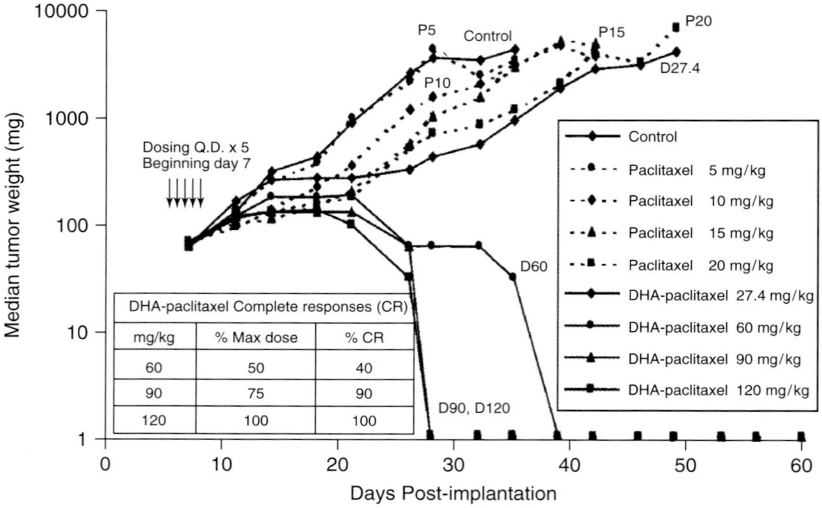

Figure 41.6 Comparison of the antitumor activity of paclitaxel and TXP in M109 mouse lung carcinoma. Both paclitaxel and TXP were injected once a day for 5 days at the indicated daily doses into the tail vein of CD2F1 mice starting on day 7 after tumor inoculation, when the tumors weighed around 65 mg. The median weight of tumors from each group of 10 animals is plotted. Histological analysis of the tissues in areas where tumors had regressed showed either normal skin or the final stages of resorption of necrotic tissue. (Reproduced from. [105] with permission.)

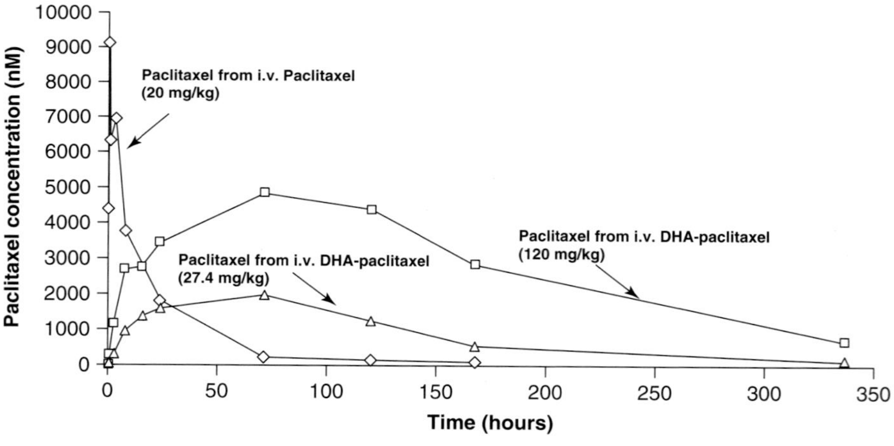

Figure 41.7 Tumor mean concentrations of paclitaxel derived from intravenous paclitaxel and intravenous TXP (DNA–paclitaxel) in the tumors of M109 tumor-bearing mice treated with intravenous paclitaxel and intravenous TXP. Both paclitaxel and TXP were injected once at the indicated doses into the tail vein of CD2F1 mice when the tumors weighed around 100 mg. The mean concentration in the M109 tumors of paclitaxel derived form each drug from 10 animals/timepoint is plotted. The lower limit of detection was 5 ng/g. (Reproduced from [105] with permission.)

maximal concentration (T_{max}), and the area under the curve (AUC) for the drug concentration through time plot. To assess the nature of the biodistribution, data for each parameter were taken from the blood plasma, muscle tissue, and tumor tissue.

When paclitaxel was administered intravenously, plasma C_{max} of 42 μM was quickly reached at a T_{max} of around 5 min and then a fast decline was observed afterwards ($T_{1/2}$ in plasma around 12 h) as the drug permeates into the surrounding tissues. The C_{max} values for muscle and tumor tissues were 7.6 and 9.2 μM, respectively, indicating little tumor specificity, and each occurred within half an hour after injection [105]. The AUC value in blood plasma was 34 μM × h, exemplifying the rapid clearance of the drug from the plasma compartment.

In stark contrast, TXP showed a marked increase in plasma distribution, with AUC values of 12.8 mM × h (AUC of paclitaxel = 61 μM × h), indicating long residency in the plasma, and a slow-release mechanism [105]. The plasma C_{max} of around 2.5 mM was reached in 30 min after injection, and TXP was distributed to tissues in 8 h with C_{max} levels of 14.9 and 107.4 μM in muscular and tumor tissues, respectively [105]. It should be noted that the high concentration of TXP in muscular tissues does not directly contribute to systemic toxicity until metabolized into the active form, since TXP possesses substantially muted cytotoxicity compared to paclitaxel.

Free paclitaxel level derived from TXP at its optimum dose reached the C_{max} of only 340 nM in muscle tissues after 120 h from injection. This data strongly suggests that the ester bond linking DHA to paclitaxel is stable in the bloodstream and its slow hydrolysis is responsible for the gradual release of the free drug *in vivo* [105]. The 22-fold lower intramuscular concentration compared to paclitaxel administration is likely to be responsible for the lack of hind-leg paralysis (typical for paclitaxel treatment) in mice treated with TXP [105]. The C_{max} of 4.8 μM for TXP-derived paclitaxel in the tumor was reached in 72 h after injection, which was around 13-fold higher than that observed in the healthy muscle tissues [105]. This indicates significant tumor specific accumulation of TXP, which is further supported by the TXP-derived paclitaxel AUC values of 1013 and 45 μM × h for tumor and healthy tissues, respectively [105]. Paclitaxel level as high as 0.73 μM was recorded in the tumor up to 336 h after the injection of TXP, which is a vast improvement to the paclitaxel administration wherein the drug becomes undetectable after 168 h [105]. These data indicate that TXP slowly releases the cytotoxic drug (paclitaxel) at relatively steady concentrations for a long period of time, which make it possible to treat even dormant or slowly dividing tumor cells.

Later studies, aimed at elucidating the major causes that contribute to TXP's unique pharmacokinetic profile, identified HSA and α_1-acid glycoprotein (AAG) binding as the major factor for TXP's extended half-life and slow release from the plasma compartment [106]. These two proteins were found to contribute equally to the plasma drug binding level of greater than 99.6%, which indicates that the TXP-derived paclitaxel concentration in blood may be insignificant [106]. *In vitro* binding constants were determined by the use of ^{3}H-DHA–pacelitaxel at varying concentrations, dilution with plasma or protein solution, 24 h dialysis at pH 7.4, and radiolabel quantification [106]. The binding affinity for TXP to both HSA and AAG was found to be $678 \pm 22.5\ \mu M^{-1}$ by this method [106]. Interestingly, the presence of the surfactant Cremophor EL had only a minor inhibitory effect on HSA binding of TXP [106]. This finding makes sharp contrast to the case of paclitaxel, wherein the HSA binding of the drug is substantially affected by the presence of Cremophor EL and indicates a much greater affinity of TXP to HSA than paclitaxel [107]. Distribution *in vivo* was determined by high-performance liquid chromatography/mass spectrometry analysis of blood and tissue extracts from patients [106]. The nonlinear elimination kinetics and drastic increase (greater than 2-fold) in plasma C_{max} and AUC on increase in dosage from 800 to 1100 mg/m^2 are explained by serum protein saturation at the high dose [106]. The capacity of binding proteins should have been exceeded at the 1100 mg/m^2 dose, which inevitably transport the nonbound drugs from the bloodstream into the peripheral tissues [106]. Therefore, almost the entirety of the administered dose appears to bind serum proteins until they become saturated at high levels, leaving the excess to be distributed to the peripheral tissue [106]. Extensive retention of TXP in the plasma compartment presumably results in prolonged exposure of the bone marrow to the drug, causing myelosuppression and neutropenia, which are two dose-limiting toxicities observed with TXP treatment in animals and humans.

41.4.3
Phase I Trials

On the basis of its early success in preclinical studies as well as its favorable pharmacokinetic and toxicity profile, TXP was advanced to phase I clinical trials in humans with the dosing schedule of a 2-h infusion every 3 weeks for a number of cancer types [105, 108]. In one study, involving 24 patients with advanced solid malignancies, a recommended dose level of 1100 mg/m^2 (containing 803 mg/m^2 paclitaxel) was established as the optimum dose for more advanced trials, which is much higher than that of 175 mg/m^2 for free paclitaxel and 260 mg/m^2 for the HSA–paclitaxel nanoparticle formulation Abraxane [73]. At this and other doses tested, myelosuppression was the major dose-limiting toxicity accompanied by grade 3/4 neutropenia, including febrile neutropenia [108]. Interestingly, no neurotoxicity was observed in any patients, which is a common dose-limiting toxicity in patients receiving weekly paclitaxel infusions [108]. No patients developed alopecia, peripheral neuropathy, or musculoskeletal toxicity greater than grade 1. Partial response was noticed in one patient, who suffered from metastatic HER-2-negative breast cancer. However, imaging studies documented stable disease after the sixth cycle of TXP treatment [108]. On average, TXP exhibited an around 7-fold longer half-life, a smaller volume of distribution by 2 orders of magnitude, and an around 300-fold slower clearance than free paclitaxel [108]. Limited blood sampling and analysis implicated HSA levels as a contributing factor to the variable pharmacokinetics values in patients receiving the same dosing schedule, which further implicates the role of albumin-binding in the unique pharmacokinetic profile of TXP.

Another phase I trial was conducted to evaluate the efficacy of a low-dose weekly dosing schedule, as it has been observed that metronomic chemotherapy can be effective in blocking angiogenesis [109]. A weekly dosage schedule of 100–600 mg/m^2 (containing 73–438 mg/m^2 paclitaxel) was examined every week for 3 out of 4 weeks based on the observations in the previous phase I study. Of the 19 evaluable patients, three had stable diseases for over 10 weeks – 1 each with esophageal (11 weeks), melanoma (16 weeks), and colon carcinoma (17 weeks) – wherein two of the three patients with stable disease had been given no prior taxane treatment [110]. At the highest dosing regimen, grade 3 hyperbilirubinemia was the dose-limiting toxicity for one patient suffering from pancreatic cancer with liver metastases and grade 1 neuropathy was observed in one patient [110]. Other common non-hematologic side-effects observed were fatigue, anorexia and nausea/vomiting. While neutropenia (including grade 3/4 in five patients) was the most frequently observed hematologic toxicity, no febrile neutropenia was detected in any patients [110]. This particular side-effect resulted in delayed dosing and dose reduction after the first cycle of treatment. Plasma concentrations of TXP remained greater than 1 μg/ml throughout the first cycle of treatment for all patients receiving 500 and 600 mg/m^2 doses and TXP remained at detectable concentrations through day 29 (i.e., 2 weeks after final drug administration) [110]. Interestingly, no significant accumulation of free paclitaxel or TXP in tissues was observed with weekly treatment at the dose levels tested. Based on the finding that longer infusions of paclitaxel are more effective in the treatment of metastatic melanoma [111], a weekly TXP treatment schedule may provide some advantage in treating this disease, which may be adapted to the treatment of other tumors.

41.4.4 Phase II/III Trials

After completion of phase I toxicity and pharmacokinetic profiling, TXP advanced to phase II clinical trials for evaluation of its efficacy against eight different tumor types, including prostate, breast, gastric, and NSCLCs as well as metastatic melanoma [112–118]. The outcomes of three of these studies are detailed below, focusing on median survival, dose-limiting toxicity, and response rate. In general, phase II trials began at the recommended dose of 1100 mg/m^2, which was lowered to 900 mg/m^2 (containing 657 mg/m^2 paclitaxel) when unacceptable toxicity was noticed. In all cases, significant activity was observed, but the results were mostly comparable to the currently used treatment methods with little if any significant improvement in efficacy.

In an open-labeled, multicenter trial for stage IIIB and IV NSCLC, TXP was evaluated as the first-line treatment [117]. Dosing was started at 1100 mg/m^2 and quickly reduced to 900 mg/m^2 after severe toxicity was observed in 10 out of the first 13 patients. The most prominent toxicity was grade 3/4 neutropenia resulting from dose-limiting myelosuppression. Of the 40 patients available for analysis of drug responses, two had partial responses and 16 had stable disease. The median survival time was 243 days, with 35% surviving more than 1 year. Although survival rates were comparable to those seen in combination with cisplatin, TXP was not recommended as a realistic therapeutic option for locally advanced and metastatic NSCLC [117].

Continuous 2-h intravenous infusion of 1100 mg/m^2 TXP every 3 weeks was investigated as the first-line treatment in patients with locally advanced or metastatic gastric or esophageal tumors in an open-label study [81]. Of the 48 patients who were evaluable for drug responses, five exhibited partial responses with a median response duration of 87 days. Median survival was 262 days and there were four deaths during the study, two of which were believed to be directly related to the drug treatment. Grade 3/4 neutropenia was observed in 93% of patients and febrile neutropenia occurred in 17% patients. In general, response rates and hematological toxicities were comparable to treatment with either docetaxel or paclitaxel as single agents. Although TXP showed a slight decrease in nonhematological side-effects as compared to paclitaxel or docetaxel, further examination of TXP as a treatment for previously untreated patients with locally advanced or metastatic gastric or esophageal adenocarcinoma was not recommended.

In the phase II study, aimed at evaluating the efficacy and safety of TXP in previously untreated malignant melanoma, 34 patients were subjected to the same treatment schedule as previously described [118]. Again, neutropenia was the primary toxicity and grade 4 was experienced by half of the patients resulting in two related deaths, while other nonhematological toxicities were minimal. Two of the 26 patients available for response evaluation exhibited partial response, while 12 showed signs of stable disease. The median duration of survival was slightly over 10 months, which is comparable to the standard single-agent treatment with dacarbazine or temozolimide. This study initiated the advancement of TXP to phase III studies in patients suffering from malignant melanoma [73].

Combination therapy of TXP with carboplatin was evaluated in a phase I/II study for patients with advanced malignant solid tumors refractory to the standard treatment [119]. Both drugs were administered on the same day every 3 weeks with carboplatin (AUC 5) and 660 or 880 mg/m^2 of TXP (containing 462 and 642 mg/m^2 paclitaxel, respectively). Of the 15 patients treated, one partial response was observed in a patient with advanced esophagogastric adenocarcinoma, while 12 patients had stable disease for a median duration of 184 days. Neutropenia was the main dose-limiting toxicity, four patients suffered from grade 3 increase in liver transaminase levels and there was one case of clinically significant neuropathy. Based on the result, phase II study for previously untreated patients using similar dosing regimens was recommended [119].

Although TXP has displayed substantially improved pharmacokinetic and toxicity profiles in animal models, the remarkable activity and tumor-specific accumulation described in early studies has not necessarily been translated into the clinic. The extended retention of TXP in blood plasma did minimize nonhematological toxicities, but the dose-limiting myelosuppression was still comparable to paclitaxel treatment and the resulting neutropenia was a serious adverse effect. Alteration of dosing schedule, new formulation, and appropriate combination therapies may allow TXP to find broader success in the clinic.

41.5
PUFA Conjugates of Second-Generation Taxoids

Paclitaxel and docetaxel are effective against breast, ovary, and lung cancers, but do not show efficacy against colon, pancreatic, melanoma, and renal cancers. Human colon carcinoma is inherently multidrug resistant due to the overexpression of P-glycoprotein (P-gp) – an effective ATP-binding cassette (ABC) transporter, which effluxes hydrophobic anticancer agents including paclitaxel and docetaxel. Accordingly, paclitaxel does not show any appreciable efficacy even against human colon cancer xenografts in mice [120]. In sharp contrast to paclitaxel, a number of new-generation taxoids show excellent activity (two to three orders of magnitude more potent than paclitaxel) against drug-resistant cancer cells, expressing multidrug resistance (MDR) phenotypes [76].

As mentioned in the preceding Section 41.4, TXP is voraciously taken up by tumor cells, internalized, and slowly hydrolyzed by esterases in the cancer cell. DHA–paclitaxel was found to be a relatively weak substrate for P-gp as compared to paclitaxel, as mentioned above. However, if the cancer cells are overexpressing P-gp and/or other ABC transporters, free paclitaxel molecules, even when released slowly, will be caught by the efflux pump(s) and eliminated from the cancer cells. Therefore, it would be beneficial to conjugate DHA to the second-generation taxoids that possess built-in P-gp-modulating ability [120, 121]. Thus, it is reasonable to anticipate that the DHA conjugates of the second-generation taxoids ("new generation DHA–taxoids") are likely to provide highly efficacious antitumor agents against drug-resistant tumors, against which TXP is not effective due to the overexpression of the ABC transporter's efflux pump(s). These drug-resistant tumors include many gastrointestinal cancers as well as lung, breast, and ovarian cancers. Also, it would be useful to examine the efficacy of PUFAs other than DHA, such as LNA (n–3) and LA (n–6), as well. Accordingly, a series of PUFA–second-generation taxoid conjugates was synthesized and evaluated their efficacy against drug-resistant as well as drug-sensitive tumor xenografts in mice [122]. Representative PUFA–second-generation taxoids are shown in Table 41.1.

41.5.1
Preclinical Study of PUFA–Second-Generation Taxoid Conjugates

Several DHA–second-generation taxoids were evaluated for their antitumor activities against drug-resistant and drug-sensitive human tumor xenografts in female severe combined immunodeficient (SCID) mice or Swiss Webster nude mice aged 6–8 weeks. Each drug treatment group or drug-free vehicle consisted of at least four or five mice per group, wherein untreated controls contained 10 mice per group. Paclitaxel or TXP was formulated with Cremophor ELP/ethanol/saline. DHA–taxoids

Table 41.1 PUFA–taxoid conjugates.

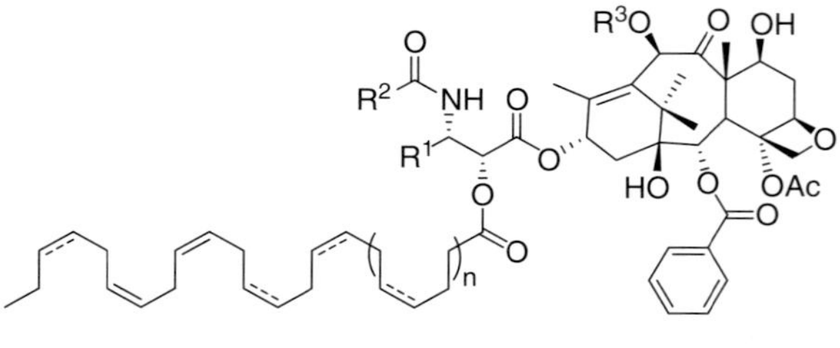

Conjugate	R^1	R^2	R^3	PUFA
DHA–paclitaxel (TXP)	Ph	Ph	Ac	22 : 6, *n*–3
DHA–docetaxel	Ph	*t*-Boc	H	22 : 6, *n*–3
DHA–SB-T-1213	$Me_2C{=}CH$	*t*-Boc	EtCO	22 : 6, *n*–3
DHA–SB-T-1103	Me_2CHCH_2	*t*-Boc	EtCO	22 : 6, *n*–3
DHA–SB-T-1214	$Me_2C{=}CH$	*t*-Boc	*c*-PrCO	22 : 6, *n*–3
DHA–SB-T-1104	Me_2CHCH_2	*t*-Boc	*c*-PrCO	22 : 6, *n*–3
DHA–SB-T-1216	$Me_2C{=}CH$	*t*-Boc	Me_2NCO	22 : 6, *n*–3
LNA–SB-T-1213	$Me_2C{=}CH$	*t*-Boc	EtCO	18 : 3, *n*–3
LA–SB-T-1213	$Me_2C{=}CH$	*t*-Boc	EtCO	18 : 3, *n*–6

and other PUFA–taxoids were formulated either with Tween 80/ethanol/saline or Solutol HS-15/ethanol/saline. DHA–SB-T-1214 was formulated by Chem Master International (*www.chemmasterint.com*) at 50 mg/ml in Solutol HS-15/EtOH (1 : 1), with L-ascorbic acid (3.9 mM) and α-tocopherol (2.0 mM). To stabilize the formulation of the DHA–taxoids and other PUFA–taxoids, small amounts of antioxidants, L-ascorbic acid, and α-tocopherol, were added. Drugs were injected intravenously via the tail vein. Each drug was administered once a day, using either a q3d × 3 or q7d × 3 schedule when the tumor size reached about 100 mm^3 in size.

41.5.1.1 DLD-1 (P-gp$^+$ Colon) Tumor Xenograft

The efficacy of DHA–SB-T-1213, DHA–SB-T-1214, DHA–SB-T-1103, and DHA–SB-T-1104 was evaluated against the paclitaxel-resistant, P-gp$^+$ DLD1 human colon tumor xenograft implanted subcutaneously in SCID mice, and compared with that of paclitaxel, TXP, DHA–docetaxel, IDN5109, and DHA–IDN5109 (Figure 41.8a) [122]. Paclitaxel and TXP were found to be totally ineffective. DHA–docetaxel and IDN5109 were better, but tumor growth delays were only 34 and 32 days. DHA–SB-T-1213 showed tumor growth delay of 68 days. In sharp contrast, DHA–SB-T-1214 caused complete regressions and cure of the DLD-1 tumor in five of five mice at the 80 mg/kg/dose (i.e., 240 mg/kg total) administered on days 5, 8, and 11 (tumor growth delay greater than 187 days). This is an exceptionally encouraging result. It was also found that the use of q7d × 3 schedule did not

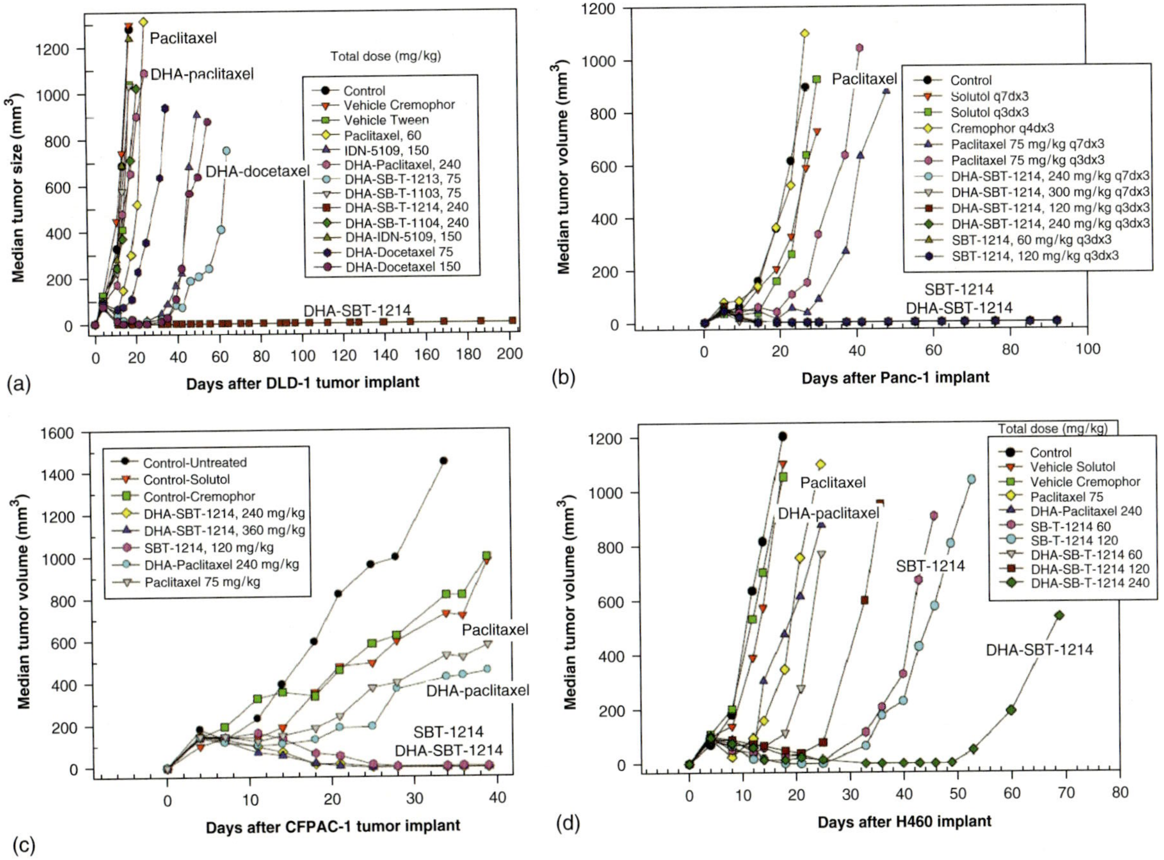

Figure 41.8 Efficacy studies of DHA–SB-T-1214 against human tumor xenografts in RPCI SCID mice or Swiss Webster nude mice: (a) DLD-1 (colon), (b) Panc-1 (pancreatic), (c) CFPAC-1 (pancreatic), and (d) H460 (NSCLC). Each drug was administered intravenously from tail vein once a day, using either a q3d × 3 or q7d × 3 schedule when the tumor size reached about 100 mm^3 in size. Total dose is indicated for each drug.

cause any weight loss. Interestingly, DHA–SB-T-1103 and DHA–SB-T-1104 were found to be ineffective, which appears to be attributed to the saturated branched alkyl group at the 3′-position of taxoids (SB-T-1213 and SB-T-1213 bear unsaturated branched alkyl groups at the same position and this is the only difference in their structures). From this study, DHA–SB-T-1214 emerged as a highly promising lead drug conjugate.

41.5.1.2 A121 (P-gp$^-$ Ovarian) Tumor Xenograft

The efficacy of paclitaxel, TXP, DHA–SB-T-1213, and DHA–SB-T-1216 was evaluated against drug-sensitive (i.e., P-gp$^-$) A121 human ovarian tumor xenograft in SCID mice [122]. As anticipated, TXP (240 mg/kg total dose) was indeed efficacious, showing greater than a 2-fold increase in tumor growth delay (186 days) as compared to paclitaxel (83 days). However, DHA–SB-T-1213 (90 mg/kg total dose) exhibited even better activity, achieving complete regression of tumor in all surviving mice (four of five) (tumor growth delay greater than 186 days). DHA–SB-T-1216 (90 mg/kg total dose) was found to be more toxic than DHA–SB-T-1213, but still had one complete regression out of five mice. The results on DLD-1 (P-gp$^+$) and A121 (P-gp$^-$) clearly indicate the dramatic negative effects of the P-gp efflux pump on the efficacy of paclitaxel as well as TXP, and in turn demonstrates the remarkable efficacy of DHA–SB-T-1214 against drug-resistant tumor xenograft, expressing MDR phenotype.

41.5.1.3 Panc-1 (Pancreatic) Tumor Xenograft

The efficacy of q7d × 3 and a q3d × 3 schedules for paclitaxel and DHA–SBT-1214 was evaluated against the human Panc-1 pancreatic tumor xenograft in RPMI SCID mice (Figure 41.8b) (Ojima, I., Zucker, S., Zimmerman, T., Berrada, K., Veith, J.M., and Bernacki, R.J., unpublished data). The results indicated that both schedules were very effective against this human pancreatic tumor xenograft (tumor growth delay greater than 90 days). The MTD for DHA–SBT-1214 appeared to be 240 mg/kg total dosage with one toxic death occurring at the 300 mg/kg total dose. All mice that received DHA–SBT-1214 achieved complete responses and essentially were cured. Paclitaxel was only weakly effective, showing tumor growth delays of 18 days with the q7d × 3 schedule and 13 days with the q3d × 3 schedule and no complete responses.

41.5.1.4 CFPAC-1 (Pancreatic) Tumor Xenograft

The efficacy of DHA–SBT-1214, paclitaxel, and DHA–paclitaxel was evaluated and compared against a human Panc-1 pancreatic tumor xenograft in Swiss Webster nude mice with the q3d × 3 schedule (Figure 41.8c) (Ojima, I., Zucker, S., Zimmerman, T., Berrada, K., Veith, J.M., and Bernacki, R.J., unpublished data.). DHA–SBT-1214 using 240 or 300 mg/kg total dose was very effective, causing complete responses and cure for five in five or four in four, respectively. Paclitaxel and TXP were much less effective with only minor tumor growth delay as compared to vehicles. SBT-1214 (120 mg/kg total dose) exhibited excellent result with tumor regressions for six in six mice and one in six was cured, but showed minor weight loss (below <4%) until day 20, while the weight loss was negligible for DHA–SBT-1214 at 240 or 300 mg/kg total dose.

41.5.1.5 H460 (NSCLC) Tumor Xenograft

The efficacy of DHA–SBT-1214, paclitaxel, TXP, and SBT-1214 was evaluated and compared against highly aggressive H460 human NSCLC tumor xenograft in RPCI SCID female mice (q3d × 3 regimen) (Figure 41.8d) (Ojima, I., Zucker, S., Zimmerman, T., Berrada, K., Veith, J.M., and Bernacki, R.J., unpublished data.). Tumor growth delays caused by paclitaxel at MTD (75 mg/kg total dose) and TXP at MTD (240 mg/kg total dose) were only 8 and 3 days, respectively. Thus, these drugs are totally ineffective. In contrast, DHA–SBT-1214 and SBT-1214 caused tumor growth delays of 55 and 34 days at about the MTD (240 and 120 mg/kg total dose, respectively), and DHA–SBT-1214 was clearly better tolerated than SBT-1214.

41.5.1.6 LNA– and LA–Second-Generation Taxoids

It has been shown that *n*–3 PUFAs such as α-LNA can be used for conjugation in place of DHA. As shown in Table 41.1, LNA (*n*–3) and LA (*n*–6) conjugates of SB-T-1213 were synthesized and evaluated against DLD-1 tumor xenograft in SCID mice [122]. The *n*–3 PUFA conjugate, LNA–SB-T-1213, achieved two out of five cures with tumor growth delay of greater than 109 days, while the corresponding *n*–6 PUFA conjugate, LA–SB-T-1213, showed very little growth inhibition (delay of only 21 days with no long-term survivors), which demonstrates the marked difference in efficacy between second-generation taxoid conjugates with *n*–3 and *n*–6 PUFAs [122]. Since LNA is much less expensive and more stable for handling than DHA, there is a potential economic merit if this *n*–3-PUFA can be used as DHA replacement without losing efficacy.

41.5.2 Cytochrome P450 Screening for Assessment of Potential Drug–Drug Interaction

Cytochrome P450 enzymes (P450s) catalyze the oxidative metabolism of a vast array of hydrophobic chemical substances, including therapeutic drugs. The inhibition of cytochrome P450s by drugs may alter drug disposition and cause adverse drug–drug interactions. In human, 57 genes encode for the different P450 enzymes. However, 89–90% of the activity of all the cytochrome P450-dependent drug metabolism is related to only five isozymes: CYP1A2, CYP2C9, CYP2C19, CYP2D6, and CYP3A4. The well-established luciferase assay clearly indicated that DHA–SB-T-1214 did not inhibit significantly any of the five major CYPs tested and IC_{50} was greater than 100 μM over the concentration range tested (0.003 nM to 100 μM), which led to the conclusion that DHA–SB-T-1214 would not cause harmful drug–drug interactions related to CYPs (Ojima, I., Zucker, S., Zimmerman, T., Berrada, K., Veith, J.M., and Bernacki, R.J., unpublished data.).

41.6
Conclusions and Perspectives

Conjugation of cytotoxic drugs to PUFAs has proven to be an effective way of improving the efficacy of many known chemotherapeutic agents *in vivo*, through HSA binding, increased tumor uptake, and decreased systemic toxicity. As PUFAs and their metabolites affect a number of cellular signaling networks in healthy and malignant tissues, the synergism observed in the coadministration of PUFAs with cytotoxic agents makes them unique components of drug conjugates. The validity of this approach to tumor-specific accumulation has been demonstrated by the promising clinical data for TXP, which has advanced to phase III human clinical trials, albeit limited to melanoma at present. However, the full potential of this approach has yet to be attained and a variety of compounds are currently at various stages in drug development. Although still in the preclinical stage, a PUFA–second-generation taxoid, especially DHA–SB-T-1214, is showing a high potential as a drug candidate in the pipeline. Judging from the substantial success of Abraxane using HSA-bound paclitaxel nanoparticle formulation, which exploits the gp60–SPARC pathway for tumor-selective accumulation of paclitaxel in tumor tissues and cells, further investigation into the effective formulations of PUFA–drug conjugates, involving HSA may provide a breakthrough in this field.

Acknowledgments

The research conducted in the authors' laboratory and described in this chapter was supported by grants from the National Cancer Institute, National Institutes of Health (**CA103314** to I.O.).

References

1. Desai, N., Yao, Z., Trieu, V., Soon-Shoing, P., Dykes, D., and Noker, P. (2003) Evidence of greater tumor and red cell partitioning and superior antitumor activity of cremophor free nanoparticle paclitaxel (ABI-007) compared to taxol. *Breast Cancer Res. Treat.*, **82** (Suppl. 1), S83, Abstract 348.
2. Ibrahim, N.K., Desai, N., Legha, S., Soon-Shiong, P., Theriault, R.L., Rivera, E., Esmaeli, B., Ring, S.E., Bedikian, A., Hortobagyi, G.N., and Ellerhorst, J.A. (2002) Phase I and pharmacokinetic study of ABI-007, a cremophor-free, protein-stabilized nanoparticle formulation of paclitaxel. *Clin. Cancer Res.*, **8**, 1038–1044.
3. Desai, N., Trieu, V., Yao, Z., Louie, L., Ci, S., Yang, A., Tao, C., De, T., Beals, B., Dykes, D., Noker, P., Yao, R., Labao, E., Hawkins, M., and Soon-Shiong, P. (2006) Increased antitumor activity, intratumor paclitaxel concentrations, and endothelial cell transport of cremophor-free, albumin-bound paclitaxel, ABI-007, compared with cremophor-based paclitaxel. *Clin. Cancer Res.*, **12**, 1317–1324.
4. Berquin, I.M., Edwards, I.J., and Chen, Y.Q. (2008) Multi-targeted therapy of cancer by omega-3 fatty acids. *Cancer Lett.*, **269**, 363–367.
5. Colquhoun, A.M., Miyake, J.A., and Benadiba, M. (2009) Fatty acids,

eicosanoids and cancer. *Nutr. Ther. Metabol.*, **27**, 105–112.

6. Pownall, H.J. and Hamilton, J. (2003) Energy translocation across cell membranes and membrane models. *Acta Physiol. Scand.*, **178**, 357–365.
7. Hirsch, D., Stahl, A., and Lodish, H.F. (1998) A family of fatty acid transporters conserved from mycobacterium to man. *Proc. Natl. Acad. Sci. USA*, **95**, 8625–8629.
8. Veerkamp, J.H. and Zimmerman, A.W. (2001) Fatty acid-binding proteins of nervous tissue. *J. Mol. Neurosci.*, **16**, 133–142.
9. Thumser, A.E., Tsai, J., and Storch, J. (2001) Collision-mediated transfer of long-chain fatty acids by neural tissue fatty acid-binding proteins (FABP): studies with fluorescent analogs. *J. Mol. Neurosci.*, **16**, 143–150.
10. Marszalek, J.R., Kitidis, C., Dararutana, A., and Lodish, H.F. (2004) Acyl-CoA synthetase 2 overexpression enhances fatty acid internalization. *J. Biol. Chem.*, **279**, 23882–23891.
11. Schley, P.D., Brindley, D.N., and Field, C.J. (2007) (*n*–3) PUFA alter raft lipid composition and decrease epidermal growth factor receptor levels in lipid rafts of human breast cancer cells. *J. Nutr.*, **137**, 548–553.
12. Foster, L.J., De Hoog, C.L., and Mann, M. (2003) Unbiased quantitative proteomics of lipid rafts reveals high specificity for signaling factors. *Proc. Natl. Acad. Sci. USA*, **100**, 5813–5818.
13. Hardman, W.E. (2004) (*n*–3) fatty acids and cancer therapy. *J. Nutr.*, **134**, 3427S–3430S.
14. Dommels, Y.E., Haring, M.M., Keenstra, N.G., Alink, G.M., van Bladeren, P.J., and van Ommen, B. (2003) The role of cyclooxygenase in *n*–6 and *n*–3 poly unsaturated fatty acid mediated effects on cell proliferation, PGE_2 synthesis and cytotoxicity in human colorectal carcinoma cell lines. *Carcinogenesis*, **24**, 385–392.
15. Rose, D.P. and Connolly, J.M. (2000) Regulation of tumor angiogenesis by dietary fatty acids and eicosanoids. *Nutr. Cancer*, **37**, 119–127.
16. Calder, P.C., Yaqoob, P., Thies, F., Wallace, F.A., and Miles, E.A. (2002) Fatty acids and lymphocyte functions. *Br. J. Nutr.*, **87**, S31–S48.
17. Brown, M.D., Hart, C.A., Gazi, E., Bagley, S., and Clarke, N.W. (2006) Promotion of prostatic metastatic migration towards human bone marrow stoma by omega 6 and its inhibition by omega 3 PUFAs. *Br. J. Cancer*, **94**, 842–853.
18. McCarthy, M.F. (1996) Fish oil may impede tumour angiogenesis and invasiveness by down-regulating protein kinase C and modulating eicosanoid production. *Med. Hypotheses*, **46**, 107–115.
19. Masoodi, M., Mir, A.A., Petasis, N.A., Serhan, C.N., and Nicolaou, A. (2008) Simultaneous lipidomic analysis of three families of bioactive lipid mediators leukotrienes, resolvins, protectins and related hydroxyl-fatty acids by liquid chromatography/electrospray ionization tandem mass spectrometry. *Rapid Commun. Mass Spectrom.*, **22**, 75–83.
20. Kroetz, D.L. and Zeldin, D.C. (2002) Cytochrome P450 pathways of arachidonic acid metabolism. *Curr. Opin. Lipidol.*, **13**, 273–283.
21. Sauer, L.A. and Dauchy, R.T. (1992) The effect of omega-6 and omega-3 fatty acids on ^{3}H-thymidine incorporation in hepatoma 7288CTC perfused in situ. *Br. J. Cancer*, **66**, 297–303.
22. Damtew, B.S. and Spagnuolo, P.J. (1997) Tumor cell–endothelial cell interactions: evidence for roles for lipoxygenase products of arachidonic acid in metastasis. *Prostagland. Leukotr. Essent. Fat. Acid.*, **56**, 295–300.
23. Calder, P.C. and Grimble, R.F. (2002) Polyunsaturated fatty acids, inflammation and immunity. *Eur. J. Clin. Nutr.*, **87**, S14–S19.
24. Sauer, L.A.B., Blask, D.E., and Dauchy, R.T. (2007) Dietary factors and growth and metabolism in experimental tumors. *J. Nutr. Biochem.*, **18**, 637–649.
25. Sauer, L.A., Dauchy, R.T., Blask, D.E., Krause, J.A., Davidson, L.K., and Dauchy, E.M. (2005) Eicosapentaenoic acid suppresses cell proliferation

in MCF-7 human breast cancer xenografts in nude rats via a pertussis toxin-sensitive transduction pathway. *J. Nutr.*, **135**, 2124–2129.

26. Serhan, C.N., Hong, S., Gronert, K., Colgan, S.P., Devchand, P.R., Mirick, G., and Moussignac, R.L. (2002) Resolvins: a family of bioactive products of omega-3 fatty acid transformation circuits initiated by aspirin treatment that counter proinflammation signals. *J. Exp. Med.*, **196**, 1025–1037.

27. Clevers, H. (2004) At the crossroads of inflammation and cancer. *Cell*, **118**, 671–674.

28. Sauer, L.A., Dauchy, R.T., and Blask, D.E. (2000) Mechanism for the antitumor and anticachectic effects of $n-3$ fatty acids. *Cancer Res.*, **60**, 5289–5295.

29. Crawford, M.G., Galli, C., Visioli, F., Renaud, S., Simopoulos, A.P., and Spector, A.A. (2000) Role of plant-derived omega-3 fatty acids in human nutrition. *Ann. Nutr. Metabol.*, **44**, 263–265.

30. Rose, D.P. and Connolly, J.M. (1990) Effects of fatty acids and inhibitors of eicosanoid synthesis on the growth of a human breast cancer cell line in culture. *Cancer Res.*, **50**, 7139–7144.

31. Badawi, A.F.A. and Archer, M.C. (1998) Effect of hormonal status on the expression of the cyclooxygenase 1 and 2 genes and prostaglandin synthesis in rat mammary glands. *Prostaglandins Other Lipid Mediat.*, **56**, 167–181.

32. Singh, J., Hamid, R., and Reddy, B.S. (1997) Dietary fat and colon cancer: modulation of cyclooxygenase-2 by types and amount of dietary fat during the postinitiation stage of colon carcinogenesis. *Cancer Res.*, **57**, 3465–3470.

33. Von Schacky, C., Kiefl, R., Marcus, A.J., Broekman, M.J., and Kaminski, W.E. (1993) Dietary $n-3$ fatty acids accelerate catabolism of leukotriene B4 in human granulocytes. *Biochim. Biophys. Acta*, **1166**, 20–24.

34. Calviello, G., Di Nicuolo, F., Gragnoli, S., Piccioni, E., Serini, S., Maggiano, N., Tringali, G., Navarra, P., Ranelletti, F.O., and Palozza, P. (2004) $n-3$ PUFAs reduce VEGF expression in human colon cancer cells modulating the COX-2/PGE2 induced ERK-1 and -2 and HIF-1α induction pathway. *Carcinogenesis*, **25**, 2303–2320.

35. Larsson, S.C., Kumlin, M., Ingelman-Sundberg, M., and Wolk, A. (2004) Dietary long-chain $n-3$ fatty acids for the prevention of cancer: a review of potential mechanisms. *Am. J. Clin. Nutr.*, **79**, 935–945.

36. Sivaraman, V.S., Wang, H., Nuovo, G.J., and Malbon, C.C. (1997) Hyper-expression of mitogen-activated kinase in human breast cancer. *J. Clin. Invest.*, **99**, 1478–1483.

37. Boucher, M.-J., Morisset, J., Vachon, P.H., Reed, J.C., Laine, J., and Rivard, N. (2000) MEK/ERK signaling pathway regulates the expression of Bcl2, BclXL and Mcl-1 and promotes survival of human pancreatic cancer cells. *J. Cell. Biochem.*, **79**, 355–369.

38. Smally, K.S.M. (2003) A pivotal role for ERK in the oncogenic behavior of malignant melanoma. *Int. J. Cancer*, **104**, 527–532.

39. Bos, J.L. (1989) Ras oncogenes in human cancer: a review. *Cancer Res.*, **49**, 4682–4689.

40. Schwartz, S.A.H., Hernandez, A., and Mark Evers, B. (1999) The role of NF-kappaB/IkappaB proteins in cancer: implications for novel treatment strategies. *Surg. Oncol.*, **8**, 143–153.

41. Bharti, A.C. and Aggarwal, B.B. (2004) Ranking the role of RANK ligand in apoptosis. *Apoptosis*, **9**, 677–690.

42. Novak, T.E., Babcock, T.A., Jho, D.H., Helton, W.S., and Espat, N.J. (2003) NF-kappa B inhibition by omega-3 fatty acids modulates LPS-stimulated macrophage TNF-alpha transcription. *Am. J. Physiol.*, **284**, L84–L85.

43. Kersten, S., Desvergne, B., and Wahli, W. (2000) Roles of PPARS in health and disease. *Nature*, **405**, 421–424.

44. Ho, T.-C., Chen, S.-L., Yang, Y.-C., Liao, C.-L., Cheng, H.-C., and Tsao, Y.-P. (2006) PEDF induces p53-mediated apoptosis through PPAR gamma signaling in human umbilical vein endothelial cells. *Cardiovasc. Res.*, **76**, 213–223.

45. Bonofiglio, D., Aquila, S., Catalano, S., Gabriele, S., Belmonte, M., Middea, E., Qui, H., Morelli, C., Gentile, M., Maggiolini, M., and Ando, S. (2006) Peroxisome proliferator-activated receptor-γ activates p53 gene promoter binding to the nuclear factor-κB sequence in human MCF7 breast cancer cells. *Mol. Endocrinol.*, **20**, 3083–3092.
46. Zand, H., Rhimipour, A., Bakhshayesh, M., Shafiee, M., Nour Mohammadi, I., and Salimi, S. (2007) Involvement of PPAR-γ and p53 in DHA-induced apoptosis in Reh cells. *Mol. Cell. Biochem.*, **304**, 71–77.
47. Diep, Q.N., Touyz, R.M., and Schiffrin, E.L. (2000) Docosahexaenoic acid, a peroxisome proliferator-activated receptor-alpha ligand, induces apoptosis in vascular smooth muscle cells by stimulation of p38 mitogen-activated protein kinase. *Hypertension*, **36**, 851–855.
48. Tuller, E.R., Brock, A.L., Yu, H., Lou, J.R., Benbrook, D.M., and Ding, W.-Q. (2009) PPARα signaling mediates the synergistic cytotoxicity of clioquinol and docosahexaenoic acid in human cancer cells. *Biochem. Pharmacol.*, **77**, 1480–1486.
49. Berger, A., Roberts, M.A., and Hoff, B. (2006) How dietary arachidonic- and docosahexaenoic-acid rich oils differentially affect the murine hepatic transcriptome. *Lipids Health Dis.*, **5**, 10.
50. Fan, Y.Y., Spencer, T.E., Wang, N., Moyer, M.P., and Chapkin, R.S. (2003) Chemopreventive $n-3$ fatty acids activate RXR-alpha in colonocytes. *Carcinogenesis*, **24**, 1541–1548.
51. Aktas, H. and Halperin, J.A. (2004) Translational regulation of gene expression by ω-3 fatty acids. *J. Nutr.*, **136**, 2487S–2491S.
52. Reddy, B.S., Simi, B., Patel, N., Alaiaga, C., and Rao, C.V. (1996) Effect of amount and types of dietary fat on intestinal bacterial 7 alpha-dehydroxylase and phosphatidylinositol-specific phospholipase C and colonic mucosal diacylglycerol kinase and PKC activities during stages of colon tumor promotion. *Cancer Res.*, **56**, 2314–2320.
53. Fang, J.L., Vaca, C.E., Valsta, L.M., and Mutanen, M. (1996) Determination of DNA adducts of alonaldehyde in humans: effects of dietary fatty acid composition. *Carcinogenesis*, **17**, 1035–1040.
54. Cosgrove, J.P., Church, D.F., and Pryor, W.A. (1987) The kinetics of the autoxidation of polyunsaturated fatty acids. *Lipids Health Dis.*, **22**, 299–304.
55. Abou-el-Ela, S.H., Prasse, K.W., Farrell, R.L., Carroll, R.W., Wade, A.E., and Bunce, O.R. (1989) Effects of D,L-2-difluoromethylornithine and indomethacin on mammary tumor promotion in rats fed high $n-3$ and/or $n-6$ fat diets. *Cancer Res.*, **49**, 1434–1440.
56. Chajes, V., Sattler, W., Stranzl, A., and Kostner, G.M. (1995) Influence of $n-3$ fatty acids on the growth of human breast cancer cells *in vitro*: relationship to peroxides and vitamin E. *Breast Cancer Res. Treat.*, **34**, 199–212.
57. Arita, K., Kobuchi, H., Utsumi, T., Takehara, Y., Akiyama, J., Horton, A.A., and Utsumi, K. (2001) Mechanism of apoptosis in HL-60 cells induced by $n-3$ and $n-6$ polyunsaturated fatty acids. *Biochem. Pharmacol.*, **62**, 821–828.
58. Grimm, H., Mayer, K., Mayser, P., and Eigenbrodt, E. (2002) Regulatory potential of $n-3$ fatty acids in immunological and inflammatory processes. *Br. J. Nutr.*, **87**, S59–S67.
59. Rose, D.P. and Connolly, J.M., (1999) Omega-3 fatty acids as cancer chemopreventive agents. *Pharmacol. Ther.*, **83**, 217–244.
60. Zhuo, Z., Zhang, L., Mu, Q., Lou, Y., Gong, Z., Shi, Y., Ouyang, G., and Zhang, Y. (2009) The effect of combination treatment with docosahexaenoic acid and 5-fluorouracil on the mRNA expression of apoptosis-related genes, including the novel gene BCL2L12, in gastric cancer cells. *In Vitro Cell. Dev. Biol. Anim.*, **45**, 69–74.
61. Yamamoto, D., Kiyozuka, Y., Adachi, Y., Takada, H., Hioki, K., and

Tsubura, A. (1999) Synergistic action of apoptosis induced by eicosapentaenoic acid and TNP-470 on human breast cancer cells. *Breast Cancer Res. Treat.*, **55**, 149–160.

62. Nakagawa, H., Yamamoto, D., Kiyozuka, Y., Tsuta, K., Uemura, Y., Hioki, K., Tsutsui, Y., and Tsubura, A. (2000) Effects of genistein and synergistic action in combination with eicosapentaenoic acid on the growth of breast cancer cell lines. *J. Cancer Res. Clin. Oncol.*, **126**, 448–454.
63. Menendez, J.A., Ropero, S., del Mar Barbacid, M., Montero, S., Solanas, M., Escrich, E., Cortes-Funes, H., and Colmer, R. (2001) Synergistic interaction between vinorelbine and gamma-linolenic acid in breast cancer cells. *Eur. J. Cancer*, **37**, 402–413.
64. Menedez, J.A., del Mar Barbacid, M., Montero, S., Sevilla, E., Escrich, E., Solanas, M., Cortes-Funes, H., and Colomer, R. (2001) Effects of gamma-linolenic acid and oleic acid on paclitaxel cytotoxicity in human breast cancer cells. *Eur. J. Cancer*, **37**, 402–413.
65. Hardman, W.E.M., Moyer, M.P., and Cameron, I.L. (2000) Dietary fish oil sensitizes A549 lung xenografts to doxorubicin chemotherapy. *Cancer Lett.*, **151**, 145–151.
66. Shao, Y., Pardini, L., and Pardini, R.S. (1995) Dietary menhaden oil enhances mitomycin C antitumor activity toward human mammary carcinoma MX-1. *Lipids*, **30**, 1035–1045.
67. DeGraffenried, L.A., Friedrichs, W.E., Fulcher, L., Fernandes, G., and Silva, J.M. (2003) Eicosapentaenoic acid restores tamoxifen sensitivity in breast cancer cells with high Akt activity. *Ann. Oncol.*, **14**, 969–970.
68. Rowinsky, E.K. (1997) The development and clinical utility of the taxane class of antimicrotubule chemotherapy agents. *Annu. Rev. Med.*, **48**, 353–374.
69. Wani, M.C., Taylor, H.L., and Wall, M.E. (1971) Plasnt antitumor agents VI. The isolation and structure of taxol: a novel antileukemic and antitumour agent from *Taxus brevifolia*. *J. Am. Chem. Soc.*, **93**, 2325–2327.
70. McGuirem, W.P., Rowinsky, E.K., Rosenshein, N.B., Grumbine, F.C., Ettinger, D.S., Armstrong, D.K., and Donehower, R.C. (1989) Taxol: a unique antineoplastic agent with significant activity in advanced ovarian epithelial neoplasms. *Ann. Intern. Med.*, **111**, 273–279.
71. Schiff, P.B., Fant, J., and Horwitz, S.B. (1980) Taxol stabilizes microtubules in mouse fibroblast cells. *Proc. Natl. Acad. Sci. USA*, **77**, 1561–1565.
72. Jordan, M.A., Toso, R.J., Thrower, D., and Wilson, L. (1993) Mechanism of mitotic block and inhibition of cell proliferation by Taxol at low concentrations. *Mol. Biol. Cell*, **10**, 947–949.
73. Hennenfent, K.L. and Govindan, R., (2006) Novel formulations of taxanes: a review. Old wine in a new bottle? *Ann. Oncol.*, **17**, 735–749.
74. Xie, Z., Guan, H., Chen, X., Lu, C., Chen, L., Hu, X., Shi, Q., and Jing, X. (2007) A novel polymer–paclitaxel conjugate based on amphiphilic triblock copolymer. *J. Control. Release*, **117**, 210–216.
75. Wang, Y., Xin, D., Liu, K., Zhu, M., and Xiang, J. (2009) Heparin–paclitaxel conjugates as drug delivery system: synthesis, self-assembly property, drug release, and antitumor activity. *Bioconjug. Chem.*, **20**, 2214–2221.
76. Ojima, I., Chen, J., Sun, L., Borell, C.P., Wang, T., Miller, M.L., Lin, S., Geng, X., Kuznetsova, L., Qu, C., Gallager, D., Zhao, X., Zanardi, I., Xia, S., Horwitz, S.B., Mallen-St. Clair, J., Guerriero, J.L., Bar-Sagi, D., Veith, J.M., Pera, P., and Bernacki, R.J. (2008) Design, synthesis, and biological evaluation of new-generation taxoids. *J. Med. Chem.*, **51**, 3203–3221.
77. Tsao, Y.P., Russo, A., Nyamuswa, G., Silber, R., and Liu, L.F. (1993) Interaction between replication forks and topoisomerase I–DNA cleavable complexes: studies in a cell-free SV40 DNA replication system. *Cancer Res.*, **53**, 5908–5914.
78. Tanizawa, A., Fujimori, A., Fujimori, Y., and Pommier, Y. (1994) Comparison of topoisomerase I inhibition, DHA damage, and cytotoxicity of

camptothecin derivatives presently in clinical trials. *J. Natl. Cancer Inst.*, **86**, 836–842.

79. Wang, Y., Li, L., Jiang, W., and Larrick, J.W. (2005) Synthesis and evaluation of a DHA and 10-hydroxycamptotecin conjugate. *Bioorg. Med. Chem.*, **13**, 5592–5599.

80. Myers, C.E. and Chabner, B.A. (1990) *Cancer Chemotherapy – Principles and Practice*, Lippincott, Philadelphia, PA.

81. Dorr, R.T. and Von Hoff, D.D. (1994) *Cancer Chemotherapy Handbook*, 2nd edn, Appleton & Lange, Norwalk, CT.

82. Fornari, F.A., Randolph, J.K., Yalowich, J.C., Ritke, M.K., and Gewitz, D.A. (1994) Interference by doxorubicin with DNA unwinding in MCF-7 breast tumor cells. *Mol. Pharmacol.*, **45**, 649–656.

83. Wang, Y., Li, L., Jiang, W., Yang, Z., and Zhang, Z. (2006) Synthesis and preliminary antitumor activity evaluation of a DHA and doxorubicin conjugate. *Bioorg. Med. Chem. Lett.*, **16**, 2974–2977.

84. Kaneko, T., Willner, D., Monkovic, I., Knipe, J.O., Braslawsky, G.R., Greenfield, R.S., and Vyas, D.M. (1991) New hydrazone derivatives of adriamycin and their immunoconjugates – a correlation between acid stability and cytotoxicity. *Bioconjug. Chem.*, **2**, 133–141.

85. Huan, M.-L., Zhou, S.-Y., Teng, Z.-H., Zhang, B.-L., Liu, X.-Y., Wang, J.-P., and Mei, Q.-B. (2009) Conjugation with α-linolenic acid improves cancer cell uptake and cytotoxicity of doxorubicin. *Bioorg. Med. Chem. Lett.*, **19**, 2579–2584.

86. Mammoto, T., Mukai, M., Mammoto, A., Yamanaka, Y., Hayashi, Y., Mashimo, T., Kishi, Y., and Nakamura, H. (2002) Intravenous anesthetic, propofol inhibits invasion of cancer cells. *Cancer Lett.*, **184**, 165–170.

87. Siddiqui, R.A., Zerouga, M., Wu, M., Castillo, A., Harvey, K., Zaloga, G.P., and Stillwell, W. (2005) Anticancer properties of propofol–docosahexaenoate and propofol–eicosapentaenoate of breast cancer cells. *Breast Cancer Res.*, **7**, R645–R654.

88. Harvey, K.A., Xu, Z., Whitley, P., Davisson, V.J., and Siddiqui, R.A. (2010) Characterization of anticancer properties of 2,6-diisopropylphenol–docasahexaenoate and analogues in breast cancer cells. *Biorg. Med. Chem.*, **10**, 1866–1874.

89. Schobert, R., Biersack, B., Knauer, S., and Ocker, M. (2008) Conjugates of the fungal cytotoxin illudin M with improved tumour specificity. *Bioorg. Med. Chem. Lett.*, **16**, 8592–8597.

90. Senzer, N., Arsenau, J., Rchards, D., Berman, B., MacDonald, J.R., and Smith, S. (2005) Irofulven demonstrates clinical activity against metastatic hormone-refractory prostate cancer in a phase 2 single-agent trial. *Am. J. Clin. Oncol.*, **28**, 36–42.

91. Alexandre, J., Raymond, E., Karci, M.O., Brain, E.C., Lokiec, F., Kahatt, C., Faivre, S., Yovin, A., Goldwasser, F., Smith, S.L., MacDonald, J.R., Misset, J.L., and Cvitkovic, E. (2004) Phase I and pharmacokinetic study of irofulven administered weekly or biweekly in advanced solid tumor patients. *Clin. Cancer Res.*, **10**, 3377–3385.

92. Anel, A., Halmos, T., Torres, J.M., Pineiro, A., Antonakis, K., and Uriel, J. (1990) Cytotoxicity of chlorambucil and chlorambucil–fatty acid conjugates against human lymphomas and normal human peripheral blood lymphocytes. *Biochem. Pharmacol.*, **40**, 1193–1200.

93. Esteban, C., Geuskens, M., and Ureil, J. (1991) Activation of an alpha-fetoprotein (AFP)/receptor autocrine loop in HT-29 human colon carcinoma cells. *Int. J. Cancer*, **49**, 425–430.

94. Amiel, S.A., Stewart, J.F., Earl, H.M., Knight, R.K., and Rubens, R.D. (1984) Adriamycin and mitomycin C as initial chemotherapy for advanced breast cancer. *Eur. J. Cancer Clin. Oncol.*, **20**, 631–634.

95. Krauss, S., Sonoda, T., and Solomon, A. (1979) Treatment of advanced gastrointestinal cancer with 5-fluorouracil and mitomycin C. *Cancer*, **43**, 1598–1603.

96. Roos, W.P. and Kaina, B. (2006) DNA damage-induced cell death by apoptosis. *Trends Mol. Med.*, **12**, 440–450.

97. Shikano, M., Onimura, K., Fukai, Y., Hori, M., Fukazawa, H., Mizuno, S., Yazawa, K., and Uehara, Y. (1998) 1a-docosahexaenoyl mitomycin C: a novel inhibitor of protein tyrosine kinase. *Biochem. Biophys. Res. Commun.*, **248**, 858–863.

98. Peters, G.J., van der Wilt, C.L., van Moorsel, C.J.A., Kroep, J.R., Bergman, A.M., and Ackland, S.P. (2000) Basis for effective combination cancer chemotherapy with antimetabolites. *Pharmacol. Ther.*, **87**, 227–253.

99. Halmos, T.M.P., Antonakis, K., and Uriel, J. (1999) Fatty acid conjugates of 2′-dexoy-5-fluorouridine as prodrugs for the selective delivery of 5-fluorouracil to tumor cells. *Biochem. Pharmacol.*, **44**, 149–155.

100. Zhang, Y.-X., Dai, G.F., Wang, L., and Tao, J.-C. (2007) Synthesis and cytotoxicity of novel fatty acid–nucleoside conjugates. *Bioorg. Med. Chem. Lett.*, **17**, 1613–1615.

101. Barnwarth, B., Labat, I., Moride, Y., and Schaeverbeke, T. (1994) Methotrexate in theumatoid arthritis: an update. *Drugs*, **47**, 25–50.

102. Kinsky, S.C., Loader, J.E., and Hashimoto, K. (1987) Inhibition of cell proliferation by putative metabolites and non-degradable analogs of methotrexate–gamma-dimyristoylphosphatidylethanolamine. *Biochim. Biophys. Acta*, **917**, 211–218.

103. Zerouga, M., Stillwell, W., and Jenski, L.J. (2002) Synthesis of a novel phosphatidylcholine conjugated to docosahexaenoic acid and methotrexate that inhibits cell proliferation. *Anti-Cancer Drugs*, **13**, 301–311.

104. Tannock, I.F. (1989) Principles of cell proliferation: cell kinetics in *Cancer: Principle and Practice of Oncology*, (eds V.T. DeVita Jr., S. Hellman, and S.A. Rosenberg), 3rd edn, Lippincott, Philadelphia, PA, pp. 3–13.

105. Bradley, M.O., Webb, N.L., Anthony, F.H., Devanesan, P., Witman, P.A., Hemamalini, S., Chander, M.C., Baker, S.D., He, L., Horwitz, S.B., and Swindell, C.S. (2001) Tumor targeting by covalent conjugation of a natural fatty acid to paclitaxel. *Clin. Cancer Res.*, **7**, 3229–3258.

106. Sparreboom, A., Wolff, A.C., Verweig, J., Zabelina, Y., van Zomeren, D.M., McIntire, G.L., Swindell, C.S., Donehower, R.C., and Baker, S.D. (2003) Disposition of docosahexaenoic acid–paclitaxel, a novel taxane, in blood: *in vitro* and clinical pharmacokinetic studies. *Clin. Cancer Res.*, **9**, 151–159.

107. Sparreboom, A., van Zuylen, L., Brouwer, E., Loos, W.J., de Bruijn, P., Gelderblom, H., Pillay, M., Nooter, K., Stoter, G., and Verweig, J. (1999) Cremophor EL-mediated alteration of paclitaxel distribution in human blood: clinical pharmacokinetic implications. *Cancer Res.*, **59**, 1454–1457.

108. Wolff, A.C., Donehower, R.C., Carducci, M.K., Carducci, M.A., Brahmer, J.R., Zabelina, Y., Bradley, M.O., Anthony, F.H., Swindell, C.S., Witman, P.A., Webb, N.L., and Baker, S.D. (2003) Phase I study of docosahexaenoic acid–paclitaxel: a taxane–fatty acid conjugate with a unique pharmacology and toxicity profile. *Clin. Cancer Res.*, **9**, 3589–3597.

109. Browder, T., Butterfield, C.E., Kraling, B.M., Shi, B., Marshall, B., O'Reilly, M.S., and Folkman, J. (2000) Antiangiogenic scheduling of chemotherapy improves efficacy against experimental drug-resistant cancer. *Cancer Res.*, **60**, 1878–1886.

110. Fracasso, P.M., Picus, J., Wildi, J.D., Goodner, S.A., Creekmore, A.N., Gao, F., Govindan, R., Ellis, M.J., Tan, B.R., Linette, G.P., Fu, C.H.H., Pentikis, H.S., Zumbrun, S.C., Egorin, M.J., and Bellet, R.E. (2009) Phase 1 and pharmacokinetic study of weekly docosahexaenoic acid–paclitaxel, Taxoprexin®, in resistant solid tumor malignancies. *Cancer Chemother. Pharmacol.*, **63**, 451–458.

111. Smith, R.E., Brown, A.M., Mamounas, E.P., Anderson, S.J., Lembersky, B.C., Atkins, J.H., Shibata, H.R., Baez, L.,

DeFusco, P.A., Divila, E., Tipping, S.J., Bearden, J.D., and Thirlwell, M.P. (1999) Randomized trial of 3-hour versus 24-hour infusion of high-dose paclitaxel in patients with metastatic or locally advanced breast cancer: National Surgical Adjuvant Breast and Bowel Project Protocol B-26. *J. Clin. Oncol.*, **17**, 3403–3411.

112. Bellet, R., Carducci, M., Petrylak, D., Kasimis, B., Irwin, D., Modiano, M., Manour, R., Axelrod, R., and Doukas, M. (2004) Phase II study of DHA–paclitaxel (TXP) as first line chemotherapy in patients with hormone refractory prostate cancer (HRPC). *Proc. Am. Soc. Clin. Oncol.*, **22**, 4657.

113. Johnston, S.R.D., Houston, S., Jones, A., Evans, T.R., and Schacter, L. (2004) Efficacy of DHA–paclitaxel (TXP) for the second-line treatment of breast cancer. *Proc. Am. Soc. Clin. Oncol.*, **22**, 65.

114. Jacobs, A., Planting, A., Ferry, D., Michell, E., Evans, T.R., Wilke, H., Hochster, H., Knuth, A., Schacter, L., and Donehower, R. (2003) Efficacy of DHA–paclitaxel (TXP) in pancreatic cancer. *Proc. Am. Soc. Clin. Oncol.*, **21**, 2981.

115. Jones, R.J., Hawkins, R.E., Eatock, M.M., Ferry, D.R., Eskens, F.A.L.M., Wilke, H., and Evans, T.R.J. (2008) A phase II open-label study of DHA–paclitaxel (Taxoprexin) by 2-h intravenous infusion in previously untreated patients with locally advanced or metastatic gastric or oesophageal adenocarcinoma. *Cancer Chemother. Pharmacol.*, **61**, 435–441.

116. Schacter, L.P., Bukowski, R.M., Carducci, M.A., Donehower, R., Dunlop, D., Evans, T.R., Gilby, E., and Johnston, S. (2004) Safety and efficacy of DHA–Paclitaxel (TXP) in non-small cell lung cancer. *Proc. Am. Soc. Clin. Oncol.*, **22**, 7111.

117. Payne, M., Ellis, P., Dunlop, D., Ranson, M., Danson, S., Schacter, L., and Talbot, D. (2006) DHA–paclitaxel (Taxoprexin) as first-line treatment in patients with stage IIIB or IV non-small cell lung cancer: report of a phase II open-label multicenter trial. *J. Thorac. Oncol.*, **1**, 984–990.

118. Modiano, M.R., Houston, S., Savage, P., Price, C., Schacter, L., and Gilby, E. (2003) Efficacy of DHA–paclitaxel (TXP) in malignant melanoma. *Proc. Am. Soc. Clin. Oncol.*, **21**, 2891.

119. Harries, M., O'Donnell, A., Scurr, M., Reade, S., Cole, C., Judson, I., Greystoke, A., Twelves, C., and Kaye, S. (2004) Phase I/II study of DHA–paclitaxel in combination with carboplatin in patients with advanced malignant solid tumors. *Br. J. Cancer*, **91**, 1651–1655.

120. Vredenburg, M.R., Ojima, I., Veith, J., Pera, P., Kee, K., Cabral, F., Sharma, A., Kanter, P., and Bernacki, R.J. (2001) Effects of orally active taxanes on P-glycoprotein modulation and colon and breast carcinoma drug resistance. *J. Natl. Cancer Inst.*, **93**, 1234–1245.

121. Ferlini, C., Distefano, M., Pignatelli, F., Lin, S., Riva, A., Bombardelli, E., Mancuso, S., Ojima, I., and Scambia, G. (2000) Antitumor activity of novel taxanes that act as cytotoxic agents and P-glycoprotein inhibitors at the same time. *Br. J. Cancer*, **83**, 1762–1768.

122. Kuznetsova, L., Chen, J., Sun, L., Wu, X., Pepe, A., Veith, J.M., Pera, P., Bernacki, R.J., and Ojima, I. (2006) Synthesis and evaluation of novel fatty acid-second-generation taxoid conjugates as promising anticancer agents. *Bioorg. Med. Chem. Lett.*, **16**, 974–977.

Part VI
Special Topics

Drug Delivery in Oncology: From Basic Research to Cancer Therapy, First Edition.
Edited by Felix Kratz, Peter Senter, and Henning Steinhagen.

42
RNA Drug Delivery Approaches

Yuan Zhang and Leaf Huang

42.1
Introduction

Small interfering RNA (siRNA) has a high potential in therapeutic applications. siRNAs are noncoding for proteins and they induce a sequence-specific messenger RNA (mRNA) degradation. Since they do not interact with DNA transcription, there is reduced concern about possible adverse gene alteration [1]. siRNA can be utilized as a therapeutic drug for gene silencing for a wide range of target proteins to potentially treat various diseases [2]. The drug siRNA molecule can target any mRNA of interest, regardless of the cellular location of the translated proteins. Furthermore, siRNA is very potent, as only a few siRNA molecules per cell are sufficient to produce effective gene silencing [3, 4].

42.2
RNA Molecules with Potential for Cancer Treatment

RNA interference (RNAi) is a process in which a specific mRNA is targeted for degradation to inhibit the synthesis of the encoded protein. Two types of small RNA molecules – microRNA (miRNA) and siRNA – are central to the RNAi function. It is known that both miRNA and siRNA participate in carcinogenesis, either inhibiting suppressor genes or stimulating oncogenes.

The initiation step of the RNAi pathway is that the double-stranded RNAs are processed into 21- to 23-nucleotide siRNAs by an RNase III-like enzyme called Dicer. Then, the siRNAs assemble into endoribonuclease-containing complexes known as RNA-induced silencing complexes (RISCs). The RISC uses the siRNA as a template for recognizing complementary mRNA. The proteins in the RISC unwind siRNA, keep the antisense strand, and degrade the sense strand. The antisense strand in the RISC recruits the corresponding mRNA in a sequence-specific manner, at which time a protein component of the RISC called Slicer cuts the mRNA in the middle of the binding region. The cut mRNA is recognized by the cell as being abnormal and is subsequently destroyed, resulting in gene silencing

Drug Delivery in Oncology: From Basic Research to Cancer Therapy, First Edition.
Edited by Felix Kratz, Peter Senter, and Henning Steinhagen.

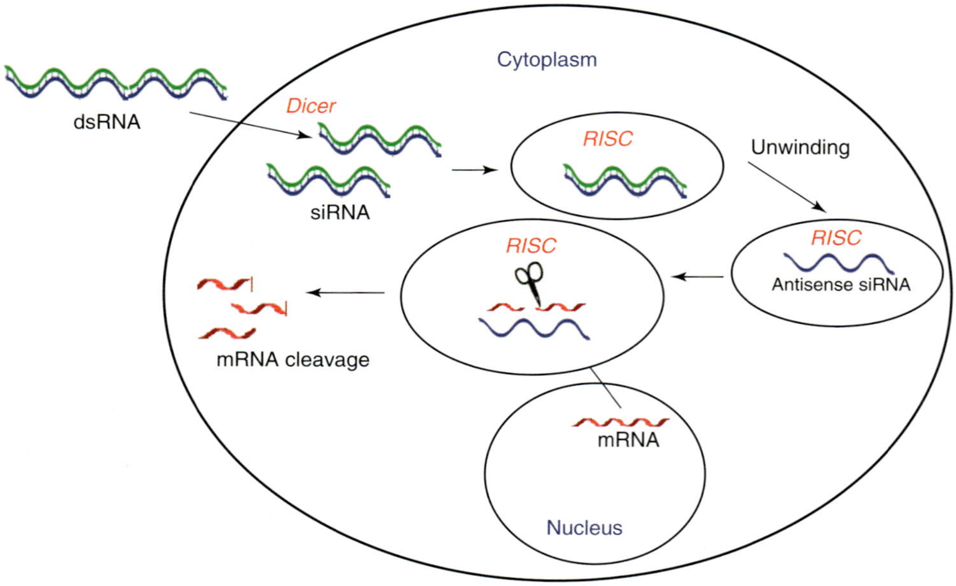

Figure 42.1 Mechanism of RNAi. (Adapted from [6].)

(Figure 42.1). As RNAi relies on the sequence-specific interaction between siRNA and mRNA, siRNA can be tailored to silence almost any gene. In addition to naturally generated siRNA from a long double-stranded RNA, siRNAs that have been chemically synthesized or created by *in vitro* transcription systems can also induce gene silencing. Moreover, the multiple administration of synthetic siRNAs achieved long-term silencing effects of the target gene without disrupting the endogenous miRNA pathways [5].

In the case of miRNA, a miRNA-induced silencing complex (miRISC) associates with the mature miRNA, and the complex binds to the 3′-untranslated region of mRNA and blocks translation. Many miRNAs form imperfectly complementary stem–loop structures on the target sense strand of mRNA, as opposed to siRNA, which requires a near-perfect match.

42.3 Chemical Modification Strategies

Although a double-stranded RNA is more stable than single-stranded RNA, unprotected siRNA can be quickly degraded in and outside the cells. In order to improve the stability of siRNA for prolonged circulation, chemical modification of siRNA has been attempted without compromising its potency. Various positions within the siRNA duplex have been chemically modified in a wide variety of ways to confer nuclease resistance (see Table 42.1).

Table 42.1 Some structures of siRNA modifications.

Sugar modification	2′-O-Me-RNA 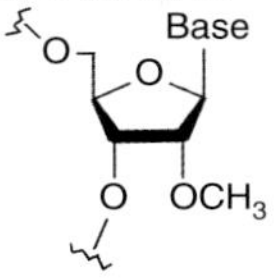	2′-O-DNP-RNA 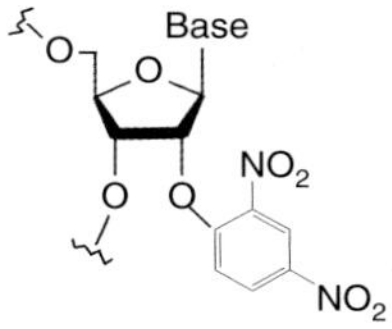
	2′F-RNA 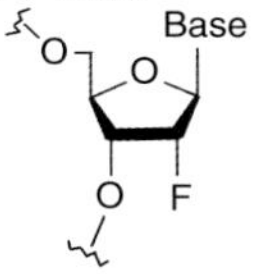	LNA 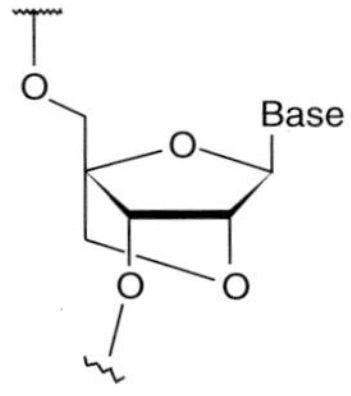
Nucleobase modification	5-Br-Ura 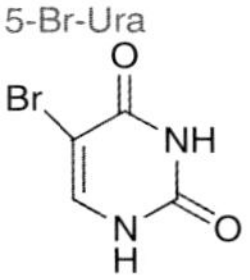	5-I-Ura 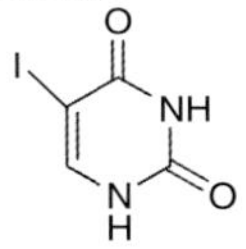
	2-thiouracil 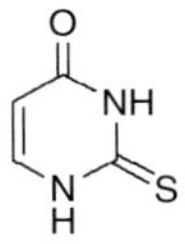	4-thiouracil 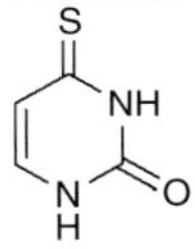
	Diaminopurine 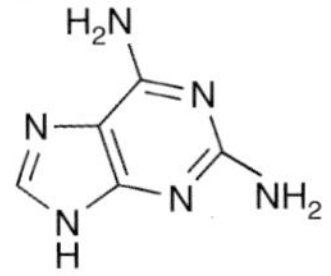	Dihydrouracil 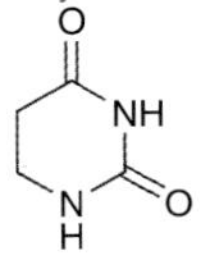
Terminal modification	Cholesterol conjugates 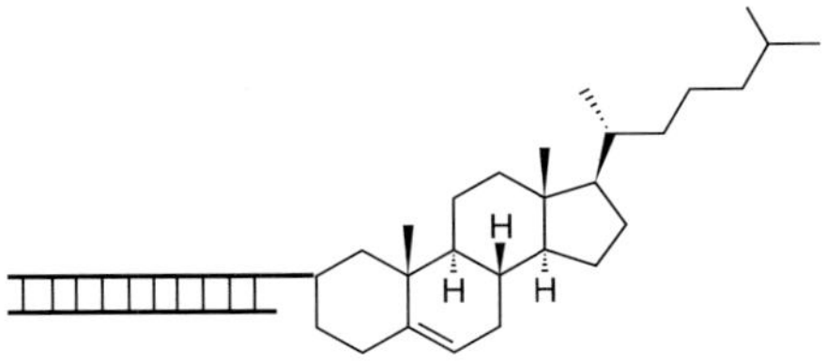	
	CPP conjugates 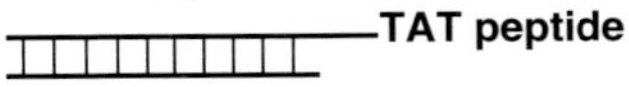	

As for increasing requirements for effective RNAi, chemical modifications can also be used to optimize potency as well, via features such as target-binding affinity by modulating hybridization on-rate and off-rate, conformational preorganization (A-form helical structure), and duplex flexibility. Part of the increase in potency may be due to the increased nuclease stability of the chemically modified siRNA.

Chemical modifications can also be used to reduce the immunostimulatory properties of siRNAs [7], which is considered a potentially dangerous off-target effect.

42.3.1 Sugar Modification

The most widely used siRNA modifications are on the sugar moiety. Early studies showed that A-form duplex structure is important, the 2′-OH is not required for active siRNA [8]. Thus, the 2′-position has been extensively modified. For example, 2′-*O*-methylation of RNA increases binding affinity and nuclease stability. Bulky 2′-substituents are not well tolerated in the siRNA duplex. The 2′-OH groups of siRNA in both strands can be converted at random into 2,4-dinitrophenyl (2′-*O*-DNP) ethers, which shows improved binding affinity, nuclease resistance, and potency. Fluorine substituent at the 2′-position can be functional and active throughout the sense and antisense strands. The 2′F-RNA-modified siRNA duplex can increase serum stability and the duplex-binding affinity. Capodici *et al.* [9] incorporated fluorinated CTP and UTP modifications into siRNA, and these fluorine-derivatized siRNAs yielded equivalent activity to unmodified siRNA. The modification could protect the siRNA from RNase A and could be delivered without the transfection reagent in the presence of serum. A fully modified siRNA composed of 2′-*O*-Me- and 2′F-RNA modified nucleotides showed 500 times more potency than the unmodified RNA [10], and significantly reduced immunostimulatory activity [11].

Locked nucleic acid (LNA) is an RNA mimic in which the ribose sugar moiety is locked by an oxymethylene bridge connecting 2′-C and 4′-C. LNA modification possesses high binding affinity and excellent specificity toward complementary DNA or RNA oligonucleotides. In addition, LNA-modified oligonucleotides improve resistance to enzymatic degradation and show high stability in biological system [12, 13]. Introduction of LNA nucleotides in siRNA (i.e., LNA-modified siRNA or siLNA) could substantially increase the thermal stability of the modified RNA duplex without compromising the efficacy of RNAi [14] and reduce the off-target gene regulation compared to the corresponding unmodified siRNA [15].

42.3.2 Nucleobase Modification

Some modified bases can be used to stabilize A–U base pairs, although the activity of the modified RNA may be somewhat reduced. Examples are 5-Br-Ura and 5-I-Ura instead of uracil, and diaminopurine instead of adenine. 2-Thiouracil, 4-thiouracil, dihydrouracil, and some uracil analogs are also used, which could increase binding affinity, potency, and specificity if placed appropriately within the duplex. For example, a 2-thiouracil base at the 3′-end of the antisense stand and a dihydrouracil base at the 3′-end of the sense strand make the modified siRNA duplex more active [16].

42.3.3 Terminal Modification

The terminal end of each strand can be modified by 5′-end chemical phosphorylation. Antisense strand phosphorylation helps to ensure high potency, especially when the strand is modified. Furthermore, various groups can be conjugated to the ends of a siRNA duplex, especially the terminal end of the sense strand. Fluorescent dyes or biotin are conjugated to the RNA terminal ends to allow biochemical studies. Cell-penetrating peptides (CPPs) are short peptides that facilitate cellular uptake of various cargos. Conjugation of CPPs via disulfide bonds and lipophilic groups such as steroids and lipids may help with siRNA delivery through improving its stability, facilitating penetration and cellular uptake. Abes *et al.* [17] and Moulton *et al.* [18] conjugated arginine-rich CPPs and penetratin to oligonucleotides for efficient delivery of nucleic acid cargos. Generally, the 5′-end of the antisense strand is most sensitive to modifications [19]. Attaching a group to an antisense 5′-phosphate does not necessarily eliminate RNAi activity [20].

42.4 Challenges in RNA Delivery

42.4.1 Chemical Stability and Structure Modification

Naked siRNAs are highly susceptible to nuclease degradation, especially *in vivo*. In order to allow siRNA to survive long enough to maintain an acceptable level in tissues, its degradation must be minimized or at least significantly delayed. Chemical modifications of siRNA have been extensively used to achieve enhanced resistance to nuclease-induced degradation [21]. Chemical modifications can be induced to the 5′- or 3′-terminus, backbone, sugar, and nucleobase of siRNA, which could increase the stability of the siRNA duplex and retain or enhance the gene-silencing activity, and in some cases also significantly reduce the immunogenicity. Effective design and modification of siRNA can also allow minimization of the potential sequence-dependent off-target effects. For example, 2′-*O*-methyl ribosyl group substitution at position 2 in the sense strand could reduce silencing of most off-target transcripts [22].

42.4.2
Extracellular Delivery Stage

The most important challenge in siRNA therapy is the issue of delivery. siRNA is negatively charged hydrophilic molecule so that it has difficulty in passing through negatively charged hydrophobic cellular membranes by passive diffusion. *In vivo* delivery of naked siRNA to appropriate disease sites remains a considerable obstacle because of rapid enzymatic digestion in the plasma and renal elimination. Limited penetration across the tumor capillary endothelium and inefficient cellular uptake by cancer cells further limit the use naked siRNA as a drug formulation [3]. Thus, developing effective *in vivo* delivery systems is critical to overcome these difficulties. The delivery vectors should be biocompatible, biodegradable, nonimmunogenic, and provide target tissue-specific distribution after systematic administration, avoiding rapid hepatic or renal clearance. Generally, nanoparticles with a mean size around 100–200 nm are ideal for tumor targeting, because they can accumulate in the tumor leaky vasculature via the enhanced permeability and retention (EPR) effect after intravenous administration. However, the circulating nanoparticles are prone to capture by the reticuloendothelial system (RES), such as liver Kupffer cells and splenic macrophages, causing a major loss of the injected dose (greater than 50%) within a few hours after intravenous injection. Thus, the nanoparticles need to have a prolonged circulation half-life and the ability to escape the surveillance of the RES, in order to encounter the leaky tumor vasculature before they are cleared from the *in vivo* circulation [23]. For the sake of improving the pharmacokinetic properties of delivery vectors after intravenous administration mentioned above, poly(ethylene glycol) (PEG) was introduced to modify the surface of nanoparticles. This hydrophilic polymer imparts a steric barrier on the surface of nanoparticles and minimizes the opsonization effect. PEGylation on the surface of the nanoparticles produces "stealth" properties – shielding the nanoparticles and helping them escape the surveillance of RES.

42.4.3
Target Cell Specificity and Uptake via Targeting Ligands

The delivery vectors need to interact with the cell membrane, internalize, and localize in the intracellular compartment before releasing the nucleic acid cargo. Although PEGylation mentioned above can largely facilitate the accumulation of nanoparticles in the tumor leaky vasculature and confer stability in the systemic circulation, it hinders the uptake of the nanoparticles by the tumor cells once they extravasate [23] because of its steric configuration coating on the outer surface of the nanoparticles. In order to solve the PEG dilemma, promote the interaction with target cells, and prevent side-effects by avoiding nonspecific binding to nondiseased cells, many cell-specific targeting ligands (e.g., small molecules, antibodies, aptamers, peptides) that can recognize unique biomarkers (e.g., antigens, receptors) on the diseased cell surface are modified on the surface of the vectors to construct functional nanoparticles.

42.4.4
Endosomal Release

In the intracellular environment, inefficient release of the nucleic acid cargo complexes from endocytic vesicles into the cytoplasm is one of the primary causes of poor gene delivery. After delivery into target cells via endocytosis, the delivery systems should promote the endosomal release of siRNA from nanoparticles into the cytoplasm, followed by the interaction of siRNA with endogenous RISC in order to be bioactive. In detail, once the delivery vectors have been internalized into cells and arrive in an endosomal compartment, two essential processes have to occur in order to achieve higher gene transfection: (i) dissociation of the nucleic acid from the delivery vector, and (ii) destabilization of the endosomal membrane to allow the release of the nucleic acid into the cytosol, which is the site of action for siRNAs, and the release process is also critical to make the other nucleic acid cargo (e.g., plasmid DNA (pDNA)) accessible for transport to the nucleus for transcription.

To overcome this obstacle, exogenous agents such as chloroquine [24] or activated adenovirus [25] were added to affect escape from the endosome and lysosomes; however, they have cellular toxicity, immunogenicity, and other side-effects that make them impractical for *in vivo* gene therapy.

Thus, a variety of stimulus-responsive nanoparticle formulations for enhancing drug endosomal release and subsequently therapeutic effect have been designed. Generally, several models have been proposed to interpret the possible mechanism of lipid/polymer-based nanoparticles disrupting the endosome membrane and fleeing from the endosome/lysosome. These accepted models include the ion-pairing model (H_{II} phase formation), the proton sponge model, and the charge–charge destabilization model [23], which will be explained in detail below.

42.5
Potential Adverse Effects of RNA Therapy

42.5.1
Induction of Immune Responses

siRNA therapy could induce "immune stimulation" – the recognition of a RNA duplex by the innate immune system. GU-rich regions in a particular sequence motif can lead to secretion of inflammatory cytokines in a cell-type- and sequence-specific manner [26]. siRNA-mediated immune induction seems to rely on the Toll-like receptor (TLR) receptors located in the endosome [27], such that the mode of delivery and hence compartmentalization of the siRNA greatly influences the cellular response. Not all siRNAs could induce immune stimulation. The stimulation of innate immune responses by siRNA may be related to a specific nucleotide sequence, or motif. The TLR-7-mediated interferon-α induction by siRNA was shown to be sequence specific [28, 29].

42.5.2
Off-Target Effect

The "off-target" effect is the inhibition of a gene not intended for silencing. It may occur because the gene shares a partial homology with the siRNA. For example, one class of siRNA off-target effects involves partial hybridization with the wrong mRNA or the sense strand can cause off-target effects if it hybridizes to an irrelevant mRNA [30]. Silencing of an off-target is clearly unwanted as the cellular consequences of altered gene activity are unknown and unpredictable [26]. Thus, one of the solutions is to increase the selective uptake of the antisense strand and decrease incorporation of the sense strand via appropriate siRNA duplex modifications. The undesired silencing of nontarget genes may lead to data misinterpretation and toxicity. Thus, the design and selection of a specific siRNA may involve consideration of internal repeated sequence, GC content, appropriate siRNA length, specific base preference in the sense strand, secondary structure, and so on. Some studies suggest that some of the off-target gene changes may be due to the delivery system itself, such as cationic lipids [31, 32]. Above all, off-targeting remains a critical issue for therapeutic applications of RNAi and tolerable levels of the off-targeting effect are required for siRNA gene therapy.

42.5.3
Saturation of Endogenous Silencing Pathway

siRNA relies on the endogenous miRNA machinery in order to achieve potent target silencing. The risk of saturating such pathways and hence perturbing the natural system has been reported [26]. siRNA resembles miRNA precursors before and after Dicer processing, so all components of the miRNA pathway might be blocked by high doses of the ectopic RNA.

42.6
RNA Delivery

Getting siRNA into cells is one of the biggest challenges of any application of RNAi (Figure 42.2). Naked siRNAs appear to be poorly transported into cells and even if there is little free siRNA that can eventually enter the cells, most would remain sequestered within endosomal/lysosomal vesicles where it may likely undergo degradation by nucleases. Therefore, in order to achieve siRNA-mediated gene silencing in cells, a feasible delivery system is required to improve cellular uptake and intracellular trafficking of the encapsulated siRNAs, facilitating their binding with the complementary mRNA in RISC in the cytosolic compartment before gene silencing.

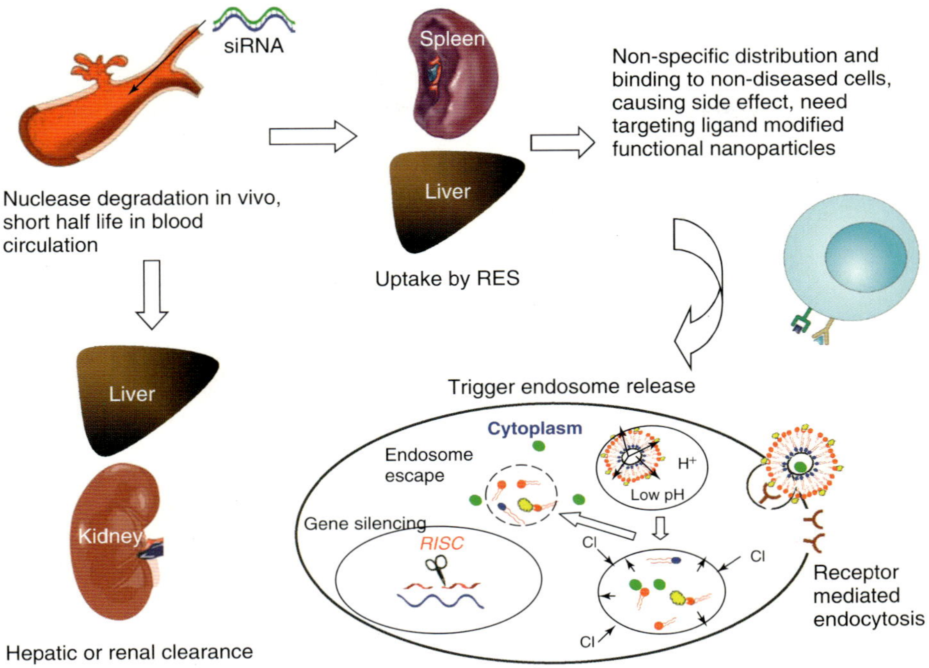

Figure 42.2 Challenges of *in vivo* siRNA delivery.

42.6.1
Physical Methods

Multiple physical and mechanical approaches have been used for *in vivo* gene delivery, which are considered the simplest ways to deliver genes *in vivo* for transfection, such as hydrodynamic intravenous injection, intraportal injection, electroporation, mechanical liver massage, particle bombardment, and so on.

42.6.1.1 Hydrodynamic Injection

Efficient gene transfer and expression can be achieved by a rapid injection of a large volume of naked DNA solution into animals via the tail vein. This hydrodynamic-based gene delivery is a simple and highly efficient procedure in gene expression to deliver and express exogenous genes in almost all major organs, especially the liver in small animals, such as mice and rats. There are two basic requirements for the hydrodynamic injection in order to achieve an appropriate hydrodynamic pressure in targeted tissues: (i) inject rapidly in 5–7 s and (ii) inject a huge volume at one time. This hydrodynamic pressure can facilitate DNA solution to transiently permeabilize the endothelium and plasma membrane of parenchyma cells, and allow efficient intracellular gene transfer. For example, naked DNA in a 2-ml volume of saline solution could be injected into mice weighing 20 g in just

5–7 s. Liu *et al.* [33] used this hydrodynamic procedure to transfect up to 40% of liver cells after a single injection of naked pDNA, showing that the level of gene expression in different organs increased with the increasing volume of the injected DNA solution and that the optimal transgene expression required an injection volume of approximately 8–12% of body weight.

Manual control of the injection speed and strength is hard to standardize, which makes the results insufficiently reliable when the experiment is performed by different individuals. In order to minimize the problem, Suda *et al.* [34] developed a computer-controlled injection device that uses real-time intravascular pressure as a regulator for the injection and can program the computer according to need. This device can self-adjust the volume needed to develop the sufficiently elevated pressure that can thereby help to achieve a successful gene transfer. The self-adjustment of the device is based on the size and anatomical structure of the selected organ of interest. This device enabled safe and effective gene delivery to mouse liver, and kidney and muscle cells in rats with plasmids or adenoviral vectors as gene carriers. Gene transfer to the liver of pigs was also successful. The study also showed that larger animals tend to require higher pressure for successful gene transfer to a given organ and that the liver shows the highest gene delivery efficiency, probably due to the high elasticity of the liver vasculature and parenchyma cells.

Although the tissue damage caused by the hydrodynamic pressure after injection can be recovered in rodents, rapid injection of a large volume of pDNA is invasive and cannot be applied to humans. A high level of gene expression achieved by this simple method may be useful to analyze the function and molecular mechanism of different genes involved in many genetic and acquired diseases within the whole animal.

42.6.1.2 **Electroporation**

Electroporation is a simple and convenient way to deliver nucleic acids (e.g., DNA) into cells. Cells act as an electrical capacitor that is generally unable to pass current. Subjecting the cells to an electric field creates transient permeable structures or micropores on the cell membrane, which last long enough after electroporation to allow penetration of pharmaceuticals or nucleic acids into the cell. Over time, the micropores on the cell membrane close and the cell becomes impermeable again. It can be applied, in principle, to any type of cells and tissues so long as the target is accessible. The advantages of electroporation include controllable tissue or cell damage, flexibility in the structure of DNA to be transfected, and the possibility of transfecting cells deep inside a specific tissue. The transfection efficiency by electroporation is many times greater than that of naked DNA and with reduced interindividual variability [35, 36].

Various devices have been designed for effective electroporation, including the electro square-wave porator, caliper electrodes, syringe electrodes, and flow-through electroporation. The caliper electrodes consist of a caliper and a pair of adjustable end-plates. The electrodes sandwich the target area and deliver electric pulses following the injection of the molecule of interest. Liu and Huang [37] invented a syringe electrode device for both DNA injection and electroporation. It applies a voltage to the syringe needle and this allows the needle to be used not only for injection, but also as an electrode. This is particularly advantageous as the electric field is applied to the same area as the injected fluid. The injected DNA can also be confined to the high-intensity region of the field, thus the required electric field strength can be reduced without compromising the transfection efficiency. Tissue damage could be minimized due to the low electric power used. Geng *et al.* [38] introduced a novel flow-through electroporation method for gene delivery into cells at a high flow rate based on disposable microfluidic chips and a direct current power supply that provides a constant voltage. With the optimal parameter design, approximately 75% of CHO cells were transfected by this method without apparent toxicity.

42.6.1.3 **Particle Bombardment**

Particle bombardment is a commonly used method for genetic transformation to a broad range of cell and tissue types. Colloid gold particles coated with DNA (microprojectiles) are shot directly into the target cells or tissues by a burst of helium gas using a biolistic device or "gene gun." The particles or macromolecules can be delivered through membranes and extracellular matrix (ECM). They can penetrate 100 μm into the skin by this method and transfect some skin Langerhan cells for antigen presentation. Particle bombardment is the only reproducible means for delivering DNA to mitochondria [39]. Therefore, the method could have a significant impact on gene expression within cytoplasmic organelles [40].

42.6.2
Chemical Vectors for RNA Delivery

42.6.2.1 **Cationic Lipids/Liposomes and Cationic Lipid Nanoparticles (Lipoplexes)**

Various cationic lipids can form complexes with negatively charged DNA or siRNA. The complexes, called lipoplexes, at suitable N/P ratios interact with cells in culture by nonspecific charge interaction, followed by endocytosis. Lipofectamine is a commonly used cationic liposome reagent for nucleic acid transfection that provides high transfection efficiency and high levels of transgene expression in a range of mammalian cell types *in vitro*. It can transfect siRNA or pDNA into cells in culture by altering the cell plasma membrane and allowing nucleic acids to gain access into the cytoplasm.

Liposomes prepared from cationic amphiphiles interact with polyanionic DNA or RNA, spontaneously forming lipoplexes driven by electrostatic interaction forces. Lipoplexes are efficient nonviral vectors to introduce nucleic acids into the desired target cells. Cationic lipid-mediated gene transfer has advantages over viral gene transfer because it is less immunogenic, easier to produce, and not oncogenic. Most studies have been performed on the synthesis and investigation of new cationic lipids for DNA or RNA complexing, used either alone or combined with a particular helper lipid, such as cholesterol and 1,2-dioleoyl-*sn*-glycero-3-phosphoethanolamine (DOPE), which are neutral lipids and can participate in bilayer formation when combined with a cationic lipid [41]. The presence of helper lipids affects the association of nucleic acids with lipoplexes [42], and can help to facilitate the release of the cargo from endosome and achieve higher transfection efficiency by promoting the inverted hexagonal H_{II} phase transition. The inverted hexagonal phase has a negative spontaneous curvature and a tendency of membranes to form an inverted micellar structure, which allows destabilizing the endosomal membrane and deassembling the lipoplex [43], resulting in concomitant release of the nucleic acid cargo from the endosome. For example, the cationic lipid 1,2-dioleoyl-3-trimethylammonium-propane (DOTAP) prefers a bilayer organization; however, mixing with a helper lipid like DOPE will affect the packing parameter and mediate fusion between the liposomes and the endosomal membrane after endocytosis, reverting to a H_{II} phase, that results in the destabilization of the endosomal membrane and release of the nucleic acid cargo to the cytosol [44–46]. The nonbilayer H_{II} phase structure is also formed due to the formation of ion pairs between cationic lipids and the anionic phospholipids in the endosome membrane [47]. Several studies have investigated the correlation between the structural properties of lipoplexes and their transfection efficiency, and revealed that lipoplexes that adopt the H_{II} phase strongly facilitate intracellular release of nucleic acid cargo from the endosomal compartment [43] and display the highest transfection efficiency [48]. Cationic lipids with multiple *cis* double bonds, small or less hydrophilic head-groups, and unsaturated bulky acyl or alkyl chains favor H_{II} phase formation and resulted in higher transfection efficiency [41, 43]. To avoid nonspecific binding *in vivo* of the positively charged lipoplex, PEG-derivatized lipids are often included to decrease the net positive charge [49], providing stealth properties that stabilize the lipoplexes. See Figure 42.3.

42.6.2.2 **Ionizable Lipids**

Recently, Alnylam Pharmaceuticals have designed some ionizable cationic lipids to formulate lipid nanoparticles (LNPs) to deliver siRNA *in vivo*, such as

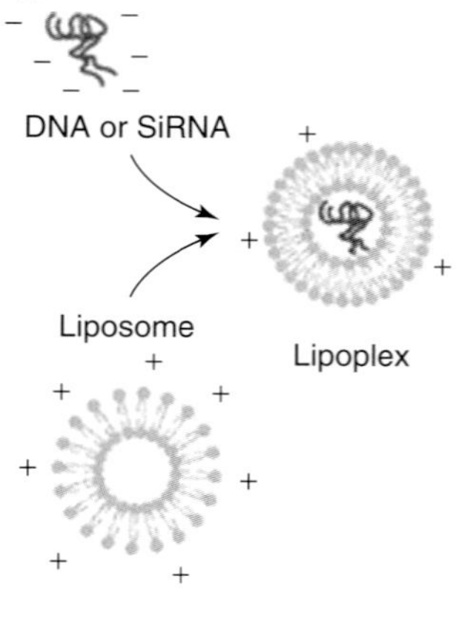

Figure 42.3 Schematic formation of lipoplexes. (Adapted from [50].)

1,2-dilinoleyloxy-3-dimethylaminopropane (DLinDMA) and other DLinDMA-based lipids. The ionizable cationic lipids contain weak basic lipid head-groups, which affect the surface charge of the particles in a pH-dependent manner, rendering them positively charged at acidic pH, but close to neutral charge at physiologic pH [51]. LNPs comprised of different lipid compositions and ratios as well as different sizes and structures have been produced using different methods, which are characterized by very high siRNA encapsulation efficiency, small uniformly sized particles as well as superior delivery capacity and therapeutic gene-silencing effects. One of the newly invented ionizable LNPs (iLNPs) termed stable nucleic acid lipid particles (SNALPs) substantially improved *in vivo* endogenous gene-silencing activity with siRNA doses as low as 0.01 mg/kg in rodents and 0.1 mg/kg in nonhuman primates [52]. The rational lipid design for SNALP-mediated delivery lies in the pK_a of the ionizable cationic lipid and the abilities of these lipids to induce the nonbilayer hexagonal H_{II} phase structure with anionic phospholipids of the endosomal membrane when protonated in the acidic pH environment in the endosome [52]. The efficient delivery mechanism of these iLNPs involves endogenous apolipoprotein E (apoE) by targeting the low-density lipoprotein receptor in hepatocytes [51]. Briefly, iLNPs behave as neutral liposomes in circulation to absorb apoE as an endogenous targeting ligand and deliver siRNA to hepatocytes in an endogenous targeting manner. The exogenous targeting approach via asialoglycoprotein receptor expressed on hepatocytes is also highly effective [51].

42.6.2.3 **Lipid-Like Delivery Molecules (Lipidoids)**

Akinc *et al.* [53] developed chemical synthesis methods based on the conjugate addition of alkyl-acrylates or alkyl-acrylamides to primary or secondary amines, to rapidly generate a substantial and diverse collection of lipid-like molecules, termed lipidoids. They are structurally distinct from other classes of lipid delivery vectors since they contained multiple protonable amine groups connected to relatively short alkyl chains. Materials with good *in vitro* and *in vivo* efficacy could be identified within the large library, including a lead material $98N_{12}$-5 that was shown to be efficacious in primates. In addition, the *in vivo* delivery efficacy of the novel lipid-like material can be affected by many parameters, such as the formulation composition, nature of PEGylation on the particle, degree of drug loading, particle size, changes in PEG lipids anchor chain length, and so on [54], resulting in distinct gene-silencing effects. The side-chains of the molecule can be further altered to obtain different capacities for hydrogen bonding, hydrophobic interactions, and protonated states, enabling the exploration of functionalized lipidoids for efficient siRNA delivery [55].

42.6.2.4 **Cationic Polymers (Polyplexes)**

Cationic polymers include natural DNA-binding proteins, such as histones, synthetic polypeptides, polyethylenimide (PEI), cationic dendrimers, and carbohydrate-based polymers such as chitosan [41]. The self-assembly of cationic polymers with nucleic acids in solution forms a particulate complex, and leads to

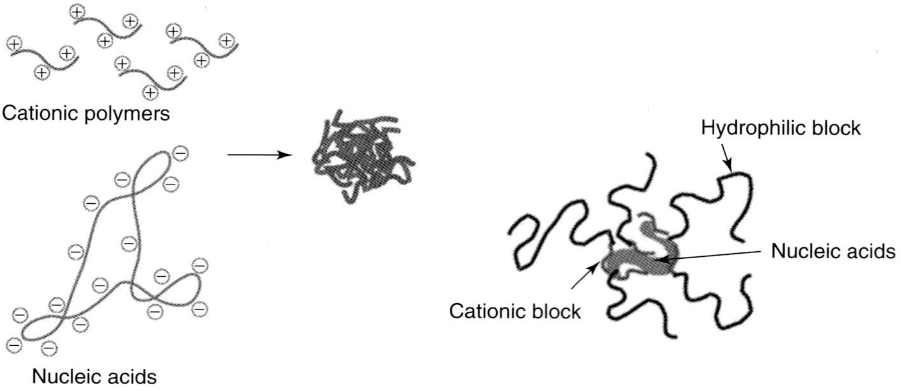

Figure 42.4 Schematic formation of polyplexes. (Adapted from [57a, b].)

a strong condensation and large size reduction of the nucleic acid drug, which is favorable to improve *in vivo* transfection efficiency [56]. See Figure 42.4.

PEI has been widely used for nonviral transfection *in vitro* and *in vivo*. PEI exists as a branched polymer and also in linear form. It is available in a broad range of molecular weights, from less than 1000 Da to 1600 kDa, and the PEIs with a molecular weight between 5 and 25 kDa are most suitable for gene transfer [58]. Higher molecular weights lead to increased cytotoxicity, probably due to aggregation of huge clusters of the cationic polymer on the outer cell membrane, which may induce necrosis [59].

Chitosan is a linear carbohydrate-based polymer comprising β-(1,4)-linked D-glucosamine and *N*-acetyl-D-glucosamine. It is widely used in the field of nonviral gene delivery due to its good biocompatibility and high positive charge density [60]. The chitosan molecular weight, salt form, and degree of deacetylation affect its gene delivery efficiency. The application of chitosan is also limited by its low water solubility, inefficient gene unpacking, and relatively low gene transfection efficiency. Thus, various chitosan derivatives have been synthesized and the structures were further modified to alter their hydrophilicity. Incorporation of negatively charged agents such as hyaluronic acid (HA) with chitosan has been shown to increase the transfection efficiency significantly due to the low density of the HA chain, which could improve the DNA release from the condensing compact nanoparticles [61]. Jiang *et al.* [62] described chitosan–PEI hybrid systems, including chitosan/PEI blend and chitosan-*graft*-PEI, to enhance the transfection efficiency of the cells owing to a proton sponge effect (see below).

Dendrimers are three-dimensional polymers that can interact with various forms of nucleic acids, such as pDNA, antisense oligonucleotides, and RNA, to form complexes that protect the nucleic acid from degradation. The cationic dendrimer condenses the anionic nucleic acids through electrostatic interaction. The positively charged dendrimer/nucleic acid complex can transfect cells by interact with the negatively charged cell membranes, although highly cationic systems are also cytotoxic. The properties of the dendrimer/nucleic acid complex depend on various factors, such as stoichiometry, concentration of dendrimer amines, and nucleic acid phosphates, as well as solvent properties like pH, salt concentration, buffer strength, and dynamics of mixing. Dendrimer-based transfection reagents could be used as routine tools for *in vitro* transfection, but *in vivo* delivery of therapeutic nucleic acids still remains a challenge.

Bartlett *et al.* [63] have developed a synthetic delivery system based on a cyclodextrin-containing polycation (CDP) that can deliver various nucleic acid payloads, including pDNA, siRNA, and ribozyme. The nucleic acid and CDP complexes formed by adamantine (AD)-containing molecules and β-cyclodextrin molecules could be attached to AD–PEG conjugates for steric stabilization and targeting ligands (AD–PEG–transferrin) for cell-specific targeting. This CDP delivery vehicle can encapsulate large amounts of payload molecules, and shows superior physicochemical and biological characterizations.

Generally, a longer polymer chain or a higher branched polymer leads to better condensation of nucleic acids. For example, low-branched PEIs with low condensation capacity require higher N/P ratios to completely condense nucleic acid payloads compared to their highly branched counterparts [59], most likely because of the lower content of primary amines in the low-branched polymers. Highly branched PEIs form smaller polyplexes and usually achieve higher transfection efficiencies, but also show greater toxicity [41]. The complex condensation can confer protection against degradation in the extracellular environment and improve cell uptake by electrostatic interactions of the polycation with the negatively charged cell surface.

Unlike cationic lipids, cationic polymers are devoid of a hydrophobic domain and hard to destabilize in the endosome by direct interaction with the endosomal membrane. Instead, cationic polymers, such as PEI, can mediate endosome disruption by the "proton sponge" effect to enhance nucleic acid cargo release [41]. The proton sponge effect arises from a large number of weak conjugated bases as proton-buffering groups (e.g., amine groups in PEI) with high buffering capabilities at pH 5–6 in acidic organelles, leading to proton absorption (sponge) and simultaneously chloride ion accumulation in the endosome, which arouses the osmotic pressure buildup in the endosome. This osmotic pressure causes swelling and/or rupture of the endosomes, and a release of the entrapped drug materials into the cytoplasm [64].

In order to achieve higher transfection efficiency, rational design of the polymer structure and systematic structure modification have been developed. The design of the proper polymers becomes a sophisticated task in terms of the different applications of polymers as gene carrier systems. The molecular weight, degree of branching, surface charge, and composition of the complexes (e.g., the ratio of polymer to nucleic acid payload) have to be optimized in order to form stable complexes and also produce desired *in vivo* release properties. Higher charge density and higher molecular weight of polymers are usually required to reach high condensation capabilities. For example, polyamidoamine dendrimers have a branched spherical shape and a high surface charge density. Their transfection

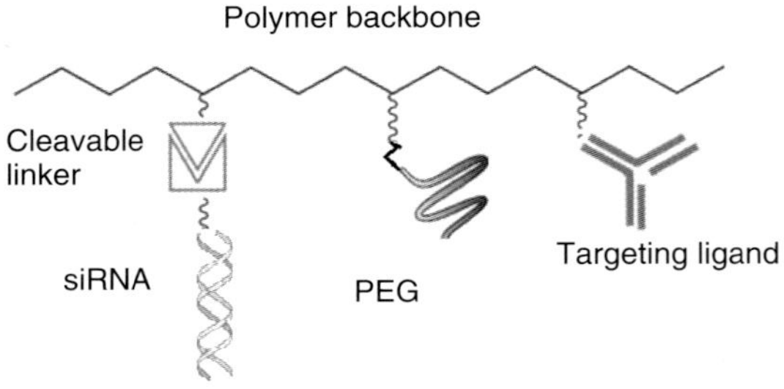

Figure 42.5 Schematic structure of polyconjugates.

ability depends on the size, shape, and number of primary amine groups on the polymer surface [65, 66].

Rozema *et al.* [67] invented a siRNA dynamic polyconjugate vehicle for the delivery of siRNA to hepatocytes both *in vitro* and *in vivo*. They use an amphipathic poly(vinyl ether) composed of butyl and amino vinyl ethers, termed PBAVE, as a latent endosomolytic agent, whose amine groups are modified with a maleic anhydride to create acid-labile maleamate bonds. These bonds reversibly mask the activity of this polymer until it reaches the acidic environment of endosomes. These bonds can be cleaved in the endosome, exposing the agent's amines and activating its endosome release capacity. The siRNA cargo is attached to PBAVE through a disulfide linkage, and the shielding agent PEG and hepatocyte targeting ligand *N*-acetylgalactosamine are attached to PBAVE by a bifunctional maleamate linkage to afford specific targeting to hepatocytes *in vivo* by intravenous injection. Using this delivery technology, two endogenous genes (*apoB* and *ppara*) in mouse liver were knocked down, consistent with the phenotypic changes of the gene functions. See Figure 42.5.

42.6.2.5 **Core/Membrane Lipid-Based Nanoparticles (Lipopolyplexes)**

The core/membrane nanoparticle "liposome–polycation–DNA" (LPD) is a DNA–protamine complex subsequently wrapped by cationic liposomes. It is further modified by postinsertion of PEG to impart a steric barrier for prolonged circulation time *in vivo* (Figure 42.6). Li *et al.* [68] developed the "LPD-I" formulation composed of protamine sulfate, DNA, and DOTAP/cholesterol liposome. The weakly immunogenic protamine sulfate condenses DNA or siRNA to form a relatively small and negatively charged complex core about 50 nm in diameter. The complex core structure has a high efficiency of encapsulation, control of particle size, controlled release of nucleic acid in cells [69], and can protect the nucleic acid cargo from enzymatic degradation by nucleases and other environmental assaults. The cationic liposome containing DOTAP wraps around the negatively charged complex core and the resulting LPD nanoparticles are slightly less than 100 nm in diameter [70]. Lee and Huang [71] developed a similar LPD gene transfer vector (LPD-II), where DNA was first complexed to polylysine to form a positively charged core. The major difference from LPD-I is that LPD-II uses pH-sensitive anionic

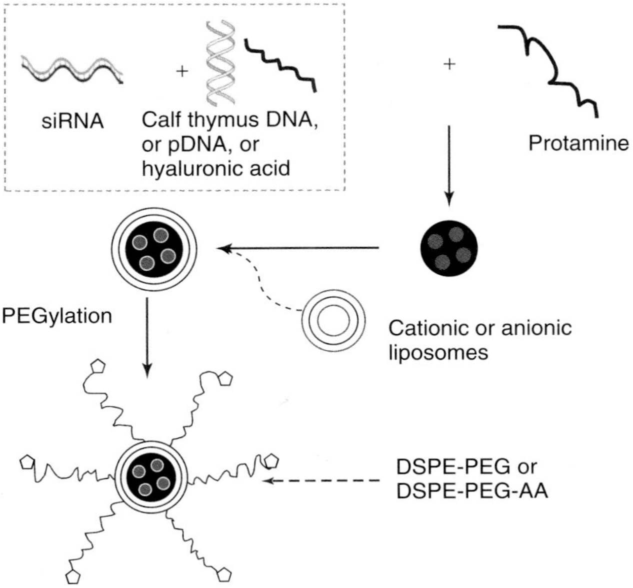

Figure 42.6 Structure and preparation scheme of LPD nanoparticles. DSPE-PEG, 1,2-distearoyl-sn-glycero-3-phosphoethanolamine-N-[methoxy (polyethylene glycol)-2000]; AA, Anisamide.

liposomes composed of DOPE/cholesteryl hemisuccinate (CHEMS) instead of cationic liposomes. Above all, the liposomes added to the LPD complexes are either made of cationic (LPD-I) or anionic (LPD-II) lipids to form lipopolyplexes. In order to increase the circulation half-life, PEG was coated outside the LPD, and targeting ligands (e.g., anisamide, folate) were also tethered to the distal end of the PEG polymer chain to achieve specific internalization, enhanced cellular uptake, and improved transfection efficiency [72, 73].

Nakamura *et al.* [69] developed a multifunctional envelope-type nanodevice (MEND) as a nonviral gene delivery for pDNA and oligodeoxynucleotides (ODNs), similar to LPD-II [71]. MEND consists of a DNA core condensed by polycation and covered with lipid membranes, and the surface of the lipid envelope can be modified with various functional devices, such as PEG for prolonged circulation, specific ligands for targeting, or fusogenic peptides for endosomal escape [74]. The lipid membrane of MEND was composed of DOPE and CHEMS without cationic lipids. Since PEG modification on the surface of the nanoparticle is undesirable for cellular uptake by interfering with the interaction with the cell membrane [23], Hatakeyama *et al.* [75] used a biological responsive PEG–peptide–lipid ternary conjugate (PEG–peptide–DOPE (PPD) conjugate) to modify the MEND gene carrier. PEG can be removed from the carriers via cleavage by a matrix metalloproteinase (MMP) that is specifically expressed in tumor tissues. The results show MEND

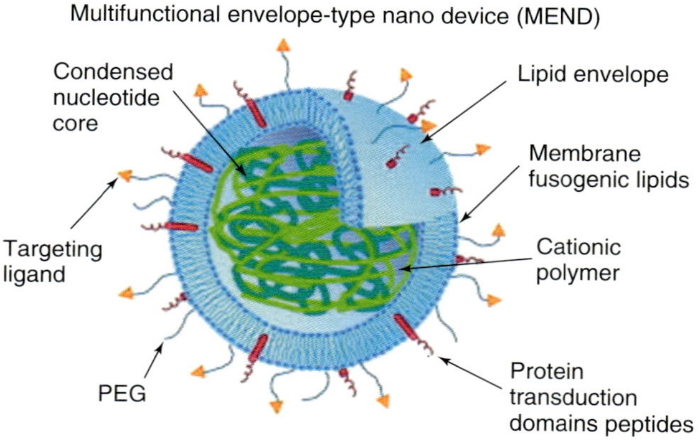

Figure 42.7 Schematic structure of MEND nanoparticle [76].

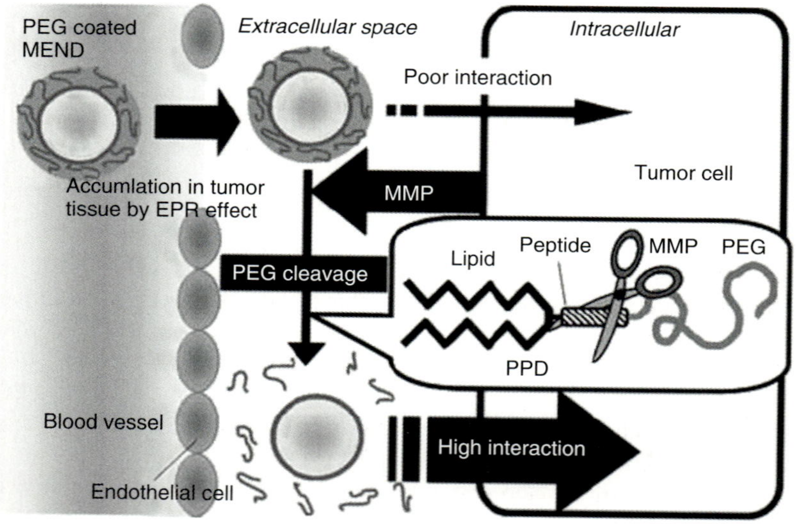

Figure 42.8 Schematic diagram illustrating the strategy of releasing the gene cargo in MEND nanoparticles by PPD modification [77].

modified with PPD is stable in systemic circulation, and can facilitate tumor accumulation and transfection (see Figures 42.7 and 42.8).

From the *xzy* confocal microscopy images by Li *et al.*, most of the siRNA was delivered intracellularly *in vivo* when formulated in anisamide targeted LPD nanoparticles (Figure 42.9c), while siRNAs only remained in the extracellular space when formulated in nontargeted nanoparticles (Figure 42.9b). Free siRNA and

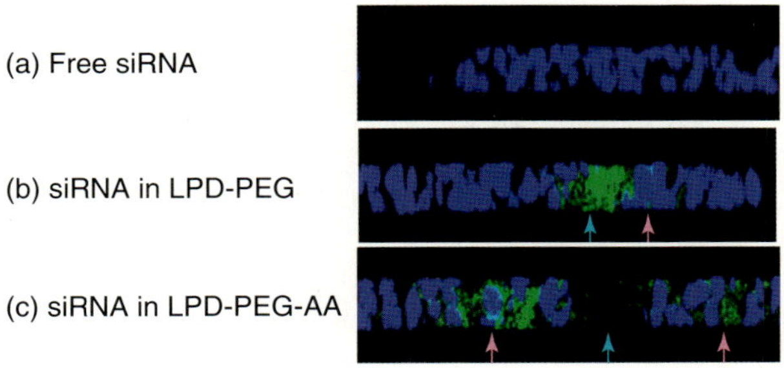

Figure 42.9 (a)–(c) Diagram illustrating the limited release of siRNA from LPD condensed core: green fluorescence is FAM™-siRNA, blue arrows indicate the extracellular space, and pink arrows indicate the intracellular uptake of siRNA [78].

nontargeted nanoparticles showed little cellular uptake (Figure 42.9a and b). However, in Figure 42.9c, the siRNA fluorescence was not distributed homogeneously; instead, there are many granular dots dispersed in the cytoplasm. The data strongly indicate that the delivered siRNA was not completely dissociated from the nanoparticles. Although LPD nanoparticles were strikingly successful in delivering siRNA via intravenous administration, most of siRNA loaded into the vector was still associated with the cores in the cytoplasm such that most of the encapsulated siRNA was not bioavailable.

In order to solve the problem regarding to the inefficient release of siRNA from LPD nanoparticles, Li *et al.* [73] developed a lipid-coated calcium phosphate (LCP) nanoparticle formulation for efficient delivery of siRNA to a xenograft tumor model by intravenous administration. Compared to the LPD nanoparticle, the previous DNA–protamine complex core was replaced by a biodegradable nanosized calcium phosphate precipitate prepared by using water-in-oil microemulsions and siRNA was entrapped in the calcium phosphate precipitate in the microemulsion. The rationale for the LCP design is that the calcium phosphate precipitate in the core of LCP nanoparticles would dissolve and deassemble at low pH in the endosome, increase the osmotic pressure, and cause endosome swelling and bursting to release the entrapped siRNA. This new formulation improved the *in vitro* silencing effect 3- to 4-fold compared to the previous LPD formulation and had decreased immunotoxicity to allow a potential application for clinical trial. The LCP nanoparticles can be further optimized by changing the precipitate core and the coating lipids. Figure 42.10 shows the formation process and the entrapped siRNA release mechanism of LCP-II nanoparticles.

42.6.2.6 **Aptamer–siRNA Chimeras**

Cancer cells usually overexpress certain surface markers [79] that can be exploited for targeted delivery of siRNA. Aptamers are single-stranded DNA, RNA, or modified nucleic acids with high binding affinity specific to their targets, which

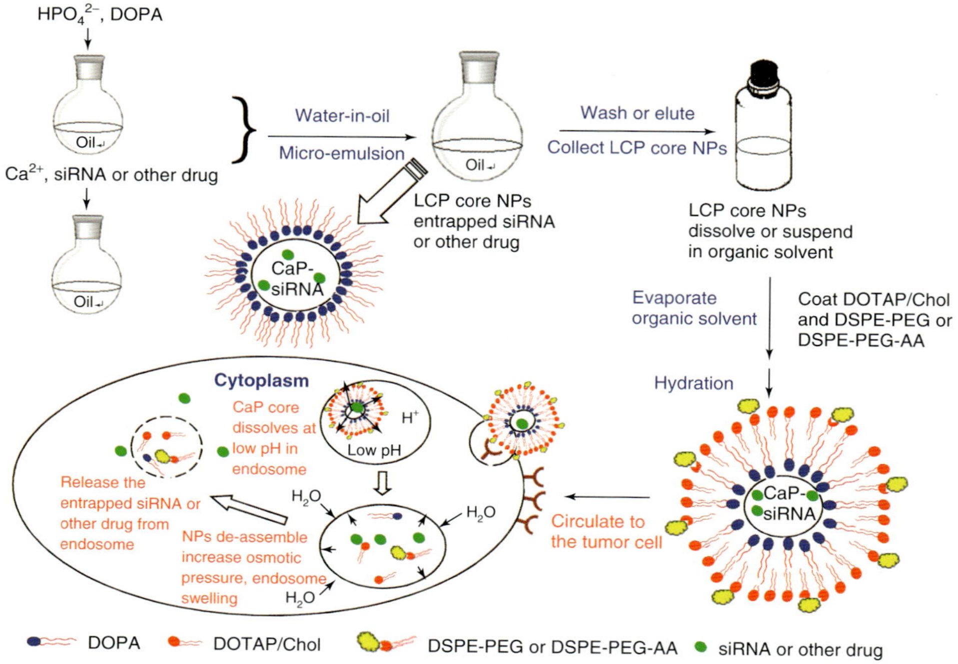

Figure 42.10 Formation process and entrapped siRNA release mechanism of LCP nanoparticles (NPs).

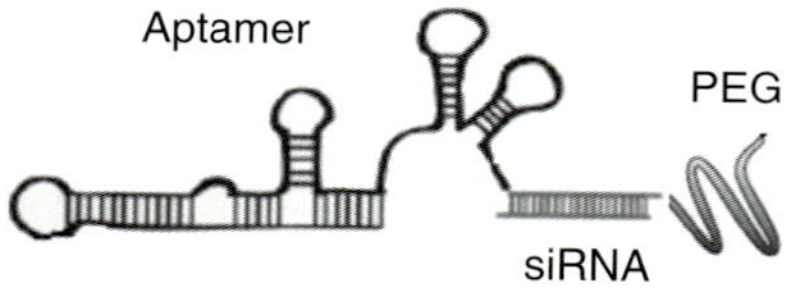

Figure 42.11 Schematic structure of aptamer–siRNA chimeras. (Adapted from [83].)

range from small molecules to proteins [80]. They have been isolated and identified for the recognition of molecular targets expressed on the surface membranes of specific cancer cells. Dassie *et al.* [81] and McNamara *et al.* [82] used aptamer–siRNA chimeras to target prostate-specific membrane antigen expressed on prostate cancer cells, triggering cell type-specific gene silencing by chimeric RNAs via the RNAi pathway. The aptamer–siRNA chimeras show specific tumor inhibition and mediate tumor regression in a xenograft model of prostate cancer, which could prove to be useful therapeutics for targeting human prostate cancer in the future. The drawback of the vector is the lack of any endosome escape mechanism in the chimera (see Figure 42.11).

42.7 Targeting Ligands

42.7.1 Aptamers

Aptamers are short single-stranded DNA or RNA oligonucleotides ranging in size from 20 to 80 bases (around 6–26 kDa) that are able to recognize and bind to their target molecules, such as proteins, phospholipids, sugars, nucleic acids and cell surface receptors, with high affinity and specificity [12, 84]. Aptamers are derived from a large random sequence pool through repeated rounds of *in vivo* selection for targets on the surface of tumor cells and *in vitro* selection using purified protein target. They can also be obtained via a process referred to as SELEX (systemic evolution of ligands by exponential enrichment) [85] to bind to various molecular targets, and even cells, tissues, and organisms. Receptor-binding RNA aptamers may help cell receptors to internalize cargos after the ligands interact with the receptors. Aptamers are also amenable to a wide variety of chemical modifications, such as radioactive or fluorescent reporters, affinity tags for molecular recognition, and ribose ring modification, which makes aptamers resistant to nuclease. Aptamers can also be covalently conjugated to nanomaterials after appropriate chemical modification. Other attractive features of aptamers in biological systems are their low toxicity, low immunogenicity [86], and long circulation half-life.

42.7.2 CPPs

CPPs (also known as protein transduction domains (PTDs)), are a class of short peptide sequences that can enter cells efficiently, either alone or linked to bulky cargos, such as peptides, proteins, oligonucleotides, pDNA, or liposomes [87, 88]. Linking the cargo macromolecule to a CPP can help to overcome the cell membrane barrier.

42.7.3 Antibodies

Antibodies and antibody fragments have been fused to various drug delivery systems as a targeting agent, so that they can selectively deliver their payload to tumor cells. Xu *et al.* [89] conjugated a single-chain monoclonal antibody fragment (scFv) that targeted to the transferrin receptor to cationic liposomes, and then mixed it with pDNA to produce a scFv–liposome–DNA complex, which enhances the transfection efficiencies both *in vitro* and *in vivo* in a variety of human tumor models. Chen *et al.* have also conjugated scFv to liposome–polycation–HA nanoparticles to deliver both siRNA and miRNA for therapy in a murine B16F10 melanoma model [90]. The siRNA delivered by the scFv targeted nanoparticles efficiently downregulated the target genes in the lung metastasis and reduced the tumor load in the lung.

42.7.4
Peptides and Proteins

Some cancer cells upregulate certain cell surface receptors that correspond to larger protein ligands, such as transferrin, which is an iron-transporting serum glycoprotein. The transferrin-modified drug delivery vectors can be efficiently taken up into cells by receptor-mediated endocytosis. Also, small immobilized peptides can be tethered on polymers as cell recognition motifs that can resist enzymatic degradation and therefore exhibit excellent long-term stability. In addition, unlike ECM proteins that normally contain many different cell recognition motifs, the small peptides represent only one single motif, so they can selectively address one particular type of cell receptor and trigger cell adhesion efficiently. Both linear peptides and cyclic peptides can be employed [91]. The Arg–Gly–Asp (RGD) sequence is one of the most effective and most often employed peptide sequences for stimulated cell adhesion, targeting to integrin family receptors on the tumor vasculature, such as $\alpha_v\beta_3$ that plays a significant role in tumor angiogenesis. Peptides containing RGD and RGD mimetics have been coupled to liposomes, polymers, other peptides, small-molecule drugs, and radiotracers for therapeutic, diagnostic imaging of tumor angiogenesis [92]. Many multivalent RGD constructs and multimeric cyclic RGD peptides have been used to increase the binding affinity and targeting capability to integrin $\alpha_v\beta_3$ [93, 94]. Multivalency not only greatly improves affinity, but also facilitates internalization via receptor-mediated endocytosis [95]. Apart from RGD-mediated delivery of small-molecule drugs, imaging agents, peptides, and proteins, RGD modification of nonviral and viral gene carriers has also been successfully exploited [96]. Similar to RGD, Asn–Gly–Arg (NGR) is another small peptide applied to target the aminopeptidase N (CD13) molecule that is overexpressed on certain tumor cells and most tumor endothelial cells [97]. Chen *et al.* [98] conjugated NGR peptide to PEGylated LPD nanoparticles for efficient delivery of siRNA and doxorubicin into solid tumors. NGR–hTNF (human tumor necrosis factor), which consists of hTNF fused with NGR peptide, showed efficient antitumor activity at low doses due to selective binding to CD13 overexpressed on tumor blood vessels, and the activity and safety of NGR–hTNF was further evaluated in a clinical study on colorectal cancer patients failing standard therapies [99]. The results showed NGR–hTNF was well tolerated in colorectal cancer patients and deserves further evaluation in combination with standard chemotherapy. Thus, both RGD and NGR have been widely used in many drug delivery systems for active tumor targeting and enhanced antitumor therapeutic effect.

42.7.5
Small-Molecular-Weight Ligands

Folate receptors are overexpressed on several types of cancers and diseased cells, but are expressed in minimal quantities in normal cells except the kidneys [100]. Thus, folate conjugation presents an effective method of targeting drug/gene carriers to cancer cells. It has been successfully applied for the receptor-specific delivery of chemotherapy agents, liposomal drug carriers, and gene transfer vectors [97]. Anisamide is a high-affinity, small-molecular-weight ligand for sigma receptors that are highly expressed on many epithelial cancer cells. It can be conjugated to lipid nanocarriers to deliver doxorubicin [101] and siRNA [102, 103] to tumors in animals. Other small molecules, such as haloperidol, SA4503, and opipramol, have also been reported as sigma receptor ligands [104]. Mukherjee *et al.* [105] reported that haloperidol-conjugated lipoplexes showed 10-fold greater delivery of DNA to breast carcinoma cells than the control lipoplexes. The advantages of small-molecular-weight ligands are their small size, convenience, relatively simple conjugation chemistry, and reduced immunogenicity.

42.8 Therapeutic Application for Treatment of Cancer

42.8.1 siRNA Therapeutic Mechanisms

Many human diseases are often caused by inappropriate endogenous or exogenous gene expression that leads to angiogenetic dysfunction. The role of angiogenesis in tumor growth is mediated by a balance of activators and inhibitors. siRNA can create new inhibitors that downregulate angiogenesis through post-transcriptional gene silencing, such as regulation of vascular endothelial growth factor receptor expression [106]. siRNA has already shown therapeutic effects in a number of animal disease models, demonstrating that antiangiogenic siRNA may play an important role in the treatment of human diseases in the near future [107]. Furthermore, siRNA targeting key elements of proliferation signal transduction pathways can prevent the development of specific human cancers. In addition, siRNAs specifically downregulating the expression of target genes can induce the induction of cell cycle arrest, apoptosis, and reduced cell proliferation *in vitro* or tumor growth *in vivo*. In addition, drug resistance in cancer cells can also be overcome by delivering c-*myc* siRNA [108].

42.8.2 Examples in Cancer Treatment of RNA Delivery Technology

Clinical trials using RNAi technology to treat human diseases were first launched in 2004 [109]. siRNA is now being evaluated for almost all types of disease and more than 13 products have entered into clinical trials. Although it is a very promising class of drug, the US Food and Drug Administration has not approved any human gene therapy product to date. Davis *et al.* [110] have finished the first siRNA clinical trial using a targeted nanoparticle delivery system invented by Calando Pharmaceuticals. This technology applied cyclodextrin polymer carriers to deliver the siRNA [88]. The synthetic delivery system tested in the clinical trail contained a

Table 42.2 RNAi drugs in clinical trials.

Company	RNAi agent	Disease	Target	RNA delivery method	Route of administration and target tissue	Trial phase
Calando	CALAA-01 [110]	solid tumors	RRM2	targeted nanoparticle delivery system	intravenous injection (systemic)	phase I
Alnylam	ALN-VSP	liver cancers and solid tumors	KSP, VEGF	liposomal conjugation	intravenous infusion (systemic)	phase I
Silence Therapeutics	Atu027/Atu093 [114]	lung cancers	PKN3	siRNA–lipoplex	intravenous injections or infusions (systemic)	phase I
Quark/Pfizer	PF-4523655/RTP-801i-14	AMD, diabetic macular degeneration	RTP801	synthetic chemically modified siRNA molecule	intravitreal injection (eye)	phase II
Alnylam	ALN-RSV01 [115]	RSV infection	nucleocapsid (N) gene of RSV genome	minimally modified, unencapsulated siRNAs	intranasal (respiratory tract)	expanded phase II
Quark	AKIi-5	ARF, AKI	TP53	chemically modified siRNA formulation	intravenous injection (systemic)	phase II
Allergan	AGN-211745 (Sirna-027) [116]	AMD and CNV infection	VEGFA, VEGFR1	sterile siRNA buffer or nuclease-free PBS	intravitreal injection (eye)	phase II
TransDerm	TD101 [117]	pachyonychia congenita	keratin 6a N171K	unmodified TD101 siRNA	intradermal injection (skin)	phase I
University of Duisburg-Essen	BCR–ABL siRNA [118]	CML	*bcr–abl*	DLS lipid solution with anionic lipoplexes	intravenous injection (systemic)	single patient
Duke University Hospital	siRNA immunotherapy	metastatic melanoma	proteasome	dendritic cell-based vaccine	intradermal injection (skin)	phase I
Opko Health	bevasiranib	wet AMD	VEGF	direct injection of siRNA to the eye	intravitreal injection (eye)	expanded phase III

AKI, acute kidney injury; AMD, age-related macular degeneration; ARF, acute renal failure; CML, chronic myeloid leukemia; CNV, choroidal neovascularization; DLS, lipid solution; KSP, kinesin spindle protein; PKN3, protein kinase N3; RRM2, M2 subunit of ribonucleotide reductase; RSV, respiratory syncytial virus; RTP801, hypoxia-inducible factor 1-responsive gene; TP53, tumor protein p53; VEGF, vascular endothelial growth factor; VEGFR-1, vascular endothelial growth factor receptor-1.

linear CDP, a human transferrin protein as the targeting ligand, hydrophilic PEG polymers to improve nanoparticle stability in the circulation, and siRNA designed to reduce the expression of RRM2 [110]. The targeted nanoparticles were designed to circulate, and then to accumulate and permeate in solid tumors after intravenous administration. Reduction of RRM2 mRNA and protein by the RRM2-specific siRNA was observed in tumor biopsies of melanoma patients. The experimental data demonstrated that siRNA administered systemically to humans can produce specific gene inhibition by an RNAi mechanism of action.

From this successful example of RNAi clinical trials, it is predictable that cancer treatment with siRNAs will be widely applicable in the near future once the challenges of targeting, potency, duration of effect, specificity, and safety issues are overcome for effective systemic delivery. Table 42.2 summarizes some ongoing clinical trials for RNAi-based therapy to cancers and a wide range of other diseases [111–113].

42.9 Conclusions

Optimal siRNA delivery vectors discussed in this chapter are widely applied to improve therapeutic nucleic acid-based transfection efficiency with limited toxic side-effects. In sum, RNAi has rapidly been recognized as an experimental tool and is expected to be used as a therapeutic treatment for various diseases.

Acknowledgments

The research in authors' laboratory has been supported by National Institutes of Health grants **CA129835** and **CA149363**.

References

1. Oh, Y.K. and Park, T.G. (2009) siRNA delivery systems for cancer treatment. *Adv. Drug Deliv. Rev.*, **61**, 850–862.
2. de Fougerolles, A. *et al.* (2007) Interfering with disease: a progress report on siRNA-based therapeutics. *Nat. Rev. Drug Discov.*, **6**, 443–453.
3. Bumcrot, D. *et al.* (2006) RNAi therapeutics: a potential new class of pharmaceutical drugs. *Nat. Chem. Biol.*, **2**, 711–719.
4. Kim, D.H. and Rossi, J.J. (2007) Strategies for silencing human disease using RNA interference. *Nat. Rev. Genet.*, **8**, 173–184.
5. John, M. *et al.* (2007) Effective RNAi-mediated gene silencing without interruption of the endogenous microRNA pathway. *Nature*, **449**, 745–747.
6. Hannon, G. (2002) RNA interference. *Nature*, **418**, 244–251.
7. Judge, A. and MacLachlan, I. (2008) Overcoming the innate immune response to small interfering RNA. *Hum. Gene Ther.*, **19**, 111–124.
8. Chiu, Y.L. and Rana, T.M. (2003) siRNA function in RNAi: a chemical modification analysis. *RNA*, **9**, 1034–1048.

9. Capodici, J., Kariko, K., and Weissman, D. (2002) Inhibition of HIV-1 infection by small interfering RNA-mediated RNA interference. *J. Immunol.*, **169**, 5196–5201.
10. Allerson, C.R. *et al.* (2005) Fully 2′-modified oligonucleotide duplexes with improved *in vitro* potency and stability compared to unmodified small interfering RNA. *J. Med. Chem.*, **48**, 901–904.
11. Judge, A.D. *et al.* (2006) Design of noninflammatory synthetic siRNA mediating potent gene silencing *in vivo*. *Mol. Ther.*, **13**, 494–505.
12. Veedu, R.N. and Wengel, J. (2010) Locked nucleic acids: promising nucleic acid analogs for therapeutic applications. *Chem. Biodivers.*, **7**, 536–542.
13. Elmen, J. *et al.* (2005) Locked nucleic acid (LNA) mediated improvements in siRNA stability and functionality. *Nucleic Acids Res.*, **33**, 439–447.
14. Braasch, D.A. *et al.* (2003) RNA interference in mammalian cells by chemically-modified RNA. *Biochemistry*, **42**, 7967–7975.
15. Mook, O.R. *et al.* (2007) Evaluation of locked nucleic acid-modified small interfering RNA *in vitro* and *in vivo*. *Mol. Cancer Ther.*, **6**, 833–843.
16. Sipa, K. *et al.* (2007) Effect of base modifications on structure, thermodynamic stability, and gene silencing activity of short interfering RNA. *RNA*, **13**, 1301–1316.
17. Abes, S. *et al.* (2007) Efficient splicing correction by PNA conjugation to an R6-Penetratin delivery peptide. *Nucleic Acids Res.*, **35**, 4495–4502.
18. Moulton, H.M. *et al.* (2007) Cell-penetrating peptide–morpholino conjugates alter pre-mRNA splicing of DMD (Duchenne muscular dystrophy) and inhibit murine coronavirus replication *in vivo*. *Biochem. Soc. Trans.*, **35**, 826–828.
19. Martinez, J. *et al.* (2002) Single-stranded antisense siRNAs guide target RNA cleavage in RNAi. *Cell*, **110**, 563–574.
20. Schwarz, D.S. *et al.* (2002) Evidence that siRNAs function as guides, not primers, in the *Drosophila* and human RNAi pathways. *Mol. Cell.*, **10**, 537–548.
21. Corey, D.R. (2007) Chemical modification: the key to clinical application of RNA interference? *J. Clin. Invest.*, **117**, 3615–3622.
22. Jackson, A.L. *et al.* (2006) Position-specific chemical modification of siRNAs reduces "off-target" transcript silencing. *RNA*, **12**, 1197–1205.
23. Li, S.D. and Huang, L. (2010) Stealth nanoparticles: high density but sheddable PEG is a key for tumor targeting. *J. Control. Release*, **145**, 178–181.
24. Wagner, E. (1998) Effects of membrane-active agents in gene delivery. *J. Control. Release*, **53**, 155–158.
25. Wagner, E. *et al.* (1992) Coupling of adenovirus to transferrin–polylysine/DNA complexes greatly enhances receptor-mediated gene delivery and expression of transfected genes. *Proc. Natl. Acad. Sci. USA*, **89**, 6099–6103.
26. Aagaard, L. and Rossi, J.J. (2007) RNAi therapeutics: principles, prospects and challenges. *Adv. Drug Deliv. Rev.*, **59**, 75–86.
27. Marques, J.T. and Williams, B.R. (2005) Activation of the mammalian immune system by siRNAs. *Nat. Biotechnol.*, **23**, 1399–1405.
28. Hornung, V. *et al.* (2005) Sequence-specific potent induction of IFN-alpha by short interfering RNA in plasmacytoid dendritic cells through TLR7. *Nat. Med.*, **11**, 263–270.
29. Judge, A.D. *et al.* (2005) Sequence-dependent stimulation of the mammalian innate immune response by synthetic siRNA. *Nat. Biotechnol.*, **23**, 457–462.
30. Jackson, A.L. *et al.* (2003) Expression profiling reveals off-target gene regulation by RNAi. *Nat. Biotechnol.*, **21**, 635–637.
31. Fedorov, Y. *et al.* (2005) Different delivery methods-different expression profiles. *Nat. Methods*, **2**, 241.
32. Omidi, Y. *et al.* (2003) Toxicogenomics of non-viral vectors for gene therapy: a microarray study of lipofectin- and oligofectamine-induced gene expression

changes in human epithelial cells. *J. Drug Target.*, **11**, 311–323.

33. Liu, F., Song, Y., and Liu, D. (1999) Hydrodynamics-based transfection in animals by systemic administration of plasmid DNA. *Gene Ther.*, **6**, 1258–1266.
34. Suda, T., Suda, K., and Liu, D. (2008) Computer-assisted hydrodynamic gene delivery. *Mol. Ther.*, **16**, 1098–1104.
35. Andre, F. and Mir, L.M. (2004) DNA electrotransfer: its principles and an updated review of its therapeutic applications. *Gene Ther.*, **11** (Suppl. 1), S33–S42.
36. Ugen, K.E. and Heller, R. (2003) Electroporation as a method for the efficient *in vivo* delivery of therapeutic genes. *DNA Cell Biol.*, **22**, 753.
37. Liu, F. and Huang, L. (2002) A syringe electrode device for simultaneous injection of DNA and electrotransfer. *Mol. Ther.*, **5**, 323–328.
38. Geng, T. *et al.* (2010) Flow-through electroporation based on constant voltage for large-volume transfection of cells. *J. Control. Release*, **144**, 91–100.
39. Johnston, S.A. *et al.* (1988) Mitochondrial transformation in yeast by bombardment with microprojectiles. *Science*, **240**, 1538–1541.
40. Klein, T.M. *et al.* (1992) Transformation of microbes, plants and animals by particle bombardment. *Biotechnology*, **10**, 286–291.
41. Tros de Ilarduya, C., Sun, Y., and Duzgunes, N. (2010) Gene delivery by lipoplexes and polyplexes. *Eur. J. Pharm. Sci.*, **40**, 159–170.
42. Simberg, D. *et al.* (2004) DOTAP (and other cationic lipids): chemistry, biophysics, and transfection. *Crit. Rev. Ther. Drug Carrier Syst.*, **21**, 257–317.
43. Tseng, Y.C., Mozumdar, S., and Huang, L. (2009) Lipid-based systemic delivery of siRNA. *Adv. Drug Deliv. Rev.*, **61**, 721–731.
44. Koltover, I. *et al.* (1998) An inverted hexagonal phase of cationic liposome-DNA complexes related to DNA release and delivery. *Science*, **281**, 78–81.
45. Simberg, D. *et al.* (2001) Phase behavior, DNA ordering, and size instability of cationic lipoplexes. Relevance to optimal transfection activity. *J. Biol. Chem.*, **276**, 47453–47459.
46. Zhou, X. and Huang, L. (1994) DNA transfection mediated by cationic liposomes containing lipopolylysine: characterization and mechanism of action. *Biochim. Biophys. Acta*, **1189**, 195–203.
47. Xu, Y. and Szoka, F.C. Jr. (1996) Mechanism of DNA release from cationic liposome/DNA complexes used in cell transfection. *Biochemistry*, **35**, 5616–5623.
48. Hafez, I.M., Maurer, N., and Cullis, P.R. (2001) On the mechanism whereby cationic lipids promote intracellular delivery of polynucleic acids. *Gene Ther.*, **8**, 1188–1196.
49. Rejman, J. *et al.* (2004) Characterization and transfection properties of lipoplexes stabilized with novel exchangeable polyethylene glycol–lipid conjugates. *Biochim. Biophys. Acta*, **1660**, 41–52.
50. Parker, A.L., Newman, C., Briggs, S., Seymour, L. and Sheridan, P.J. (2003) Nonviral gene delivery: techniques and implications for molecular medicine. *Expert Reviews in Molecular Medicine*, **5** (21), 1–15.
51. Akinc, A. *et al.* (2010) Targeted delivery of RNAi therapeutics with endogenous and exogenous ligand-based mechanisms. *Mol. Ther.*, **18**, 1357–1364.
52. Semple, S.C. *et al.* (2010) Rational design of cationic lipids for siRNA delivery. *Nat. Biotechnol.*, **28**, 172–176.
53. Akinc, A. *et al.* (2008) A combinatorial library of lipid-like materials for delivery of RNAi therapeutics. *Nat. Biotechnol.*, **26**, 561–569.
54. Akinc, A. *et al.* (2009) Development of lipidoid-siRNA formulations for systemic delivery to the liver. *Mol. Ther.*, **17**, 872–879.
55. Mahon, K.P. *et al.* (2010) Combinatorial approach to determine functional group effects on lipidoid-mediated siRNA delivery. *Bioconjug. Chem.*, **21**, 1448–1454.
56. Curiel, D.T. *et al.* (1991) Adenovirus enhancement of transferrin-polylysine-mediated gene

delivery. *Proc. Natl. Acad. Sci. USA*, **88**, 8850–8854.
57. (a) Pack, D.W. *et al.* (2005) Design and development of polymers for gene delivery. *Nat. Rev. Drug Discov.*, **4**, 581–593; (b) Duncan, R., Ringsdorf, H., and Satchi-Fainaro, R. (2006) Polymer Therapeutics: Polymers as Drugs, Drug and Protein Conjugates and Gene Delivery Systems: Past, Present and Future Opportunities. *Adv. Polym. Sci.*, **192**, 1–8.
58. Neu, M., Fischer, D., and Kissel, T. (2005) Recent advances in rational gene transfer vector design based on poly(ethylene imine) and its derivatives. *J. Gene Med.*, **7**, 992–1009.
59. Fischer, D. *et al.* (1999) A novel non-viral vector for DNA delivery based on low molecular weight, branched polyethylenimine: effect of molecular weight on transfection efficiency and cytotoxicity. *Pharm Res.*, **16**, 1273–1279.
60. Weecharangsan, W. *et al.* (2008) Evaluation of chitosan salts as non-viral gene vectors in CHO-K1 cells. *Int. J. Pharm.*, **348**, 161–168.
61. Duceppe, N. and Tabrizian, M. (2009) Factors influencing the transfection efficiency of ultra low molecular weight chitosan/hyaluronic acid nanoparticles. *Biomaterials*, **30**, 2625–2631.
62. Jiang, H.L. *et al.* (2008) Efficient gene delivery using chitosan-polyethylenimine hybrid systems. *Biomed. Mater.*, **3**, 025013.
63. Bartlett, D.W. and Davis, M.E. (2007) Physicochemical and biological characterization of targeted, nucleic acid-containing nanoparticles. *Bioconjug. Chem.*, **18**, 456–468.
64. Yezhelyev, M.V. *et al.* (2008) Proton-sponge coated quantum dots for siRNA delivery and intracellular imaging. *J. Am. Chem. Soc.*, **130**, 9006–9012.
65. Bielinska, A. *et al.* (1996) Regulation of *in vitro* gene expression using antisense oligonucleotides or antisense expression plasmids transfected using starburst PAMAM dendrimers. *Nucleic Acids Res.*, **24**, 2176–2182.
66. Kukowska-Latallo, J.F. *et al.* (1996) Efficient transfer of genetic material into mammalian cells using Starburst polyamidoamine dendrimers. *Proc. Natl. Acad. Sci. USA*, **93**, 4897–4902.
67. Rozema, D.B. *et al.* (2007) Dynamic PolyConjugates for targeted *in vivo* delivery of siRNA to hepatocytes. *Proc. Natl. Acad. Sci. USA*, **104**, 12982–12987.
68. Li, S. *et al.* (1998) Characterization of cationic lipid–protamine–DNA (LPD) complexes for intravenous gene delivery. *Gene Ther.*, **5**, 930–937.
69. Nakamura, Y. *et al.* (2007) Octaarginine-modified multifunctional envelope-type nano device for siRNA. *J. Control. Release*, **119**, 360–367.
70. Li, S. and Huang, L. (1997) *In vivo* gene transfer via intravenous administration of cationic lipid–protamine–DNA (LPD) complexes. *Gene Ther.*, **4**, 891–900.
71. Lee, R.J. and Huang, L. (1996) Folate-targeted, anionic liposome-entrapped polylysine-condensed DNA for tumor cell-specific gene transfer. *J. Biol. Chem.*, **271**, 8481–8487.
72. Brown, M.D. *et al.* (2000) Preliminary characterization of novel amino acid based polymeric vesicles as gene and drug delivery agents. *Bioconjug. Chem.*, **11**, 880–891.
73. Li, J. *et al.* (2010) Biodegradable calcium phosphate nanoparticle with lipid coating for systemic siRNA delivery. *J. Control. Release*, **142**, 416–421.
74. Kamiya, H., Akita, H., and Harashima, H. (2003) Pharmacokinetic and pharmacodynamic considerations in gene therapy. *Drug Discov. Today*, **8**, 990–996.
75. Hatakeyama, H. *et al.* (2007) Development of a novel systemic gene delivery system for cancer therapy with a tumor-specific cleavable PEG-lipid. *Gene Ther.*, **14**, 68–77.
76. Kogure, K. *et al.* (2008) Multifunctional envelope-type nano device (MEND) as a non-viral gene delivery system. *Adv. Drug Deliv. Rev.*, **60**, 559–571.
77. Hatakeyama, H. *et al.* (2007) Development of a novel systemic gene

delivery system for cancer therapy with a tumor-specific cleavable PEG-lipid. *Gene Ther.*, **14**, 68–77.

78. Li, SD. *et al.* (2008) Tumor-targeted delivery of siRNA by self-assembled nanoparticles. *Mol. Ther.*, **16**, 163–169.
79. Espina, V. *et al.* (2005) Pathology of the future: molecular profiling for targeted therapy. *Cancer Invest.*, **23**, 36–46.
80. Wilson, D.S. and Szostak, J.W. (1999) *In vitro* selection of functional nucleic acids. *Annu. Rev. Biochem.*, **68**, 611–647.
81. Dassie, J.P. *et al.* (2009) Systemic administration of optimized aptamer–siRNA chimeras promotes regression of PSMA-expressing tumors. *Nat. Biotechnol.*, **27**, 839–849.
82. McNamara, J.O. II *et al.* (2006) Cell type-specific delivery of siRNAs with aptamer–siRNA chimeras. *Nat. Biotechnol.*, **24**, 1005–1015.
83. Lares, M.R., Rossi, J.J., and Ouellet, D.L. (2010) RNAi and small interfering RNAs in human disease therapeutic applications. *Trends Biotechnol.*, **28**, 570–579.
84. Wang, K.Y. *et al.* (1993) A DNA aptamer which binds to and inhibits thrombin exhibits a new structural motif for DNA. *Biochemistry*, **32**, 1899–1904.
85. Stoltenburg, R., Reinemann, C., and Strehlitz, B. (2007) SELEX – a (r)evolutionary method to generate high-affinity nucleic acid ligands. *Biomol. Eng.*, **24**, 381–403.
86. Drolet, D.W. *et al.* (2000) Pharmacokinetics and safety of an anti-vascular endothelial growth factor aptamer (NX1838) following injection into the vitreous humor of rhesus monkeys. *Pharm. Res.*, **17**, 1503–1510.
87. Khalil, I.A. *et al.* (2006) High density of octaarginine stimulates macropinocytosis leading to efficient intracellular trafficking for gene expression. *J. Biol. Chem.*, **281**, 3544–3551.
88. Mae, M. and Langel, U. (2006) Cell-penetrating peptides as vectors for peptide, protein and oligonucleotide delivery. *Curr. Opin. Pharmacol.*, **6**, 509–514.
89. Xu, L. *et al.* (2002) Systemic tumor-targeted gene delivery by anti-transferrin receptor scFv-immunoliposomes. *Mol. Cancer Ther.*, **1**, 337–346.
90. Chen, Y. *et al.* (2010) Nanoparticles modified with tumor-targeting scFv deliver siRNA and miRNA for cancer therapy. *Mol. Ther.*, **18**, 1650–1656.
91. Gurrath, M. *et al.* (1992) Conformation/activity studies of rationally designed potent anti-adhesive RGD peptides. *Eur. J. Biochem.*, **210**, 911–921.
92. Haubner, R.H. *et al.* (2003) Radiotracer-based strategies to image angiogenesis. *Q. J. Nucl. Med.*, **47**, 189–199.
93. Wang, L. *et al.* (2009) Improving tumor-targeting capability and pharmacokinetics of ^{99m}Tc-labeled cyclic RGD dimers with PEG_4 linkers. *Mol. Pharm.*, **6**, 231–245.
94. Kok, R.J. *et al.* (2002) Preparation and functional evaluation of RGD-modified proteins as $alpha_v beta_3$ integrin directed therapeutics. *Bioconjug. Chem.*, **13**, 128–135.
95. Boturyn, D. *et al.* (2004) Template assembled cyclopeptides as multimeric system for integrin targeting and endocytosis. *J. Am. Chem. Soc.*, **126**, 5730–5739.
96. Temming, K. *et al.* (2005) RGD-based strategies for selective delivery of therapeutics and imaging agents to the tumour vasculature. *Drug Resist. Updat.*, **8**, 381–402.
97. Sudimack, J. and Lee, R.J. (2000) Targeted drug delivery via the folate receptor. *Adv. Drug Deliv. Rev.*, **41**, 147–162.
98. Chen, Y., Wu, J.J., and Huang, L. (2010) Nanoparticles targeted with NGR motif deliver c-*myc* siRNA and doxorubicin for anticancer therapy. *Mol. Ther.*, **18**, 828–834.
99. Santoro, A. *et al.* (2010) Phase II study of NGR–hTNF, a selective vascular targeting agent, in patients with metastatic colorectal cancer after failure of standard therapy. *Eur. J. Cancer*, **46**, 2746–2752.

100. Lee, R.J. and Low, P.S. (1994) Delivery of liposomes into cultured KB cells via folate receptor-mediated endocytosis. *J. Biol. Chem.*, **269**, 3198–3204.
101. Banerjee, R. *et al.* (2004) Anisamide-targeted stealth liposomes: a potent carrier for targeting doxorubicin to human prostate cancer cells. *Int. J. Cancer*, **112**, 693–700.
102. Chono, S. *et al.* (2008) An efficient and low immunostimulatory nanoparticle formulation for systemic siRNA delivery to the tumor. *J. Control. Release*, **131**, 64–69.
103. Li, S.D., Chono, S., and Huang, L. (2008) Efficient oncogene silencing and metastasis inhibition via systemic delivery of siRNA. *Mol. Ther.*, **16**, 942–946.
104. Maurice, T. and Su, T.P. (2009) The pharmacology of sigma-1 receptors. *Pharmacol. Ther.*, **124**, 195–206.
105. Mukherjee, A. *et al.* (2005) Haloperidol-associated stealth liposomes: a potent carrier for delivering genes to human breast cancer cells. *J. Biol. Chem.*, **280**, 15619–15627.
106. Hadj-Slimane, R. *et al.* (2007) Short interfering RNA (siRNA), a novel therapeutic tool acting on angiogenesis. *Biochimie*, **89**, 1234–1244.
107. Lu, P.Y., Xie, F.Y., and Woodle, M.C. (2003) siRNA-mediated antitumorigenesis for drug target validation and therapeutics. *Curr. Opin. Mol. Ther.*, **5**, 225–234.
108. Chen, Y. *et al.* (2010) Targeted nanoparticles deliver siRNA to melanoma. *J. Invest. Dermatol.*, **130**, 2790–2798.
109. Siomi, M.C. (2009) Short interfering RNA-mediated gene silencing; towards successful application in human patients. *Adv. Drug Deliv. Rev.*, **61**, 668–671.
110. Davis, M.E. *et al.* (2010) Evidence of RNAi in humans from systemically administered siRNA via targeted nanoparticles. *Nature*, **464**, 1067–1070.
111. Lopez-Fraga, M., Martinez, T., and Jimenez, A. (2009) RNA interference technologies and therapeutics: from basic research to products. *BioDrugs*, **23**, 305–332.
112. Phalon, C., Rao, D.D., and Nemunaitis, J. (2010) Potential use of RNA interference in cancer therapy. *Expert. Rev. Mol. Med.*, **12**, e26.
113. Nguyen, T. *et al.* (2008) RNAi therapeutics: an update on delivery. *Curr. Opin. Mol. Ther.*, **10**, 158–167.
114. Aleku, M. *et al.* (2008) Atu027, a liposomal small interfering RNA formulation targeting protein kinase N3, inhibits cancer progression. *Cancer Res.*, **68**, 9788–9798.
115. Tiemann, K. and Rossi, J.J. (2009) RNAi-based therapeutics – current status, challenges and prospects. *EMBO Mol. Med.*, **1**, 142–151.
116. Kleinman, M.E. *et al.* (2008) Sequence- and target-independent angiogenesis suppression by siRNA via TLR3. *Nature*, **452**, 591–597.
117. Leachman, S.A. *et al.* (2010) First-in-human mutation-targeted siRNA phase Ib trial of an inherited skin disorder. *Mol. Ther.*, **18**, 442–446.
118. Koldehoff, M. *et al.* (2007) Therapeutic application of small interfering RNA directed against *bcr–abl* transcripts to a patient with imatinib-resistant chronic myeloid leukaemia. *Clin. Exp. Med.*, **7**, 47–55.

43
Local Gene Delivery for Therapy of Solid Tumors

Wolfgang Walther, Peter M. Schlag, and Ulrike Stein

43.1
Introduction

Cancer still represents a disease of high incidence, which explains why a high percentage of experimental as well as clinical gene therapeutic efforts are aimed at cancer therapy [1] (Figure 43.1). Different viral and nonviral vector systems have been developed for this ambitious goal, with improved safety, delivery, and gene expression features [2]. In addition, great efforts have been made for efficient and selective gene delivery to treat cancer [3]. The most prominent systems are viral, liposomal, and physical delivery technologies, designed for gene transfer into the respective tumor tissues (Figure 43.2). The major challenge for cancer gene therapy is the fact that cancer is a systemic disease, due to metastasis formation. Thus, numerous approaches are dealing with the problems associated with proper tumor targeting for systemic gene delivery [2, 3]. Particularly for clinical cancer gene therapy, poor selectivity and inefficiency in vector application are the major obstacles for successful gene therapy. In this context, a growing number of gene therapeutic approaches have focused on local gene delivery to treat cancer [4]. This strategy has shown some applicability in clinical settings for improved control of cancer by avoiding the problems of systemic gene delivery.

43.2
Gene Therapeutic Strategies for Cancer Treatment

Five major strategies have been developed for the treatment of cancer by gene therapy (Table 43.1 and Figure 43.3), aiming at either introduction of tumor suppressor genes (A; gene correction therapy), improving the antitumoral immune response (B; immunogene therapy), directly killing the tumor cells by suicide genes (C; suicide gene therapy) or oncolytic viruses (D; virotherapy), or employing interference with oncogene expression by, for example, small interfering RNA (siRNA) or short hairpin RNA (shRNA) technology (E; gene suppression therapy)

Drug Delivery in Oncology: From Basic Research to Cancer Therapy, First Edition.
Edited by Felix Kratz, Peter Senter, and Henning Steinhagen.

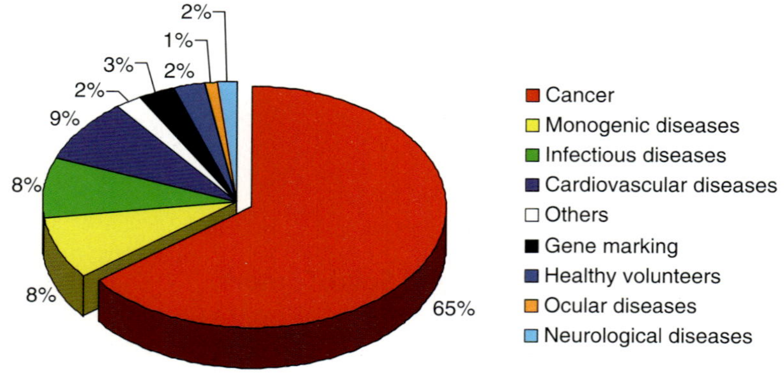

Figure 43.1 Percentages of gene therapy clinical trials worldwide treating different diseases. The highest proportion is represented by cancer gene therapy trials (*www.wiley.com/legacy/wileychi/genmed/clinical/*).

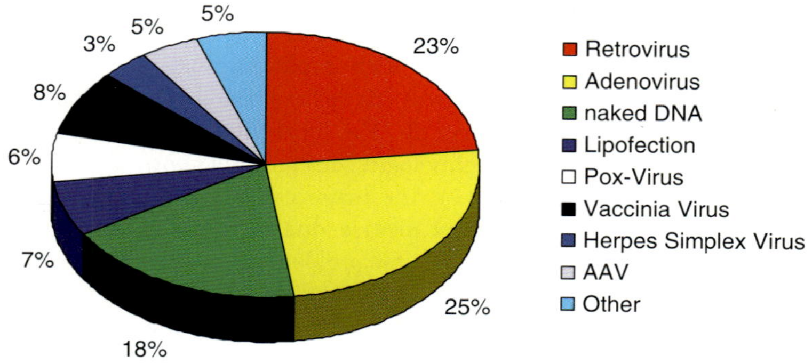

Figure 43.2 Percentages of the different vector systems used in clinical gene therapy applications worldwide. The highest proportion is represented by retroviral (including lentiviral) and adenoviral vectors, followed by use of naked DNA, mostly plasmid-based vectors (*www.wiley.com/legacy/wileychi/genmed/clinical/*).

[1]. All these strategies are under intense experimental investigation and have already entered clinical trials with varying success (Table 43.2).

43.2.1
Gene Correction Therapy

Gene correction therapy aims at the restoration of mutated tumor suppressor genes or cellular oncogenes. This is based on the knowledge that development of tumors is caused by the accumulation of mutational changes leading to inactivation of tumor

Table 43.1 Major strategies and representative transgenes used for experimental and clinical cancer gene therapy approaches (*www.clinicaltrials.gov*).

Strategy	Transgenes	Clinical trial: gene and phase
(A) Gene correction therapy/restoration of normal gene function	tumor suppressor genes/cell cycle regulatory genes: e.g., p53, RB-1, *mda-7*, FUS1, 101F6, NPRL2, FHIT, $p21^{CIP1}$, $p16^{INK1}$	p53: I, II
(B) Immunogene therapy	cytokine genes: IFN-α, IFN-β, IFN-γ, IL-2, -4, -7, -10, -12, GM-CSF, G-CSF, TNF-α	IFN-β: I, II; IL-12: I, II; GM-CSF: I, II; TNF-α: I, II, III;
	genes coding for costimulatory molecules or HLA-determinants: e.g., B7-1, B7-2	B7-1: III
	genes encoding tumor antigens for tumor vaccination: e.g., CEA, PSA, gp100	CEA: II, III; PSA: II; gp100: I
	genes encoding engineered tumor-specific T-cell receptor (Toll-like receptors)	
Tumor cell killing		
(C) by suicide genes	GDEPT: e.g., HSV-*tk*, CD, nitroreductase	HSV-*tk*: I, II; CD: I
(D) by oncolytic viruses (virotherapy)	ONYX-015, HSV-1, Newcastle disease virus, reovirus, measles virus	ONYX-015: I, II, III; HSV-1: I, II; reovirus: I, II, III
(E) Gene suppression therapy	siRNA for interference with genes controlling growth signaling; with oncogenes (e.g., TGF-β, EGFR, PKC-α, STAT-3, H-*ras*, K-*ras*, BCR–ABL) or angiogenesis (e.g., VEGF, FAK)	
	hammerhead ribozymes against: multidrug resistance genes (e.g., MDR-1, MRP-1)	
	antisense oligonucleotides for interference with oncogene expression (e.g., c-*myc*, H-*ras*, *raf*, Bcl-2)	Bcl-2: I, II; B-*raf*: I

CEA, carcinoembryonic antigen; EGFR, epidermal growth factor receptor; FAK, focal adhesion kinase; G-CSF, granulocyte colony-stimulating factor; MDR-1, multidrug resistance gene 1; MRP-1, multidrug resistance-related protein 1; PKC, protein kinase C; RB-1, retinoblastoma gene 1; TGF, transforming growth factor; VEGF, vascular endothelial growth factor; see text for other abbreviations.

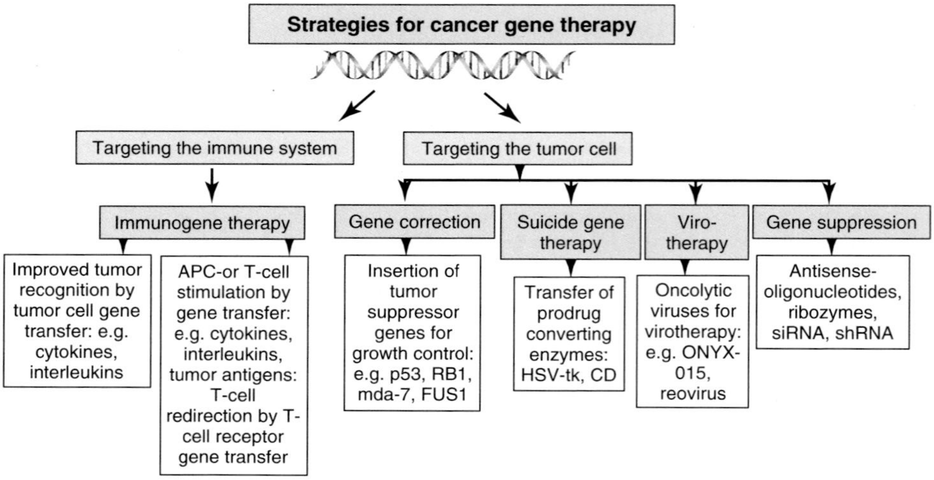

Figure 43.3 Schematic representation of the five major strategies used in cancer gene therapy. Immunogene therapy aims at the restoration and stimulation of the patient's immune system to improve antitumoral defense mechanisms. This approach targets cancer as a systemic disease. The direct killing of tumor cells or inhibition of their malignant growth is targeted by gene correction therapy, suicide gene therapy, oncolytic virotherapy, or gene suppression approaches.

suppressor genes or activation of oncogenes [5]. Although this affects a complex network, making it a challenging task to repair all mutations, some of them are crucial for the maintenance and progression of the tumor, as is shown for p53 [6]. Therefore, restoration of the normal controlling function of such key regulator genes could inhibit tumor growth. Such an approach has been extensively explored for replacement of mutated p53 with wild-type p53 (wt-p53) to inhibit tumor growth and to induce apoptosis. The restoration of wt-p53 function has been tested *in vitro, in vivo,* and in clinical studies using adenovirus vectors (Advexin®/INGN 201 from Introgen or Gendicine® from SiBiono) for gene transfer [7, 8]. In particular, gene correction therapy is combined in different studies with chemotherapy or radiation to improve therapeutic efficacy.

43.2.2
Immunogene Therapy

The strategy to activate the immune response against cancer cells is defined as immunogene therapy [9]. This therapeutic concept is based on the observation that many cancers develop strategies to escape immune surveillance mechanisms by downregulation of molecules involved in the immune response, such as loss of class I antigen on tumor cells, lack of costimulatory signals, and secretion of immune inhibitory cytokines. To overcome these mechanisms or to restore efficient antitumoral defense mechanisms, several strategies of immunogene therapy have been explored: cytokine gene transfer to autologous or allogeneic tumor cells,

Table 43.2 Overview of selected representative gene therapy trials (*www.clinicaltrials.gov*).

Cancer	Gene	Mode of action	Institution	Trial ID/phase
HNC	p53	radiosensitization of tumors by adenoviral p53 gene transfer	Southwest Oncology Group	NCT00017173/II
Breast	p53	chemosensitization of tumors by adenoviral p53 gene transfer	Introgen Therapeutics	NCT00044993/II
Neuroblastoma	IL-2	autologous neuroblastoma cells engineered to express IL-2 to induced immune response	Baylor College of Medicine	NCT00048386/I/II
Kidney	B 7-1	autologous kidney cancer cells adenovirally transduced with B 7-1 to build an immune response	H. Lee Moffitt Cancer Center and Research Institute	NCT00031564/II
B-cell lymphoma	IFN-γ	intratumoral adenoviral gene transfer for induction of immune response and tumor eradication	Transgene	NCT00394693/II
Colorectal	IFN-β	intratumoral adenoviral gene transfer for induction of immune response	Biogen Idec	NCT00107861/I/II
Pancreas	TNF-α	TNFerade adenoviral intratumoral transduction for chemo- and radiosensitization	GenVec	NCT00051467/III
Prostate	GM-CSF	allogenic prostate cancer vaccine engineered to express GM-CSF	Providence Health & Services	NCT00122005/I/II
Breast	CEA	replication-incompetent vaccinia and fowlpox viruses engineered to express CEA to induce immune response	National Cancer Institute	NCT00052351/II

(*continued overleaf*)

Table 43.2 (*continued*).

Cancer	Gene	Mode of action	Institution	Trial ID/phase
Ovarian	HSV-*tk*	introduction of the HSV-*tk* gene for sensitization toward ganciclovir as prodrug	John Stoddard Cancer Center	NCT00005025/II
Solid tumors	HSV-1	use of engineered HSV as oncolytic virus to kill cancer cells	Children's Hospital Medical Center, Cincinnati	NCT00931931/I
HNC	reovirus	use of engineered reovirus for oncolysis of tumors	Oncolytics Biotech	NCT01166542/III
Colorectal	anti-Bcl-2 oligo	use of antisense oligonucleotide to Bcl-2 to sensitize tumors to chemotherapy	San Antonio Cancer Institute	NCT00004870/I/II
Neoplasms	anti-B-*raf* oligo	use of antisense oligonucleotide to Bcl-2 to sensitize tumors to radiotherapy	Neopharm	NCT00024661/I

to antigen-presenting cells (APCs) or T-cells, costimulation with B7-1 or B7-2, vaccination against tumor-associated antigens, or redirecting T-cells to the tumor by T-cell receptor gene transfer [10, 11] (Table 43.1).

43.2.3 Suicide Gene Therapy

Suicide gene therapy (also called gene-directed enzyme prodrug therapy (GDEPT)) was developed for the direct killing of tumor cells (Table 43.1). In this gene therapeutic strategy cancer cells are transduced with enzyme-encoding genes, which convert nontoxic prodrugs into cytotoxic metabolites [12]. Meanwhile, numerous such genes have been isolated, which are mainly of viral or bacterial origin, such as herpes simplex virus thymidine kinase (HSV-*tk*), cytosine deaminase (CD), nitroreductase, or cytochrome P450 2B [12, 13]. *In vitro, in vivo*, and clinical studies have shown their effectiveness in different tumors, such as colon cancer, prostate cancer, glioblastoma, and melanoma [2]. In suicide gene therapy the surrounding cells, which do not express the respective suicide gene, are also killed by the "bystander effect" [14, 15]. This effect turned out to be an important factor for efficacy of prodrug therapy. In this context is has been shown in animal studies that tumor regression was achieved in mice bearing colorectal cancer xenografts after treatment with 5-fluorouracil, although only 2% of the tumor contains CD-expressing cells and 98% nontransfected wild-type cells [14].

43.2.4 Virotherapy

Another approach for direct tumor cell killing uses oncolytic viruses in the strategy called virotherapy. These viruses are able to specifically replicate in tumor cells, causing tumor cell lysis. As a result of this lysis mature viral particles can infect neighboring cells, amplifying the therapeutic effect. The first oncolytic virus developed and tested in clinical trials was the adenovirus-derived ONYX-015, which selectively acts in cells with defective p53 [16]. Further developments led to the clinical use of ONYX-015 for combination with chemo- or radiotherapy. HSV represents another established oncolytic system for cancer therapy. The neurotropism of HSV was employed for oncolytic therapies of glioblastoma using engineered HSV-1 variants [17]. Meanwhile, other oncolytic viruses, such as Newcastle disease virus, reovirus, or measles virus, have also come into focus for virotherapies and are being tested in clinical applications [18, 19].

43.2.5 Gene Suppression

The suppression of gene expression in tumor cells is a fast-evolving field of research activity. This approach targets the post-transcriptional process in tumor cells to specifically downregulate genes involved in the development, growth, and progression of cancer cells [20]. To achieve this, either antisense deoxyoligonucleotides, ribozymes, siRNA, or shRNA technologies are used to specifically interfere with gene expression, in particular with expression of oncogenes (Table 43.1). The advantage of these technologies is the high sequence specificity for the transcript target, leading to interruption of the expression of those particular genes that are essential for tumor survival or oncogenic potential.

43.3
Vectors for Cancer Gene Therapy

For gene therapy, effective gene delivery is one important component that is decisive for efficient therapeutic outcome. In cancer gene therapy viral and nonviral vector systems are used to deliver and express the desired transgenes (Table 43.3 and Figure 43.4). Numerous experimental and clinical studies have shown that the choice of vector for the specific application and tumor entity is crucial for successful gene therapy. In this regard, vecterology has made important steps toward the improvement of transfer efficiencies, selectivity of transgene expression by targeting viral and nonviral vectors, and using tumor-specific or regulatable promoters.

Table 43.3 Viral, nonviral, and bacterial vectors used for cancer gene therapy.

		Uses in strategies
Viral vectors		
RNA virus	retroviral vectors Newcastle disease virus vectors reovirus vectors measles virus vectors adenoviral vectors	suicide, immunogene, gene replacement, virotherapy
DNA virus	adeno-associated virus vectors HSV vectors vaccinia virus vectors	suicide, gene replacement, virotherapy, immunogene, virotherapy
Nonviral vectors	liposomal systems (liposome, lipoplex) plasmid DNA siRNA/shRNA ribozymes antisense oligonucleotides DNA or RNA aptamers	immunogene, suicide gene, gene replacement, gene suppression
Bacterial vectors	anaerobic bacteria (*Clostridium*, *Salmonella*, *Bifidobacterium* spp.)	suicide

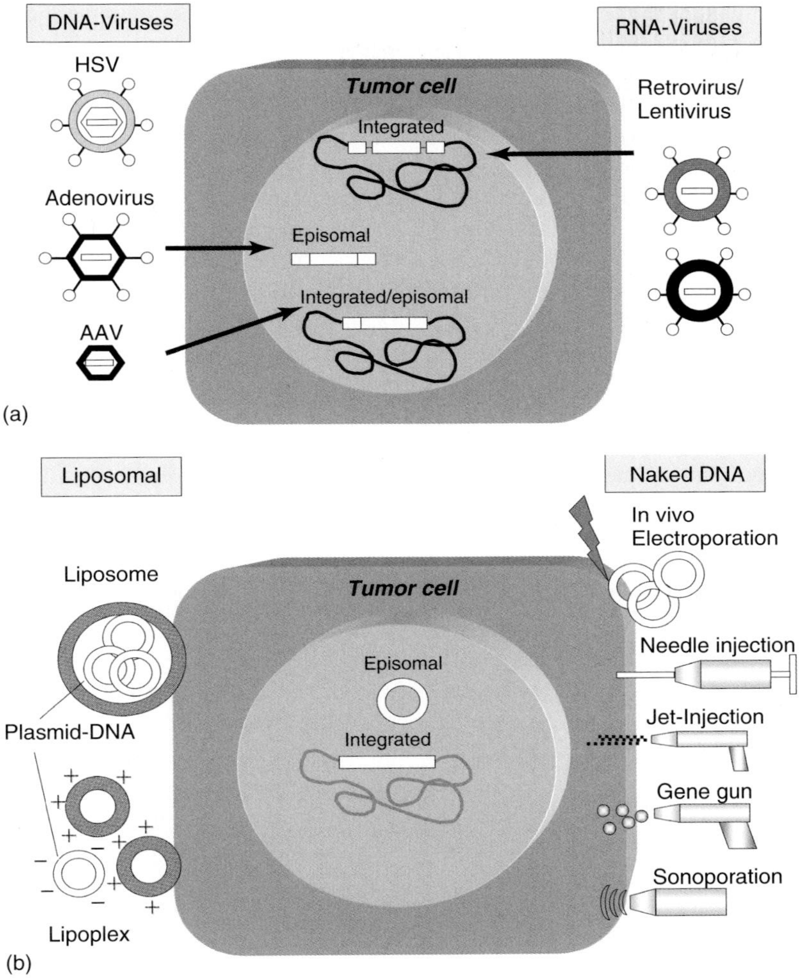

Figure 43.4 Schematic representation of viral and nonviral vector systems for gene transfer. (a) Viral vectors are based on RNA or DNA viruses and permit high transfer efficiencies with efficient transgene expression. Retrovirus vectors are particularly suited for long-term gene expression due to their efficient integration into the host genome. (b) Nonviral gene transfer uses either liposomal transfer systems or naked DNA. For transfer of naked DNA, physical transfer technologies are used, such as electroporation, jet-injection, gene gun, or sonoporation.

43.3.1
Viral Vectors

Viral vectors are still the most efficient gene transfer vehicles, since they infect high proportions of cells and have great cargo capacities for transgene insertion [21]. The majority of studies that employ viral vectors are focused on their improvement for a safe and targeted gene transfer to efficiently express the transgenes in tumors. In particular, the reduction of potential side-effects of viral vector application to humans, such as immunogenicity, toxicities, homologous recombination, or insertional mutagenesis, is of importance for their safe clinical application [21]. Since cancer gene therapy is applied to cancers of different entities possessing various biological properties, viral vectors have been adapted to their specific applications. Numerous different viral vector systems were developed for *ex vivo* and *in vivo* gene transfer, which are mainly derived from murine or human RNA and DNA viruses. In contrast the most commonly used vectors are developed from retroviruses, including lentiviruses, adenoviruses, HSV, vaccinia virus, and adeno-associated virus (Table 43.3). Meanwhile, many more different virus vector systems are under development, such as human cytomegalovirus, Epstein–Barr virus, poxviruses, and foamy virus, which have started to enter clinical applications [22].

Retroviral vectors are derived from RNA viruses that use reverse transcriptase for transcription of their viral RNA genome into a double-stranded DNA, which is then stably inserted into the host DNA (Figure 43.4). Members of this class of RNA viruses are the murine leukemia virus and lentivirus, which provided the platforms for virus vector engineering. Retroviral vectors are frequently and widely used systems in gene therapy due to their efficient gene transfer in dividing and even resting cells, and effective transgene expression [21, 22] (Figure 43.2).

Adenoviruses are the most commonly used DNA viruses for cancer gene therapy (Figures 43.2 and 43.4). These vectors achieve high-level transgene expression combined with high gene transfer efficacy of the recombinant virus particles associated with broad tissue tropism in humans. Clinical trials use adenoviral vectors for transfer of the HSV-*tk* suicide gene to treat head and neck cancer (HNC), non-small-cell lung cancer (NSCLC), ovarian cancer, prostate cancer, and brain tumors. Furthermore, adenoviral vectors are also employed for the gene transfer of immunostimulatory cytokine genes (granulocyte macrophage colony-stimulating factor (GM-CSF) or interleukin (IL)-2) and for the transfer of wt-p53 to restore normal p53 function [23]. Apart from using adenovirus vectors as delivery systems for transgenes, replication-competent oncolytic adenoviral vectors, such as ONYX-015, were generated lacking the E1B 55-kDa gene, which normally binds and inactivates wt-p53 for efficient viral replication. The mutant adenovirus ONYX-015 therefore only replicates in p53-deficient tumor cells, leading to tumor cell lysis in association with virus spread within the tumor [24]. The spectrum of oncolytic vectors has been broadened by other oncolytic viruses, such as HSV, Newcastle disease virus, reovirus, or measles vectors, which were developed to specifically eradicate tumors [18, 25, 26].

43.3.2
Nonviral Vectors

Liposomal systems, such as liposomes, lipoplexes, or naked DNA, are predominantly used in nonviral gene therapy [1]. In liposomal transfer systems DNA is complexed with cationic lipids or enclosed in liposomal microspheres (Figure 43.4). Currently, about 7% of all gene therapy trials use liposomal systems for gene delivery (Figure 43.2). Clinically, lipofection is either applied systemically, by local injection, or delivered as an aerosol (e.g., as done for gene transfer to the lungs) [27]. Examples of formulations with high efficiency for cellular entry and low toxicity are DC-cholesterol/DOPE (1,2-dioleoyl-*sn*-3-phosphoethanolamine)- or DMRIE/DOTMA (*N*-(1,2-dimyristyloxyprop-3-yl)-*N,N*-dimethyl-*N*-hydroxyethyl ammonium bromide/*N*-(2,3-dioleyloxy)propyl)-*N,N,N*-trimethylammonium chloride)-based liposomal systems, which are therefore widely used in clinical cancer gene therapy trials [28].

The nonviral transfer of naked DNA is an applicable alternative to liposomal or viral gene transfer technologies. This is supported by the fact that 18% of all gene therapy trials are based on naked DNA gene transfer [1]. The studies that use naked DNA technologies are mainly aimed at immunostimulation of the host's antitumoral defense mechanisms. For these intradermal, intratumoral, or intramuscular applications, the use of naked DNA has shown efficiency as a cancer vaccine in different animal models [29–33]. Particularly for improved local delivery of naked DNA, various physical procedures are employed *in vivo*, such as needle and syringe injection, particle bombardment ("gene gun"), sonoporation, hydrodynamics procedures, *in vivo* electroporation, or jet-injection [34–37] (Figure 43.4).

43.3.3 Bacterial Vectors

Apart from viral and nonviral vectors, bacterial vectors have experienced a tremendous development for use in cancer gene therapy. It has been known for more than 50 years that facultative and obligate anaerobic bacteria selectively replicate in anaerobic area of tumors, leading to tumor necrosis [38]. Based on this, bacterial vectors derived from *Clostridium*, *Salmonella*, and *Bifidobacterium* were designed for therapeutic purposes. It has been shown that application of these bacteria causes bacterial growth in hypoxic tumor regions, and induces tumor necrosis, inhibits angiogenesis, and stimulates antitumor immunity [39]. The antitumoral features of bacterial vectors were broadened by using them as delivery systems for suicide genes, such as HSV-*tk*, CD, or nitroreductase, and cytokine genes, such as tumor necrosis factor (TNF)-α or IL-2, to improve their therapeutic efficacies [40–43]. More recent developments employ bacterial vectors for tumor-targeted delivery of specific siRNAs to interfere with β-catenin or Stat-3 expression in tumors [44, 45]. Due to their ability of specific tumor targeting, bacterial vectors have already entered clinical trials for tumor treatment [46].

43.4 Local Application of Gene Therapy

Clinical gene therapy trials demonstrated that efficient gene delivery is a crucial factor and the major hurdle for clinically applicable cancer gene therapy. Hitting high percentages of tumor cells is particularly important, since unaffected surviving tumor cells can re-emerge and cause recurrent disease after incomplete therapy. Currently, systemic application of viral or nonviral gene therapy vectors is still accompanied by many obstacles. These include insufficient tumor-specific vector targeting and uncontrolled vector spread, in association with possible systemic side-effects. To achieve the desired therapeutic outcome for cancer gene therapy, local gene transfer has come into focus. Almost 20% of all cancer gene therapy trials use local gene transfer for viral or nonviral vectors to ensure efficient tumor-targeted transgene expression, to bypass the numerous hurdles that exist for systemic tumor-targeted gene delivery. Despite the fact that local gene therapy is only partially useful to target cancer as a metastasizing disease (except strategies of local gene transfer in the context of immunogene therapy), such an approach is an important step to approach the clinical applicability of cancer gene therapy. Thus, in many clinical gene therapy trials vectors (virus particles, liposomes, naked DNA, etc.) are applied intratumorally or in close vicinity to the tumor site. The concept of optimal local cancer gene therapy implies the local therapeutic antitumoral effect in association with possible bystander effects for the benefit of cancer patients. Therefore, a large number of clinical gene therapies are performed as intratumoral, peritumoral, or intralesional applications of virus, liposomal, or other nonviral vectors.

43.4.1
Specific Strategies for Local Gene Delivery

A variety of specific strategies have been developed for local gene delivery for different tumor entities. In this regard, clinical experiences exist for brain tumors, breast, colon, lung, HNC, malignant melanoma, prostate, bladder, and ovarian cancer. Gene therapy of brain tumors, in particular of malignant glioblastomas, favors stereotactic vector application into the tumor site or the intralesional cavity during or shortly after surgery to eradicate remaining tumor cells [47, 48]. For this, retroviral, adenoviral, HSV-derived, and genetically engineered virus producer cells are used to infect tumor cells *in situ* or, alternatively, in nonviral applications liposomal systems are employed. These local applications were performed for transduction or transfection of suicide (HSV-*tk*)-expressing vectors for glioblastoma therapy. In addition to these approaches, oncolytic viruses, such as ONYX-015 or HSV-1, were locally applied for brain tumor virotherapy [49, 50]. All these stereotactic gene therapies for brain tumors generated limited but measurable success of the generation of stable disease and partially prolonged patient survival [51].

Clinical gene therapy trials for breast cancer applied wt-p53-expressing adenovirus or liposomal transfer of the E1A gene intratumorally or intralesionally to suppress tumorigenicity and to promote tumor apoptosis [52]. Similarly, colon cancer or liver metastases of colon cancer were treated by the local administration of the desired vector system. In the majority, intratumoral needle injection was employed to apply adenoviruses, DNA–liposome complexes, or naked DNA to express suicide (HSV-*tk*, CD) or tumor suppressor (wt-p53) genes. These studies revealed the tight correlation between sufficiently high levels of transgene expression and therapeutically relevant antitumor effects.

Clinical gene therapy trials for NSCLC preferably use the local instillation of DNA–liposome complexes or of adenoviruses, mostly for the introduction of the wt-p53 gene. These procedures were performed by computed tomographic guidance for flexible needle bronchoscopic injection or bronchoalveolar lavage [53, 54]. Partially stable disease could be achieved in NSCLC patients in these trials. However, local wt-p53 gene transfer studies for NSCLC were more encouraging when combined with radiation.

HNC is also treated by local introduction of wt-p53-expressing nonviral vectors or adenoviruses. Furthermore, HNC has been treated frequently by intratumoral injection of the oncolytic adenovirus ONYX-015, which generated partial or even complete responses [55]. The combination of local application of ONYX-015 and chemotherapy could further improve therapeutic efficiencies [56]. Due to the high oncolytic capacity, ONYX-015 has also been used widely for the local treatment of ovarian and pancreatic cancers by intratumoral or intraperitoneal injections [57, 58].

For malignant melanoma particularly the skin lesions represent accessible targets for local gene therapy. In this context, numerous clinical trials of melanoma gene therapy use direct intratumoral injection of nonviral naked plasmid DNA, DNA–liposome complexes, or adenoviral vectors to express the HSV-*tk* suicide gene, the wt-p53 tumor suppressor, or IL-12 [59–61]. These studies showed varying success due to great variations in transfer efficiencies observed in the treated patients. More promising approaches represent the intratumoral or peritumoral injections of DNA/lipid formulations for expression of costimulatory molecules (human lymphocyte antigen (HLA)-B7, interferon (IFN)-γ), which led to local tumor regression and partial or complete responses associated with an increase in tyrosinase or MAGE-A1 antibodies in the patients [62, 63].

Prostate cancer is preferably targeted by intratumoral injection gene delivery in clinical studies, using adenoviral vectors or liposomal systems to express suicide (HSV-*tk* or fusion HSV-*tk*/CD) or cytokine genes. In several local gene therapy studies reduction in serum prostate-specific antigen (PSA) level has been observed, indicating a reduction in tumor progression [64–66]. Gene therapy for bladder cancer frequently uses intravesical gene transfer, in which mostly adenoviral vectors are employed either for wt-p53 gene or for suicide gene expression. A major barrier for gene delivery in bladder cancer, however, is the glycosaminoglycan layer on the bladder mucosa, which can interfere with adenovirus entry. Thus, current efforts focus on the modification of adenovirus fibers to improve viral infectivity [67].

In contrast to the different intratumoral gene deliveries, ovarian cancer is rather treated by intraperitoneal gene transfer to apply the desired viral or nonviral liposomal vectors close to the tumor for the expression of wt-p53, E1A [68, 69]. Since gene transfer in this tumor only showed limited success, other approaches focus on the intraperitoneal instillation of oncolytic adenovirus or measles virus for improved eradication of the tumor [70, 71].

In summary, clinical trials that use local gene delivery mostly employ intratumoral or intralesional and, in some the cases, peritumoral transfer. In specific applications, intravesical, intraperitoneal, and intrapleural gene delivery is used. All these applications aim at local control or reduction of the tumor mass of a particular tumor type by inducing tumor cell killing or provoking local attraction of antitumor immune responses.

43.4.2
Technologies for Local Gene Delivery

During the last two decades physical gene transfer technologies have come into focus. They represent an applicable approach for local gene delivery of nonviral but also of viral vectors (Table 43.4). For local vector delivery, most clinical gene therapy studies use needle injection, stereotactic injection, or instillation independently of the tumor entity. The advantage of these routes of administration is that they do not require further technical equipment. However, other methods of application emerge for their use in clinical trials. In this context, a growing arsenal of novel and efficient physical delivery technologies is under development for local *in vivo* gene transfer. These technologies are intended to improve transfer efficiency mostly for nonviral vectors, to achieve transgene expression at therapeutically relevant level [72].

The simplest method for delivery is intratumoral needle injection of the desired vector either as naked DNA, DNA–liposome formulation, or viral particle. Apart

Table 43.4 Physical methods for local gene delivery.

Method of gene delivery	Vectors transferred
Intratumoral syringe/needle injection	viral vectors, DNA–liposome complexes, naked plasmid DNA, oligonucleotides, siRNA
Hydrodynamic injection procedure, injection via artery or vein	naked plasmid DNA, siRNA, viral vectors
Organ perfusion (intravenous vector application by venal occlusion)	DNA–liposome complexes, naked plasmid DNA, viral vectors
In vivo electroporation	naked plasmid DNA, RNA, oligonucleotides, siRNA
Ballistic gene delivery/gene gun for dermal, intratumoral or intramuscular application	naked plasmid DNA
Jet-injection for intratumoral application	Naked plasmid DNA, DNA–liposome complexes, adeno-associated virus particles, siRNA
Ultrasound-mediated delivery (sonoporation/sonotransfection)	naked plasmid DNA, DNA–liposome complexes
Osmotic pump	DNA–liposome complexes
Laser beam transduction	naked plasmid DNA

from application of virus vectors or liposomes, it has been shown that simple needle injection is sufficient for transfection of naked DNA into muscle tissue, whereas this technique is largely inefficient for gene delivery to other tissues, including tumors. Major drawbacks of needle injection are the quantitative seepage of the injected DNA solution and frequently observed restriction of transfection areas to the needle track. Therefore, numerous studies focused on the modification of this procedure for optimization of transfer efficiencies, particularly for nonviral systems [73, 74]. One such modification is the development of the hydrodynamics-based procedure to deliver large volumes of naked DNA-containing solutions of more than 1 ml. These are injected either directly into the tissue or applied by artery or vein injections within few seconds [73–75]. Although the efficiency of this procedure has been demonstrated in several *in vivo* studies, at its current stage it will be rather limited to the perfusion of specific tumor-bearing organs or specific parts or regions of the targeted organ for local or locoregional gene delivery.

The use of electrical fields for the generation of electropores in cell membranes and its use for gene transfer led to the development of *in vivo* electroporation technology. This physical delivery method was shown to significantly enhance gene transfer efficiencies in different *in vivo* models and meanwhile was shown to be applicable for clinical use [72, 76, 77]. In fact, this method is mostly combined with intratumoral DNA needle injection to facilitate cellular entry of the vector, and has been extensively and successfully tested for intratumoral gene transfer [78, 79].

The "gene gun" (ballistic bombardment gene delivery) uses DNA-coated microparticles (gold or tungsten) for nonviral transfection into different tissues. These particles are propelled into the target tissue by pressurized gas. This ballistic gene transfer generates only limited DNA penetration into the tissue and does not reach deeper areas. Therefore, most studies that use ballistic delivery for nonviral gene transfer aim at immunostimulation or DNA vaccination approaches to target different areas in the skin, including APC populations [80]. This has been exploited for local epidermal delivery of gp100 and GM-CSF-expressing nonviral vectors to treat melanoma patients [81].

Apart from other established nonviral delivery systems, jet-injection has developed to an applicable technology, which allows gene transfer into different tissue types with deeper penetration of the naked DNA. Jet-injection is based on the needleless application of fluid jets by pressurized air with high velocity into the target tissue, leading to dispersed penetration of comparatively low volumes. This method can achieve *in vivo* transfer efficiencies comparable with *in vivo* electroporation or liposomal gene transfer [37].

There are certainly many other new and promising techniques for gene delivery under development, such as sonoporation and laser beam-aided transfection (Table 43.4), which might also enter clinical testing. In addition, variations or combinations of the aforementioned different physical delivery methods are being tested, which might lead to improved transfer efficiencies, particularly in local gene delivery approaches.

43.4.3
Jet-Injection Technology for Local Cancer Gene Therapy

In the context of local gene delivery for treatment of cancer, we focused on the employment of the needleless jet-injection technology. Jet-injection was originally developed for needleless injection of insulin and is used for local application of various drugs, as well as for immunization [82, 83]. Meanwhile, jet-injection has also been developed to an applicable physical gene delivery system [84]. In the last decade we established the low-volume Swiss-Injector® (EMS Medical, Nyon, Switzerland), which uses compressed air to eject small volumes of up to 10 μl of naked plasmid DNA-containing solutions at high speed (greater than 300 m/s). The pulse of the liquid jet permits precise and deep penetration into tissues with broad intratumoral liquid dispersion. In our studies jet-injection has demonstrated efficiency for *in vivo* gene transfer in various tumor models. Therapeutic *in vivo* experiments using jet-injection transfer of the CD suicide gene demonstrated antitumor effects [85]. In these *in vivo* studies human colon carcinoma-bearing mice were jet-injected with the CD gene harboring vector plasmid. Analyses of the jet-injected tumor revealed strong CD expression for the entire observation time. The tumor volumes of control and treatment groups were measured during the treatment with the prodrug 5-fluorocytosine. Growth inhibition in association with massive necrosis was seen in the CD-gene transduced, 5-fluorocytosine-treated tumors compared to the non-jet-injected control group, which lasted for the entire observation time. Jet-injection technology was also successfully used for the intratumoral application of a heat-inducible TNF-α-expressing vector [86]. The jet-injection of the naked vector DNA led to heat-induced TNF-α expression and to therapeutic effects. This was reflected by the significant tumor growth inhibition of the jet-injected animals if heat-induced TNF-α expression was combined with cytostatic drug treatment. In a different therapeutic approach, jet-injection was employed for intratumoral application of shRNA-expressing plasmid vectors to reverse *mdr1*-mediated multidrug resistance in tumors [87]. The application of anti-*mdr1* shRNA-expressing vector DNA into *mdr1*-overexpressing tumors led to sustained downregulation of *mdr1* expression at the mRNA and protein level. This reversed the resistant tumors to the sensitive phenotype, which then responded to subsequent cytostatic drug treatment by reduction in tumor growth.

43.4.4
Clinical Application of Local Jet-Injection Gene Therapy

Based on our preclinical jet-injection studies, we performed a phase I clinical trial to evaluate the safety and efficiency of local intratumoral jet-injection. We performed β-galactosidase (LacZ) reporter gene transfer into skin metastases of melanoma and breast cancer patients [88]. The patients received jet-injections into a single cutaneous lesion (Figure 43.5). In the clinical study, safety monitoring was done and plasmid DNA distribution and LacZ mRNA expression were analyzed, complemented by Western blot, immunohistochemistry, and X-gal stain of

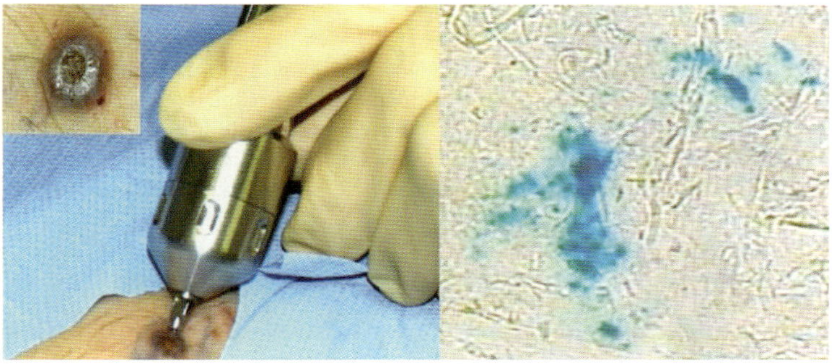

(a) (b)

Figure 43.5 Clinical application of local nonviral gene transfer of naked plasmid DNA by using the low-volume jet-injection technology. (a) Intratumoral application by jet-injection directly into a skin metastasis from melanoma; the inset shows the application site shortly after five jet-injections. (b) Detection of β-galactosidase reporter gene expression by X-gal staining (blue areas) in the tumor tissue after jet-injection gene transfer (original magnification × 100).

LacZ protein expression. Systemic plasmid clearance was monitored at different timepoints before and after jet-injection in blood samples. The trial revealed that jet-injection was safely performed with no side-effects. Plasmid DNA, LacZ mRNA, and protein expression were detected in all treated lesions. Low-level systemic plasmid DNA distribution was detected shortly after jet-injection with a peak 30 min after application, followed by rapid DNA clearance within hours.

This clinical gene transfer trial demonstrated the safety and applicability of local nonviral jet-injection of plasmid DNA, which leads to efficient transgene expression. The data from this trial support the feasibility of jet-injection gene transfer for cancer gene therapy, particularly if local control of the disease is anticipated.

43.5 Conclusions

Cancer is still the most prominent target for gene therapeutic efforts (64% of all gene therapy trails). Clinical gene therapy trials, however, clearly revealed that success in cancer gene therapy depends on efficient and targeted gene transfer to ensure effective transgene expression in the tumor. Due to the existing obstacles for safe and tumor-targeted systemic gene delivery, many clinical trials rely on local gene transfer approaches for more direct intervention of the tumor. In fact, local cancer gene therapy can be beneficial for local disease control, to reduce tumor mass, to sustain vital organ function affected by cancer, or to effectively induce antitumoral immune response mechanisms. In addition, local cancer gene therapy could be advantageous in a multimodality concept for its combination with other, established conventional therapies, such as chemo- or radiotherapy, by improving their therapeutic efficacies.

References

1. Edelstein, M.L., Abedi, M.R., and Wixon, J. (2007) Gene therapy clinical trials worldwide to 2007 – an update. *J. Gene Med.*, **9**, 833–842.
2. Gillet, J.P., Macadangdang, B., Fathke, R.L., Gottesmann, M.M., and Kimchi-Sarfati, C. (2009) The development of gene therapy: from monogenic recessive disorders to complex diseases such as cancer. *Methods Mol. Biol.*, **542**, 5–54.
3. Dachs, G.U., Dougherty, G.J., Stratford, I.J., and Chaplin, D.J. (1997) Targeting gene therapy to cancer: a review. *Oncol. Res.*, **9**, 313–325.
4. Vile, R.G., Rssell, S.J., and Lemoine, N.R. (2000) Cancer gene therapy: hard lessons and new courses. *Gene Ther.*, **7**, 2–8.
5. Weinstein, I.B. and Joe, A.K. (2006) Mechanism of disease: oncogene addiction – a rationale for molecular targeting in cancer therapy. *Nat. Clin. Pract. Oncol.*, **3**, 448–457.
6. Pisters, L.L., Pettaway, C.A., Troncoso, P., McDonnell, T.J., Stephens, L.C., Wood, C.G., Do, K.A., Brisbay, S.M., Wang, X., Hossan, E.A., Evans, R.B., Soto, C., Jacobson, M.G., Parker, K., Merritt, J.A., Steiner, M.S., and Logothetis, C.J. (2004) Evidence that transfer of functional p53 protein results in increased apoptosis in prostate cancer. *Clin. Cancer Res.*, **10**, 2587–2593.
7. Gabrilovich, D.I. (2006) INGN 201 (advexin). Adenoviral p53 gene therapy for cancer. *Expert. Opin. Biol. Ther.*, **6**, 823–832.
8. Swisher, S.G., Roth, J.A., Komaki, R., Gu, J., Lee, J.J., Hicks, M., Ro, J.Y., Hong, W.K., Merritt, J.A., Ahrar, K., Atkinson, N.E., Correa, A.M., Dolormente, M., Dreiling, L., El-Naggar, A.K., Fossella, F., Francisco, R., Glisson, B., Grammer, S., Herbst, R., Huaringa, A., Kemp, B., Khuri, F.R., Kurie, J.M., Liao, Z., McDonnell, T.J., Morice, R., Morello, F., Munden, R., Papadimitrakopoulou, V., Pisters, K.M., Putnam, J.B. Jr., Sarabia, A.J., Shelton, T., Stevens, C., Shin, D.M., Smythe, W.R., Vaporciyan, A.A., Walsh, G.L., and Yin, M. (2003) Induction of p53-regulated genes and tumor regression in lung cancer patients after intratumoral delivery of adenoviral p53 (INGN 201) and radiation therapy. *Clin. Cancer Res.*, **9**, 93–101.
9. Xue, S.A. and Strauss, H.J. (2007) Enhancing immune responses for cancer therapy. *Cell. Mol. Immunol.*, **4**, 173–184.
10. Thomas, S., Hart, D.P., Xue, S.A., Cesco-Gaspere, M., and Strauss, H.J. (2007) T-cell receptor gene therapy for cancer: the progress to date and future objectives. *Expert Opin. Biol. Ther.*, **7**, 1207–1218.
11. Sobol, R.E. (2006) The rationale for prophylactic cancer vaccines and need for a paradigm shift. *Cancer Gene Ther.*, **13**, 725–731.
12. Walther, W. and Stein, U. (1999) Therapeutic genes for cancer gene therapy. *Mol. Biotechnol.*, **13**, 21–28.
13. Fillat, C., Carrio, M., Cascante, A., and Sangro, B. (2003) Suicide gene therapy mediated by the herpes simplex virus thymidine kinase gene/ganciclovir system: fifteen years of application. *Curr. Gene Ther.*, **3**, 13–26.
14. Huber, B.E., Austin, E.A., Richards, C.A., Davis, S.T., and Good, S.S. (1994) Metabolism of 5-fluorocytosine to 5-fluorouracil in human colorectal tumor cells transduced with cytosine deaminase gene: significant antitumor effects when only a small percentage of tumor cells express cytosine deaminase. *Proc. Natl. Acad. Sci. USA*, **91**, 8302–8306.
15. Burrows, F.J., Gore, M., Smiley, W.R., Kanemitsu, M.Y., Jolly, D.J., Read, S.B., Nicholas, T., and Kruse, C.A. (2002) Purified herpes simplex virus thymidine kinase retroviral particles: III. Characterization of bystander killing mechanisms in transfected tumor cells. *Cancer Gene Ther.*, **9**, 87–95.
16. Crompton, A.M. and Kirn, D.H. (2007) From ONYX-015 to armed vaccinia viruses: the education and evolution of oncolytic virus development. *Curr. Cancer Drug Targets*, **7**, 133–139.

17. Barzon, L., Zanusso, M., Colombo, F., and Palú, G. (2006) Clinical trials of gene therapy, virotherapy, and immunotherapy for malignant gliomas. *Cancer Gene Ther.*, **13**, 539–554.
18. Hotte, S.J., Lorence, R.M., Hirte, H.W., Polawski, S.R., Bamat, M.K., O'Neil, J.D., Roberts, M.S., Groene, W.S., and Major, P.P. (2007) an optimized clinical regimen for the oncolytic virus PV701. *Clin. Cancer Res.*, **13**, 977–985.
19. Marcato, P., Shmulevitz, M., Pan, D., Stoltz, D., and Lee, P.W. (2007) Ras transformation mediates reovirus oncolysis by enhancing virus uncoating, particle infectivity, and apoptosis-dependent release. *Mol. Ther.*, **15**, 1522–1530.
20. Verreault, M., Webb, M.S., Ramsey, E.C., and Bally, M.B. (2006) Gene silencing in the development of personalized cancer treatment: the targets, the agents and the delivery systems. *Curr. Gene Ther.*, **6**, 505–533.
21. Lotze, M.T. and Kost, T.A. (2002) Viruses as gene delivery vectors: application to gene function, target validation, and assay development. *Cancer Gene Ther.*, **9**, 692–699.
22. Walther, W. and Stein, U. (2000) Viral vectors for gene transfer: a review of their use in the treatment of human diseases. *Drugs*, **60**, 249–271.
23. Fukazawa, T., Matsuoka, J., Yamatsuji, T., Maeda, Y., Durbin, M.L., and Naomoto, Y. (2010) Adenovirus-mediated cancer gene therapy and virotherapy. *Int. J. Mol. Med.*, **25**, 3–10.
24. Heise, C., Sampson-Johannes, A., Williams, A., McCormick, F., Von Hoff, D.D., and Kirn, D.H. (1997) ONYX-015, an E1B gene-attenuated adenovirus, causes tumor-specific cytolysis and antitumoral efficacy that can be augmented by standard chemotherapeutic agents. *Nat. Med.*, **3**, 639–645.
25. Varghese, S. and Rabkin, S.D. (2002) Oncolytic herpes simplex virus vectors for cancer virotherapy. *Cancer Gene Ther.*, **9**, 967–978.
26. Norman, K.L., Coffey, M.C., Hirasawa, K., Demetrick, D.J., Nishikawa, S.G., DiFrancesco, L.M., Strong, J.E., and Lee, P.W. (2002) Reovirus oncolysis of human breast cancer. *Hum. Gene Ther.*, **13**, 641–652.
27. Orson, F.M., Kinsey, B.M., Bhogal, B.S., Song, L., Densmore, C.L., and Barry, M.A. (2003) Targeted delivery of expression plasmids to the lung via macroaggregated polyethylenimine-albumin conjugates. *Methods Mol. Med.*, **75**, 575–590.
28. Templeton, N.S., Lasic, D.D., Frederick, P.M., Strey, H.H., Roberts, D.D., and Pavlakis, G.N. (1997) Improved DNA:liposome complexes for increased systemic delivery and gene expression. *Nat. Biotechnol.*, **15**, 647–652.
29. Rakhmilevich, A.L., Turner, J., Ford, M.J., McCabe, D., Sun, W.H., Sondel, P.H., Grota, K., and Yang, N.-S. (1996) Gene gun-mediated skin transfection with interleukin 12 gene results in regression of established primary and metastatic murine tumors. *Proc. Natl. Acad. Sci. USA*, **93**, 6291–6296.
30. Liu, M.A. and Ulmer, J.B. (2000) Gene based vaccines. *Mol. Ther.*, **1**, 497–500.
31. Turner, J.G., Tan, J., Crucian, B.E., Sullivan, D.M., Ballester, O.F., Dalton, W.S., Yang, N.-S., Burkholder, J.K., and Yu, H. (1998) Broadened clinical utility of gene gun-mediated granulocyte-macrophage colony-stimulating factor cDNA-based tumor cell vaccines as demonstrated with a mouse myeloma model. *Hum. Gene Ther.*, **9**, 1121–1130.
32. Davis, H.L., Demeneix, B.A., Quantin, B., Coulombe, J., and Whalen, R.G. (1993) Plasmid DNA is superior to viral vectors for direct gene transfer into adult mouse skeletal muscle. *Hum. Gene. Ther.*, **4**, 733–740.
33. Heinzerling, L., Feige, K., Rieder, S., Akens, M.K., Dummer, R., Stranzinger, G., and Moelling, K. (2001) Tumor regression induced by intratumoral injection of DNA coding for human interleukin 12 into melanoma metastases in grey horses. *J. Mol. Med.*, **78**, 692–702.
34. Yang, N.-S., Burkholder, J., Roberts, B., Martinell, B., and McCabe, D. (1990) *In vivo* and *in vitro* gene transfer to

mammalian cells by particle bombardment. *Proc. Natl. Acad. Sci. USA*, **87**, 9568–9572.

35. Somiari, S., Glasspool-Malone, J., Drabick, J.J., Gilbert, R.A., Heller, R., Jaroszeski, M., and Malone, R.W. (2000) Theory and *in vivo* application of electroporative gene delivery. *Mol. Ther.*, **2**, 178–187.
36. Nozaki, T., Ogawa, R., Feril, L.B., Kagiya, G., Fuse, H., and Kondo, T. (2003) Enhancement of ultrasound-mediated gene transfection by membrane modification. *J. Gene Med.*, **5**, 1046–1055.
37. Walther, W., Stein, U., Fichtner, I., Malcherek, L., Lemm, M., and Schlag, P.M. (2001) Non-viral *in vivo* gene delivery into tumors using a novel low volume jet-injection technology. *Gene Ther.*, **8**, 173–180.
38. Möse, J.R. and Möse, G. (1964) Oncolysis by clostridia. I. Activity of *Clostridium butyricum* (M-55) and other nonpathogenic clostridia against the Ehrlich carcinoma. *Cancer Res.*, **24**, 212–216.
39. Sznol, M., Lin, S.L., Bermudes, D., Zheng, L.M., and King, I. (2000) Use of preferentially replicating bacteria for the treatment of cancer. *J. Clin. Invest.*, **105**, 1027–1030.
40. Theys, J., Landuyt, W., Nuyts, S., Van Mellaert, L., van Oosterom, A., Lambin, P., and Anné, J. (2001) Specific targeting of cytosine deaminase to solid tumors by engineered *Clostridium acetobutylicum*. *Cancer Gene Ther.*, **8**, 294–297.
41. Pawelek, J.M., Low, K.B., and Bermudes, D. (1997) Tumor-targeted salmonella as a novel anticaner vector. *Cancer Res.*, **57**, 4537–4544.
42. Theys, J., Pennington, O., Dubois, L., Anlezark, G., Vaughan, T., Mengesha, A., Landuyt, W., Anné, J., Burke, P.J., Dûrre, P., Wouters, B.G., Minton, N.P., and Lambin, P. (2006) Repeated cycles of *Clostridium*-directed enzyme prodrug therapy result in sustained antitumour effects *in vivo*. *Br. J. Cancer*, **95**, 1212–1219.
43. Barbé, S., Van Mellaert, L., Theys, J., Geukens, N., Lammertyn, E., Lambin, P., and Anné, J. (2005) Secretory production of biologically active rat interleukin-2 by *Clostridium acetobutylicum* DSM792 as a tool for anti-tumor treatment. *FEMS Microbiol. Lett.*, **246**, 67–73.
44. Xiang, S., Fruehauf, J., and Li, C.J. (2006) Short hairpin RNA-expressing bacteria elicit RNA interference in mammals. *Nat. Biotechnol.*, **24**, 697–702.
45. Zhang, L., Gao, L., Zhao, L., Guo, B., Ji, K., Tian, Y., Wang, J., Yu, H., Hu, J., Kalvakolanu, D.V., Kopecko, D.J., Zhao, X., and Xu, D.Q. (2007) Intratumoral delivery and suppression of prostate tumor growth by attenuated *Salmonella enterica* serovar *typhimurium* carrying plasmid-based small interfering RNAs. *Cancer Res.*, **67**, 5859–5864.
46. Cunningham, C. and Nemunaitis, J. (2001) A phase I trial of genetically modified *Salmonella typhimurium* expressing cytosine deaminase (TAPET-CD, VNP20029) administered by intratumoral injection in combination with 5-fluorocytosine for patients with advanced or metastatic cancer. Protocol no. CL-017. Version: April 9, 2001. *Hum. Gene Ther.*, **12**, 1594–1596.
47. Ram, Z., Culver, K.W., Oshiro, E.M., Viola, J.J., DeVroom, H.L., Otto, E., Long, Z., Chiang, Y., McGarrity, G.J., Muul, L.M., Katz, D., Blaese, R.M., and Oldfield, E.H. (1997) Therapy of malignant brain tumors by intratumoral implantation of retroviral vector-producing cells. *Nat. Med.*, **3**, 1354–1361.
48. Immonen, A., Vapalahti, M., Tyynela, K., Hurskainen, H., Sandmair, A., Vanninen, R., Langford, G., Murray, N., and Yla-Herttuala, S. (2004) AdvHSV-*tk* gene therapy with intravenous ganciclovir improves survival in human malignant glioma: a randomised, controlled study. *Mol. Ther.*, **10**, 967–972.
49. Rainov, N.G. (2000) A phase III clinical evaluation of herpes simplex virus type 1 thymidine kinase and ganciclovir gene therapy as an adjuvant to surgical resection and radiation in adults with previously untreated glioblastoma multiforme. *Hum. Gene Ther.*, **11**, 2389–2401.

50. Chiocca, E.A., Abbed, K.M., Tatter, S., Louis, D.N., Hochberg, F.H., Barker, F., Kracher, J., Grossman, S.A., Fisher, J.D., Carson, K., Rosenblum, M., Mikkelsen, T., Olson, J., Markert, J., Rosenfeld, S., Nabors, L.B., Brem, S., Phuphanich, S., Freeman, S., Kaplan, R., and Zwiebel, J. (2004) A phase I open-label, dose-escalation, multi-institutional trial of injection with an E1B-attenuated adenovirus, ONYX-015, into the peritumoral region of recurrent malignant gliomas, in the adjuvant setting. *Mol. Ther.*, **10**, 958–966.
51. Lawler, S.E., Peruzzi, P.P., and Chiocca, E.A. (2006) Genetic strategies for brain tumor therapy. *Cancer Gene Ther.*, **13**, 225–233.
52. Hortobagyi, G.N., Hung, M.C., and Lopez-Berestein, G. (1998) A Phase I multicenter study of E1A gene therapy for patients with metastatic breast cancer and epithelial ovarian cancer that overexpresses HER-2/*neu* or epithelial ovarian cancer. *Hum. Gene Ther.*, **9**, 1775–1798.
53. Roth, J.A., Swisher, S.G., Merritt, J.A., Lawrence, D.D., Kemp, B.L., Carrasco, C.H., El-Naggar, A.K., Fossella, F.V., Glisson, B.S., Hong, W.K., Khurl, F.R., Kurie, J.M., Nesbitt, J.C., Pisters, K., Putnam, J.B., Schrump, D.S., Shin, D.M., and Walsh, G.L. (1998) Gene therapy for non-small cell lung cancer: a preliminary report of a phase I trial of adenoviral p53 gene replacement. *Semin. Oncol.*, **25**, 33–37.
54. Swisher, S.G., Roth, J.A., Nemunaitis, J., Lawrence, D.D., Kemp, B.L., Carrasco, C.H., Connors, D.G., El-Naggar, A.K., Fossella, F., Glisson, B.S., Hong, W.K., Khuri, F.R., Kurie, J.M., Lee, J.J., Lee, J.S., Mack, M., Merritt, J.A., Nguyen, D.M., Nesbitt, J.C., Perez-Soler, R., Pisters, K.M., Putnam, J.B. Jr., Richli, W.R., Savin, M., Schrump, D.S., Shin, D.M., Shulkin, A., Walsh, G.L., Wait, J., Weill, D., and Waugh, M.K. (1999) Adenovirus-mediated p53 gene transfer in advanced non-small-cell lung cancer. *J. Natl. Cancer Inst.*, **91**, 763–771.
55. Nemunaitis, J., Khuri, F., Ganly, I., Arseneau, J., Posner, M., Vokes, E., Kuhn, J., McCarty, T., Landers, S., Blackburn, A., Romel, L., Randlev, B., Kaye, S., and Kirn, D. (2001) Phase II trial of intratumoral administration of ONYX-015, a replication-selective adenovirus, in patients with refractory head and neck cancer. *J. Clin. Oncol.*, **19**, 289–298.
56. Khuri, F.R., Nemunaitis, J., Ganly, I., Arseneau, J., Tannock, I.F., Romel, L., Gore, M., Ironside, J., MacDougall, R.H., Heise, C., Randlev, B., Gillenwater, A.M., Bruso, P., Kaye, S.B., Hong, W.K., and Kirn, D.H. (2000) A controlled trial of intratumoral ONYX-015, a selectively-replicating adenovirus, in combination with cisplatin and 5-fluorouracil in patients with recurrent head and neck cancer. *Nat. Med.*, **6**, 879–885.
57. Heise, C., Ganly, I., Kim, Y.T., Sampson-Johannes, A., Brown, R., and Kirn, D. (2000) Efficacy of a replication-selective adenovirus against ovarian carcinomatosis is dependent on tumor burden, viral replication and p53 status. *Gene Ther.*, **7**, 1925–1929.
58. Hecht, J.R., Bedford, R., Abbruzzese, J.L., Lahoti, S., Reid, T.R., Soetikno, R.M., Kirn, D.H., and Freeman, S.M. (2003) A phase I/II trial of intratumoral endoscopic ultrasound injection of ONYX-015 with intravenous gemcitabine in unresectable pancreatic carcinoma. *Clin. Cancer Res.*, **9**, 555–561.
59. Heinzerling, L., Burg, G., Dummer, R., Maier, T., Oberholzer, P.A., Schultz, J., Elzaouk, L., Pavlovic, J., and Moelling, K. (2005) Intratumoral injection of DNA encoding human interleukin 12 into patients with metastatic melanoma: clinical efficacy. *Hum. Gene Ther.*, **16**, 35–48.
60. Klatzmann, D., Cherin, P., Bensimon, G., Boyer, O., Coutellier, A., Charlotte, F., Boccaccio, C., Salzmann, J.L., and Herson, S., Study Group on Gene Therapy of Metastatic Melanoma (1998) A phase I/II dose-escalation study of herpes simplex virus type 1 thymidine kinase "suicide" gene therapy for metastatic melanoma. *Hum. Gene Ther.*, **9**, 2585–2594.
61. Dummer, R., Bergh, J., Karlsson, Y., Horowitz, J.A., Mulder, N.H., Huinink, D.T.B., Burg, G., Hofbauer, G., and

Osanto, S. (2000) Biological activity and safety of adenoviral vector-expressed wild-type p53 after intratumoral injection in melanoma and breast cancer patients with p53-overexpressing tumors. *Cancer Gene Ther.*, **7**, 1069–1076.
62. Stopeck, A.T., Hersh, E.M., Akporiaye, E.T., Harris, D.T., Grogan, T., Unger, E., Warneke, J., Schluter, S.F., and Stahl, S. (1997) Phase I study of direct gene transfer of an allogeneic histocompatibility antigen, HLA-B7, in patients with metastatic melanoma. *J. Clin. Oncol.*, **15**, 341–349.
63. Fujii, S., Huang, S., Fong, T.C., Ando, D., Burrows, F., Jolly, D.J., Nemunaitis, J., and Hoon, D.S. (2000) Induction of melanoma-associated antigen systemic immunity upon intratumoral delivery of interferon-gamma retroviral vector in melanoma patients. *Cancer Gene Ther.*, **7**, 1220–1230.
64. Herman, J.R., Adler, H.L., Aguilar-Cordova, E., Rojas-Martinez, A., Woo, S., Timme, T.L., Wheeler, T.M., Thompson, T.C., and Scardino, P.T. (1999) In situ gene therapy for adenocarcinoma of the prostate: a phase I clinical trial. *Hum. Gene Ther.*, **10**, 1239–1249.
65. Freytag, S.O., Khil, M., Stricker, H., Peabody, J., Menon, M., DePeralta-Venturina, M., Nafziger, D., Pegg, J., Paielli, D., Brown, S., Barton, K., Lu, M., Aguilar-Cordova, E., and Kim, J.H. (2002) Phase I study of replication-competent adenovirus-mediated double suicide gene therapy for the treatment of locally recurrent prostate cancer. *Cancer Res.*, **62**, 4968–4976.
66. DeWeese, T.L., van der Poel, H., Li, S., Mikhak, B., Drew, R., Goemann, M., Hamper, U., DeJong, R., Detorie, N., Rodriguez, R., Haulk, T., DeMarzo, A.M., Piantadosi, S., Yu, D.C., Chen, Y., Henderson, D.R., Carducci, M.A., Nelson, W.G., and Simons, J.W. (2001) A phase I trial of CV706, a replication-competent, PSA selective oncolytic adenovirus, for the treatment of locally recurrent prostate cancer following radiation therapy. *Cancer Res.*, **61**, 7464–7472.
67. Irie, A. (2003) Advances in gene therapy for bladder cancer. *Curr. Gene Ther.*, **3**, 1–11.
68. Wen, S.F., Mahavni, V., Quijano, E., Shinoda, J., Grace, M., Musco-Hobkinson, M.L., Yang, T.Y., Chen, Y., Runnenbaum, I., Horowitz, J., Maneval, D., Hutchins, B., and Buller, R. (2003) Assessment of p53 gene transfer and biological activities in a clinical study of adenovirus-p53 gene therapy for recurrent ovarian cancer. *Cancer Gene Ther.*, **10**, 224–238.
69. Madhusudan, S., Tamir, A., Bates, N., Flanagan, E., Gore, M.E., Barton, D.P., Harper, P., Seckl, M., Thomas, H., Lemoine, N.R., Charnock, M., Habib, N.A., Lechler, R., Nicholls, J., Pignatelli, M., and Ganesan, T.S. (2004) A multicenter Phase I gene therapy clinical trial involving intraperitoneal administration of E1A–lipid complex in patients with recurrent epithelial ovarian cancer overexpressing HER-2/*neu* oncogene. *Clin. Cancer Res.*, **10**, 2986–2996.
70. Vasey, P.A., Shulman, L.N., Campos, S., Davis, J., Gore, M., Johnston, S., Kirn, D.H., O'Neill, V., Siddiqui, N., Seiden, M.V., and Kaye, S.B. (2002) Phase I trial of intraperitoneal injection of the E1B-55-kd-gene-deleted adenovirus ONYX-015 (dl1520) given on days 1 through 5 every 3 weeks in patients with recurrent/refractory epithelial ovarian cancer. *J. Clin. Oncol.*, **20**, 1562–1569.
71. Galanis, E., Hartmann, L.C., Cliby, W.A., Long, H.J., Peethambaram, P.P., Barrette, B.A., Kaur, J.S., Haluska, P.J. Jr., Aderca, I., Zollman, P.J., Sloan, J.A., Keeney, G., Atherton, P.J., Podratz, K.C., Dowdy, S.C., Stanhope, C.R., Wilson, T.O., Federspiel, M.J., Peng, K.W., and Russell, S.J. (2010) Phase I trial of intraperitoneal administration of an oncolytic measles virus strain engineered to express carcinoembryonic antigen for recurrent ovarian cancer. *Cancer Res.*, **70**, 875–878.
72. Wells, D.J. (2004) Gene therapy progress and prospects: electroporation and other physical methods. *Gene Ther.*, **11**, 1363–1369.
73. Liu, F., Song, Y.K., and Liu, D. (1999) Hydrodynamics-based transfection

in animals by systemic administration of plasmid DNA. *Gene Ther.*, **6**, 1258–1266.

74. Zhang, G., Song, Y.K., and Liu, D. (2000) Long-term expression of human alpha1-antitrypsin gene in mouse liver achieved by intravenous administration of plasmid DNA using hydrodynamics-based procedure. *Gene Ther.*, **7**, 1344–1349.

75. Suda, T. and Liu, D. (2007) Hydrodynamic gene delivery: its principles and applications. *Mol. Ther.*, **12**, 2063–2069.

76. Yamashita, Y., Shimada, M., Hasegawa, H., Minagawa, R., Rikimaru, T., Hamatsu, T., Tanaka, S., Shirabe, K., Miyazaki, J., and Sugimachi, K. (2001) Electroporation-mediated interleukin-12 gene therapy for hepatocellular carcinoma in the mice model. *Cancer Res.*, **61**, 1005–1012.

77. Tjelle, T.E., Rabussay, D., Ottensmeier, C., Mathiesen, I., and Kjeken, R. (2008) Taking electroporation-based delivery of DNA vaccination into humans: a generic clinical protocol. *Methods Mol. Biol.*, **423**, 497–507.

78. Heller, L.C. and Coppola, D. (2002) Electrically mediated delivery of vector plasmid DNA elicits an antitumor effect. *Gene Ther.*, **9**, 1321–1325.

79. Wells, D.J. (2010) Electroporation and ultrasound enhanced non-viral gene delivery *in vitro* and *in vivo*. *Cell Biol. Toxicol.*, **26**, 21–28.

80. Seigne, J., Turner, J., Diaz, J., Hackney, J., Pow-Sang, J., Helal, M., Lockhart, J., and Yu, H. (1999) Feasibility study of gene gun mediated immunotherapy for renal cell carcinoma. *J. Urol.*, **162**, 1259–1263.

81. Cassaday, R.D., Sondel, P.M., King, D.M., Macklin, M.D., Gan, J., Warner, T.F., Zuleger, C.L., Bridges, A.J., Schalch, H.G., Kim, K.M., Hank, J.A., Mahvi, D.M., and Albertini, M.R. (2007) A phase I study of immunization using particle-mediated epidermal delivery of genes for gp100 and GM-CSF into uninvolved skin of melanoma patients. *Clin. Cancer Res.*, **13**, 540–549.

82. Weller, C. and Linder, M. (1966) Jet injection of insulin vs the syringe-and-needle method. *J. Am. Med. Assoc.*, **195**, 844–847.

83. Baxter, J. and Mitragotri, S. (2006) Needle-free liquid jet injections: mechanisms and applications. *Expert Rev. Med. Devices*, **3**, 565–574.

84. Mitragotri, S. (2006) Current status and future prospects of needle-free liquid jet injectors. *Nat. Rev. Drug Discov.*, **5**, 543–548.

85. Walther, W., Stein, U., Fichtner, I., Aumann, J., Arlt, F., and Schlag, P.M. (2005) Nonviral jet-injection gene transfer for efficient *in vivo* cytosine deaminase suicide gene therapy of colon carcinoma. *Mol. Ther.*, **12**, 1176–1184.

86. Walther, W., Arlt, F., Stein, U., Fichtner, I., and Schlag, P.M. (2007) Heat-inducible *in vivo* gene therapy of colon carcinoma by human mdr1 promoter regulated TNF-α expression. *Mol. Cancer Ther.*, **6**, 235–243.

87. Stein, U., Stege, A., Walther, W., and Lage, H. (2008) Complete *in vivo* reversal of the multidrug resistance (MDR) phenotype in a breast cancer model by jet-injection of anti-MDR1 short hairpin RNA-encoding plasmid DNA. *Mol. Ther.*, **16**, 178–186.

88. Walther, W., Siegel, R., Kobelt, D., Knösel, T., Dietel, M., Bembenek, A., Aumann, J., Schleef, M., Baier, R., Stein, U., and Schlag, P.M. (2008) Nonviral intratumoral jet-injection gene transfer in metastatic melanoma and breast cancer: results of phase I clinical trial. *Clin. Cancer Res.*, **14**, 7545–7553.

44
Viral Vectors for RNA Interference Applications in Cancer Research and Therapy

Henry Fechner and Jens Kurreck

44.1
Introduction

Despite recent progress, treatment of cancer, cardiovascular diseases, and viral infections remains a major challenge in modern medicine. Biologics have come to supplement the traditional approach of developing small-molecular-weight compounds. In particular, monoclonal antibodies that are obtained from genetically engineered mice to produce human-like antibodies that no longer elicit strong immune responses have become a valuable new class of anticancer drugs. The antibody Herceptin® and similar antibodies that work by targeting the HER2 receptor and that are employed to treat metastatic breast cancer represent one of the most successful developments in molecular medicine.

In addition to monoclonal antibodies, nucleic acid-based approaches hold great promise to offer new therapeutic options. In the late 1970s the concept of antisense oligonucleotides was introduced: antisense oligonucleotides are approximately 15- to 20-nucleotide long single-stranded DNA molecules or modified derivatives thereof that bind to a complementary target RNA by Watson–Crick base pairing [1–3]. Through the activation of RNase H or a steric blockade of the ribosome this duplex formation prevents the synthesis of the encoded protein. The technology thus offers the theoretical potential to be applicable to any disease caused by the expression of a deleterious gene (e.g., an oncogene). Disappointingly, antisense approaches never could fulfill these expectations. Efficient cellular delivery, potency, and toxicity remained major challenges that could not be satisfactorily solved.

The hopes were fueled again with the discovery of catalytically active RNAs, known as ribozymes [4]. Most of the naturally occurring ribozymes are active in *cis* (i.e., they cleave their own RNA molecule). It was, however, quickly shown that ribozymes can be redesigned to cleave in *trans* (i.e., target RNA). Hammerhead and hairpin ribozymes were developed and clinically testing against virus infections and cancer [5]. However, again, the outcome of the clinical trials was disappointing due to the low potency of ribozymes *in vivo*.

With the advent of RNA interference (RNAi; an evolutionary conserved mechanism for post-transcriptional gene silencing in eukaryotic cells mediated by

Drug Delivery in Oncology: From Basic Research to Cancer Therapy, First Edition.
Edited by Felix Kratz, Peter Senter, and Henning Steinhagen.

double-stranded RNA molecules), gene-silencing technologies now have a new chance for the long-awaited breakthrough. RNAi was originally described in the nematode *Caenorhabditis elegans*, in which long double-stranded RNA molecules were found to inhibit the expression of a homologous gene [6]. The RNA molecules are initially processed by the nuclease Dicer into so-called small or short interfering RNAs (siRNAs), which are 21–23 nucleotides in length. These siRNA molecules are then loaded into a multimeric protein complex – the RNA-induced silencing complex (RISC). In the process of RISC loading one of the two siRNA strands, named the passenger strand, is discarded while the other strand guides the RISC to the target RNA. Subsequently, the Argonaute 2 (Ago2) protein, which is the major component of the RISC (along with the antisense strand of the siRNA), cleaves the target RNA, thereby initiating its final degradation (for reviews, see [7, 8]).

The great potential of RNAi was immediate recognized by the scientific community. Craig Mello and Andrew Fire were awarded the 2006 Nobel Prize for Medicine or Physiology only 8 years after publication of their milestone discovery. The technology has also rapidly become a standard method in most molecular biology laboratories – a development that is comparable to that of the polymerase chain reaction (PCR). In addition, RNAi has already made its way into the clinic [9] (Table 44.1).

The potential of RNAi in the field of cancer research and therapy was rapidly noticed [11]. In basic research laboratories RNAi is widely used for the inhibition of a specific gene and analysis of the resulting loss-of-function phenotype. It can even be employed to investigate the function of closely related gene products, which cannot be inhibited specifically by small-molecule drugs. For example, hypoxia-inducible factor (HIF) is known to play an important role in tumor angiogenesis. The specific functions of the two closely related subunits, HIF-1α and HIF-2α, however, were not fully understood. RNAi technology allowed the selective inhibition of each of the two subunits. Analysis of downstream targets of HIF revealed that most of the genes tested were responsive only to HIF-1α, with the exception of erythropoietin, which is dependent on HIF-2α [12].

In addition to research applications, RNAi holds great promise as a therapy against cancer. The most straightforward strategy is to inhibit cellular factors such as oncogenes that mediate the uncontrolled proliferation of cells. Furthermore, RNAi can be employed to block angiogenesis (e.g., by targeting vascular endothelial growth factor (VEGF)). As a consequence the tumor will not be supplied with sufficient oxygen and nutrients. Another strategy is to target genes that are known to be involved in metastasis, since in most cases the primary tumor can be surgically removed and the metastases represent the major problem. As an example, RNAi-mediated silencing of phosphatidylinositol 3-kinase resulted in a significant reduction in the formation of metastases, but not in tumor size, in an orthotopic metastatic mouse model for human prostate cancer [13]. Furthermore, RNAi can be employed to resensitize tumor cells against chemotherapeutics. Induction of the multidrug resistance (*mdr*) gene is one of the major causes for chemotherapeutic treatment failure in cancer patients. Silencing of *mdr* was shown to restore sensitivity to drugs transported by the encoded P-glycoprotein [14].

Table 44.1 RNAi in ongoing and completed clinical trials to treat cancer (based on [10]).

Company	RNAi agent	Name	Disease	Target	Trial phase
Calando Pharmaceuticals	unmodified siRNA	CALAA-01	solid tumors	RRM2	I
Alnylam Pharmaceuticals	modified siRNA	ALN-VSP	liver cancers and solid tumors	KSP, VEGF	I
Silence Therapeutics	modified siRNA	Atu027	lung cancers	PKN3	I
Benitec/City of Hope	shRNA, decoy and ribozyme from lentiviral vector	pHIV7-shl-TAR-CCR5RZ	HIV lymphoma	HIV, CCR5	I
University of Duisburg Essen	unmodified siRNA	BCR–ABL siRNA	chronic myeloid leukemia	*bcr–abl*	single patient
Senetek	double-stranded RNA	ATN-RNA	glioblastoma multiforme	Tenascin-C	I
Gradalis	shRNA	FANG	advanced cancer	furin	I
Hadassah Medical Organization	siRNA in SV40 vector	SV40/BCR–ABL	chronic myeloid leukemia	*bcr–abl*	I
Duke University Hospital	unmodified siRNA	siRNA immunotherapy	metastatic melanoma	proteasome	I

In the meantime, RNAi has made the step from basic cancer research to clinical application. The first clinical RNAi cancer trial aimed at the treatment of patients with glioblastoma multiforme [15]. These brain tumors are currently almost untreatable and thus new forms of therapy are urgently needed. An RNAi treatment against Tenascin-C, which is strongly expressed in brain tumor tissue, succeeded in preventing the re-emergence of operatively removed glioblastoma in several patients [15]. In a second trial Calando Pharma employed a targeted nanoparticle to deliver an unmodified siRNA against the M2 subunit of the ribonucleotide reductase in a phase I study for the treatment of solid tumors. Analysis of the treated patients not only revealed successful tumor targeting with the nanoparticle, but a special rapid amplification of cDNA ends (RACE)-PCR approach also provided evidence for the first time that RNAi was induced in humans after systemic delivery of the siRNA [16]. Moreover, a highly modified siRNA against the expression of the protein kinase N3 formulated as a lipoplex (a complex of a nucleic acid and lipid bilayer structures used as a nonviral vehicle for delivery – the term lipoplex is generally used to differentiate from liposomes which embed the cargo) was developed for clinical testing by the company Silence Therapeutics. Another phase I trial was conducted at Duke University in which RNAi was employed to treat metastatic melanoma [9]. Monocytes of patients were treated *ex vivo* with siRNAs targeting inducible immunoproteasome subunits. After differentiation to dendritic cells, mRNAs encoding melanoma antigens were transfected into the cells. The siRNA knockdown of the proteasome enhances melanoma antigen presentation of the dendritic cells [17], thereby provoking a stronger immune response against the melanoma cells in these patients. A summary of completed and currently ongoing clinical trials based on RNAi to treat cancer is given in Table 44.1.

44.2 Plasmid Expression of Short Hairpin RNAs

Chemically synthesized siRNAs elicit transient silencing of the target gene only. In contrast to model organisms like *C. elegans*, the human genome does not encode an RNA-dependent RNA polymerase, which allows amplification of the silencing signal. Therefore, silencing vanishes after several days due to degradation of the siRNAs and, in rapidly dividing cells, by dilution of the effector through cell division. For example, siRNA-mediated silencing of phospholamban in cardiac myocytes resulted in a rapid decrease in mRNA levels, which reached a nadir by 12 h, but returned to the normal level after 4 days [18]. The time course of the silencing, however, is strongly dependent on factors such as the cell type, duration of cell division, and so on.

In order to overcome this restriction, several groups simultaneously came up with the idea to generate double-stranded RNAs continuously by intracellular expression (reviewed in [19, 20]). These expression systems not only extend the duration of RNAi-mediated gene silencing, they also open up opportunities for completely new application strategies. As outlined above, delivery is a major challenge for successful RNAi applications. The development of expression systems for double-stranded RNAs immediately suggested the use of viral vectors, which had already been applied in gene therapeutic settings for many years. The high efficiency of RNAi led to the justified hope that a combination of RNAi and gene therapy might bring new success to the field of molecular medicine [21]. Vector expression, furthermore, allows directed induction of RNAi, thereby increasing the safety and specificity of the approach.

In the most commonly used expression systems, the double-stranded RNA is generated as a small or short hairpin RNA (shRNA). The expression is controlled by an RNA polymerase III (Pol III) promoter (usually the U6 or H1 promoter). Type III RNA polymerases are optimized to generate large amounts of short RNA molecules without a cap or poly(A) tail. The transcribed shRNA consists of a sense strand, a loop, and a complementary antisense strand. After its export from the nucleus to the cytoplasm, the RNase Dicer cleaves the shRNA into an siRNA (Figure 44.1). As described above, the siRNA is then loaded into RISC. In this process, one of the two strands of the siRNA is discarded, while the other strand guides RISC to the target RNA, which is cleaved by the Ago2 protein.

Plasmids containing shRNA expression cassettes can easily be transfected into cells. The most widely used strategy for this purpose is the formation of lipoplexes consisting of cationic lipids and the nucleic acids to be delivered into cells. Alternatively, liposomes or other delivery agents such as polyethylenimine can be employed. Usually shRNAs expressed from plasmids work longer than chemically synthesized siRNAs. In addition, plasmid systems allow the selection of stably transfected cells, in which the target gene can be downregulated for several months. Brummelkamp *et al.* demonstrated that the expression of the tumor suppressor p53 was inhibited virtually to completion in stably transfected cells even after 2 months in culture [22].

RNAi is not only considered to be a new strategy to treat cancer, but is also being developed as a new antiviral approach. The main problem in long-term inhibition of viruses by means of RNAi is the emergence of resistant escape mutants that contain nucleotide substitutions in the siRNA target site. As a countermeasure, the combination of two or more shRNA expression cassettes in one plasmid has been suggested [23, 24]. We have recently developed a cloning strategy making use of compatible sticky ends generated from different restriction sites, which allows the easy combination of several shRNA expression cassettes [25]. Alternatively, long hairpin RNAs can be produced, which consist of multiple siRNAs [26]. Dicer will then cleave the extended shRNAs into effective siRNAs.

The concept of combining shRNAs has been successfully employed against viruses, but its potential for cancer therapy has not been widely recognized to date. As outlined above, RNAi can be directed against a number of cancer targets: proliferative or angiogenic factors, drug resistance genes, genes involved in metastasis, and so on. The anticancer effect of an RNAi approach can be expected to be enhanced by a combination of shRNAs targeting at least two cancer targets, such as a proliferative and an angiogenic factor. Tiemann *et al.* recently developed

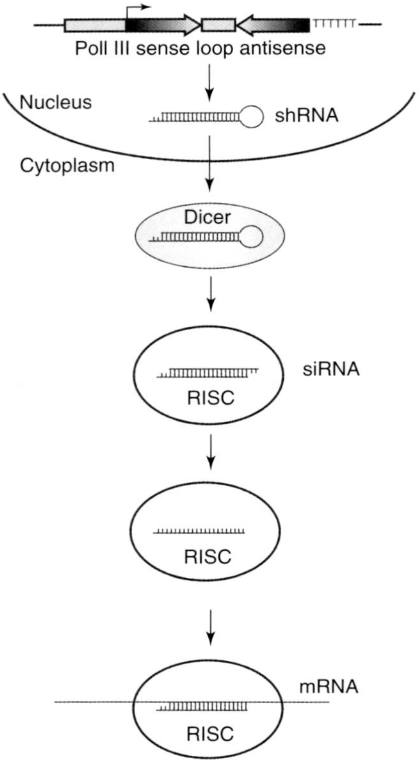

Figure 44.1 RNAi pathway of plasmid-derived shRNAs. In the most widely used systems, shRNAs are expressed under control of Pol III promoters. After being exported from the nucleus to the cytoplasm, the shRNA is processed by Dicer to give the mature siRNA, which is incorporated into RISC. After removal of the passenger strand, the remaining strand guides RISC to the target mRNA and induces its cleavage by the Ago2 protein.

dual-targeting siRNA, in which both strands are deliberately designed to separately target different mRNAs (e.g., Bcl-2 and Myc) [27]. The design of dual-targeting siRNAs and their delivery to tumor cells after systemic application, however, is demanding. The use of multiple shRNA expression systems can therefore be considered as an attractive alternative.

In the systems described so far, shRNAs are expressed under control of RNA Pol III promoters. A major disadvantage of this approach is that Pol III promoters induce ubiquitous expression of the encoded shRNA at very high, sometimes deleterious levels. Alternatively, shRNAs can be expressed under control of polymerase II (Pol II) promoters by simulating the expression of microRNAs (miRNAs; short double-stranded RNA molecules, usually 21–23 nucleotides long, that are endogenously expressed and act as natural post-transcriptional regulators of gene expression). To this end, the naturally occurring miRNA is replaced by an artificial

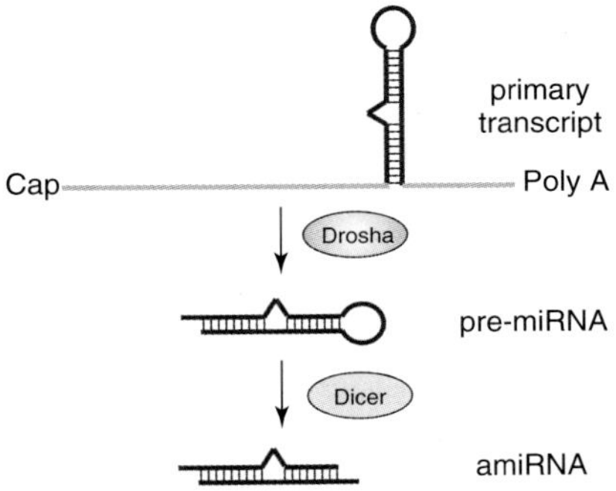

Figure 44.2 Artificial miRNAs. Artificial miRNAs are expressed as parts of long RNAs from Pol II promoters, which contain a cap at the 5′-end and a poly(A) tail at the 3′-end. In the nucleus, Drosha cleaves the pre-miRNA out of the primary transcript. The pre-miRNAs is exported to the cytoplasm and further processed into the mature amiRNA. (Modified from [20].)

shRNA in the sequence context of the miRNA. The resulting double-stranded RNA is referred to as a miRNA-type shRNA or artificial miRNA (amiRNA). Pol II first generates a long transcript, which is processed by Drosha to give the pre-miRNA (Figure 44.2). Similar to shRNAs, these pre-miRNAs are exported to the cytoplasm and processed by Dicer into the mature amiRNAs, which are incorporated into RISC [28].

The application of amiRNAs has several advantages as compared to the use of conventional shRNAs. First of all, they allow the expression of a protein-encoding sequence upstream of the miRNA. For example, reporters like Green Fluorescent Protein (GFP) can be used to follow transfection/transduction of target cells by the amiRNA expression construct. Alternatively, transgenes for therapeutic purposes can be expressed together with the amiRNA. Secondly, several amiRNAs can be expressed as a single transcript in a polycistronic manner [29]. This strategy can either be used to prevent viral escape or to silence more than one endogenously expressed gene as described above. Finally, the expression of amiRNAs under control of Pol II promoters allows the use of tissue-specific promoters, thereby potentially reducing undesired side-effects. In one of the first applications of this technology, an amiRNA against the transcription factor Wilm's tumor 1 was expressed under the control of the proximal promoter of the murine gene *Rhox5* [30]. This expression system restricted the RNAi effect to the nurse cells of the testis.

Tissue-specific promoters are normally weaker than the ubiquitous Pol III promoters. Since RNAi is a highly efficient process, the expression of amiRNAs from Pol II promoters is usually sufficient to elicit gene silencing without inducing strong side-effects. It was, for example, shown that expression of amiRNAs under control of a liver-specific Pol II promoter drastically reduced liver damage that was observed after U6-mediated shRNA expression, as will be discussed in more detail below [31].

To date no clear consensus has emerged with regard to whether vector-expressed shRNAs are immunostimulatory. Factors such as the hairpin length, sequence, and structure may all contribute to an induction of the interferon (IFN) response. It was, for example, shown that the presence of an AA dinucleotide near the transcription start site can induce an IFN response – an effect that can be avoided by preserving the wild-type U6 promoter sequence [32]. Furthermore, reduction of the hairpin length to 19 nucleotides was found to prevent the induction of the oligoadenylate synthase I – a classic IFN target gene [33]. Altogether, some studies encountered problems with the IFN response, while others did not. Currently, the rules for avoiding an IFN response remain to be completely defined (for more details on this topic, see [34]) and it is thus essential to confirm experimentally that shRNAs used for functional gene studies or therapy mediate RNAi-specific silencing rather than nonspecific effects. It should be noted, however, that experiences from the past have shown that highly specific tools are not always the most effective in cancer therapy. Sometimes unexpected "off-target effects" have proven to be most important for successful applications.

44.3 Conditional RNAi Systems

As in other therapies, the safe application of RNAi requires precise titration of gene product dosage, intermittent or pulsatile treatment, and defined termination in order to prevent side-effects [35]. Whereas this assessment seems at least in part less relevant to tumor cell treatment, where generally the maximal silencing of tumor genes is favored, it is an important aspect with respect to the nonspecific expression of an shRNA in normal cells. All currently available viral vectors used in cancer gene therapy transduce, in addition to the target tumor cells, healthy nontarget cells to a certain extent. In addition, conventional shRNA expression systems using constitutively active Pol III promoters result in permanent shRNA expression in both cancer and normal cells. This will become a problem in cases in which the silenced gene is essential for normal cell function. Moreover, it has been shown that very strong shRNA expression can induce severe side-effects due to saturation of the miRNA pathway [36]. The development of regulatable expression systems for tight control of shRNA expression will thus be of fundamental importance for therapeutic applications of RNAi in humans.

In principle, two types of conditional RNAi have been established. The first class comprises *irreversible* systems, namely the Cre–loxP [37] and the flippase recognition target (FRT)/flippase recombination enzyme (FLP) system [38]. They produce a permanent phenotype generated either by induction or repression of the shRNA expression. The second class comprises *reversible* systems. Here, the expression of the shRNA can be switched on and off, thereby producing a temporary, reversible knockdown phenotype. Tetracycline (Tet)-, LacR-, and ecdysone-based expression cassettes are the most important systems for reversible induction of RNAi [39–42].

44.3.1
Irreversible Conditional Systems

Among the irreversible systems, the Cre–loxP system was most extensively evaluated for conditional RNAi [43, 44]. In this system, inactivation of shRNA expression can be achieved either by separation of the distal site enhancer (DSE) and proximal site enhancer (PSE) elements of the Pol III promoter by a loxP flanked stuffer sequence [43] or by separation of sense and antisense strands of the shRNA by positioning DNA stuffer sequences between loxP sites into the shRNA loop structure [45]. In both cases, the reconstitution of a functional shRNA expression cassette occurs after elimination of the stuffer by Cre recombinase. Alternative systems for conditional repression of RNAi by using the Cre–loxP system have been developed as well [44]. Site-specific recombination approaches based on the Cre–loxP and FLP/FRT systems are popular for nonreversible induction of gene expression in the mouse genome to study gene functions [46], but their application for cancer gene therapy is rare [47]. A major disadvantage of these systems is that they can only be switched on once, while the reversible inducible systems allow repetitive on and off cycles. They therefore seem to better fulfill the major requirements of a therapeutic application (e.g., regulation of shRNA expression within the therapeutic window).

44.3.2
Reversible Systems

The reversible RNAi systems available to date are based on approaches developed in the last 20 years for the inducible expression of transgenes. In these systems, a drug-dependent transactivator and transrepressor protein, respectively, activates or suppresses transcription regulated by a response promoter. Reversible systems can be further divided into "On" and "Off" systems. For therapeutic applications, the "On" systems seem to be better suited as the expression of the transgene/shRNA is induced after application of the drug and can simply be switched off by withdrawal of the effector. The reverse situation in "Off" systems would make it necessary to add the drug permanently after finishing therapy to prevent shRNA expression.

The first and currently most widely used reversible gene expression system adapted for gene silencing is the Tet-inducible system [48]. It combines various desirable properties, including highly inducible expression levels, low background activity, fast onset kinetics after addition of the well defined, relatively nontoxic inducer drugs Tet and doxycycline (Dox) as well as rapid reversal of induction after their withdrawal [49]. Three different variants of the basic configuration of the Tet system were developed for the regulation of shRNA expression from Pol III promoters. They are characterized by epigenetic suppression, steric hindrance, and the use of new transactivators [50].

The epigenetic suppression is based on the inhibition of the H1, U6, or $tRNA^{val}$ promoter activity by a Tet-controlled transcriptional silencer (tTS) [51, 52] (Figure 44.3a), which is a fusion protein consisting of the Krüppel-associated box (KRAB) domain derived from the human *Kox1* gene and the Tet repressor (TetR).

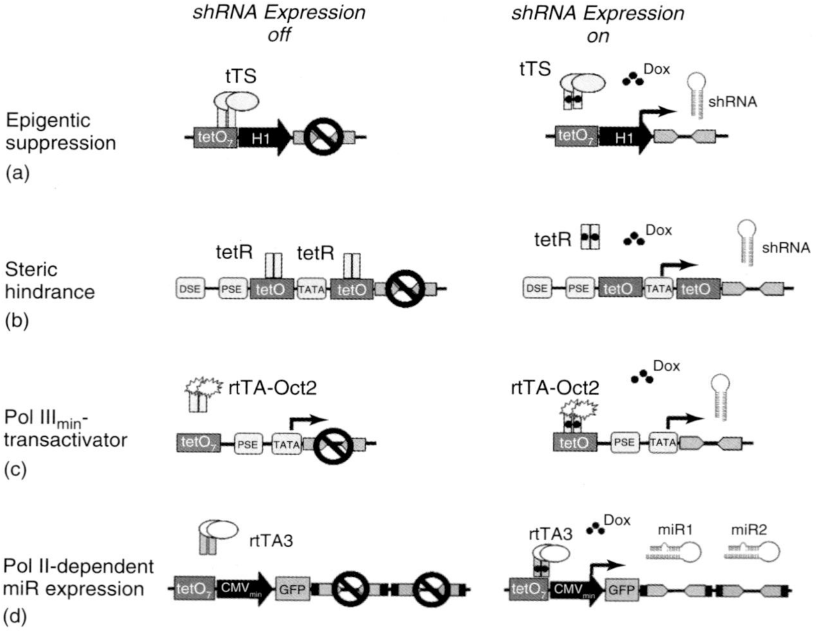

Figure 44.3 Tet-inducible systems. (a) Dox-dependent epigenetic suppression of Pol III promoter. The tTS binds to a $tetO_7$ sequence located upstream of the Pol III promoter in the absence of Dox, resulting in suppression of shRNA transcription. In the presence of Dox, tTS is released and generation of shRNA is switched on. (b) Dox-dependent steric hindrance of Pol III promoters. The tetR binds to a tetO in the absence of Dox. The tetOs are located between the PSE element and the TATA box and between the TATA box and the transcriptional start site (US/DS-type). Binding of tetR prevents expression of the shRNA. In the presence of Dox, the tetR no longer interacts with the tetO and the shRNA is expressed. (c) Pol III_{min} transactivator system. A reverse Tet-controlled transcriptional transactivator (rtTA-$Oct2^Q$) binds to a $tetO_7$ in the presence of Dox and transactivates a minimal Pol III promoter leading to shRNA transcription. In the absence of Dox, rtTA-$Oct2^Q$ is unable to bind to $tetO_7$ and the shRNA is not transcribed. (d) Inducible Pol II-dependent amiRNA expression. The rtTA3 binds to the $tetO_7$ in the presence of Dox and transactivates a minimal CMV (cytomegalovirus) promoter, leading to expression of both a GFP marker gene and amiRNAs from the same transcript. In the absence of Dox, the rtTA3 is unable to bind to the $tetO_7$ and expression of GFP and the amiRNAs is turned off. (Modified from [50].). rtTA-$Oct2^Q$ and rtTA3, reverse tetracycline-controlled transcriptional transactivator; tTS, tetracycline-controlled transcriptional silencer; TATA, TATA box; tetR, tetracycline repressor; H1, Pol III promoter H1; CMV_{min}, minimal CMV promoter; TetO, tet-operon; $tetO_7$, repeat of seven tetO.

Alternatively the KRAB domain can be fused to a mutated TetR DNA-binding domain (rtTR) that binds – other than tTS – to the Tet operator sequence (tetO) in the presence of Dox making it possible to switch off shRNA expression in the presence of Dox [52]. Szulc *et al.* furthermore directly compared the tTS-dependent Tet-On system and the rtTR-KRAB-dependent Tet-Off system using a single lentiviral vector. Both variants exhibited tight and efficient control of shRNA expression, and enabled time- and dose-dependent as well as reversible knockdown of marker gene expression *in vitro* [52].

Steric hindrance of shRNA expression by the Tet system is achieved by binding of TetR to a tetO that is located in the Pol III promoter. The system has a permanent "Off" status in the absence of the inducer drug, but becomes activated after addition of the inducer (Figure 44.3b). The three basic systems developed to date have insertions of one tetO sequence just upstream of the transcriptional start site (DS-type) or between the PSE and the TATA box (US-type), or represent a combination of both through insertion of one tetO sequence between the PSE and the TATA box and a second tetO sequence upstream of the transcriptional start site (US/DS-type) [39]. It is important to assure that the tetO sequences do not affect the position of the individual promoter elements relative to each other or with respect to the transcriptional start site, as the distance between essential elements, but not the intervening sequence itself, seems to be critical for their function. Several studies revealed significant drawbacks of steric hindrance-based Tet systems. The main bottlenecks are the relatively high leakiness of the uninduced state and a comparably low rate of induction [53, 54].

As the VP16 transactivator domain traditionally located in the Tet-regulated transactivators is incapable of inducing shRNA expression from Pol III promoters, a new Tet-regulatable transactivator was generated by replacing the three minimal VP16-derived activation domains located in the transactivator rtTA2-M2 [55] by Oct-2^{Q} (Q $\rightarrow$ A) domains [56]. Furthermore, all regulatory and response elements were inserted into one lentiviral vector genome (Figure 44.3c). This system silenced the target gene after administration of Dox by about 90%. The concentration of Dox required for full induction of shRNA expression, however, was approximately 10-fold higher than that needed in a similar Pol II promoter transactivator system. Since high concentrations of Dox may induce side-effects, this requirement for elevated Dox doses will significantly reduce the suitability of the system for *in vivo* applications.

Due to the difficulties in developing new Pol III promoter-dependent inducible RNAi system, several groups have developed Pol II promoter-dependent inducible shRNA expression systems. The basis for this approach was the generation of shRNAs as amiRNAs as described above, allowing their expression from Pol II promoters. Tests of the Dox-inducible Pol II promoter system in the context of Tet-On and Tet-Off systems revealed that it works well in various configurations [42, 57] (Figure 44.3d). Moreover, in these inducible systems a marker gene can be coexpressed with the amiRNA, which allows direct monitoring of the amiRNA expression status and all components of the Tet system can be inserted in one vector genome. Further details of systems for conditional RNAi are summarized in [58].

Tumor regression upon silencing of several procancerous genes has been demonstrated in various studies employing Tet-inducible shRNA expression [39, 52, 59]. In one study, an inducible RNAi vector containing a Tet-responsive derivative of the H1 promoter was employed for the conditional delivery of an shRNA directed against the human polo-like kinase-1 (Plk1) which is overexpressed in a broad spectrum of human tumors. Exposure of HeLa cells that stably expressed the TetR to Dox resulted in a strong repression of Plk1 mRNA and Plk1 protein expression to 3 and 14%, respectively, compared to the normal levels. Plk1 expression was unaffected in the absence of Dox. As a result of Plk1 depletion, cell proliferation strongly decreased. The *in vitro* results were confirmed *in vivo* in a xenotransplantation mouse model. After administration of Dox, Plk1 expression was downregulated and tumor growth was significantly inhibited [39]. In another approach, Hoeflich *et al.* developed an inducible shRNA xenograft model to examine the *in vivo* efficacy of inhibiting the oncogenic protein BRAF (a member of the RAF serine/threonine kinase family) by inducible shRNA delivery [59]. To this end, they used a lentiviral vector system for transfection of melanoma cells with a TetR regulator protein and H1-TetO Tet-inducible promoter driving the shRNA targeting BRAF. Subcutaneous application of the vector-transduced tumor cells resulted in a pronounced tumor growth. Following induction of anti-BRAF shRNA expression by application of Dox, the tumor volume distinctly decreased within 5 days and after 2 weeks the tumor volume had grossly regressed. Moreover, the system was inducible, reversible, and tightly regulated *in vivo*.

44.4
Viral Vectors for shRNA Delivery

The concept of using modified viruses as vectors for the delivery of genes with therapeutic purposes into humans has been investigated since the late 1980s, and more than 1500 clinical trials were carried out between 1990 and 2010. After a long period with many setbacks, some very promising results have been obtained in the last few years as reflected by a the title of a commentary in the *New England Journal of Medicine*: "Gene therapy fulfilling its promise" [60]. As vehicles for gene delivery, viral vectors are usually replication deficient (i.e., essential components are removed so that they cannot produce progeny virus and therefore cannot harm the patient or the environment). Exceptions, which will be discussed in detail below, are oncolytic viruses, which are designed to replicate specifically in tumor cells. Although many types of viruses have been used for gene delivery, three types of vectors currently dominate preclinical and clinical development: retrovirus vectors, adenovirus vectors, and adeno-associated virus (AAV) vectors. The basic principle of the generation of viral vectors is similar: a shuttle plasmid containing the shRNA expression cassette and some essential viral components and DNA encoding helper functions (such as capsid proteins and polymerases) are cotransfected into packaging cells to produce the viral vector. Details of the specific procedures for the production of the different types of vectors are outlined in Figure 44.4.

It has become clear that no single vector will be suitable for all indications. The choice of vector type depends on the targeted tissue and the specific therapeutic

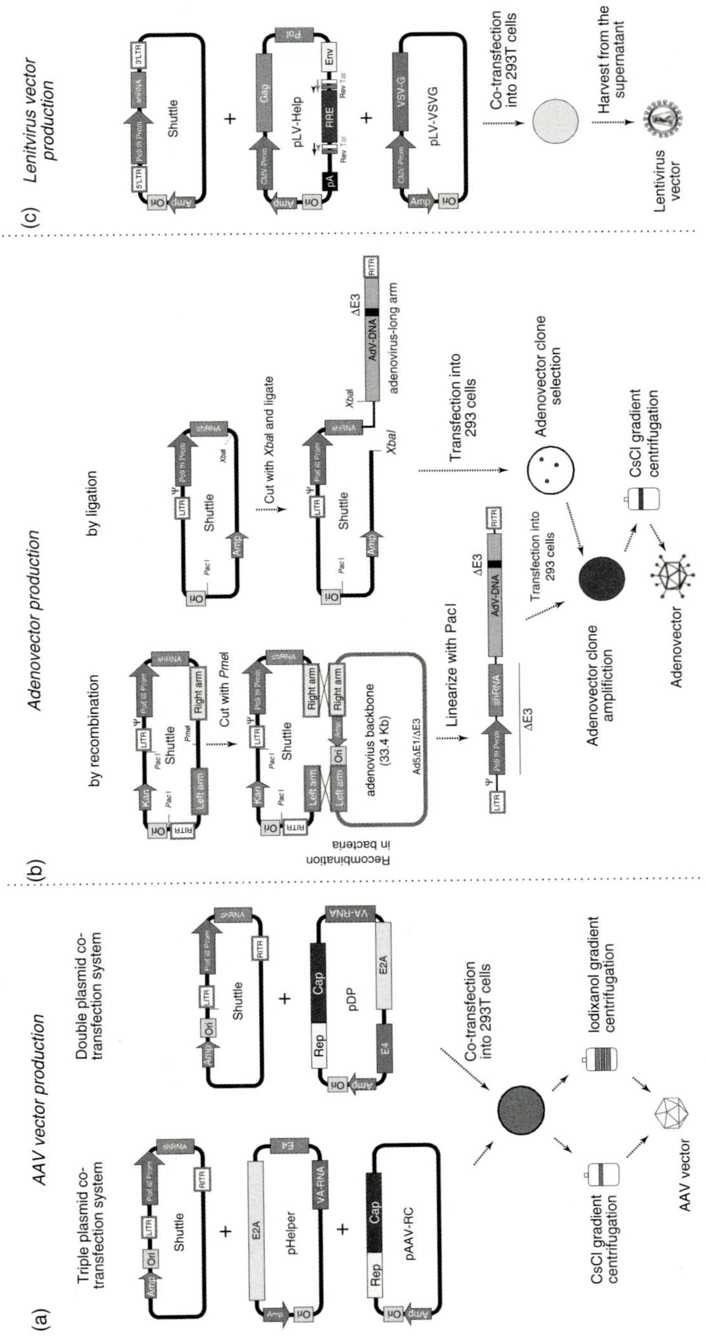
(a)
AAV vector production
Triple plasmid co-transfection system
Double plasmid co-transfection system
Shuttle
pHelper
pAAV-RC
pDP
Amp
Ori
LITR
Pol III Prom
shRNA
RITR
E2A
VA-RNA
E4
Rep
Cap
+
Co-transfection into 293T cells
CsCl gradient centrifugation
Iodixanol gradient centrifugation
AAV vector
(b)
Adenovector production
by recombination
by ligation
Kan
Pac I
PmeI
Left arm
Right arm
Cut with PmeI
Recombination in bacteria
adenovius backbone (33.4 Kb)
Ad5ΔE1/ΔE3
Linearize with PacI
ΔE3
AdV-DNA
Cut with XbaI and ligate
XbaI
adenovirus-long arm
Transfection into 293 cells
Adenovector clone selection
Adenovector clone amplifiction
Adenovector
(c)
Lenitvirus vector production
5'LTR
3'LTR
CMV Prom
Gag
Pol
RRE
Env
Rev
Tat
pA
VSV-G
pLV-Help
pLV-VSVG
Co-transfection into 293T cells
Harvest from the supernatant
Lentivirus vector

Figure 44.4 Production of viral vectors. (a) AAV vector production. Triple-plasmid cotransfection system: shRNA containing plasmid AAV shuttle, the plasmid pHelper containing adenoviral helper functions, and the plasmid pAAV-RC containing Rep and Cap genes from AAV are cotransfected into 293T cells. Recombinant AAVs are purified from cells and cell culture supernatant by CsCl or iodixanol gradient centrifugation. Double-plasmid cotransfection system: in contrast to the triple-plasmid cotransfection system, adenoviral helper functions and AAV Rep and Cap genes are expressed from one plasmid. (b) Adenoviral vector production. By recombination: the shRNA is cloned into an adenoviral shuttle plasmid that contains adenovirus sequences that are complementary to adenovirus sequences located in the left and right site of the adenovirus. The adenoviral shuttle plasmid is linearized with *PmeI* and cotransfected with a ΔE1/ΔE3 adenovirus backbone-carrying plasmid into bacteria. Recombinants are selected and transfected into 293A cells to produce recombinant adenoviral vectors. The vectors are purified from the lysed cell culture by CsCl gradient centrifugation. By ligation: the shRNA is cloned into an adenoviral shuttle plasmid containing a singular *XbaI* site. The shuttle plasmid is linearized with *XbaI*, ligated to *XbaI*-digested ΔE1/ΔE3 adenovirus mutant (*XbaI* site at nucleotide position 3333 of adenovirus 5), and transfected into 293 cells. Adenovirus clones are selected and further amplified in 293 cells. Purification of recombinant adenovirus is carried out as described above. (c) Lentiviral vector production. The shRNA-containing shuttle plasmid is cotransfected into 293 cells with two helper plasmids: LV helper that expresses LV genes and pLV-VSVG that expresses the G-protein of the vesicular stomatitis virus envelope gene. LV vectors can be harvested from the cell culture supernatant.

←

Table 44.2 Summary of the main properties of viral vectors.

	Retrovirus vector	Adenovirus vector	AAV vector
Transduction of proliferating cells	yes	yes	yes
Transduction of quiescent cells	no – onco-retrovirus; yes – lentivirus	yes	yes
Genomic integration	yes	no	no (or as a rare event)
Replication	no	no – adenovirus vector; yes – oAdVs	no
Potential risks	insertional mutagenesis	immune reaction, cytotoxicity	cytotoxicity

use. The most important properties of the different vector types are summarized in Table 44.2, while further details will be discussed in the following subsections.

44.4.1 Retroviral Vectors

Retroviral vectors were the first vehicles to deliver therapeutic genes into patients. A main characteristic of retroviruses is their integration into the host genome as a proviral DNA. Thus, retroviral vectors permanently express the transgene and are well suited to treat chronic diseases. The downside of this advantage is the risk of insertional mutagenesis.

The class of retroviruses can be divided into two subgroups: onco-retroviruses and lentiviruses (a genus of the retrovirus family, characterized by a long incubation period; letiviruses are able to replicate in nondividing cells and HIV belongs to the lentivirus genus). Onco-retroviruses cannot transduce quiescent cells and have therefore been employed primarily *ex vivo* for transduction of cells of the hematopoietic system. To this end, cells (e.g., hematopoietic stem cells) are obtained from the patient and transduced with the viral vector in tissue culture dishes. Cells that were successfully treated are then reinfused into the patient. A prominent example for this approach is the treatment of patients (mainly children) suffering from severe combined immunodeficiency disorder (SCID). Children suffering from X-chromosomal linked SCID were treated with onco-retroviruses delivering the correct version of the mutated γc IL receptor gene. Initial enthusiasm about the success of the treatment was stalled when several of the children developed leukemia as a consequence of the treatment [61]. Further analysis revealed that the retrovirus vector had integrated in the proximity of the LMO2 protooncogene promoter and led to strong expression of the gene. A second trial, in which 10 patients with SCID due to the lack of adenosine deaminase (ADA) were treated with a retroviral vector containing the *ADA* gene was more successful [62]: all patients were alive after a median follow-up of 4 years. Nine patients had immune reconstitution with increased T-cell counts and normalization of T-cell function and eight patients no longer required enzyme-replacement therapy. The differences in the outcome of the two studies are not fully understood, but they may be related to the time of immune recovery, which is markedly longer in the case of ADA-SCID.

These signs of success are accompanied by the development of safer designs of retroviral vectors and new vector types [60]. While in most studies to date the vectors were derived from murine γ-retroviruses, which tend to integrate close to the transcriptional control elements of cellular genes, newer vectors are being developed from lentiviruses. These vectors are not only safer, they also transduce quiescent as well as proliferating cells, thereby increasing the therapeutic range. Furthermore, self-inactivating vectors have been developed to eliminate the strong long terminal repeat enhancer. Instead of using viral promoters, the promoters of cellular genes are often used in modern vectors in order to reduce the risk of activating genes adjacent to the integration site. These and further measures will help to make retroviral delivery a safer approach in the near future.

Due to the high transduction efficiency of retroviral vectors, they are valuable tools for research purposes. Genome-wide libraries based on shRNA or amiRNA expression have been set up [63], and lentiviral vectors with shRNAs against any human or murine gene are commercially available. Furthermore, large-scale approaches can be used to identify new targets for cancer therapy. In one genome-wide screen an essential survival pathway in malignant glioma was elucidated [64]. More than 62 000 shRNAs directed against around 28 000 mouse genes were divided into pools and packaged into retrovirus particles. The vectors were used to stably

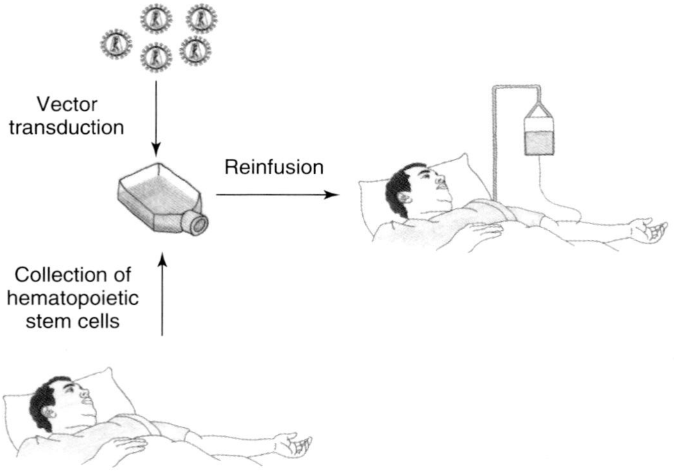

Figure 44.5 Scheme for the treatment of HIV patients using lentiviral vectors to transduce anti-HIV shRNA-encoding viral vectors into hematopoietic stem cells. After stimulation, the hematopoietic stem cells are collected from the patient. Subsequently, they are treated *ex vivo* with the lentiviral vector encoding the shRNA expression cassette. Finally, the protected cells are reinfused into the patient. (Modified from [66].)

transduce a malignant glioma cell line and identify transcriptional regulators of the activating transcription factor-5, which plays a key role in promoting cell survival.

In the first clinical RNAi trial based on a viral vector, a lentivirus vector was used to deliver an expression cassette encoding an shRNA, a decoy, and a ribozyme *ex vivo* into hematopoietic progenitor cells derived from AIDS patients [65, 66] (Figure 44.5). Transfected cells were successfully engrafted in all four infused patients and no severe toxicities were observed. Expression at low levels from the lentiviral vector was detected for up to 24 months.

Although methods for efficient *in vivo* delivery of shRNA expression cassettes by retroviral vectors remain to be developed, some studies have already employed this type of vector to knock down cancer-related genes. For example, the oncogenic K-ras^{V12} allele was specifically silenced by retrovirus vector-mediated RNAi [67]. The *RAS* genes are frequently mutated in human cancers, particularly in pancreatic and colon carcinoma. An shRNA that specifically inhibits the mutant K-ras^{V12} allele, while leaving the wild-type K-*ras* allele untouched, reduced anchorage-independent growth and tumorigenicity of human pancreatic carcinoma cells. The treatment also prevented tumor growth of subcutaneously injected tumor cells in athymic nude mice.

In a more recent *in vivo* study, a lentivirus vector encoding an expression cassette with an shRNA against VEGF-C was employed to transduce breast cancer cells in a murine xenograft model [68]. The RNAi treatment stably reduced VEGF-C mRNA and protein expression. In the xenograft model, the tumor volume was significantly smaller in the VEGF-C siRNA group than in the control group.

Furthermore, inhibition of lymphangiogenesis and suppression of lymph node metastasis were observed.

44.4.2 Adenoviral Vectors and Oncolytic Adenoviruses

Human adenoviruses cause acute respiratory infections, pharyngitis, and conjunctivitis, and have also been associated with gastroenteritis and pneumonia in young children as well as with myocarditis. More than 50 different serotypes of human adenoviruses have been identified to date [69]. The adenovirus is a nonenveloped, icosahedral virus of 60–90 nm in diameter with a linear, double-stranded DNA genome of about 36 kb. The adenoviral genome remains episomal in infected cells. Adenoviruses have been considered as suitable vectors for gene therapeutic applications for several reasons. First of all they have a low pathogenicity in humans and exploit a broad tissue tropism. Furthermore, they enable fast and strong transgene expression after entering the target cells. In contrast to onco-retroviruses, adenoviruses can transduce both quiescent and proliferating cells. Moreover, the adenovirus genome can easily be genetically modified. By deletion of adenoviral genes foreign DNA of up to 8 kb (first- and second-generation adenovectors) and more than 30 kb (third-generation "gutless" adenovectors), respectively, can be packed into a vector. The major drawback of adenovirus vectors results from the induction of a strong cytotoxic T-lymphocyte-mediated immune response. Triggering of the immune system leads to rapid clearance of vector-transduced cells and thus restricts transgene expression to a short duration of only a few weeks [70]. Gutless vectors, however, lacking all adenoviral genes have been shown to possess considerably reduced toxicity and immunogenicity *in vivo*. Long-term stability of more than 10 months *in vivo* has been reported [71].

Adenoviruses as therapeutic tools can be differentiated into two classes according to their ability to replicate: the first class comprises replication deficient adenoviral vectors, while the second class consists of adenoviruses that possess replication competence in tumor cells, but are unable to replicate in normal cells. The latter viruses are also known as oncolytic adenoviruses (oAdVs), or restricted or conditional replication-competent adenoviruses [72].

For the generation of replication-deficient adenoviral vectors, deletion of the E1A gene is a common feature. This gene is the first adenoviral gene expressed in the viral replication cycle and is therefore essential for virus replication. Replication-deficient adenoviral vectors can be employed as delivery vehicles for transgenes and have been used in roughly a quarter of all gene therapy trials that have been conducted to date (according to the Wiley database "Gene Therapy Clinical Trials Worldwide, *http://www.wiley.com/legacy/wileychi/genmed/clinical/*). Likewise, adenovirus vectors can be employed to deliver shRNA expression cassettes. The number of studies using adenoviral vectors for RNAi-mediated anticancer applications, however, is limited. In one example, intratumoral administration of an adenoviral vector with an shRNA against Skp2 efficiently inhibited growth of established subcutaneous tumors on NOD/SCID mice [73]. In a second, more recent example, an shRNA against the X-linked inhibitor of apoptosis protein (XIAP) was delivered into xenograft tumors by an adenoviral vector [74]. The RNAi treatment resulted in a retardation of tumor growth, which was associated with enhanced apoptosis.

For the majority of adenovirus-based anticancer applications, oAdVs have been employed, since their efficiency seems to be distinctly higher than that of replication-deficient adenovirus vectors [75]. The major reason for the higher efficiency is the improved tumor penetration of oAdVs, which results directly from replication and spreading of oAdV progeny from a primarily infected tumor cell to neighboring noninfected cells.

The application of oAdVs requires strict restriction of virus replication to tumor cells. This safety feature can be achieved in several ways. The first approach is to delete genes involved in deregulation of the cell cycle. For example, deletion of the gene encoding the E1B-55K protein [76] or the complete E1B gene [77] as well as of E1A binding sites to the retinoblastoma protein [78] have been shown to be suitable to abrogate virus replication in normal cells without affecting replication competence in cancer cells. A second way to restrict virus replication to tumor cells comprises the use of tumor cell-specific promoters to drive essential adenoviral genes (in most cases E1A) [79, 80]. A third strategy has been developed only recently. It is based on a miRNA-mediated blockade of oAdV replication, which is cell type specific. In these oAdVs multiple copies of target sequences with full complementary to a cellular miRNA are inserted into the 3′-untranslated region of the adenoviral E1A gene. Binding of the miRNA to its target site results in RNAi-mediated degradation of the E1A mRNA and inhibition of oAdV replication [81, 82]. For example, Cawood *et al.* inserted four copies of the target site of the liver specific miR-122 into the adenovirus genome and achieved a 50-fold reduction of hepatic adenovirus replication. The viro-oncolytic potency of the oAdV in cancer cells, however, was unaffected [82]. Transductional detargeting and retargeting is the fourth strategy to restrict oAdV replication to tumor cells. It can be achieved (i) by the use of heterologous targeting ligands that are bispecific in binding to the adenovirus fiber knob domain and a tumor-associated antigen; (ii) by incorporation of targeting ligands into capsid proteins; or (iii) by genetic incorporation of fiber/knob chimeras in which the adenovirus fiber knob is replaced by another adenovirus knob or in which the entire adenovirus fiber is replaced with an artificial fiber and knob structure [83].

In addition to these four main strategies, which aim to spatially restrict virus replication, drug-inducible oAdVs have been developed for temporal restriction of oAdVs [77, 84]. In these oAdVs the E1A gene was placed under control of a Dox- or rapamycin-inducible promoter. Although virus replication and tumor cell destruction were tightly regulated *in vitro* and *in vivo* the possible application of these oAdVs in cancer gene therapy suffers from the fact that cotransduction of one (rapamycin-regulated oAdV) or even two (Tet-regulated oAdV) additional oAdVs expressing a drug-inducible transactivator or a drug-inducible transactivator and silencer, respectively, was necessary. This disadvantage has been overcome in novel regulatable oAdVs either by use of improved components of the Tet-On gene expression system [85] or by employment of tamoxifen-regulated E1A chimeras [86], so that in these oAdVs all regulatory components of the inducible system are located in one vector genome.

In clinical trials, oAdVs have been shown to be safe. In most cases only mild, tolerable side-effects were observed. In terms of efficiency, up to 70% of cancer patients can profit from oAdV cancer therapy [87, 88]. Despite these encouraging clinical data, the efficiency of first-generation oAdVs as mono agents or in combination with chemo- and radiotherapy was unsatisfactorily. Therefore, several efforts are currently being undertaken to further increase oAdV efficiency. The most promising approach is the delivery of antitumor genes by oAdVs. The delivery of apoptotic, cell killing, tumor suppressor, and antiangiogenetic genes, as well as of death ligands and immunmodulators, to cancer cells has been shown to result in significant improvement of anticancer efficiency of oAdVs (for review, see [89]). The use of these so-called "armed" oAdVs has meanwhile become a standard procedure to increase oAdV efficacy in cancer gene therapy.

A rather new approach is the utilization of RNAi to improve the viro-oncolytic activity of oAdV. In one of the first studies in this respect, K-*ras* shRNAs were delivered by the oAdV ONYX-411. Daily intratumoral injections of the virus significantly improved blockade of growth of subcutaneous pancreatic cancer xenografts in nude mice by 85.5% compared to the parental ONYX-411 control and, moreover, led to complete suppression of tumor growth in three out of five mice [90]. Further studies have demonstrated that the delivery of shRNAs directed against VEGF [91], IL-8 [92], XIAP [93], Bcl-2 [94], or the human telomerase reverse transcriptase [95] can improve antitumor efficiency of oAdVs as well. Therefore, arming of oAdVs with shRNA expression cassettes against oncogenic factors is a promising strategy to enhance antitumor efficiency. It should be noted that similar approaches can be developed for other oncolytic viruses, such as the reovirus or herpes simplex virus.

44.4.3 Vectors Based on AAVs

AAVs are small nonenveloped viruses with a diameter of about 20 nm that contain a linear single-stranded DNA molecule with a genome size of about 4.8 kb. The genome encodes two genes (*rep* and *cap*) that are embedded between two inverted terminal repeats (ITRs; repetitive elements at the end of the virus genome), and encode four nonstructural (Rep) and three structural (VP) proteins [96]. AAVs are characterized by broad tissue tropism and are not currently known to cause any pathogenicity in humans.

AAV vectors contain only the ITRs of the virus at the 5′- and 3′-end, whereas the *rep* and *cap* gene sequences are deleted [97]. As a consequence, AAV vectors are replication deficient. Furthermore, removal of *rep* and *cap* genes enlarges the space for addition of foreign genes to about 4.4 kb. In general, shRNA expression cassettes are less than 1 kb in size, allowing insertion of four to five complete cassettes into one vector genome. Alternatively, the space for foreign genes allows coexpression of an shRNA and a transgene from the same vector genome simultaneously. This may be advantageous from the view of therapeutic efficiency if the shRNA and the transgene act additively or synergistically. Alternatively, coexpression of a reporter gene offers the possibility of monitoring AAV-mediated shRNA delivery into the target tissue [98].

Recombinant AAV vectors differ from their parental AAVs in that they do not integrate their DNA into the host genome [99]. The episomal state of the AAV vector reduces or eliminates the risk of insertional mutagenesis, which is one of the most important drawbacks of retrovirus vectors (see above). In addition, the small size of AAV vectors seems to be an important advantage regarding their use as vehicles to deliver shRNA expression cassettes into a tumor, as it is likely that small virus vectors can more easily pass the endothelial barrier of blood vessels and distribute throughout the tumor tissue than larger vectors derived, for example, from adeno- or retroviruses [7].

For many gene therapeutic applications, including cancer gene therapy, fast and strong shRNA expression is essential. Unfortunately, conventional AAV vectors need several days to reach maximal expression of their transgene *in vitro* and several weeks after application *in vivo*. Great progress has been made with the development of a new AAV vector type forming a double-stranded genome by incomplete replication. These self-complementary (sc) AAV vectors enabled strong transgene expression within 24 h *in vitro* and a few days *in vivo* [100]. It is important to note that the reduction of packaging capacity for foreign genes in scAAV vectors to about 2.2 kb does not affect the suitability of AAV vectors for insertion of shRNA expression cassettes due to their small size as mentioned above.

Until several years ago AAV vectors were exclusively generated from the AAV serotype 2. These vectors, however, suffer from a limited tissue specificity of transduction *in vivo* [101]. An extended analysis carried out by Gao *et al.* revealed the occurrence of more than 100 different AAV variants in humans and nonhuman primates [102]. Based on this knowledge, next-generation AAV vectors, so-called pseudotyped AAV vectors, were developed that helped to overcome the bottleneck of conventional AAV2 vectors. Pseudotyped vectors contain the transgene expression cassette flanked by the ITRs derived from the genome of serotype 2, while their genome is packaged into a capsid of another AAV serotype. AAV vectors with capsids from serotypes 1–10 are currently most commonly used in experimental research and clinical applications. As the capsid of a serotype determines the tissue tropism, pseudotyped AAV vectors can be used to deliver the vector DNA more specifically and with higher efficiency to a given target tissue. For example, AAV2/9 vectors can efficiently transduce the heart in mice, rats, and nonhuman primates [103, 104], whereas AAV2/8 vectors transduce the liver with high efficiency [105].

To date, no systematic analyses have been performed to determine the transduction efficiency of the serotypes for different tumor entities, but based on the currently available data preferences of specific serotypes for certain tumors can be assumed. Wu *et al.* showed that AAV2/5 vectors transduced A549 lung carcinoma cells much more efficiently than serotypes 1, 2, or 6–10 [106], and Harding *et al.*

reported that pseudotyped vectors with capsids from serotypes 6–8 had a higher efficiency of transduction of glioblastoma tumors in mice than AAV2 vectors [107].

The availability of different AAV serotypes has an additional advantage: patients treated with an AAV vector may have antibodies directed against the AAV serotype from a previous AAV infection or develop antibodies following the AAV vector administration. As a consequence, administration and readministration of the same serotype is likely to result in low transduction efficiency and transgene expression [108]. An easy way to overcome this limitation is to switch the AAV serotype by simply packaging the vector genome into the capsid of another serotype.

It should be noted that high doses of AAV vectors carrying an shRNA expression cassette can exert severe side-effects. In a highly recognized study, 49 different shRNA expressing AAV vectors were tested in mice, 36 of which caused liver damage, which in 23 cases was fatal [36]. Toxicity was due to oversaturation of components (Exportin-5 and RISC) of the endogenous miRNA pathway. In the same study, the authors demonstrated that no side-effects occur at a lower concentration of the vector, while protection from hepatitis B virus was achieved in an animal model for up to 1 year.

Several promising reports on the development of AAV vectors for the expression of antitumor shRNAs have already been published in the last few years. In one of the most recent studies, the suitability of AAV vector-mediated RNAi with shRNAs directed against the androgen receptor was investigated as a potential treatment of prostate cancer [109]. The antitumor efficiency was analyzed in a preclinical mouse xenograft tumor model and tumor growth was found to be significantly suppressed by intratumoral injection of the AAV vector. Most interestingly, systemic delivery of the vector eliminated xenografts within 10 days. Further analysis revealed that the anti-androgen receptor-shRNA reduced the expression of androgen receptor-regulated cellular survival genes and caused a strong apoptotic response. In another approach, Li *et al.* developed an AAV vector expressing an shRNA directed against angiogenin and investigated its potential for treatment of human lung cancer [110]. *In vitro* investigations showed distinct reduction of angiogenin protein expression in human lung squamous cancer cells 72 h after anti-angiogenin-shRNA treatment. More importantly, application of the vector in a lung cancer mouse model *in vivo* resulted in a remarkable reduction in the mass and volume of the tumors compared to the controls, which was furthermore accompanied by reduction of microvessel density, higher percentage of apoptotic cells, and lower proliferating cell nuclear antigen index. These data demonstrate that shRNA expressing AAV vectors can be considered valuable tools for cancer treatment.

44.5 Outlook

Without doubt, RNAi has revolutionized research in the field of life sciences within just a few years. The opportunity to specifically inhibit a gene with high efficiency offers new pathways for functional genomics studies. RNAi has therefore become a standard method in most molecular biology laboratories around the world. The success story of RNAi has also caught the attention of the pharmaceutical industry, and led to billion dollar deals between big pharma and biotech companies [111]. The translation of this research method into a clinically applicable approach has already begun, but faces numerous challenges. One of the major hurdles is efficient delivery of the short double-stranded RNA molecules into the target cells. Experience in the field of gene therapy offers strategies to begin to overcome these problems. Due to the many setbacks with gene therapeutic approaches, however, there is a pronounced skepticism toward the use of viral vectors in many pharmaceutical companies. It will therefore be necessary to show that combining new viral vectors with improved safety features and the highly efficient RNAi methodology will have the potential to become a valuable new therapeutic options for the treatment of cancer and other severe diseases, for which not satisfactory cure exists to date.

Acknowledgments

The authors wish to thank Erik Wade for careful proofreading and valuable comments, and Rebecca Troll for help with Figure 44.5.

References

1. Kurreck, J. (2003) Antisense technologies. Improvement through novel chemical modifications. *Eur. J. Biochem.*, **270**, 1628–1644.
2. Crooke, S.T. (2004) Progress in antisense technology. *Annu. Rev. Med.*, **55**, 61–95.
3. Zamecnik, P.C. and Stephenson, M.L. (1978) Inhibition of Rous sarcoma virus replication and cell transformation by a specific oligodeoxynucleotide. *Proc. Natl. Acad. Sci. USA*, **75**, 280–284.
4. Kruger, K., Grabowski, P.J., Zaug, A.J., Sands, J., Gottschling, D.E., and Cech, T.R. (1982) Self-splicing RNA: autoexcision and autocyclization of the ribosomal RNA intervening sequence of *Tetrahymena*. *Cell*, **31**, 147–157.
5. Schubert, S. and Kurreck, J. (2004) Ribozyme- and deoxyribozyme-strategies for medical applications. *Curr. Drug Targets*, **5**, 667–681.
6. Fire, A., Xu, S., Montgomery, M.K., Kostas, S.A., Driver, S.E., and Mello, C.C. (1998) Potent and specific genetic interference by double-stranded RNA in *Caenorhabditis elegans*. *Nature*, **391**, 806–811.
7. Grimm, D. (2009) Small silencing RNAs: state-of-the-art. *Adv. Drug Deliv. Rev.*, **61**, 672–703.
8. Kurreck, J. (2009) RNA interference: from basic research to therapeutic applications. *Angew. Chem. Int. Ed. Engl.*, **48**, 1378–1398.
9. Tiemann, K. and Rossi, J.J. (2009) RNAi-based therapeutics – current status, challenges and prospects. *EMBO Mol. Med.*, **1**, 142–151.
10. Phalon, C., Rao, D.D., and Nemunaitis, J. (2010) Potential use of RNA interference in cancer therapy. *Expert Rev. Mol. Med.*, **12**, e26.
11. Pai, S.I., Lin, Y.Y., Macaes, B., Meneshian, A., Hung, C.F., and Wu, T.C. (2006) Prospects of RNA interference therapy for cancer. *Gene Ther.*, **13**, 464–477.
12. Warnecke, C., Zaborowska, Z., Kurreck, J., Erdmann, V.A., Frei, U.,

Wiesener, M., and Eckardt, K.U. (2004) Differentiating the functional role of hypoxia-inducible factor (HIF)-1alpha and HIF-2alpha (EPAS-1) by the use of RNA interference: erythropoietin is a HIF-2alpha target gene in Hep3B and Kelly cells. *FASEB J.*, **18**, 1462–1464.

13. Czauderna, F., Santel, A., Hinz, M., Fechtner, M., Durieux, B., Fisch, G., Leenders, F., Arnold, W., Giese, K., Klippel, A. *et al.* (2003) Inducible shRNA expression for application in a prostate cancer mouse model. *Nucleic Acids Res.*, **31**, e127.
14. Wu, H., Hait, W.N., and Yang, J.M. (2003) Small interfering RNA-induced suppression of MDR1 (P-glycoprotein) restores sensitivity to multidrug-resistant cancer cells. *Cancer Res.*, **63**, 1515–1519.
15. Zukiel, R., Nowak, S., Wyszko, E., Rolle, K., Gawronska, I., Barciszewska, M.Z., and Barciszewski, J. (2006) Suppression of human brain tumor with interference RNA specific for tenascin-C. *Cancer Biol. Ther.*, **5**, 1002–1007.
16. Davis, M.E., Zuckerman, J.E., Choi, C.H., Seligson, D., Tolcher, A., Alabi, C.A., Yen, Y., Heidel, J.D., and Ribas, A. (2010) Evidence of RNAi in humans from systemically administered siRNA via targeted nanoparticles. *Nature*, **464**, 1067–1070.
17. Dannull, J., Lesher, D.T., Holzknecht, R., Qi, W., Hanna, G., Seigler, H., Tyler, D.S., and Pruitt, S.K. (2007) Immunoproteasome down-modulation enhances the ability of dendritic cells to stimulate antitumor immunity. *Blood*, **110**, 4341–4350.
18. Watanabe, A., Arai, M., Yamazaki, M., Koitabashi, N., Wuytack, F., and Kurabayashi, M. (2004) Phospholamban ablation by RNA interference increases Ca2+ uptake into rat cardiac myocyte sarcoplasmic reticulum. *J. Mol. Cell. Cardiol.*, **37**, 691–698.
19. Shi, Y. (2003) Mammalian RNAi for the masses. *Trends Genet.*, **19**, 9–12.
20. Fechner, H. and Kurreck, J. (2008) Vector-mediated and viral delivery of short hairpin RNAs in *Therapeutic Oligonucleotides* (ed. J. Kurreck), Royal Society of Chemistry, Cambridge, pp. 267–295.
21. Grimm, D. and Kay, M.A. (2007) RNAi and gene therapy: a mutual attraction. *Hematol. Am. Soc. Hematol. Educ. Program.*, **2007**, 473–481.
22. Brummelkamp, T.R., Bernards, R., and Agami, R. (2002) A system for stable expression of short interfering RNAs in mammalian cells. *Science*, **296**, 550–553.
23. Schubert, S., Grunert, H.P., Zeichhardt, H., Werk, D., Erdmann, V.A., and Kurreck, J. (2005) Maintaining inhibition: siRNA double expression vectors against coxsackieviral RNAs. *J. Mol. Biol.*, **346**, 457–465.
24. ter Brake, O., Konstantinova, P., Ceylan, M., and Berkhout, B. (2006) Silencing of HIV-1 with RNA interference: a multiple shRNA approach. *Mol. Ther.*, **14**, 883–892.
25. Rothe, D., Wajant, G., Grunert, H.P., Zeichhardt, H., Fechner, H., and Kurreck, J. (2010) Rapid construction of adeno-associated virus vectors expressing multiple short hairpin RNAs with high antiviral activity against echovirus 30. *Oligonucleotides*, **20**, 191–198.
26. Liu, Y.P., von Eije, K.J., Schopman, N.C., Westerink, J.T., ter Brake, O., Haasnoot, J., and Berkhout, B. (2009) Combinatorial RNAi against HIV-1 using extended short hairpin RNAs. *Mol. Ther.*, **17**, 1712–1723.
27. Tiemann, K., Hohn, B., Ehsani, A., Forman, S.J., Rossi, J.J., and Saetrom, P. (2010) Dual-targeting siRNAs. *RNA*, **16**, 1275–1284.
28. Zeng, Y., Wagner, E.J., and Cullen, B.R. (2002) Both natural and designed micro RNAs can inhibit the expression of cognate mRNAs when expressed in human cells. *Mol. Cell.*, **9**, 1327–1333.
29. Chung, K.H., Hart, C.C., Al-Bassam, S., Avery, A., Taylor, J., Patel, P.D., Vojtek, A.B., and Turner, D.L. (2006) Polycistronic RNA polymerase II expression vectors for RNA interference based on BIC/miR-155. *Nucleic Acids Res.*, **34**, e53.
30. Rao, M.K. and Wilkinson, M.F. (2006) Tissue-specific and cell type-specific

RNA interference *in vivo*. *Nat. Protoc.*, **1**, 1494–1501.

31. Giering, J.C., Grimm, D., Storm, T.A., and Kay, M.A. (2008) Expression of shRNA from a tissue-specific pol II promoter is an effective and safe RNAi therapeutic. *Mol. Ther.*, **16**, 1630–1636.
32. Pebernard, S. and Iggo, R.D. (2004) Determinants of interferon-stimulated gene induction by RNAi vectors. *Differentiation*, **72**, 103–111.
33. Fish, R.J. and Kruithof, E.K. (2004) Short-term cytotoxic effects and long-term instability of RNAi delivered using lentiviral vectors. *BMC Mol. Biol.*, **5**, 9.
34. Couto, L.B. and High, K.A. (2010) Viral vector-mediated RNA interference. *Curr. Opin. Pharmacol.*, **10**, 534–542.
35. Rivera, V.M., Clackson, T., Natesan, S., Pollock, R., Amara, J.F., Keenan, T., Magari, S.R., Phillips, T., Courage, N.L., Cerasoli, F. Jr. *et al.* (1996) A humanized system for pharmacologic control of gene expression. *Nat. Med.*, **2**, 1028–1032.
36. Grimm, D., Streetz, K.L., Jopling, C.L., Storm, T.A., Pandey, K., Davis, C.R., Marion, P., Salazar, F., and Kay, M.A. (2006) Fatality in mice due to oversaturation of cellular microRNA/short hairpin RNA pathways. *Nature*, **441**, 537–541.
37. Sternberg, N. and Hamilton, D. (1981) Bacteriophage P1 site-specific recombination. I. Recombination between loxP sites. *J. Mol. Biol.*, **150**, 467–486.
38. Voutev, R. and Hubbard, E.J. (2008) A "FLP-Out" system for controlled gene expression in *Caenorhabditis elegans*. *Genetics*, **180**, 103–119.
39. Kappel, S., Matthess, Y., Zimmer, B., Kaufmann, M., and Strebhardt, K. (2006) Tumor inhibition by genomically integrated inducible RNAi-cassettes. *Nucleic Acids Res.*, **34**, 4527–4536.
40. Wu, R.H., Cheng, T.L., Lo, S.R., Hsu, H.C., Hung, C.F., Teng, C.F., Wu, M.P., Tsai, W.H., and Chang, W.T. (2007) A tightly regulated and reversibly inducible siRNA expression system for conditional RNAi-mediated gene silencing in mammalian cells. *J. Gene Med.*, **9**, 620–634.
41. Gupta, S., Schoer, R.A., Egan, J.E., Hannon, G.J., and Mittal, V. (2004) Inducible, reversible, and stable RNA interference in mammalian cells. *Proc. Natl. Acad. Sci. USA*, **101**, 1927–1932.
42. Wiederschain, D., Wee, S., Chen, L., Loo, A., Yang, G., Huang, A., Chen, Y., Caponigro, G., Yao, Y.M., Lengauer, C. *et al.* (2009) Single-vector inducible lentiviral RNAi system for oncology target validation. *Cell Cycle*, **8**, 498–504.
43. Coumoul, X., Li, W., Wang, R.H., and Deng, C. (2004) Inducible suppression of Fgfr2 and Survivin in ES cells using a combination of the RNA interference (RNAi) and the Cre–loxP system. *Nucleic Acids Res.*, **32**, e85.
44. Ventura, A., Meissner, A., Dillon, C.P., McManus, M., Sharp, P.A., Van Parijs, L., Jaenisch, R., and Jacks, T. (2004) Cre–lox-regulated conditional RNA interference from transgenes. *Proc. Natl. Acad. Sci. USA*, **101**, 10380–10385.
45. Fritsch, L., Martinez, L.A., Sekhri, R., Naguibneva, I., Gerard, M., Vandromme, M., Schaeffer, L., and Harel-Bellan, A. (2004) Conditional gene knock-down by CRE-dependent short interfering RNAs. *EMBO Rep.*, **5**, 178–182.
46. Feil, R. (2007) Conditional somatic mutagenesis in the mouse using site-specific recombinases. *Handb. Exp. Pharmacol.*, **178**, 3–28.
47. Ghatak, S., Hascall, V.C., Berger, F.G., Penas, M.M., Davis, C., Jabari, E., He, X., Norris, J.S., Dang, Y., Markwald, R.R. *et al.* (2008) Tissue-specific shRNA delivery: a novel approach for gene therapy in cancer. *Connect. Tissue Res.*, **49**, 265–269.
48. van de Wetering, M., Oving, I., Muncan, V., Pon Fong, M.T., Brantjes, H., van Leenen, D., Holstege, F.C., Brummelkamp, T.R., Agami, R., and Clevers, H. (2003) Specific inhibition of gene expression using a stably integrated, inducible small-interfering-RNA vector. *EMBO Rep.*, **4**, 609–615.
49. Toniatti, C., Bujard, H., Cortese, R., and Ciliberto, G. (2004) Gene therapy

progress and prospects: transcription regulatory systems. *Gene Ther.*, **11**, 649–657.

50. Poller, W. and Fechner, H. (2010) Development of novel cardiovascular therapeutics from small regulatory RNA molecules – an outline of key requirements. *Curr. Pharm. Des.*, **16**, 2252–2268.

51. Wiznerowicz, M. and Trono, D. (2003) Conditional suppression of cellular genes: lentivirus vector-mediated drug-inducible RNA interference. *J. Virol.*, **77**, 8957–8961.

52. Szulc, J., Wiznerowicz, M., Sauvain, M.O., Trono, D., and Aebischer, P. (2006) A versatile tool for conditional gene expression and knockdown. *Nat. Methods*, **3**, 109–116.

53. Lin, X., Yang, J., Chen, J., Gunasekera, A., Fesik, S.W., and Shen, Y. (2004) Development of a tightly regulated U6 promoter for shRNA expression. *FEBS Lett.*, **577**, 376–380.

54. Matthess, Y., Kappel, S., Spankuch, B., Zimmer, B., Kaufmann, M., and Strebhardt, K. (2005) Conditional inhibition of cancer cell proliferation by tetracycline-responsive, H1 promoter-driven silencing of PLK1. *Oncogene*, **24**, 2973–2980.

55. Urlinger, S., Baron, U., Thellmann, M., Hasan, M.T., Bujard, H., and Hillen, W. (2000) Exploring the sequence space for tetracycline-dependent transcriptional activators: novel mutations yield expanded range and sensitivity. *Proc. Natl. Acad. Sci. USA*, **97**, 7963–7968.

56. Amar, L., Desclaux, M., Faucon-Biguet, N., Mallet, J., and Vogel, R. (2006) Control of small inhibitory RNA levels and RNA interference by doxycycline induced activation of a minimal RNA polymerase III promoter. *Nucleic Acids Res.*, **34**, e37.

57. Shin, K.J., Wall, E.A., Zavzavadjian, J.R., Santat, L.A., Liu, J., Hwang, J.I., Rebres, R., Roach, T., Seaman, W., Simon, M.I. *et al.* (2006) A single lentiviral vector platform for microRNA-based conditional RNA interference and coordinated transgene expression. *Proc. Natl. Acad. Sci. USA*, **103**, 13759–13764.

58. Lee, S.K. and Kumar, P. (2009) Conditional RNAi: towards a silent gene therapy. *Adv. Drug Deliv. Rev.*, **61**, 650–664.

59. Hoeflich, K.P., Gray, D.C., Eby, M.T., Tien, J.Y., Wong, L., Bower, J., Gogineni, A., Zha, J., Cole, M.J., Stern, H.M. *et al.* (2006) Oncogenic BRAF is required for tumor growth and maintenance in melanoma models. *Cancer Res.*, **66**, 999–1006.

60. Kohn, D.B. and Candotti, F. (2009) Gene therapy fulfilling its promise. *N. Engl. J. Med.*, **360**, 518–521.

61. Hacein-Bey-Abina, S., Von Kalle, C., Schmidt, M., McCormack, M.P., Wulffraat, N., Leboulch, P., Lim, A., Osborne, C.S., Pawliuk, R., Morillon, E. *et al.* (2003) LMO2-associated clonal T cell proliferation in two patients after gene therapy for SCID-X1. *Science*, **302**, 415–419.

62. Aiuti, A., Cattaneo, F., Galimberti, S., Benninghoff, U., Cassani, B., Callegaro, L., Scaramuzza, S., Andolfi, G., Mirolo, M., Brigida, I. *et al.* (2009) Gene therapy for immunodeficiency due to adenosine deaminase deficiency. *N. Engl. J. Med.*, **360**, 447–458.

63. Moffat, J. and Sabatini, D.M. (2006) Building mammalian signalling pathways with RNAi screens. *Nat. Rev. Mol. Cell Biol.*, **7**, 177–187.

64. Sheng, Z., Li, L., Zhu, L.J., Smith, T.W., Demers, A., Ross, A.H., Moser, R.P., and Green, M.R. (2010) A genome-wide RNA interference screen reveals an essential CREB3L2–ATF5–MCL1 survival pathway in malignant glioma with therapeutic implications. *Nat. Med.*, **16**, 671–677.

65. DiGiusto, D.L., Krishnan, A., Li, L., Li, H., Li, S., Rao, A., Mi, S., Yam, P., Stinson, S., Kalos, M. *et al.* (2010) RNA-based gene therapy for HIV with lentiviral vector-modified $CD34^+$ cells in patients undergoing transplantation for AIDS-related lymphoma. *Sci. Transl. Med.*, **2**, 36ra43.

66. Hannon, G.J. and Rossi, J.J. (2004) Unlocking the potential of the human

genome with RNA interference. *Nature*, **431**, 371–378.
67. Brummelkamp, T.R., Bernards, R., and Agami, R. (2002) Stable suppression of tumorigenicity by virus-mediated RNA interference. *Cancer Cell*, **2**, 243–247.
68. Guo, B., Zhang, Y., Luo, G., Li, L., and Zhang, J. (2009) Lentivirus-mediated small interfering RNA targeting VEGF-C inhibited tumor lymphangiogenesis and growth in breast carcinoma. *Anat. Rec.*, **292**, 633–639.
69. Russell, W.C. (2009) Adenoviruses: update on structure and function. *J. Gen. Virol.*, **90**, 1–20.
70. Yang, Y., Li, Q., Ertl, H.C., and Wilson, J.M. (1995) Cellular and humoral immune responses to viral antigens create barriers to lung-directed gene therapy with recombinant adenoviruses. *J. Virol.*, **69**, 2004–2015.
71. Morral, N., O'Neal, W., Rice, K., Leland, M., Kaplan, J., Piedra, P.A., Zhou, H., Parks, R.J., Velji, R., Aguilar-Cordova, E. *et al.* (1999) Administration of helper-dependent adenoviral vectors and sequential delivery of different vector serotype for long-term liver-directed gene transfer in baboons. *Proc. Natl. Acad. Sci. USA*, **96**, 12816–12821.
72. Bauerschmitz, G.J., Barker, S.D., and Hemminki, A. (2002) Adenoviral gene therapy for cancer: from vectors to targeted and replication competent agents. *Int. J. Oncol.*, **21**, 1161–1174.
73. Sumimoto, H., Yamagata, S., Shimizu, A., Miyoshi, H., Mizuguchi, H., Hayakawa, T., Miyagishi, M., Taira, K., and Kawakami, Y. (2005) Gene therapy for human small-cell lung carcinoma by inactivation of Skp-2 with virally mediated RNA interference. *Gene Ther.*, **12**, 95–100.
74. Dai, Y., Qiao, L., Chan, K.W., Yang, M., Ye, J., Zhang, R., Ma, J., Zou, B., Lam, C.S., Wang, J. *et al.* (2009) Adenovirus-mediated down-regulation of X-linked inhibitor of apoptosis protein inhibits colon cancer. *Mol. Cancer Ther.*, **8**, 2762–2770.
75. Suzuki, K., Fueyo, J., Krasnykh, V., Reynolds, P.N., Curiel, D.T., and Alemany, R. (2001) A conditionally replicative adenovirus with enhanced infectivity shows improved oncolytic potency. *Clin. Cancer Res.*, **7**, 120–126.
76. Heise, C., Sampson-Johannes, A., Williams, A., McCormick, F., Von Hoff, D.D., and Kirn, D.H. (1997) ONYX-015, an E1B gene-attenuated adenovirus, causes tumor-specific cytolysis and antitumoral efficacy that can be augmented by standard chemotherapeutic agents. *Nat. Med.*, **3**, 639–645.
77. Fechner, H., Wang, X., Srour, M., Siemetzki, U., Seltmann, H., Sutter, A.P., Scherubl, H., Zouboulis, C.C., Schwaab, R., Hillen, W. *et al.* (2003) A novel tetracycline-controlled transactivator–transrepressor system enables external control of oncolytic adenovirus replication. *Gene Ther.*, **10**, 1680–1690.
78. Heise, C., Hermiston, T., Johnson, L., Brooks, G., Sampson-Johannes, A., Williams, A., Hawkins, L., and Kirn, D. (2000) An adenovirus E1A mutant that demonstrates potent and selective systemic anti-tumoral efficacy. *Nat. Med.*, **6**, 1134–1139.
79. Huang, Q., Zhang, X., Wang, H., Yan, B., Kirkpatrick, J., Dewhrist, M.W., and Li, C.Y. (2004) A novel conditionally replicative adenovirus vector targeting telomerase-positive tumor cells. *Clin. Cancer Res.*, **10**, 1439–1445.
80. Nettelbeck, D.M., Rivera, A.A., Balague, C., Alemany, R., and Curiel, D.T. (2002) Novel oncolytic adenoviruses targeted to melanoma: specific viral replication and cytolysis by expression of E1A mutants from the tyrosinase enhancer/promoter. *Cancer Res.*, **62**, 4663–4670.
81. Ylosmaki, E., Hakkarainen, T., Hemminki, A., Visakorpi, T., Andino, R., and Saksela, K. (2008) Generation of a conditionally replicating adenovirus based on targeted destruction of E1A mRNA by a cell type-specific MicroRNA. *J. Virol.*, **82**, 11009–11015.
82. Cawood, R., Chen, H.H., Carroll, F., Bazan-Peregrino, M., van Rooijen, N., and Seymour, L.W. (2009) Use of tissue-specific microRNA to control

pathology of wild-type adenovirus without attenuation of its ability to kill cancer cells. *PLoS Pathog.*, **5**, e1000440.

83. Mathis, J.M., Stoff-Khalili, M.A., and Curiel, D.T. (2005) Oncolytic adenoviruses – selective retargeting to tumor cells. *Oncogene*, **24**, 7775–7791.
84. Chong, H., Ruchatz, A., Clackson, T., Rivera, V.M., and Vile, R.G. (2002) A system for small-molecule control of conditionally replication-competent adenoviral vectors. *Mol. Ther.*, **5**, 195–203.
85. Fechner, H., Wang, X., Pico, A.H., Wildner, J., Suckau, L., Pinkert, S., Sipo, I., Weger, S., and Poller, W. (2007) A bidirectional Tet-dependent promotor construct regulating the expression of E1A for tight control of oncolytic adenovirus replication. *J. Biotechnol.*, **127**, 560–574.
86. Sipo, I., Wang, X., Hurtado Pico, A., Suckau, L., Weger, S., Poller, W., and Fechner, H. (2006) Tamoxifen-regulated adenoviral E1A chimeras for the control of tumor selective oncolytic adenovirus replication *in vitro* and *in vivo*. *Gene Ther.*, **13**, 173–186.
87. Nemunaitis, J., Cunningham, C., Buchanan, A., Blackburn, A., Edelman, G., Maples, P., Netto, G., Tong, A., Randlev, B., Olson, S. *et al.* (2001) Intravenous infusion of a replication-selective adenovirus (ONYX-015) in cancer patients: safety, feasibility and biological activity. *Gene Ther.*, **8**, 746–759.
88. Pesonen, S., Helin, H., Nokisalmi, P., Escutenaire, S., Ribacka, C., Sarkioja, M., Cerullo, V., Guse, K., Bauerschmitz, G., Laasonen, L. *et al.* (2010) Oncolytic adenovirus treatment of a patient with refractory neuroblastoma. *Acta Oncol.*, **49**, 117–119.
89. Cody, J.J. and Douglas, J.T. (2009) Armed replicating adenoviruses for cancer virotherapy. *Cancer Gene Ther.*, **16**, 473–488.
90. Zhang, Y.A., Nemunaitis, J., Samuel, S.K., Chen, P., Shen, Y., and Tong, A.W. (2006) Antitumor activity of an oncolytic adenovirus-delivered oncogene small interfering RNA. *Cancer Res.*, **66**, 9736–9743.
91. Yoo, J.Y., Kim, J.H., Kwon, Y.G., Kim, E.C., Kim, N.K., Choi, H.J., and Yun, C.O. (2007) VEGF-specific short hairpin RNA-expressing oncolytic adenovirus elicits potent inhibition of angiogenesis and tumor growth. *Mol. Ther.*, **15**, 295–302.
92. Yoo, J.Y., Kim, J.H., Kim, J., Huang, J.H., Zhang, S.N., Kang, Y.A., Kim, H., and Yun, C.O. (2008) Short hairpin RNA-expressing oncolytic adenovirus-mediated inhibition of IL-8: effects on antiangiogenesis and tumor growth inhibition. *Gene Ther.*, **15**, 635–651.
93. Pan, Q., Liu, B., Liu, J., Cai, R., Liu, X., and Qian, C. (2008) Synergistic antitumor activity of XIAP-shRNA and TRAIL expressed by oncolytic adenoviruses in experimental HCC. *Acta Oncol.*, **47**, 135–144.
94. Zhang, H., Wang, H., Zhang, J., Qian, G., Niu, B., Fan, X., Lu, J., Hoffman, A.R., Hu, J.F., and Ge, S. (2009) Enhanced therapeutic efficacy by simultaneously targeting two genetic defects in tumors. *Mol. Ther.*, **17**, 57–64.
95. Zheng, J.N., Pei, D.S., Sun, F.H., Zhang, B.F., Liu, X.Y., Gu, J.F., Liu, Y.H., Hu, X.L., Mao, L.J., Wen, R.M. *et al.* (2009) Inhibition of renal cancer cell growth by oncolytic adenovirus armed short hairpin RNA targeting hTERT gene. *Cancer Biol. Ther.*, **8**, 84–91.
96. Grimm, D. and Kleinschmidt, J.A. (1999) Progress in adeno-associated virus type 2 vector production: promises and prospects for clinical use. *Hum. Gene Ther.*, **10**, 2445–2450.
97. Grimm, D., Pandey, K., and Kay, M.A. (2005) Adeno-associated virus vectors for short hairpin RNA expression. *Methods Enzymol.*, **392**, 381–405.
98. Gorbatyuk, M., Justilien, V., Liu, J., Hauswirth, W.W., and Lewin, A.S. (2007) Suppression of mouse rhodopsin expression *in vivo* by AAV mediated siRNA delivery. *Vision Res.*, **47**, 1202–1208.

99. McCarty, D.M., Young, S.M. Jr., and Samulski, R.J. (2004) Integration of adeno-associated virus (AAV) and recombinant AAV vectors. *Annu. Rev. Genet.*, **38**, 819–845.
100. McCarty, D.M., Fu, H., Monahan, P.E., Toulson, C.E., Naik, P., and Samulski, R.J. (2003) Adeno-associated virus terminal repeat (TR) mutant generates self-complementary vectors to overcome the rate-limiting step to transduction *in vivo*. *Gene Ther.*, **10**, 2112–2118.
101. Nakai, H., Thomas, C.E., Storm, T.A., Fuess, S., Powell, S., Wright, J.F., and Kay, M.A. (2002) A limited number of transducible hepatocytes restricts a wide-range linear vector dose response in recombinant adeno-associated virus-mediated liver transduction. *J. Virol.*, **76**, 11343–11349.
102. Gao, G., Vandenberghe, L.H., Alvira, M.R., Lu, Y., Calcedo, R., Zhou, X., and Wilson, J.M. (2004) Clades of adeno-associated viruses are widely disseminated in human tissues. *J. Virol.*, **78**, 6381–6388.
103. Fechner, H., Sipo, I., Westermann, D., Pinkert, S., Wang, X., Suckau, L., Kurreck, J., Zeichhardt, H., Muller, O., Vetter, R. *et al.* (2008) Cardiac-targeted RNA interference mediated by an AAV9 vector improves cardiac function in coxsackievirus B3 cardiomyopathy. *J. Mol. Med.*, **86**, 987–997.
104. Suckau, L., Fechner, H., Chemaly, E., Krohn, S., Hadri, L., Kockskamper, J., Westermann, D., Bisping, E., Ly, H., Wang, X. *et al.* (2009) Long-term cardiac-targeted RNA interference for the treatment of heart failure restores cardiac function and reduces pathological hypertrophy. *Circulation*, **119**, 1241–1252.
105. Pacak, C.A., Mah, C.S., Thattaliyath, B.D., Conlon, T.J., Lewis, M.A., Cloutier, D.E., Zolotukhin, I., Tarantal, A.F., and Byrne, B.J. (2006) Recombinant adeno-associated virus serotype 9 leads to preferential cardiac transduction *in vivo*. *Circ. Res.*, **99**, e3–e9.
106. Wu, J.Q., Zhao, W.H., Li, Y., Zhu, B., and Yin, K.S. (2007) Adeno-associated virus mediated gene transfer into lung cancer cells promoting CD40 ligand-based immunotherapy. *Virology*, **368**, 309–316.
107. Harding, T.C., Dickinson, P.J., Roberts, B.N., Yendluri, S., Gonzalez-Edick, M., Lecouteur, R.A., and Jooss, K.U. (2006) Enhanced gene transfer efficiency in the murine striatum and an orthotopic glioblastoma tumor model, using AAV-7- and AAV-8-pseudotyped vectors. *Hum. Gene Ther.*, **17**, 807–820.
108. Nathwani, A.C., Gray, J.T., McIntosh, J., Ng, C.Y., Zhou, J., Spence, Y., Cochrane, M., Gray, E., Tuddenham, E.G., and Davidoff, A.M. (2007) Safe and efficient transduction of the liver after peripheral vein infusion of self-complementary AAV vector results in stable therapeutic expression of human FIX in nonhuman primates. *Blood*, **109**, 1414–1421.
109. Sun, A., Tang, J., Terranova, P.F., Zhang, X., Thrasher, J.B., and Li, B. (2010) Adeno-associated virus-delivered short hairpin-structured RNA for androgen receptor gene silencing induces tumor eradication of prostate cancer xenografts in nude mice: a preclinical study. *Int. J. Cancer*, **126**, 764–774.
110. Li, B.L., Zhang, G.X., Hou, X.L., Tan, M.W., Yuan, Y., Liu, X.H., Gong, D.J., and Huang, S.D. (2009) Recombinant adeno-associated virus mediated RNA interference of angiogenin expression inhibits cell growth of human lung adenocarcinoma. *Chin. J. Tuber. Resp. Dis.*, **32**, 188–192.
111. Haussecker, D. (2008) The business of RNAi therapeutics. *Hum. Gene Ther.*, **19**, 451–462.

45
Design of Targeted Protein Toxins

Hendrik Fuchs and Christopher Bachran

45.1
Introduction

45.1.1
Basic Idea

The basic idea of targeted protein toxins is analogous to the delivery of small-molecule drugs or radioisotopes, namely to design chimeric molecules that consist of one component that binds to a disease-specific cell surface target molecule and another that confers cytotoxicity. For small drugs and radioisotopes this is realized, for instance, in gemtuzumab ozogamicin (Mylotarg®) and ibritumomab tiuxetan (Zevalin®), respectively (see other chapters on antibody-based systems in this volume). Whereas small drugs stoichiometrically inhibit only one target molecule per drug molecule and radioisotopes decay during their action, protein toxins exhibit the advantage of nonstoichiometric enzymatic amplification. Each of them is able to affect thousands of substrate molecules, resulting in a high potency. As is known from drug or radio conjugates, the targeting moiety and toxin can be joined covalently *in vitro* by chemical conjugation; however, in contrast, it can also be expressed as a fusion protein generated by recombinant DNA technology provided that the targeting moiety is also a protein. This is usually a monoclonal antibody (mAb), a derivative thereof, a growth factor, or a cytokine, but it can in principle be any molecule with targeting properties (e.g., an aptamer). After selective binding to disease cells, targeted toxins are internalized and released into the cytosol. The mechanism of cytosolic transfer mainly depends on the nature of the toxin and is essentially understood only for a few toxins. Once inside the cytosol, the enzymatic reaction stops vital metabolic pathways, which finally results in cell death (Figure 45.1). Typical targets of these protein toxins include the eukaryotic elongation factor-2, and different RNAs and proteins involved in apoptosis. In order to enhance specificity and cytosolic uptake, a number of additional functional elements were designed to complement the basic idea. The elevated expression of certain matrix metalloproteases (MMPs) in the tumor environment is utilized to activate the toxins on site,

Drug Delivery in Oncology: From Basic Research to Cancer Therapy, First Edition.
Edited by Felix Kratz, Peter Senter, and Henning Steinhagen.

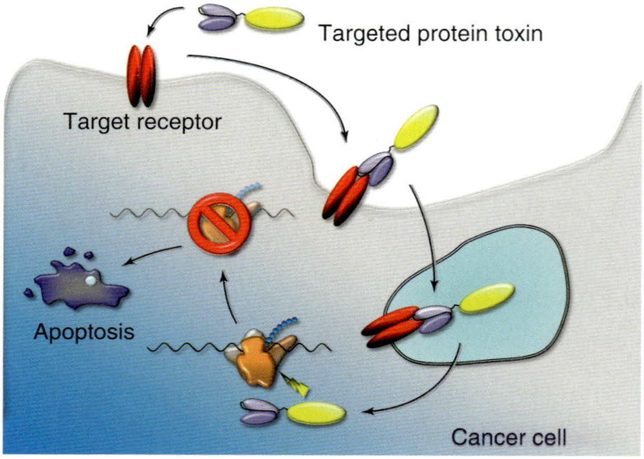

Figure 45.1 Initial idea of targeted protein toxins. A protein toxin is linked (either chemically or expressed as fusion protein) to an antibody to achieve binding to a tumor-specific receptor. Later, only a part of the protein toxin was utilized and scFv fragments were more commonly used. The conjugate is internalized into endosomal compartments and passes the endosomal membrane to access the cytosol. The first protein toxins in targeted protein toxins were diphtheria toxin and *Pseudomonas* exotoxin A, which both inactivate protein synthesis. The breakdown of the cellular processes results in the initiation of apoptosis.

while cell-penetrating peptides (CPPs) are designed for optimized membrane transfer into the cytosol, and cleavable bonds are introduced to release the enzyme and ensure unidirectionality of the cellular uptake. In some cases, additional compounds that facilitate endosomal escape of the drug were applied in parallel.

The most widely used generic name for targeted toxins is "immunotoxins" since antibodies or antibody fragments are frequently selected as targeting ligands for tumor surface antigen receptors. Even though this name is sometimes employed for all targeted toxins, the generic application is strictly incompatible due to the heterogeneous sources of the targeting moiety. A number of further names, however, have been created in the last decades – depending on the ligand and the type of linkage – including immunoconjugates, growth factor toxin fusions, growth factor toxin conjugates, cytotoxins, cytokine toxin fusions, cytokine toxin conjugates, ligand toxin fusions, ligand toxin conjugates, chimeric toxins, and targeted toxins. When the toxic moiety is not originally described as a toxin, terms such as immunokinases and immunoRNases are also used. The term "targeted toxin," presumably first used by Murphy *et al.* in 1988 for an interleukin (IL)-2 diphtheria toxin-related fusion protein [1], appears to be both meaningful and enclosing, and may also be suitable for generic use in the future. To exclude small molecules or radioisotopes, the term can be further specified by writing it as "targeted protein toxins."

45.1.2
Cell Death

Although the death of the tumor cell is the ultimate goal, the method of achieving this goal is not arbitrary. Uncontrolled cell death that results in colliquation, tyromatosis, or coagulative necrosis is not desired since detrimental and fatal consequences for the organism are possible. In contrast, apoptosis is the process of programmed cell death that can be triggered by either extracellular or intracellular signals. Cells are degraded in a controlled and systematic manner with no damage to neighboring cells – an action that naturally occurs billions of times a day in the human body. A further degradation process is autophagy, which is characterized by digestion of the cell's own components through the lysosomal machinery. Dependent on environmental parameters, autophagy can function to promote cell survival or cell death. It is a tumor suppressor process and induction of the autophagic machinery can cause cell demise in apoptosis-resistant cancer. Thus, this metabolic pathway can act either to prevent or to promote carcinogenesis, as well as to modulate the response to anticancer therapies, including toxin-induced apoptosis. Autophagy and apoptosis share common stimuli and signaling pathways, so that the final fate – life or death – depends on the cell response (reviewed in [2]). Typically, the primary target of a toxin is not directly involved in necrosis, apoptosis, or autophagy, but in general they are processes that are vital for the cells. For instance, diphtheria toxin ADP-ribosylates eukaryotic elongation factor-2, which results in the block of protein synthesis; however, this does not allow prediction of the secondary effects that are responsible for the type of cell death. Moreover, in a number of studies a couple of determined parameters indicated induction of apoptosis while others did not for the same cell line, implying that the cellular response to targeted protein toxins is more complex than anticipated. As discussed later, the choice of toxin is one of the most important decisions in the design of targeted protein toxins not only with regard to the mechanism of cell death, but also for other aspects, such as immunogenicity and cytosolic uptake.

45.1.3
Combination with Other Therapy Strategies

Although targeted protein toxins can be highly effective, it is expected, on the one hand, that large quantities of solid tumor tissue cannot be easily eliminated. Penetration of massive tumors is restricted, the maximal dose of the toxins is limited, and rapid necrotic destruction of large tumor masses can lead to serious adverse events. On the other hand, the targeting moiety allows tracing of small tumor cell clusters or even single tumor cells. Thus, targeted protein toxins are particularly suitable for the treatment of relapses, residuals, and metastases as well as inaccessible, disseminated, and hematopoietic tumors. In this respect, a combination with other strategies is advisable. For instance, targeted protein toxins can be applied as accompanying treatment for surgery or directly combined

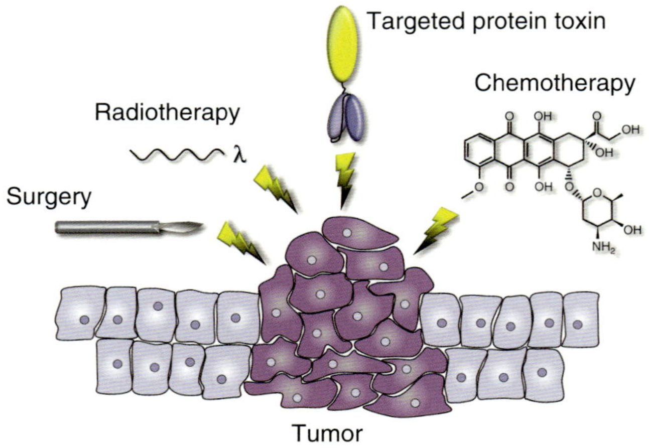

Figure 45.2 Combination of targeted protein toxins with conventional therapy approaches. In several studies, protein toxins were combined with chemotherapeutics in order to increase the impact of the treatment on tumor growth. The combination with radiotherapy is less common; however, a number of studies proved the beneficial effect of these combinations. It is furthermore intended to use targeted protein toxin therapies for follow-up treatments after initial surgery that removes the mass of a tumor, before the molecular treatment eliminates residual tumor cells and metastases.

with radio- or chemotherapy (Figure 45.2). A number of preclinical and a few clinical studies have been reported in the literature, most of them showing additive or synergistic effects. For example, a targeted toxin composed of IL-13 and *Pseudomonas* exotoxin A showed synergistic cytotoxicity when combined with the cytotoxic drug gemcitabine in an orthotopic mouse model of human pancreatic ductal adenocarcinoma [3]. Furthermore, nude mice bearing mesothelin-expressing xenografts treated with a combination of radiation and SS1P, a targeted toxin described in more detail at the end of this chapter (Section 45.3.2.3), had a statistically significant prolongation in time to tumor doubling or tripling compared with SS1P or radiation alone [4].

45.2 Rationale for the Respective Drug Delivery Concept

45.2.1 Design

45.2.1.1 Domains

A targeted protein toxin consists of different functional domains (Figure 45.3). Structurally, these domains can be part of a single peptide chain or spread over two or multiple chains. A number of natural toxins possess a cell-binding domain, which does not target tumor cells, but instead, depending on the toxin,

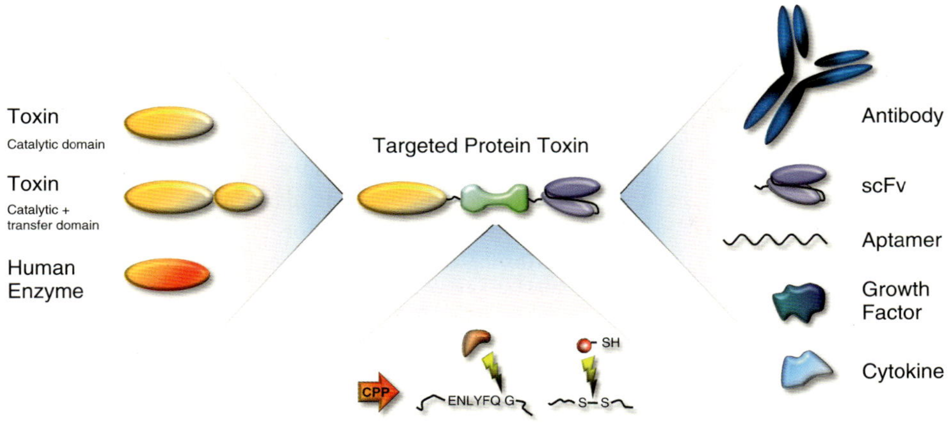

Figure 45.3 Different domains of targeted protein toxins. Described is an example for a targeted protein toxin, where several examples for the toxic moiety, a linker, and the targeting moiety are depicted. The toxic moiety can either be the catalytic domain of a bacterial or plant toxin, the catalytic domain and the translocation domain of these toxins (some RIPs do not contain a translocation domain), or a human enzyme. Some targeted protein toxins contain an artificial linker comprising CPPs or cleavable linkers (either reducible linkers or enzymatic cleavable linkers). The targeting moiety may either be a full-length antibody, a scFv (as an example of several antibody derivates such as Fab, dsFv, or bisFv that are described in more detail in other chapters in this volume), an aptamer, a growth factor, or a cytokine. Aptamers and full-length antibodies are only suitable for chemical conjugation to protein toxins.

different protein or glycan structures expressed on various normally differentiated cells. In addition to the cell-binding domain, these toxins are typically composed of a membrane transfer domain that mediates cytosolic uptake and a catalytic domain that is the fundamental part of each toxin. In the simplest case of a tumor-targeted protein toxin, a tumor antigen-binding domain (e.g., an antibody) is linked to the toxin regardless of the toxin's own cell-binding domain. It is intended to suppress undesired effects of this domain by steric hindrance or dominant competition due to a higher binding affinity of the tumor antigen-binding domain. To prevent problems with the toxin's cell-binding domain, toxins are used that either naturally lack this domain or the domain is removed by chemical or recombinant methods.

Several toxins lack a membrane transfer domain since they are naturally produced as a suicide protein directly inside the target cell (e.g., to repel a virus attack) or to enter cells by supporting proteins, such as perforin. To overcome this dilemma, CPPs (also known as protein transduction domains or Trojan peptides) are used as membrane transfer domains. These short peptides that vary considerably in sequence facilitate the transport of cargo molecules across membranes. By coupling them to various biological compounds, either chemically or through recombinant

DNA techniques, the uptake of effector molecules can be considerably improved (reviewed in [5]).

Further domains for supplementing the efficacy of targeting proteins are composed of cleavable bonds designed for a variety of purposes. These domains can be either represented by short peptides consisting of protease-specific recognition motifs or by chemical bonds that are cleaved under particular environmental conditions (e.g., at the acidic pH of endosomes or reducing potential of the cytosol). Aims of the cleavage include activation of the toxin, endosomal release of the targeting moiety, or cytosolic release of the membrane transfer domain (see below).

45.2.1.2 **Targeting Moieties**

The targeting moieties of a targeted toxin can, in principle, be of any kind of chemical structure; however, proteins as targeting moieties have the advantage that the whole drug can be generated as a fusion protein in bacterial or eukaryotic expression systems. Advanced non-protein-based targeting moieties are, for instance, aptamers (see Chapter 39, Aptamer Conjugates). Protein-based targeting can be mediated by antibodies or fragments thereof, or by any protein that recognizes a suitable tumor cell-specific surface receptor; however, since the toxic moiety of targeted protein toxins is only active inside the cell, simple binding is not sufficient. The targeting moiety must therefore be directed to a receptor that is constitutively endocytosed or internalized after ligand binding. Beyond antibodies, ILs and growth factors are the most often used ligands in targeting toxins. For more information on targeting, see the corresponding chapters in this volume.

One method to improve target cell specificity in targeted toxins is the use of a bispecific ligand. Such a fusion protein called DT2219ARL consists of a catalytically active fragment of diphtheria toxin and two scFv ligands recognizing CD19 and CD22. Genetic alterations included reverse orienting $V_H - V_L$ domains and adding stabilizing linkers [6]. *In vivo*, these improvements resulted in long-term tumor-free survivors measured in a bioluminescent xenograft imaging model. A similar fusion protein contains a fragment of *Pseudomonas* exotoxin A instead of diphtheria toxin (Figure 45.4) [7]. Alternatively antibody fragments can be replaced by natural ligands against tumor-specific surface receptors. Both human epidermal growth factor (EGF) and IL-4 cytokines were cloned onto the same single-chain molecule with truncated exotoxin A. The fusion protein was significantly effective against established systemic human breast cancer and prevented metastatic spread [8].

45.2.1.3 **Toxins**

The protein toxins used in tumor targeting were initially derived from particular bacteria or plants. Within the last years, vertebrate and, in particular, human enzymes utilized as toxins have gained more and more attention (Figure 45.5). The first described toxin with regard to a targeted tumor therapy was diphtheria toxin from *Corynebacterium diphtheriae*. In 1970, Moolten and Cooperband described the selective destruction of target cells by diphtheria toxin conjugated to antibodies directed against tumor cell surface antigens [9]. The toxin belongs to the class of

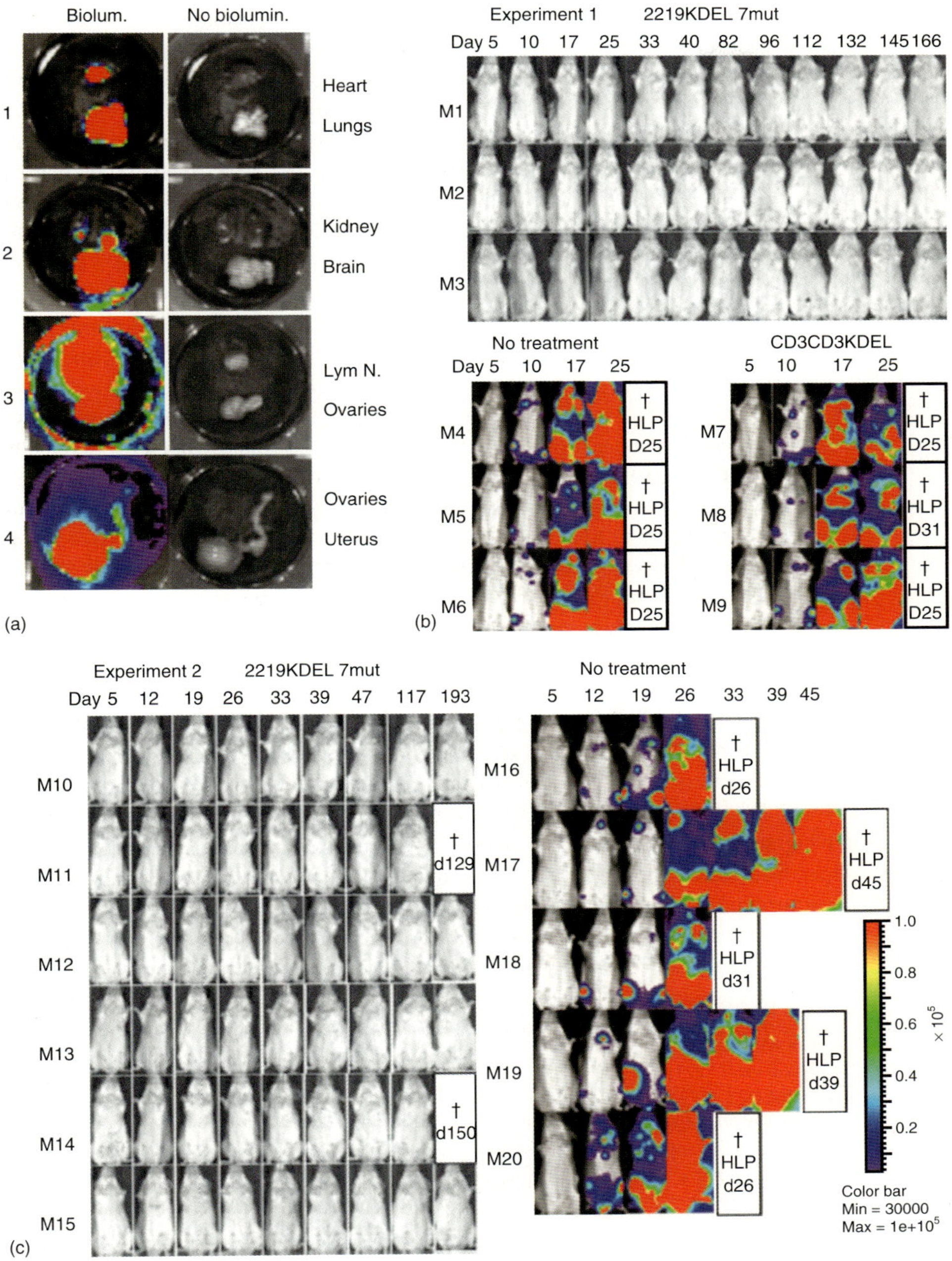
Biolum.
No biolumin.
Heart
Lungs
Kidney
Brain
Lym N.
Ovaries
Ovaries
Uterus
1
2
3
4
(a)
Experiment 1 2219KDEL 7mut
Day 5 10 17 25 33 40 82 96 112 132 145 166
M1
M2
M3
No treatment
Day 5 10 17 25
M4
M5
M6
† HLP D25
† HLP D25
† HLP D25
CD3CD3KDEL
5 10 17 25
M7
M8
M9
† HLP D25
† HLP D31
† HLP D25
(b)
Experiment 2 2219KDEL 7mut
Day 5 12 19 26 33 39 47 117 193
M10
M11
M12
M13
M14
M15
† d129
† d150
No treatment
5 12 19 26 33 39 45
M16
M17
M18
M19
M20
† HLP d26
† HLP d45
† HLP d31
† HLP d39
† HLP d26
1.0
0.8
0.6
0.4
0.2
× 10^5
Color bar
Min = 30000
Max = 1e+10^5
(c)

ADP-ribosylating enzymes and transfers ADP-ribose from nicotinamide adenine dinucleotide to the N^1 nitrogen of the imidazole ring in diphthamide, an unusually modified histidine at amino acid position 715 of the mammalian elongation factor-2 [10]. At least two further proteins catalyze exactly the same reaction – the long-known exotoxin A from *Pseudomonas aeruginosa* and the recently discovered cholix toxin from *Vibrio cholerae* [11]. ADP-ribosylation of elongation factor-2 prevents the interaction with its binding cavern in the 60S ribosomal subunit, which results in protein synthesis arrest. Although even today the full-length toxins have been successfully tested *in vitro* and *in vivo* [12], most of the described targeted proteins contain more or less a truncated toxin without the natural binding domain to reduce undesirable cell binding. This was first published a decade after Moolten and Copperband's publication by Blythman *et al.* who conjugated a mAb to the isolated A-chain of diphtheria toxin [13]. Corresponding exotoxin A fragments from *P. aeruginosa* are called PE40 and PE38, and have been applied in a number of clinical trials (see Section 45.3.2).

Another bacterial toxin that came into focus for targeted tumor therapies is anthrax toxin. The mechanism and application of anthrax toxin are completely different from diphtheria toxin and exotoxin A. Anthrax toxin is composed of three separate proteins (protective antigen, lethal factor, and edema factor). Protective antigen is cleaved and thus activated by furin after binding to its surface receptor and forms an oligomer (a heptamer or an octamer) to which both lethal factor and edema factor bind [14, 15]. The complex is endocytosed, and the low pH triggers the insertion of protective antigen into the membrane to form a pore that promotes the delivery of edema factor and lethal factor into the cytosol. Edema factor is a calcium- and calmodulin-dependent adenylate cyclase. It increases cAMP levels, thus interfering with cellular water homeostasis and intracellular signaling pathways, causing edema. Owing to its less localized effect this toxin is not applied to tumor targeting. Lethal factor is a zinc-dependent metalloprotease cleaving off the N-termini of several mitogen-activated protein kinase kinases. The resulting block in signal transduction leads to apoptosis. Anthrax toxin has been rendered tumor specific by conversion of the furin cleavage site within protective antigen into MMP and urokinase cleavage sites [16]. These enzymes are secreted in a tumor-specific manner, resulting in localized activation of protective antigen. In addition, fusion proteins of lethal factor (only the protective antigen-binding N-terminus)

Figure 45.4 Selective efficacy of a bispecific targeted toxin (2219KDEL7mut) consisting of an anti-CD22 scFv, an anti-CD19 scFv, and a truncated *Pseudomonas* exotoxin A (PE38). SCID mice were injected intravenously with Raji-luc lymphoma cells. To determine the metastatic ability of these cells, (a) shows representative mouse organs imaged on day 25 with bioluminescent imaging (left) and the same organ without bioluminescence (right). (b) and (c) Mice M1–M3 and M10–M15 were treated intraperitoneally with three courses of 2219KDEL7mut, whereas mice M4–M6 and M16–M20 were untreated. Mice M7–M9 received treatment with the identical dose and schedule, but with an irrelevant control, Bic3, that recognizes human T-cells and was synthesized by fusing two repeating scFvs against human CD3ϵ to DT390. HLP, hind limb paralysis. (Reproduced with permission from [7].)

Table 45.1 List of plant RIPs tested in targeted toxins for tumor therapy.

Toxin name	Type	Plant	Experimental stage of derived targeted toxins[a]
Abrin	II	*Abrus precatorius* L.	mouse melanoma model
Bouganin[b]	I	*Bougainvillea spectabilis* Wild.	human xenograft mouse model
Bryodin	I	*Bryonia dioica* L.	mouse and rat (toxicity)
Dianthin	I	*Dianthus caryophyllus* L.	cell culture
Ebulin	II	*Sambucus ebulus* L.	cell culture
Gelonin	I	*Gelonium multiflorum* A. Juss.	phase I
Luffin	I	*Luffa aegyptiaca* Mill.	cell culture
Momorcochin	I	*Momordica cochinchinensis* Spreng.	cell culture
Momordin	I	*Momordica charantia* L.	human xenograft mouse model
Moschatin	I	*Cucurbita moschata* Duchesne	cell culture
Nigrin b	II	*Sambucus nigra* L.	cell culture
Pokeweed antiviral protein	I	*Phytolacca americana* L.	phase I
Ricin[c]	II	*Ricinus communis* L.	phase II
Saporin	I	*Saponaria officinalis* L.	phase I
Trichosanthin	I	*Trichosanthes kirilowii* Maxim.	cell culture

[a] Most advanced stage for use as a cancer-targeted agent known until mid 2010.
[b] Used as the derivative de-bouganin, where T-cell epitopes were removed.
[c] Used as derivatives with blocked natural galactose binding sites, as ricin toxin A-chain or as deglycosylated ricin toxin A-chain.

with the catalytic domain of exotoxin A were applied for tumor-targeting approaches [17].

A number of homologous plant enzymes represent the second important group of toxins. These are the ribosome-inactivating proteins (RIPs) found in different dicots (Table 45.1). A few of them have already been tested as part of targeted toxins in clinical trials (see Section 45.3.2). RIPs are subdivided into type I species consisting of a single catalytic A-chain of 26–32 kDa, and type II species comprising a catalytic A-chain and a lectin-binding B-chain of approximately 31–36 kDa that associates with specific cell surface carbohydrate groups (reviewed in [18]). The A-chain cleaves a specific *N*-glycosidic bond in the mammalian 28S ribosomal RNA, resulting in the release of adenine [19]. Since this residue is required to bind eukaryotic elongation factor-1 and -2, the modification also results in the arrest of protein biosynthesis. Since RIPs of type I naturally lack a cell-binding domain that

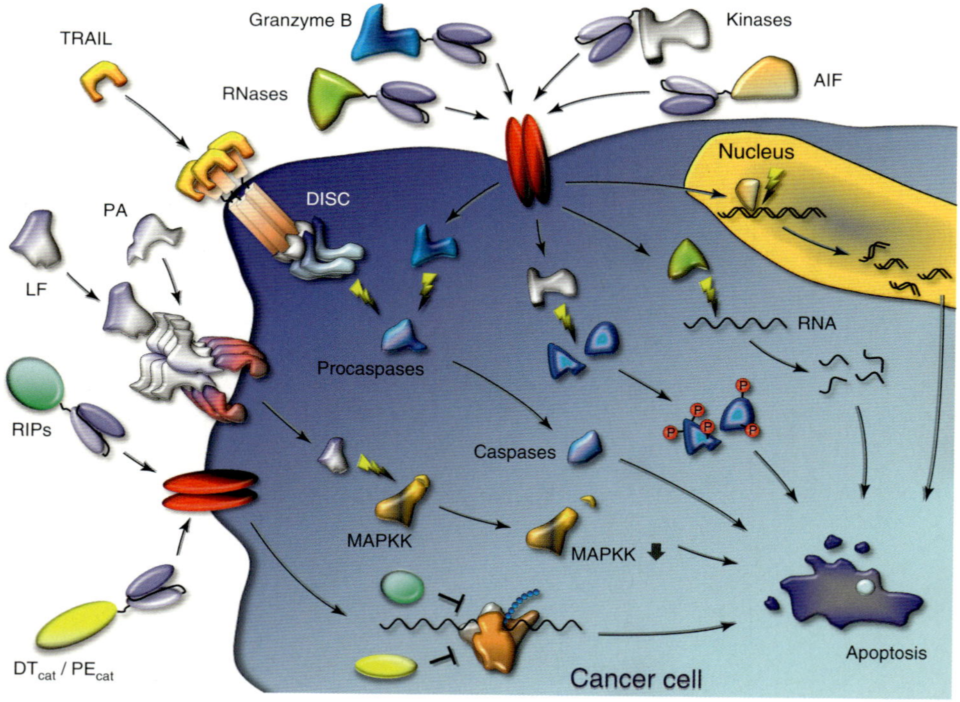

Figure 45.5 Mechanisms of action for the toxic moieties of targeted protein toxins. This overview depicts the intracellular targets for the bacterial, plant, and human enzymes utilized in targeted protein toxins described in this chapter. Several enzymes and toxins have further targets not shown in this overview for clarity. Most enzymes are presented as a fusion with a scFv as an example for the utilization in targeted protein toxins. DT, diphtheria toxin; LF, lethal factor of anthrax toxin; MAPKK, mitogen-activated protein kinase kinase; PA, protective antigen of anthrax toxin; PE, *Pseudomonas* exotoxin A; see text for other abbreviations.

can cause undesired cell binding, they are in this respect ideal for the design of targeted toxins; however, in contrast to type II, they do not possess a membrane transfer mechanism, which results in an impaired cytosolic uptake. Ricin is the best investigated type II RIP. It possesses such a high cytotoxicity that it cannot be applied as natural full-length protein; however, a modified full-length toxin and its isolated A-chain were successfully tested in targeted proteins. Alternative type II RIPs are ebulin and nigrin b, which are about 10 000-fold less toxic for cells than ricin, but exhibit a similar enzymatic activity on ribosomal RNA once inside the cytosol [20]. Shiga toxins are bacterial toxins that catalyze the same reaction as plant RIPs, but are rarely used as the toxic moiety in targeted drugs. Notably, the B subunit of Shiga toxins can act as the targeting moiety since the natural receptor, glycosphingolipid Gb3, is overexpressed in membranes of certain tumor cells [21].

A further group of toxins is represented by aspergillins – fungal endonucleases that cleave 28S ribosomal RNA directly next to the adenosine that is depurinated by plant RIPs [19, 22]. These fungal RIPs are small proteins of approximately 17 kDa and bear no relation to plant RIPs. Although a few aspergillins such as α-sarcin and clavin were tested as targeted toxins in cell culture [23, 24], they never gained the importance of plant RIPs.

Despite their high toxicity and their membrane transfer potential, all nonhuman proteins exhibit the disadvantage of being immunogenic, as discussed later in Section 45.2.2.3. This raised the question whether human proteins with toxic potential are suitable to act in targeted tumor therapies. Proapoptotic proteins appear to be the best candidates, including proteins involved in germ defense and developmental apoptosis. Indeed, the proapoptotic serine protease granzyme B that is released from cytoplasmic granules of cytotoxic T-cells and natural killer cells, the RNase angiogenin, apoptosis-inducing factor (AIF), and others are human proteins that have been tested as toxic moieties in targeted strategies. Granzyme B possesses a caspase-like ability to cleave substrates at key aspartic acid residues, and can thus activate several procaspases and directly cleave downstream caspase substrates such as the inhibitor of caspase-activated DNase. In addition, there are also caspase-independent pathways. Granzyme B can damage non-nuclear structures such as mitochondria, and can rapidly translocate to the nucleus where it cleaves poly(ADP-ribose) polymerase and nuclear matrix antigen (reviewed in [25]).

Angiogenin induces angiogenesis by activating vessel endothelial and smooth muscle cells, and triggering a number of biological processes. It has been reported that angiogenin exerts ribonucleolytic activity, induces basement membrane degradation, is involved in signal transduction, and translocates into the nucleus of target cells directly. Angiogenin belongs to the RNase superfamily with a 33% sequence homology to the pancreatic RNase A (reviewed in [26]). Although the ribonucleolytic activity is more than 10^5 times lower than that of RNase A, angiogenin was successfully tested *in vitro* in targeted toxins [27]. Mutations of residue Glu117 in angiogenin greatly increase its RNase activity up to 30-fold [28], which may improve the efficacy of angiogenin-based antitumor drugs. Another member of the

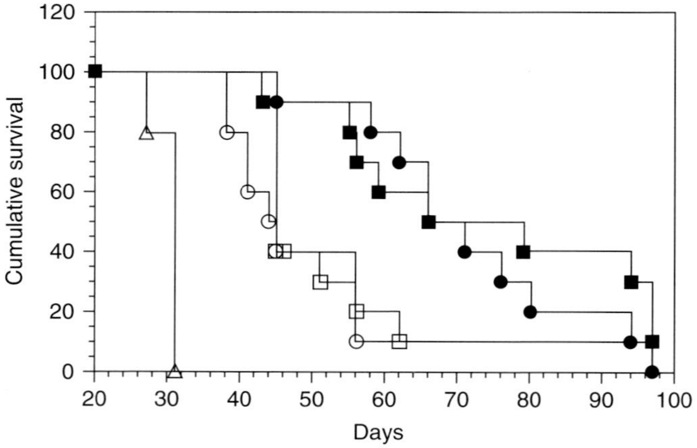

Figure 45.6 Treatment of aggressive minimal and advanced Daudi lymphoma disease with a targeted RNase generated by covalent linkage of a monoclonal anti-CD22 antibody (LL2) and an amphibian RNase (ranpirnase). A mixture of uncoupled LL2 and ranpirnase served as control. Daudi lymphoma cells (5×10^6 cells) were injected intravenously, followed 1 or 7 days later with daily intravenous injections for 5 consecutive days of phosphate-buffered saline (open triangles), 80 μg LL2 and 20 μg ranpirnase (open circles and squares, treatment days 1–5 and 7–11, respectively), or 100 μg LL2–ranpirnase conjugate (solid circles and squares, treatment days 1–5 and 7–11, respectively). Both groups of mice treated with LL2–ranpirnase conjugate survived significantly longer than mice treated with phosphate-buffered saline ($P < 0.0001$) or a mixture of LL2 plus ranpirnase ($P < 0.0002$) [30].

pancreatic RNase A superfamily is ranpirnase, originally isolated from oocytes of the northern leopard frog (*Rana pipiens*). Ranpirnase degrades intracellular RNAs such as tRNA and double-stranded RNA, and thereby suppresses protein synthesis (reviewed in [29]). Although not a human protein, ranpirnase alone was successfully tested in a clinical phase III trial [29] and its immunoconjugates were effective in preclinical animal models (Figure 45.6) [30].

AIF plays an important role in caspase-independent programmed cell death (summarized in [31]). It is translated as a 67-kDa precursor molecule that harbors two putative mitochondrial localization signals. On mitochondrial import, the first 52 amino acids are cleaved off, resulting in a 62-kDa form that is retained in the mitochondrial intermembrane space. On stimulation of cell death, AIF is further cleaved to a 57-kDa protein and released into the cytosol, from where it translocates to the nucleus and interacts with cyclophilin A to form an active DNase. A truncated AIF derivative ($AIF_{\Delta 100}$) that lacks the mitochondrial import signal of the protein is enzymatically active and induces cell death accompanied by clear signs of apoptosis [31]. Further ideas that aim to directly trigger apoptosis include the use of the tumor suppressor protein death-associated protein kinase 2 (DAPK2) and of tumor necrosis factor-related apoptosis-inducing ligand (TRAIL). DAPK2 is a calcium/calmodulin-regulated proapoptotic serine/threonine kinase that is downregulated in various tumor cells, including Hodgkin's lymphoma-derived tumor cell lines as well as malignant kidney and intestinal epithelial cells [32, 33]. A recombinant DAPK2 that exhibits constitutive kinase activity with enhanced proapoptotic function was tested as a targeted fusion protein, and shown to inhibit cell proliferation and induce apoptotic cell death in DAPK2-negative target cells [32]. TRAIL can initiate the formation of the proapoptotic death-inducing signaling complex (DISC) by binding to one of its two cognate proapoptotic receptors, TRAIL receptor-1 and -2. Processing of caspase-8/10 at the DISC triggers the caspase cascade, which finally results in apoptotic cell death. Variants of TRAIL selective for either TRAIL receptor-1 or -2 and agonistic antibodies have been designed to selectively kill tumor cells. To increase tumor sensitivity, TRAIL receptor ligands have already been combined with various therapies in preclinical models (reviewed in [34]). Targeting with TRAIL or agonistic antibodies is different from the other presented strategies insofar as the toxic and targeting moiety are represented by the same domain.

45.2.1.4 **Toxin Delivery**

Most of the toxins that are tested for targeted therapies act in the cytosol or nucleus. To deliver these toxins to their final destination, several steps are required, including binding to the cell surface, internalization, vesicular transport, and membrane transfer to the cytosol. Whereas binding and internalization are predominantly determined by the targeting moiety and the natural behavior of targeted receptor, trafficking and cytosolic uptake are typically guided by the properties of the toxin. As already mentioned, bacterial toxins and type II RIPs possess an intrinsic translocation domain in their B-chain, while type I RIPs and vertebrate toxins do not. Thus, in the majority of cases, diphtheria toxin and *Pseudomonas* exotoxin A are administered in a truncated form with the cell-binding domain removed and the membrane transfer domain retained (Figure 45.3). Ricin, however, is so toxic that the utilization of solely the A-chain is strongly preferred. Alternatively, the galactose binding site of the B-chain can be blocked. Although the A-chain of the bacterial and plant toxins alone and the vertebrate toxins exhibit a slight cytotoxicity due to unspecific membrane transfer by unknown mechanisms, it is at least sufficient to observe a target cell-specific effect since increased efficacy is of strong importance. Based on this situation, the development of strategies to enhance cytosolic delivery of protein toxins is an ongoing challenge.

There are two principal techniques to improve the cytosolic accumulation of an active toxin. The first technique is the insertion of additional elements directly into the targeted toxin. This can comprise peptides with new functions or chemical modifications. The second technique is the combined application of the targeted toxin together with other substances that support toxin delivery. The chemical nature of these additives is principally variable; however, it must fulfill the requirements to be approved as a drug.

CPPs are derived from parts of various proteins from diverse origins, including viral, bacterial, insect, and mammalian, or are artificially designed. These peptides are generally 10–16 amino acids in length, with a maximum of about 45 amino acids. They are structurally completely different from each other with no consensus sequence (reviewed in [35] and see Chapter 37 for a detailed description). The most widely studied CPP is the protein transduction domain TAT from the HIV-1 transcriptional activator protein Tat. Other examples include the *Drosophila melanogaster* homeotic transcription protein Antennapedia (penetratin), the herpes simplex virus structural protein VP22, a sequence derived from human Kaposi fibroblast growth factor, the synthetic peptides transportan and SynB1, a motif from the PreS2 domain of hepatitis B virus surface antigen (TLM), the short amphipathic peptide Pep-1, and nuclear localization signals. This section only deals with the particular use of CPPs in targeted protein toxins. CPPs are not cell specific by themselves, but the specificity mediated by the targeting moiety is retained in targeted toxins equipped with such a peptide. Snyder *et al.* linked a chemokine receptor-4 ligand to two different anticancer peptides via TAT and demonstrated an enhancement of tumor cell killing *in vitro* [36]. In another study three different CPPs were fused to the type I RIP dianthin. Two of them proved to be able to increase the cytotoxicity in conjugation with transferrin in comparison to a transferrin–dianthin conjugate [37]. A fusion protein of the type I RIP saporin and the EGF that contains the CPP, designated "TLM," exhibited increased antitumor efficacy in a breast cancer model in mice (Figure 45.7) [38]. TLM was also successfully used in a targeted toxin composed of an anti-CD64 scFv and angiogenin [27].

To further improve drug delivery, the utilization of CPPs can be supplemented by further peptides that support drug activation, release, or accumulation. Particular MMPs are often enriched in the environment of a tumor. Peptides representing a MMP recognition motif can therefore be used for tumor site-specific activation. Such a peptide can, for instance, link a polycationic CPP to a neutralizing polyanion. Uptake into cells is inhibited until the linker is proteolyzed [39]. Alternatively, a CPP can be activated after target receptor-mediated endocytosis. Cleavage of recognition motifs for furin-like proteases can result in the exposure of the CPP inside the endosomes [40]. An increase in efficacy can also be achieved when only the furin-site is exerted without a CPP, which is probably caused by the resulting drug release [41, 42]; however, this must be tested for the individual case since the addition of either one of two furin cleavage sites to a targeted gelonin was less efficient in a xenograft tumor model compared to a flexible noncleavable linker [43]. Further strategies to increase the cytotoxicity of targeted toxins include the use of the translocation motif of diphtheria toxin or *Pseudomonas* exotoxin A instead of a CPP demonstrated for ricin and granzyme B, and cellular protein retention signals such as REDLK and KDEL as shown for ricin and RNases (reviewed in [44]). Regardless of the internalization mechanism, a drug should accumulate within the cell to achieve maximum toxicity. A promising strategy to achieve intracellular trapping is the inclusion of a cleavable peptide that, once cleaved inside the cytosol, converts the drug to a membrane-impermeable protein by getting rid of any motif or domain used for membrane translocation. This was shown *in vitro* and *in vivo* for a saporin-based targeted toxin containing different cytosolic cleavage motifs [38, 45]. An analogous procedure describes the insertion of a natural organelle-specific cleavage recognition site of the mitochondrial malate dehydrogenase signal sequence. Cleavage results in mitochondrial cargo accumulation, making this approach suitable for use with targeted toxins that mediate their toxic effects inside mitochondria [46]. Another strategy is the utilization of a protease-cleavable disulfide-forming peptidic loop between two parts of the fusion protein [47].

In addition to recombinant fusion proteins, chemically conjugated or modified toxins are equally accepted. Where chemical coupling is used as the preparation method, a disulfide bridge may fulfill the role of a cytosolic cleavable peptide and an acid-cleavable hydrazone bond that of an endosomal cleavable peptide.

As mentioned above, several methods were developed for the improvement of drug uptake by combining the application of targeted toxins with other substances that achieve transport of the toxic moiety into the cytosol. Lysosomic agents (e.g., chloroquine) accumulate in the lysosomes, increase the lysosomal pH, and thus promote the transport of ricin-containing targeted toxins into the cytosol. The use of retinoic acid had the strongest effects, increasing cytotoxicity more than 10 000-fold. These effects appear to be restricted to ricin since saporin does not enter the lysosomal pathway [48, 49]. Efficient delivery systems for toxins other than ricin were also discovered. The phosphoinositide 3-kinase inhibitor

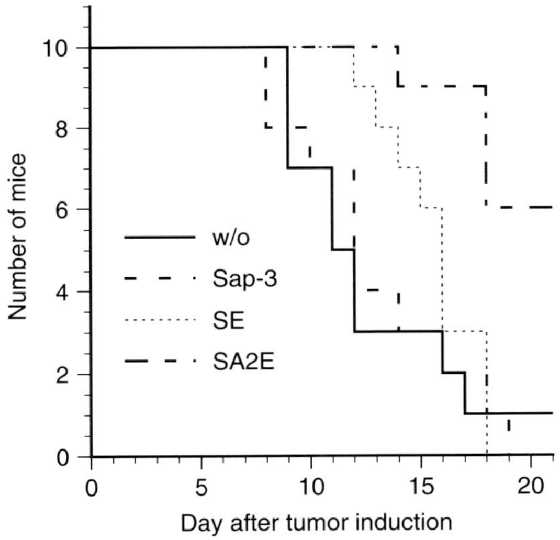

Figure 45.7 Treatment of adenocarcinoma with targeted saporin. BALB/c mice were inoculated at their right flank with 1.25×10^5 syngeneic mammary adenocarcinoma TSA cells transfected with the human EGFR. Mice were treated on days 0, 3, 6, and 11 by subcutaneous injection of 5 μg of either the RIP saporin (Sap-3) alone, a fusion protein (SE) of saporin and EGF, or a similar fusion protein (SA2E) containing in addition a CPP and cleavable peptides for improved endosomal escape. Untreated mice (w/o) served as control. The individual course of tumor growth is shown by a Kaplan–Meyer curve referring to a tumor volume less than 5 μl. The *P*-values were calculated according to Breslow–Wilcoxon and are, compared to untreated mice, 0.79 for treatment with Sap-3, 0.038 for SE, and less than 0.001 for SA2E. The *P*-value for SA2E compared to SE is 0.003. (Reproduced with permission from [38].)

wortmannin increased the cytotoxicity of targeted toxins containing *Pseudomonas* exotoxin A, saporin, or gelonin, both *in vitro* and *in vivo* [50]. Saponins are plant glycosides containing a steroid or triterpene core structure to which one or two glycans are attached. Particular saponins increase the target specific cytotoxicity of fusions consisting of EGF and saporin, dependent on the cell line, up to more than 100 000-fold *in vitro* and up to 300-fold *in vivo* [51, 52]. Photochemical internalization is a further technology for the release of endocytosed macromolecules into the cytosol and is based on the activation by light of photosensitizers located in endocytic vesicles to induce the release of macromolecules from the endocytic vesicles. Photochemical internalization was shown to stimulate intracellular delivery of a large variety of macromolecules, including type I RIPs, and was successfully tested for several targeted protein toxins, including fusions of EGF and saporin, cetuximab and saporin, as well as MOC31 (an antibody against cluster 2 epithelial antigen) and gelonin (reviewed in [44, 53]).

45.2.2
Obstacles and Circumvention

The production and application of targeted protein toxins has revealed a number of drug-related problems. Continuous efforts demonstrated that most of the obstacles can at least be partially circumvented by taking corresponding steps. This section will only present a selection of the most prominent cases without raising a claim to completeness.

45.2.2.1 Production

Independent of whether the targeting and toxic moieties are chemically linked or designed as a fusion protein, the proteins must be expressed by a suitable host system. There are a number of expression systems, including bacteria, yeast, insects, and mammalian cells. This section cannot present a comprehensive overview on protein expression, but instead will focus on a selection of some major problems. Production of the toxin in the natural host is critical. The corresponding bacteria are pathogenic, planting is time-consuming and sophisticated, and human cell lines suffer from the toxic effects. Heterologous expression in a foreign species is linked to general problems, such as different frequency in the use of certain codons, no or modified post-translational modifications, wrong protein folding, low solubility, and undesirable cleavage. In addition, toxicity for the host and the development of a reliable purification procedure may also be critical.

Although all these aspects describe general difficulties, there is no general solution since the individual sequence of each targeted toxin determines each of its properties and the exchange of a single amino acid can alter the physicochemical properties completely. Thus, solutions presented here can be suitable to solve problems with similar or even completely different proteins, and yet may fail for homologous or even identical proteins when, for instance, expressed in another strain of the same host. To compensate for different codon usage that often results in slow synthesis or premature termination, the codons of interest can be mutated according to the usage of the host; however, this can require ambitious work or the expensive resynthesis of the complete cDNA. Alternatively, there are a number of host strains available that possess additional genes to provide those aminoacyl-tRNAs, which are naturally rarely expressed in the host organism. Post-translational modifications may be required for particular functions of the protein or can essentially influence its folding, and thus solubility, stability, and half-life. While particular functions mediated by covalent alterations typically cannot be restored by alternative procedures, but only by the choice of another more suitable host, general properties such as correct folding, good solubility, and prevented cleavage can be achieved by coexpression of chaperones or intramolecular chaperone-mediated folding (reviewed in [54, 55]), expression in eukaryotes to support folding of glycoproteins (reviewed in [56]), and point mutations at preferred protease recognition motifs [45]. Toxicity may be reduced by expression of inactive toxin precursors that can be activated (e.g., due to proteolytic cleavage or induced conformational changes), by coexpression of inhibiting peptides or proteins such as intrabodies, or by microinjection of neutralizing antibodies [57]. An interesting finding was the benefit resulting from PDZ domains. These domains share a common structural motif of 80–90 amino acids found in signaling proteins of almost all living organisms. PDZ is an acronym combining the first letters of three proteins ((i) postsynaptic density protein-95, official name: DLG4 – disks, large homolog-4 (*Drosophila*); (ii) DLG1 – disks, large homolog 1 (*Drosophila*); (iii) zona occludens protein 1, official name: TJP1 – tight junction protein-1), which were first discovered to possess this domain. In general, PDZ domains bind to a short C-terminal region of other specific proteins. The production of the type I RIP saporin in a soluble form was greatly enhanced by adding the sequence for a PDZ-binding domain at the C-terminus and coexpression of this targeted toxin with a PDZ domain. The increase of production was not due to protection from bacterial intoxication; instead, it was from a stabilization effect during biosynthesis. The purified targeted toxin is stable and yet surprisingly nontoxic to free ribosomes, while being fully active against human cancer cells [58]. A further technique to avoid host toxicity is the secretion of the toxic product. Codon usage optimization and toxin secretion greatly increased the expression levels of an active saporin fused to the N-terminal fragment of human urokinase as targeting moiety in a yeast expression system [59]. Purification of the proteins can be facilitated by additional purification tags, such as a hexahistidine. If the tag bears the risk to impair the tolerance to the drug, the tag can be removed by proteolytic cleavage of a protease recognition motif placed between the drug and the tag.

45.2.2.2 **Biological Half-Life**

The production and purification of a stable targeted toxin does not imply that this protein exhibits an appropriate biological half-life. The bioavailability of the drug is in particular threatened by proteolytic cleavage, degradation by the liver, and renal clearance. Since proteases of a bacterial or fungal host are different from those of the treated animal or human patient, cleavage of the targeted toxin may occur even when never previously observed. Beyond the removal of critical protease recognition motifs [60], masking the protein by covalently attached poly(ethylene glycol) (PEG) molecules is an alternate strategy to protect the protein. This technique, known as PEGylation, is also valuable to decrease immunogenicity (see Section 45.2.2.3) and can prevent renal clearance due to the increase in the size of the molecule (reviewed in [61, 62]). The insertion of additional glycosylation sites can also increase the half-life and biological activity of proteins [63]; however, the exposure of terminal galactose residues results in rapid clearance of glycoproteins from the circulation through hepatocyte asialoglycoprotein receptors. Since terminal sialylation prevents binding to this receptor and subsequent degradation, cell culture conditions that ensure a high degree of sialylation are therefore advantageous in this respect. The half-life of protein toxins in addition may be positively influenced by the choice of site and type of application. An intratumoral injection can result in rapid depletion of the targeted toxin from the blood due to the high number of target receptors in the tumor tissue, therefore preventing degradation by the liver or renal clearance.

45.2.2.3 **Immunogenicity**

Proteins that are not the body's own molecules underlie the attacks of the immune system. This can result in the inactivation of the applied drugs by neutralizing antibodies or, in the worst case, in anaphylactic shock. A simple way to counteract against the immune response is the accompanying application of immunosuppressive drugs; however, this impairs the body's resistance against infections. Furthermore, this technique combats the effect rather than the cause. Therefore, it appears more suitable to mask or remove immunogenic epitopes, or to develop techniques that avoid these critical epitopes from scratch. PEGylation was shown to reduce the immunogenicity of a variety of protein drugs (reviewed in [61]). As described above, PEGylation is also advantageous for protein solubility, stability, and biological half-life, and can be coupled by site-directed procedures to obtain uniform products. Thus, it appears to be a valuable tool for targeted protein toxins. Site-directed PEGylation of trichosanthin, a type I RIP suitable for cancer treatment, led to a 3- to 4-fold decrease in immunogenicity [64]. Similar results were obtained for LMB-2, a recombinant targeted toxin composed of a scFv fragment of an antibody to the IL-2 receptor α subunit fused to truncated *Pseudomonas* exotoxin A (referred to as PE38) [65]. Another method to reduce immunogenicity is the removal of immunogenic epitopes by site-directed mutagenesis. To eliminate most of the identified B-cell epitopes, and thus allow more treatment cycles and increase efficacy, Onda *et al.* inserted eight mutations into the targeted toxin BL22 that is composed of an anti-CD22 Fv fused to PE38 [66]. The new targeted protein toxin is significantly less immunogenic in three strains of mice, and yet retains full cytotoxic and antitumor activities. Analogously, Oh *et al.* inserted seven mutations into *Pseudomonas* exotoxin A [8] and Cizeau *et al.* removed the T-cell epitopes from the type I RIP bouganin [41]. In order to principally avoid the existence of immunogenic epitopes, the tendency of the newest developments is the design of humanized targeted toxins (reviewed in [67]). This means that in the best case all parts of the fusion protein are of human origin, which essentially reduces immunogenicity, if present at all, to neoepitopes that have arisen from the bridging regions of the different moieties. Concerning the targeting moiety, animal antibodies can be humanized or human antibodies can be developed by phage-display as detailed in the relevant chapters on antibody-based systems in this volume. Alternatively, human ligands such as growth factors or cytokines can be employed. As described in Section 45.2.1.3, certain human proteases, RNases, or kinases can be used as the toxic moiety, which reduces the likelihood of an immune response. Fusions of a human antibody or ligand with a human toxin appear thus to be ideal; however, as discussed above, these targeted toxins lack a membrane transfer domain and other functional elements that improve the efficacy of the drug.

45.2.2.4 **Tumor Penetration**

Whereas hematopoietic malignancies are easily accessible for targeted protein toxins, solid tumors exhibit a strong barrier. Therefore, the decisive property is the size of the drug. Regrettably, there are opposing effects that determine the efficacy of the fusion protein. A larger size is advantageous to benefit from the enhanced permeability and retention (EPR) effect, which is the property by which certain sizes of molecules tend to accumulate in tumor tissue much more than they do in normal tissues (see Chapter 3). As discussed above, a larger size is also valuable in preventing renal clearance. However, the toxins in targeted protein drugs are effective in the cytosol and must therefore overcome the cellular membrane. Transport by natural translocation motifs of the toxin and by CPPs is better the smaller the protein is. One technique to fulfill both conditions is the use of endosomal cleavable peptides that are susceptible to proteases naturally located inside the endosomes. Cleavage of these peptides results in the release of the large ligand after endocytosis of the toxin. Another important issue is the tumor stroma that is characterized by distorted blood vessels and activated connective tissue cells producing a collagen-rich matrix, which is accompanied by elevated interstitial fluid pressure, indicating a transport barrier between tumor tissue and blood. Oldberg *et al.* showed that the collagen-binding proteoglycan fibromodulin controls stroma structure and fluid balance in experimental carcinoma [68]. This finding can be the basis for further developments since targeted modulations of the fluid balance in carcinoma can increase the response to cancer therapeutic agents.

45.2.2.5 **Undesirable Effects**

Beyond immunogenicity a number of further off-target effects are observed after treatment with targeted toxins. Most of the effects are a consequence of general toxicity to normal cells, particularly liver cells, and include necrotic lesions, fever, nausea, hypoalbuminemia, and elevated levels of alanine transaminase and aspartate transaminase. The mechanisms of general toxicity are difficult to understand, as demonstrated by deletions introduced into a PE38-based targeted toxin to reduce proteolytic susceptibility of a protease-sensitive cluster. Surprisingly, mice tolerated doses of the protease-resistant protein that were at least 10-fold higher than lethal doses of the parent molecule [60]. The major nonspecific and dose-limiting toxicity associated with a couple of targeted toxins is the vascular leak syndrome characterized by fluid leakage from capillaries, a fall in serum albumin, fluid retention, edema, and weight gain. Baluna *et al.* identified a motif present in both the ricin A-chain and human IL-2 (the targeting moiety in some targeting toxins), which caused nonspecific binding to integrin receptors on vascular endothelial cells [69]. Nevertheless, endothelial cell damage caused by high concentrations of targeted toxins can usually be managed by adequate hydration of patients. To avoid damage to nontarget cells, which causes the undesired effects, the main objectives in this regard include further improvement of cell target specificity (e.g., by bispecific ligands, removal or blocking of nonspecific binding motifs, increase of cytosolic uptake after target cell binding, and better purification strategies to minimize byproducts).

45.3 Examples

A large number of targeted toxins are in preclinical and clinical development. The examples presented here are selected on the basis of innovation, variation, progress, and success, but can only provide a brief insight into the multifarious world of strategies. Fungal toxins are not considered since they are rarely tested. Tables provide a comprehensive overview on targeted toxins in clinical trials.

45.3.1 Preclinical Development

45.3.1.1 Drugs Based on Bacterial Toxins

Since bacterial toxins represent the first group of proteins used in targeted toxins, they have already been tested in a number of clinical trials. Novel developments typically focus on improvements of successfully applied toxins and on the optimization of the targeting moiety. An exception to this is anthrax toxin, which came into focus for tumor treatment at the beginning of this century.

A continuous development can be described for RFB4 (dsFv)–PE38 also known as BL22, a recombinant targeted toxin containing an anti-CD22 dsFv antibody fused to truncated *Pseudomonas* exotoxin A consisting of amino acids 253–364 and 381–613 (see below in Figure 45.16). The binding moiety of this molecule was further improved; the Fv was mutated and antibody phage-display was used to isolate mutant phage that bound better to CD22. In the resulting HA22, residues SSY in heavy chain CDR3 have been mutated to THW. HA22 has a 5- to 10-fold increase in cytotoxic activity on various $CD22^+$ cell lines and is up to 50 times more cytotoxic to cells from patients with chronic lymphocytic leukemia and hairy cell leukemia [70]. BL22 and HA22 are described in more detail as an example for clinical development below. Since HA22 has a proteolytic susceptibility to lysosomal proteases within a limited segment of PE38, deletion mutants were generated. One mutant, HA22-LR, lacks all identified cleavage sites in domain

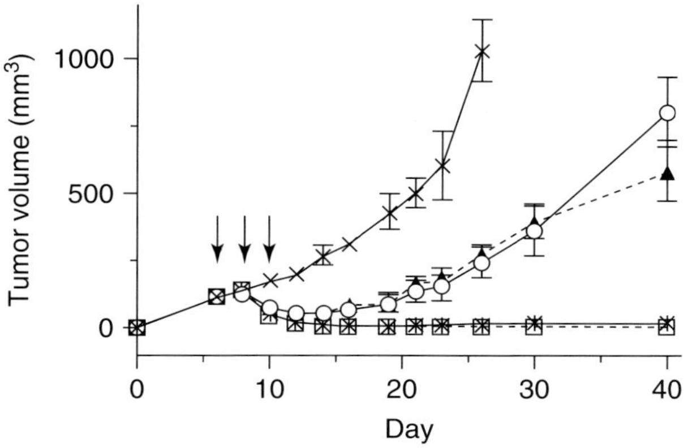

Figure 45.8 Antitumor activity of HA22 and HA22-LR. HA22 is a recombinant targeted toxin containing an anti-CD22 dsFv antibody fused to truncated *Pseudomonas* exotoxin A (PE38). HA22-LR is a mutant that lacks all identified cleavage sites in domain II of PE38, resulting in resistance to lysosomal degradation. The tolerated doses for HA22-LR are at least 10-fold higher than for HA22. SCID mice with CA46 xenograft tumors were treated every other day 3 times (on days 6, 8, and 10) intravenously with phosphate-buffered saline (times symbols), 0.3 mg/kg HA22 (open circles), or HA22-LR at 1.0 (closed triangles), 1.75 (open squares), or 2.5 (asterisks) mg/kg. Arrows indicate days when treatment was administered. Tumor size was measured over the course of 40 days. Points represent the mean tumor size of all mice in the treatment group. Error bars show the 95% confidence interval of each mean value from [60].

II, is resistant to lysosomal degradation, and retains biologic activity. HA22-LR killed chronic lymphocytic leukemia cells more potently and uniformly, and mice tolerated doses at least 10-fold higher than lethal doses of HA22, and these higher doses exhibited markedly enhanced antitumor activity (Figure 45.8) [60]. As PE38 is a bacterial protein, patients frequently produce antibodies that neutralize its activity, therefore preventing retreatment. Certain B-cell epitopes are already removed by the deletion of the major part of domain II in HA22-LR and further mutations of six residues in domain III resulted in removal of most B-cell epitopes [71]. This improved targeted toxin, HA22-LR-6X, is cytotoxic to several lymphoma cell lines, has very low nonspecific toxicity, and retains potent antitumor activity in mice with CA46 lymphomas. Three major histocompatibility complex-divergent strains of mice immunized with 5-μg doses of HA22-LR-6X elicited significantly lower antibody responses than HA22 or other mutants with fewer epitopes removed. Even large doses of HA22-LR-6X (50 μg) induced markedly lower antibody responses than 5 μg of HA22, indicating that high doses can be administered with low immunogenicity.

Another example for the improvement of targeted protein toxins is based on the prolongation of the intracellular retention time after endocytosis. The transferrin receptor is overexpressed on glioblastoma multiforme – the most common and lethal primary brain tumor. A major limitation of transferrin-based therapeutics is

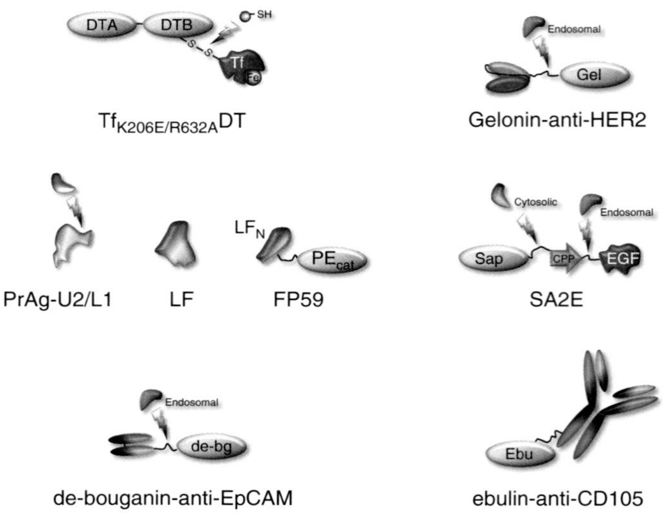

Figure 45.9 Examples for bacterial and plant toxin-related targeted protein toxins. All depicted targeted protein toxins are described in detail in the text. Cleavage sites by endosomal or cytosolic proteases as well as reducible sites are labeled. de-bg, deglycosylated bouganin; DTA and DTB, A- and B-chain of diphtheria toxin; Ebu, ebulin; Gel, gelonin; LF$_N$, N-terminal fragment of lethal factor; PE, *Pseudomonas* exotoxin A; Sap, saporin; Tf, transferrin; see text for other abbreviations.

the rapid recycling of endocytosed ferri-transferrin after release of the two bound iron ions. Two transferrin double mutants (K206E/R632A and K206E/K534A), in which iron is locked into each of the two homologous lobes, were conjugated to diphtheria toxin (Figure 45.9). After treatment of a monolayer culture of glioma cells, these conjugates showed an enhanced cellular association as well as enhanced delivery of diphtheria toxin in comparison to conjugates with wild-type transferrin. Treatment of glioblastoma cell U87: EGFRvIII xenografts with toxin conjugates containing mutant transferrin resulted in pronounced tumor regression in nude mice [72]. The utilized cell line expresses EGFRvIII, a constitutively active mutant variant of the EGF receptor (EGFR), which leads to more rapid proliferation than the typical U87 cell line. Each tumor received 0.25 μg of the conjugates every other day starting at day 0 and ending on day 6.

A strategy different from classical targeted toxins is applied by the use of anthrax toxin (Figure 45.9). Here, protective antigen of anthrax toxin was mutated to be activated by MMP-2 instead of the widely expressed furin [17]. This mutation resulted in specific tumor cell killing only of tumor cells overexpressing MMP-2. The mutant protective antigen was designated as PrAg-L1. In a further study another tumor-associated protease, urokinase plasminogen activator, was utilized, resulting in specific activation of the mutant PrAg-U2 on various tumor cells [73]. Further modifications of the intermolecular binding sites within protective antigen permitted the generation of intermolecular complementing protective antigens,

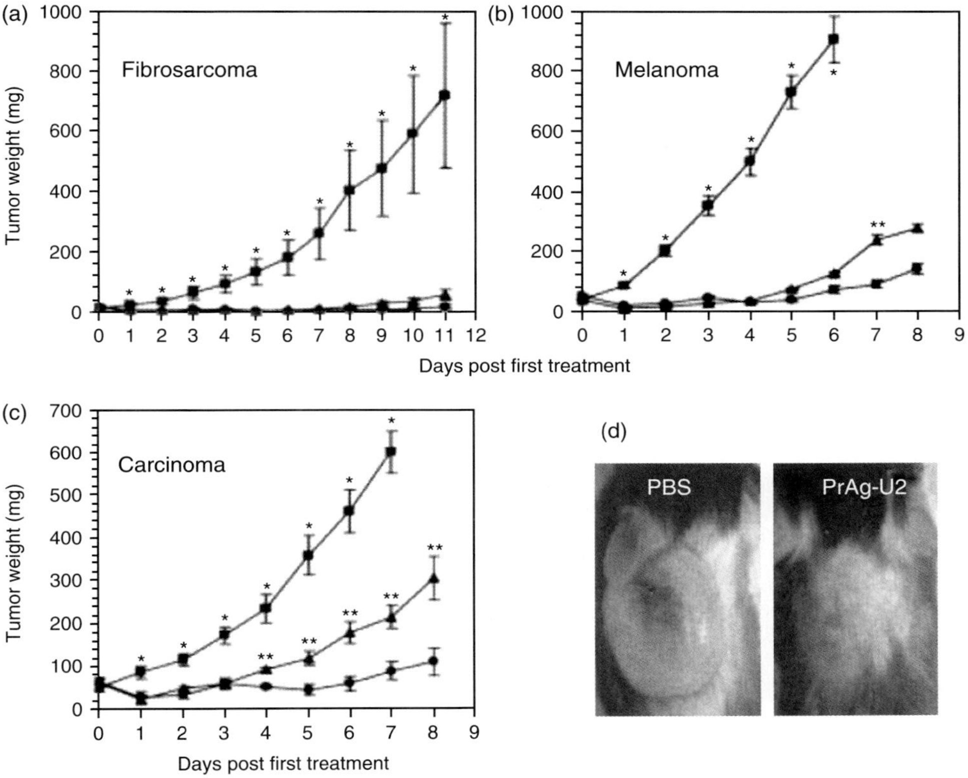

Figure 45.10 Tumor growth inhibition by the combination of anthrax toxin protective antigen variant PrAgU2 and the fusion protein of anthrax toxin lethal factor N-terminus and *Pseudomonas* exotoxin A catalytic domain (FP59) in C57BL/6J mice. The study was performed in mice that were injected intradermally with 0.3×10^6 murine T241 fibrosarcoma cells (a), 0.5×10^6 murine B16-BL6 melanoma cells (b), and 0.5×10^6 murine Lewis lung carcinoma cells (c). Treatment was initiated when the tumors had reached a size ranging from 0.05 to 0.5% of total body mass. The drugs were administered intradermally either once (on day 0) or twice (on day 0 and day 3). Mice were treated with phosphate-buffered saline on day 0 and day 3 (filled squares), 15 μg PrAgU2 and 5 μg FP59 on day 0 and phosphate-buffered saline on day 3 (filled triangles), or PrAgU2 and FP59 on both day 0 and day 3 (filled circles). Both treatment regimen significantly reduced tumor growth (*significance ($P < 0.05$) of phosphate-buffered saline treatment versus single treatment with PrAg-U2; **significance ($P < 0.05$) of the single treatment with PrAg-U2 at day 0 versus treatment with PrAg-U2 on both day 0 and day 3). The data points indicate the mean tumor weight, the bars denote the standard error. (d) Representative example of the appearance of T241 fibrosarcoma-bearing mice 14 days after phosphate-buffered saline treatment (PBS; left) or PrAgU2/FP59 treatment (right). (Reproduced with permission from [74].)

which result in activation only upon dual cleavage by MMP-2 and urokinase plasminogen activator [16]. The toxic component for these studies was wild-type lethal factor, which proved to effectively inhibit tumor growth *in vivo*. Other studies were performed with a fusion of the N-terminal 254 amino acids of lethal factor and the domain III of *Pseudomonas* exotoxin A (Figure 45.10) [74, 75].

45.3.1.2 **Drugs Based on Plant Toxins**

Targeted drugs based on plant protein toxins are typically improved by the same general strategies as applied to bacterial toxins; however, in contrast to them, there is a high number of known toxins (Table 45.1) and more are continuously being discovered. This results in a large variety of targeted toxins with different advantageous properties. Bouganin, a type I RIP isolated from the leaf of *Bougainvillea spectabilis* Wild., was mutated to remove the T-cell epitopes while preserving the biological activity of the wild-type molecule. This variant, referred to as de-bouganin, was genetically linked to either the N- or C-terminal end of either the heavy or light chain of an antiepithelial cell adhesion molecule Fab moiety (Figure 45.9). The peptidic linker contained a furin proteolytic site. Only constructs with de-bouganin at the C-terminus of the targeting moiety were expressed at full length. The targeted toxins bound and selectively killed target cell lines with a greater potency than many commonly used chemotherapeutic agents. *In vivo* efficacy was demonstrated using a human tumor xenograft model in SCID mice with the majority of the mice treated being tumor free at the end of the study (Figure 45.11) [41].

The goal of another study was to characterize a series of anti-HER2/*neu* constructs to identify how different antibodies and linker choices affect specificity and cytotoxicity. The targeted toxins contain either the human scFv antibody C6.5 or the murine scFv antibody e23 fused to the type I RIP gelonin via one of either a noncleavable linker or two linkers containing furin cleavage sites (Figure 45.9). The fusion proteins with the noncleavable linker retained the specificity of the original antibodies as well as the biological activity of gelonin and displayed similar cytotoxicity against different carcinoma cells. In contrast to other studies presented in this chapter, the introduction of a cleavable linker did not result in any benefit. The constructs exhibited very similar intracellular gelonin release, cytotoxic kinetics, and induction of autophagic cell death *in vitro*. Tumor inhibition in SKOV-3 ovarian tumor xenografts was more efficient with constructs containing the noncleavable linker than with those containing furin linkers [43].

Further studies using the type I RIP saporin shed light on the combined use of CPPs, cleavable peptides, and enhancer substances (Figure 45.9). Herein, a multifunctional molecular adapter that links the toxic and targeting moiety was developed. It was designed to improve endosomal escape, retain the toxin inside the cytosol, and detoxify the drug after cell death, and consists of an endosomal cleavable peptide, the translocation motif from the PreS2 domain of hepatitis B virus surface antigen, and a cytosolic cleavable peptide. Saporin was linked either directly or via the adapter to EGF as the targeting moiety [45]. After optimizing the molecular adapter *in vitro*, the fusion protein was tested in different mouse tumor models. The lethal toxicity for BALB/c mice was 3 times less for the adapter-containing toxin

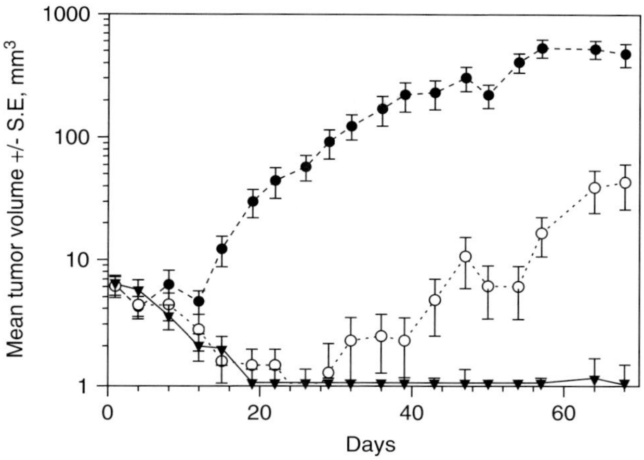

Figure 45.11 Treatment of human ovarian tumor xenografts in SCID mice with VB6-845-C_L. This targeted toxin is composed of a T-cell epitope-depleted variant of the type I RIP bouganin and an antiepithelial cell adhesion molecule Fab moiety. The genetic linkage occurred to the C-terminal end of the light chain via a peptidic linker containing a furin proteolytic site. NIH OVCAR-3 human ovarian tumors (1 mm^3) were subcutaneously implanted into the flank of female CB.17 SCID mice. After day 8 of implantation at an approximate tumor size of 5 mm^3, 15 mice per dose were injected with either formulation buffer (filled circles) or VB6-845-C_L at 10 (open circles) or 20 mg/kg (filled triangles) for 5 consecutive days for 3 weeks, and then received maintenance dosing on Monday and Friday for 4 weeks. VB6-845-C_L was administered in a bolus injection via the tail vein until day 26 when due to tail swelling, route of administration was changed to intraperitoneal for the remaining seven doses. In the 20 mg/kg cohort, 12 out of 15 mice were tumor-free at the end of the study (25 days after the last dose), which was statistically significant from the untreated group (log-rank test $P < 0.001$) [41].

(SA2E) than for the corresponding toxin without adapter (SE) and severe side-effects were drastically reduced. In a syngeneic mouse mammary adenocarcinoma model with cells expressing the human target receptor, SA2E-treated mice exhibited 71% regression in tumor weight with an almost complete suppression in 60% of the cases, whereas SE only led to 33% regression (Figure 45.7) [38]. In a second model, application of SA2E resulted in up to 60% reduction of primary human cervical cancer xenografts in SCID beige mice [76]. Further improvement was achieved by a combined application of SA2E with the triterpenoid composite saponinum album from *Gypsophila paniculata,* which enhances the specific cytotoxicity on tumor target cells up to 385 000-fold, whereas nontarget cells are affected less than 1000-fold, thus broadening the therapeutic window (Figure 45.12) [52]. In the BALB/c mouse tumor model mentioned above, this highly synergistic effect resulted in 94% tumor volume reduction although a 50-fold lower SA2E concentration compared to treatment without saponinum album was used. Side-effects were only moderate and reversible [51].

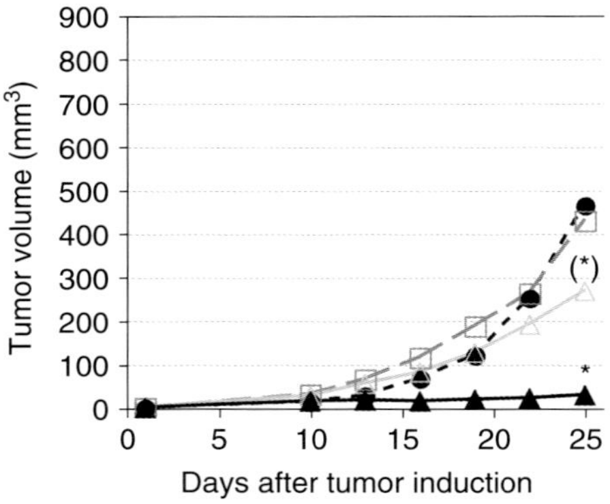

Figure 45.12 Progress of tumor growth in BALB/c mice after treatment with SA2E in combination with saponinum album (see Figure 45.7 for details concerning the tumor model and the targeted toxin SA2E). Saponinum album is a natural composite of glycosylated triterpenoids from the ornamental flower *G. paniculata* L. Saponinum album was injected subcutaneously in the neck and SA2E 1 h later subcutaneously in the vicinity of the tumor in the right flank. Each group was treated 6 times with the indicated drugs, beginning on day 4 after tumor inoculation (ongoing every 3 days) and the experiment ended on day 25. Only mice with developing tumors were used for the experiment. Data points represent the mean tumor volume of mock-treated BALB/c mice (closed circles, $n = 7$) and mice treated with 0.1 μg SA2E alone (open triangles, $n = 10$), 30 μg saponinum album alone (open squares, $n = 13$), and the combination of both in the same concentrations (closed triangles, $n = 10$). Statistical significance in comparison to mock-treated mice was $P = 0.051$ for SA2E alone and $P = 0.001$ for the combination treatment. (Reproduced with permission from [51].)

The low *in vivo* toxicity of the type II RIP ebulin-1 as compared to ricin makes this protein to an interesting candidate for targeted toxins. Since CD105 is being considered as a potential target for the antivascular therapy of tumors, ebulin-1 was chemically linked to the mouse antihuman CD105 mAb 44G4 (Figure 45.9). The conjugation does not affect the activity of ebulin-l. The targeted toxin displays cytotoxicity on human $CD105^+$ cells in the lower nanomolar range whereas cells lacking human CD105 were 100- to 300-fold less sensitive. Antibody-free ebulin-1 was effective in the micromolar range [77].

45.3.1.3 **Drugs Based on Human Proteins**

As detailed above, human proteins play an important role in the development of targeting toxins due to the predicted absence of immunogenicity; however, strong efforts are necessary to improve cytosolic uptake since human toxins lack a natural membrane transfer mechanism. A promising toxin candidate is granzyme B – a human serine protease originating from cytotoxic granules of $CD8^+$ T-lymphocytes and natural killer cells. Granzyme B was genetically fused to H22 (Figure 45.13) – a humanized anti-CD64 scFv antibody recognizing cells of certain subtypes of acute myeloid leukemia. The fusion protein bound specifically to $CD64^+$ cells and proteolytic activity was identical to that of free granzyme B.

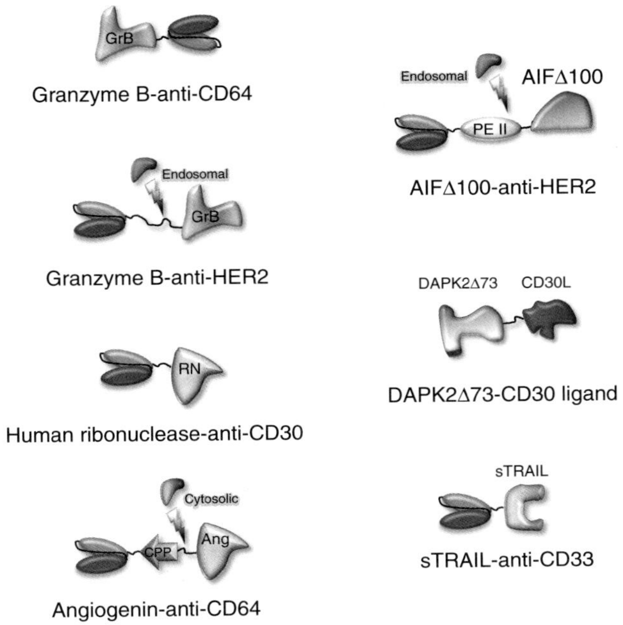

Figure 45.13 Examples for human enzyme-related targeted protein toxins. All depicted targeted protein toxins are described in detail in the text. Cleavage sites by endosomal or cytosolic proteases are labeled. $AIF_{\Delta 100}$, AIF lacking the first 100 amino acids; Ang, angiogenin; CD30L, CD30 ligand; $DAPK2_{\Delta 73}$, DAPK2 lacking the first 73 amino acids; GrB, granzyme B; PE II, *Pseudomonas* exotoxin A domain II; RN, RNase; see text for other abbreviations.

Target cell-specific cytotoxicity was observed in the lower nanomolar range and apoptosis was observed in primary $CD64^+$ acute myeloid leukemia cells, whereas $CD64^-$ acute myeloid leukemia cells remained unaffected [78]. Domain II of *Pseudomonas* exotoxin A has been shown to facilitate the translocation into the cytoplasm and can transport heterologous molecules into target cells. Since the full-length domain may elicit a host immune response, Zhang *et al.* tried to identify the minimal translocation motif and used this fragment as the linker between the anti-HER2/*neu* scFv antibody e23 and granzyme B (Figure 45.13). Notably, the fusion protein that contains only the furin cleavage site of domain II still induced apoptosis of HER2-positive breast adenocarcinoma SK-BR-3 cells. Moreover, this sequence is virtually identical to the essential part of domain II in HA22-LR described above. Delivery of the recombinant protein by intramuscular injection of lipofectamine-encapsulated plasmids led to an apparent tumor regression in a nude mouse xenograft SK-BR-3 model [42].

RNases form another group of enzymes suitable for humanized protein drugs. A targeted toxin composed of human pancreatic RNase fused to an anti-CD30 scFv antibody was designed to treat Hodgkin's lymphoma and anaplastic large

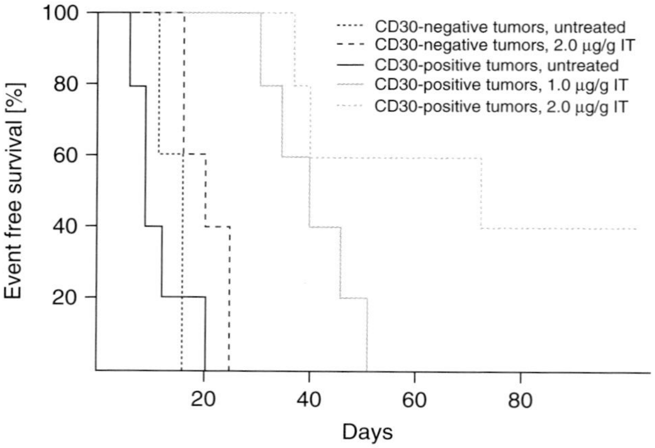

Figure 45.14 *In vivo* evaluation of a targeted RNase. Ber-H2-scFv-hpRNase is a targeted toxin composed of an anti-CD30 scFv antibody fused to the human pancreatic RNase. The tumor model was similar to that described in Figure 45.7 with the difference that TSA cells were transfected with human CD30 as target antigen. For tumor induction 5×10^6 cells were subcutaneously injected in 10- to 12-week-old BALB/c mice. Ber-H2-scFv-hpRNase (1.0 or 2.0 μg/g) or phosphate-buffered saline (untreated) was administered intraperitoneally (i.p.) at day 0 and 2. The Kaplan–Meyer plot shows event-free survival defined as a tumor volume less than 1 ml. The graph shows the data of one representative experiment out of three independent experiments. Five mice were included in each experiment per treatment arm. Two mice, inoculated with $CD30^+$ tumor cells, did not develop a tumor greater than 1 ml following application of 2.0 μg/g body weight. Reduction in tumor growth was statistically significant ($P < 0.05$) for 1.0 μg/g compared to untreated controls and for 2.0 compared to 1.0 μg/g [79].

cell lymphoma, which exhibit strong CD30 expression (Figure 45.13). The fusion protein showed CD30-specific binding and ribonucleolytic activity resistant to the inhibitor RNasin. It revealed CD30-specific antitumor activity *in vivo* as demonstrated in BALB/c mice that were challenged with $CD30^+$ syngeneic tumor cells or, as a control, $CD30^-$ cells (Figure 45.14) [79]. Another example of an RNase-based targeted toxin is a fusion protein composed of the anti-CD64 scFv H22 described above, genetically fused to the human RNase angiogenin (Figure 45.13). As angiogenin lacks a dedicated translocation domain, the CPP-containing, cleavable adapter that was defined above for the type I RIP-based targeted toxin SA2E was incorporated in the angiogenin fusion protein. Although insertion of the adapter increased the cytotoxicity by up to 20-fold, serum stability was markedly reduced. Therefore, a modified adapter variant lacking the endosomal cleavable peptide was designed, and showed significantly higher cytotoxicity than the adapter-free toxin and superior serum stability [27].

AIF is a mitochondrial flavoprotein that is an important mediator of caspase-independent programmed cell death. Two targeted toxins were designed containing the truncated AIF derivative $AIF_{\Delta 100}$ that lacks the mitochondrial import signal (Figure 45.13). In both drugs the targeting moiety was the anti-HER2/*neu* scFv antibody FRP5; one fusion protein harbored in addition the translocation domain II of *Pseudomonas* exotoxin A to facilitate endosomal escape. Potent cell killing activity was strictly dependent on the expression of HER2 on the target cell surface, but was only observed in the presence of the endosomolytic reagent chloroquine for the domain II-containing targeted toxin, and not for the direct fusion of $AIF_{\Delta 100}$ and FRP5 [31].

DAPK2 is a calcium/calmodulin-regulated proapoptotic kinase that acts as a tumor suppressor. To determine whether selective reconstitution of DAPK2 catalytic activity in DAPK2-depleted cells can induce apoptosis, Tur *et al.* created a fusion protein comprising a human CD30 ligand and a constitutively active human DAPK2 calmodulin-deletion mutant (Figure 45.13). The authors demonstrated that this fusion protein induces apoptosis specifically in $CD30^+$ and DAPK2-negative tumor cells *in vitro* and significantly prolonged overall survival in a disseminated Hodgkin's lymphoma xenograft SCID mouse model (Figure 45.15) [80].

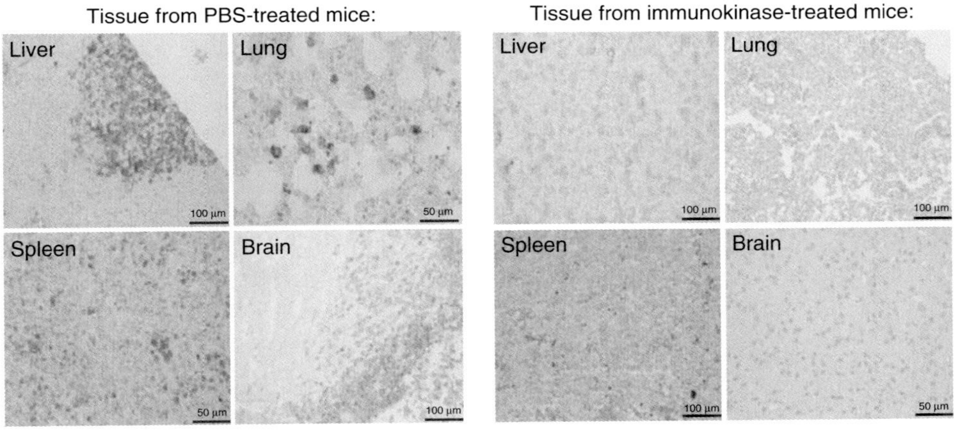

Figure 45.15 Treatment of disseminated tumors by a targeted kinase. DAPK2 has proapoptotic and tumor-suppressive functions, but expression in various cancer cell lines is low or completely blocked. $DAPK2_{\Delta 73}$ is a tumor-targeting fusion protein developed by combining CD30 ligand with a constitutively active version of DAPK2. In SCID mice, the intravenous injection of Hodgkin's lymphoma-derived L540 cells resulted in disseminated growth of tumor cells within 5–6 weeks. Antitumor treatment started one day after tumor challenge by administering the maximum tolerable dose of 70 μg per mouse. The overall survival rate (eight out of 10 mice survived longer than 175 days) was significantly higher ($P = 0.028$) than of controls treated with phosphate-buffered saline (PBS; mean survival 55 days) or a nonspecific targeted kinase (mean survival 60 days). The figure depicts immunohistochemical analyses of selected organ sections from the control group (phosphate-buffered saline) and the $DAPK2_{\Delta 73}$ ("immunokinase")-treated group. Many $CD30^+$ cells were observed after staining with a monoclonal anti-CD30 antibody in control sections, while no evidence of disseminated tumor cells is present in sections of treated mice. (Reproduced with permission from [80].)

The last example for the drugs based on human proteins is a fusion construct of an anti-CD33 scFv antibody and the soluble TRAIL (sTRAIL) (Figure 45.13). The efficacy of this fusion protein was compared with gemtuzumab ozogamicin (Mylotarg), which is an anti-CD33 antibody chemically coupled to a highly cytotoxic calicheamicin (see other chapters in this volume). The sTRAIL fusion protein was up to 30-fold more active on acute myeloid leukemia cells than gemtuzumab ozogamicin. Moreover, it showed potent antileukemia activity toward $CD33^+$ chronic myelogenous leukemia cells when treatment was combined with the tyrosine kinase inhibitor imatinib (Gleevec®/Glivec®). *Ex vivo* treatment of patient-derived $CD33^+$ acute myeloid leukemia tumor cells with the sTRAIL fusion resulted in potent apoptosis induction that was enhanced by valproic acid, mitoxantrone and 17-(allylamino)-17-demethoxygeldanamycin. Normal $CD33^+$ monocytes were fully resistant to prolonged treatment with the sTRAIL fusion protein, whereas treatment with gemtuzumab ozogamicin resulted in substantial cytotoxicity [81].

45.3.2 Clinical Development

By the end of the first decade of this century more than 40 targeted protein toxins had been or were being tested in clinical trials. All employed toxins are either ADP-ribosylating proteins derived from bacteria (Tables 45.2 and 45.3) or RIPs derived from plants (Table 45.4). One member of the RNase family, ranpirnase from the northern leopard frog, is also being tested in clinical phase III, yet without a conjugated targeted moiety. Since ranpirnase immunoconjugates were effective in preclinical animal models and ranpirnase, although not human, is a representative member of the newly developed toxins in protein-based targeted drugs, it is presented as an example in this chapter.

45.3.2.1 Denileukin Diftitox

Denileukin diftitox (Ontak®) is the first and, until 2010, sole targeted protein toxin approved by the US Food and Drug Administration (FDA), in February 1999, for the treatment of cutaneous T-cell lymphoma (CTCL) on condition to provide further data from clinical studies. It is composed of the catalytic and membrane transfer domain of diphtheria toxin and IL-2 as targeting moiety for malignant T-lymphocytes (Figure 45.16). Preclinical data showed that 90% of treated animals exhibited no evidence of malignancy in a histological analysis (Figure 45.17). A phase III, placebo-controlled, randomized trial was designed to investigate efficacy and safety of two doses of denileukin diftitox in patients with stage IA/III, CD25 assay-positive CTCL [82]. Patients ($n = 144$) with biopsy-confirmed, CD25 assay-positive CTCL were randomly assigned to a dose of 9 μg/kg/day ($n = 45$), 18 μg/kg/day ($n = 55$), or placebo infusions ($n = 44$), administered for 5 consecutive days every 3 weeks for up to eight cycles. The overall response rate was 44% for all participants treated with verum ($n = 100$; 10% complete response and 34% partial response) compared with 16% for placebo-treated patients (2% complete response and 14% partial response). According to the authors, this

Table 45.2 Targeted diphtheria toxin variants in clinical trials for tumor therapy.

Name	Molecular target	Binding moiety	Amino acids of the toxin	Indication
A-dmDT390-bisFv (UCHT1)	CD3ϵ	recombinant bivalent scFv antibody	1–390 mutated	T-cell lymphomas, T-cell leukemias
DT2219ARL	CD19, CD22	recombinant bispecific scFv antibody	1–390	B-cell lymphomas, B-cell leukemias
Denileukin diftitox, Ontak® (DAB_{389}IL2)	IL-2 receptor	IL-2	1–387	CTCL, non-Hodgkin's lymphoma (B- or T-cell), chronic lymphocytic leukemia
DAB_{486}IL2	IL-2 receptor	IL-2	1–485	lymphoma, leukemia
DT388-IL3	IL-3 receptor	IL-3	1–389	acute myeloid leukemia, chronic myeloid leukemia
DAB_{389}EGF	EGFR-1	EGF	1–387	carcinoma
DT388-GM-CSF	granulocyte macrophage colony-stimulating factor receptor	granulocyte macrophage colony-stimulating factor	1–388	acute myeloid leukemia
Tf-CRM107	transferrin receptor	transferrin	complete mutated	brain and central nervous system tumors

study [82] documents for the first time that responses in CTCL treatment can be observed in patients receiving placebo, probably reflecting the waxing and waning of skin lesions that have been described in CTCL patients. Further analysis of placebo responses indicated significantly shorter progression-free survival and lesser benefits as measured by secondary and supporting endpoints addressing clinical benefit. The overall response rate was higher in the 18- versus 9-μg/kg/day group (49 versus 38%, respectively), and both doses were significantly superior to placebo. Progression-free survival was significantly longer (median greater than 2 years) for verum compared to placebo (median 124 days). Rates of moderately severe and severe adverse events were slightly higher in the verum groups, whereas

Table 45.3 Targeted *Pseudomonas* exotoxin A variants in clinical trials for tumor therapy.

Name	Molecular target	Binding moiety	Amino acids of the toxin	Indication
dsFv (RFB4)–PE38 (BL22, CAT-3888)	CD22	dsFv	253–364, 381–613	non-Hodgkin's lymphoma (B- or T-cell), chronic lymphocytic leukemia, hairy cell leukemia
dsFv (RFB4 mutant)–PE38 (HA22, CAT-8015)	CD22	dsFv	253–364, 381–613	hairy cell leukemia, chronic lymphocytic leukemia, prolymphocytic leukemia, small lymphocytic lymphoma
LMB-2	CD25	scFv	253–364, 381–613	non-Hodgkin's lymphoma (B- or T-cell), leukemias
IL-4(38–37)–PE38KDEL (NBI-3001)	IL-4 receptor	IL-4, mutated	253–364, 381–613 mutated	brain, central nervous system, kidney and breast tumors, NSCLC
IL13–PE38QQR (cintredekin besudotox)	IL-13 receptor	IL-13	253–364, 381–613 mutated	brain, central nervous system, and renal tumors
TP40	EGFR-1	transforming growth factor-α	253–613 mutated	bladder cancer, carcinoma *in situ*
TP38	EGFR-1	transforming growth factor-α	253–364, 381–613	brain and central nervous system tumors
MR1-1 (dsFv)–PE38KDEL	EGFRvIII	dsFv	253–364, 381–613 mutated	brain tumors
erb38	HER2	dsFv	253–364, 381–613	breast cancer, ovarian cancer
scFv (FRP5)-ETA	HER2	scFv	253–613	breast cancer
LMB-1	Lewis Y	mAb	253–364, 381–613	adenocarcinoma
LMB-9	Lewis Y	dsFv	253–364, 381–613	adenocarcinoma
LMB-7	Lewis Y	scFv	253–364, 381–613	adenocarcinoma
BR96(scFv)-PE40	Lewis Y	scFv	253–613	adenocarcinoma
OVB3-PE	Ovarian cancer antigen	mAb	complete	ovarian cancer
SS1 (dsFv)-PE38 (SS1P)	Mesothelin	dsFv	253–364, 381–613	mesothelioma, ovarian cancer

dsFv, disulfide-linked Fv antibodies.

Table 45.4 Targeted RIP variants in clinical trials for tumor therapy.

Name	Molecular target	Binding moiety	RIP[a]	Indication
Anti-CD6-bR	CD6	mAb	ricin, blocked	CTCL
Anti-CD7-dgA	CD7	mAb	ricin, dgA	T-cell non-Hodgkin's lymphoma
TXU-PAP	CD7	mAb	pokeweed antiviral protein	T-cell non-Hodgkin's lymphoma
Anti-B4-bR	CD19	mAb	ricin, blocked	B-cell non-Hodgkin's lymphoma
HD37-dgA (IMTOX-19)[b]	CD19	mAb	ricin, dgA	B-cell non-Hodgkin's lymphoma, acute lymphocytic leukemia
B43-PAP	CD19	mAb	pokeweed antiviral protein	acute lymphocytic leukemia
RFB4-dgA (IMTOX-22)[b]	CD22	mAb	ricin, dgA	B-cell non-Hodgkin's lymphoma, acute lymphocytic leukemia, chronic lymphocytic leukemia
RFB4-Fab′-dgA	CD22	Fab	ricin, dgA	B-cell non-Hodgkin's lymphoma
RFT5-dgA (IMTOX-25)	CD25	mAb	ricin, dgA	Hodgkin's disease, CTCL, melanoma
K_i-4.dgA	CD30	mAb	ricin, dgA	Hodgkin's disease
BER-H2-Sap6	CD30	mAb	saporin	Hodgkin's disease
Hum-195/rGel	CD33	mAb	gelonin	acute myeloid leukemia, chronic myeloid leukemia
Anti-My9-bR	CD33	mAb	ricin, blocked	acute myeloid leukemia
N901-bR	CD56	mAb	ricin, blocked	small-cell lung cancer
Anti-CEA-bR	carcinoembryonic antigen	mAb	ricin, blocked	colorectal cancer
454A12-rRA	transferrin receptor	mAb	ricin A	cerebrospinal fluid cancer
260F9-rRTA	55-kDa breast cancer antigen	mAb	ricin A	breast cancer
XomaZyme-791	72-kDa cancer antigen	mAb	ricin A	colorectal cancer
XomaZyme-Mel	melanoma antigen	mAb	ricin A	melanoma

[a] Ricin blocked, galactose-binding sites of the B-chain are blocked; ricin A, ricin A-chain only; ricin dgA, deglycosylated ricin A-chain only.
[b] HD37-dgA combined with RFB4-dgA known as Combotox.

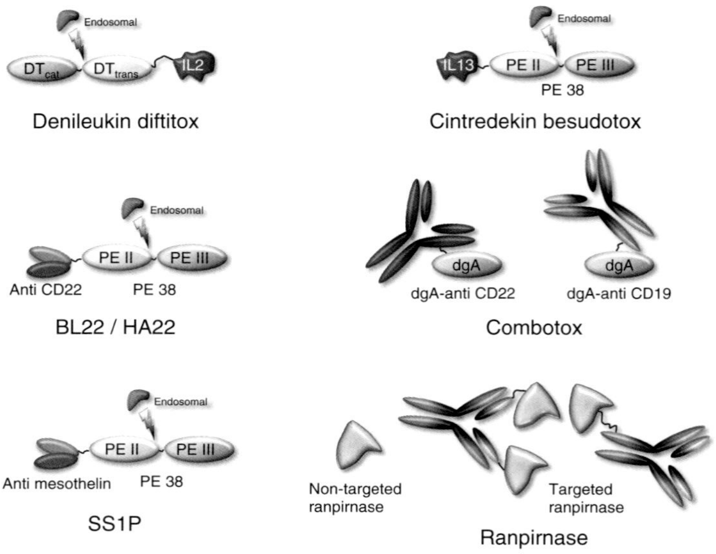

Figure 45.16 Examples of targeted protein toxins in clinical trials. All depicted targeted protein toxins are described in detail in the text. Cleavage sites by endosomal proteases are labeled. dgA, deglycosylated ricin A-chain; DT, diphtheria toxin; PE38 (PE II and III), *Pseudomonas* exotoxin A domains II and III; see text for other abbreviations.

moderate and mild adverse events were similar to placebo. No statistical differences were observed for drug-related serious adverse events. It can be concluded that denileukin diftitox had a significant and durable effect on the overall response rate and on progression-free survival with an acceptable safety profile in patients with early- and late-stage CTCL.

In another study, denileukin diftitox was tested for the treatment of advanced relapsed non-small-cell lung cancer (NSCLC) [83]. It was a multicenter phase II trial in patients with Eastern Cooperative Oncology Group performance status 0–2, stage IIIB/IV at diagnosis, who had failed at least one previous chemotherapy regimen. Denileukin diftitox was infused at 18 μg/kg/day for 5 days, every 21 days for one to six cycles. Among 41 patients enrolled, 44% had stable disease, 24% progressive disease, and 32% were not evaluable for response as they received less than two treatment cycles. The median time to disease progression was 1.8 months and median survival was 5.8 months. The median follow-up time was 16.1 months. One death from myocarditis verified at autopsy was attributed to treatment. One grade 4 toxicity (vascular leak syndrome) was encountered and 18 grade 3 toxicities, primarily gastrointestinal, vascular leak syndrome, and constitutional symptoms. Thus, in contrast to CTCL, denileukin diftitox at the current dose schedule has limited activity in patients with previously treated NSCLC, manifested by disease control without impact on survival.

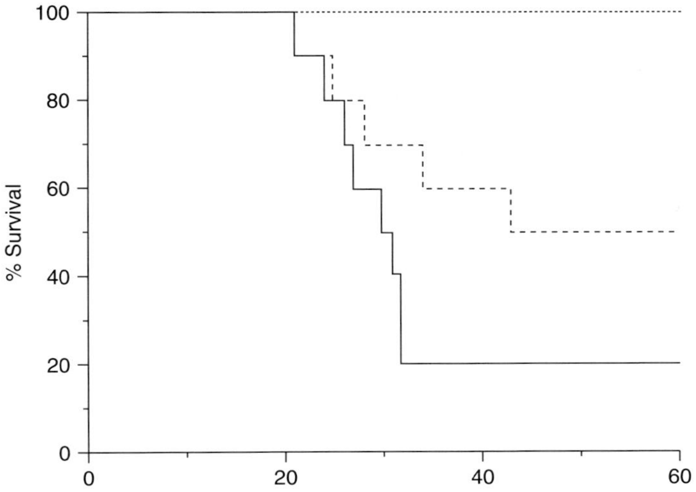

Figure 45.17 Impact of IL-2 receptor-targeted toxin treatment on survival of CP3-tumor-bearing animals. CP3 cells were derived from C57BL/6 mouse cytotoxic T-lymphocyte CTLL-2 cells by retroviral transfection with human IL-2 and selection for fast-growing variants. On day 0, three groups of 10 C57BL/6 mice were injected in the tail vein with 10^6 CP3 cells. On days 1–10, the mice received a daily intravenous injection of either 10 μg $DAB_{486}IL2$ (dashed line), 5 μg of $DAB_{389}IL2$ (denileukin diftitox) (dotted line), or Tris-buffered saline as control (solid line). The toxic moieties of the targeted proteins consist of differently sized fragments of diphtheria toxin (see Table 45.2). The animals were monitored to day 60 as illustrated by the Kaplan–Meyer curves and then killed. A histological analysis demonstrated that 90% of the $DAB_{389}IL2$-treated animals showed no evidence of malignancy upon microscopic examination while one of the two surviving buffer-treated controls had microscopic tumors. (Reproduced with permission from [84] Bacha (1991).)

45.3.2.2 **BL22/HA22**

CD22 is an inhibitory coreceptor of the B-cell receptor and plays a critical role in establishing signaling thresholds for B-cell activation. It is a member of the sialic acid-binding Ig-like lectin (Siglec) family and binds sialic acid residues with $\alpha 2$–6 linkages. CD22 is expressed on B-cell progenitors and more strongly on mature B-cells. Huang *et al.* showed that neoplastic cells in B-cell chronic lymphoproliferative disorders exhibit aberrant CD22 expression in 70% of cases, including chronic lymphocytic leukemia, mantle cell lymphoma, marginal zone lymphoma, hairy cell leukemia, and follicular lymphoma [85]. Thus, CD22 is a promising target for such diseases and an important alternative to the B-lymphocyte antigen CD20, which is targeted by approved antibodies or conjugated antibodies (e.g., rituximab (Rituxan®/MabThera®) and ibritumomab tiuxetan (Zevalin®)).

As described in more detail in Section 45.3.1.1, BL22 and HA22 are anti-CD22 targeted toxins based on *Pseudomonas* exotoxin A, while HA22 is a direct advancement of BL22 (Figure 45.16). A phase II trial in chemoresistant hairy cell leukemia was conducted with BL22 and patients who had relapsed/refractory hairy cell leukemia [86]. Patients were stratified into three groups: response to cladribine less than 1 year, those with a response lasting 1–4 years or no response, and uncontrolled infection. They received 40 μg/kg BL22 every other day for three doses on cycle 1. Patients achieving hematologic remission were observed; those without hematologic remission were retreated at 30 μg/kg every other day for three doses every 4 weeks beginning at least 8 weeks after cycle 1. In total, 36 patients were enrolled for the study. The response after one cycle (25% complete response and 25% partial response) improved when 56% were retreated (47% complete response and 25% partial response). The patients with baseline spleen height (the maximum vertical distance across the splenic hilum) lower than 200 mm ($n = 22$) had higher complete response (64 versus 21%) and overall response rates (95 versus 36%) compared to 14 patients with spleens either absent or higher than 200 mm. The only serious toxicity was reversible grade 3 hemolytic uremic syndrome, not requiring plasmapheresis, in two patients (6%). High neutralizing antibodies were observed in four patients (11%) and prevented retreatment. In conclusion, BL22 exhibited high efficacy in hairy cell leukemia and best responses were achieved after cladribine failure before the patients developed massive splenomegaly or underwent splenectomy. BL22 was also tested in $CD22^+$ hematologic malignancies of childhood [87]. Phase I trial cohorts were treated at escalating doses and schedules ranging from 10 to 40 μg/kg every other day for three or six doses repeated every 21 or 28 days. Treatment was associated with an acceptable safety profile, adverse events were rapidly reversible, and no maximum tolerated dose was defined.

HA22 is a high-affinity derivative of BL22 that displays higher CD22-binding and inhibitory activity due to mutation of three amino acids. Adult hairy cell leukemia patients who previously received at least two systemic therapies and had cytopenias or symptomatic splenomegaly requiring treatment were enclosed in a multicenter, dose-escalation, phase I study [88]. A standard 3 + 3 dose-escalation design was employed at doses of 5, 10, 20, 30, 40, and 50 μg/kg. HA22 was administered intravenously on days 1, 3, and 5 of each 28-day cycle for up to a total of 10 cycles. Three patients out of 26 enrolled at each of the 5, 10, 20, and 30 μg/kg dose levels, four patients at the 40 μg/kg dose level, and 10 patients at the 50 μg/kg dose level. Patients were heavily pretreated (e.g., 14 received prior rituximab). No dose-limiting toxicities were observed and a maximum tolerated dose was not achieved. Expanded enrollment at 50 μg/kg was undertaken to better characterize the safety profile and antitumor activity. The most common drug-related toxicities were grade 2 or lower severity. Four patients developed grade 2 vascular leak syndrome and one treatment-related serious adverse event occurred (a reversible grade 2 hemolytic uremic syndrome that was reported in the 30 μg/kg dose cohort). Antidrug antibodies developed in 10 patients (39%). Among the 26 patients treated, the objective response rate was 73% with a complete response rate of 35% and a partial response rate of 39%. Responses were observed at all dose levels. Specific objective response rates at the 5, 10, 20, 30, 40, and 50 μg/kg/dose cohorts were 100, 100, 33, 33, 75, and 80%, respectively. At the time of the data presentation, the authors reported no relapse of the patients achieving a complete response. Four of nine patients with complete response had a duration of more than 12 months at this time. These data demonstrate that HA22 is a promising new product candidate for patients with advanced hairy cell leukemia.

45.3.2.3 SS1P

Mesothelin is a tumor differentiation antigen that is normally present on the mesothelial cells lining the pleura, peritoneum, and pericardium. It is, however, highly expressed in several human cancers, including malignant mesothelioma, pancreatic, ovarian, and lung adenocarcinoma. The limited mesothelin expression in normal tissues and high expression in many cancers makes it an attractive candidate for cancer therapy [89]. SS1P is a mesothelin-targeting toxin that is composed of a disulfide-linked Fv antibody directed against mesothelin and the exotoxin A fragment PE38 (Figure 45.16). In a phase I trial patients were treated who had mesothelioma, ovarian, or pancreatic cancer, which were recurrent or unresectable despite standard therapy, and were mesothelin-positive by immunohistochemistry [90]. SS1P was given by continuous infusion for 10 days and cycles could be repeated at 4-week intervals in the absence of neutralizing antibodies or progressive disease. The patients ($n = 24$) received 4, 8, 12, 18, and 25 μg/kg/day × 10, five of them received a second cycle. The maximum tolerated dose was 25 μg/kg/day × 10, where one of six patients had dose-limiting toxicity due to reversible vascular leak syndrome. Immunogenicity was observed in 75% of patients. One patient had a partial response; nonmajor responses included cessation of ascites and independence from paracentesis, resolution of masses by positron emission tomography, and improved pain and range of motion. In summary, SS1P was well tolerated and showed evidence of modest clinical activity. Combination with chemotherapy may result in better benefit.

45.3.2.4 Cintredekin Besudotox

Cintredekin besudotox is an example of a *Pseudomonas* exotoxin A-based drug bearing an IL as targeting moiety (see Table 45.3) (Figure 45.16). In a phase III study, convection-enhanced delivery of this drug was compared with Gliadel wafers, which are polymers loaded with carmustine (a mustard gas-related compound) [91]. Patients with glioblastoma multiforme at first recurrence were randomized 2 : 1 to receive cintredekin besudotox or Gliadel wafers. The targeted toxin (0.5 μg/ml) was administered over 96 h with a flow rate of 0.75 ml/h via two to four intraparenchymal catheters placed after tumor resection. The median survival of 296 enrolled patients was 36 weeks for cintredekin besudotox and 35 weeks for Gliadel wafers. For the efficacy-evaluable population, the median survival was 45 weeks for cintredekin besudotox and 40 weeks for Gliadel wafers; however, the difference was not statistically significant. The adverse events profile was similar in both arms, except that pulmonary embolism was higher in the cintredekin besudotox arm (8 versus 1%). Further investigations are required to determine the final outcome of this targeted protein toxin.

45.3.2.5 Combotox

Combotox is a 1 : 1 mixture of two targeted toxins prepared from the deglycosylated ricin A-chain conjugated to mAbs directed against either CD22 (RFB4) or CD19 (HD37) (Figure 45.16). In a phase I dose-escalation study using Combotox in children ($n = 17$) with refractory or relapsed B-lineage acute lymphoblastic leukemia, patients were treated at four dose levels: 2, 4, 5, and 6 mg/m^2 [92]. The maximum tolerated dose was 5 mg/m^2 and graft-versus-host disease defined the maximum tolerated dose. Three patients experienced complete remission. Six additional patients experienced a decrease of more than 95% in their peripheral blood blast counts, and one patient experienced a decrease of 75%. Thus, Combotox can be safely administered to children with refractory leukemia and has clinically important anticancer activity as a single agent.

45.3.2.6 Ranpirnase

Ranpirnase (Onconase®) is not a targeted toxin, but instead represents a novel generation of mammalian toxins. It was tested in a nude mouse A549 human lung cancer xenograft model. At single doses of 5–10 mg/kg, ranpirnase was significantly and effectively tumoricidal, reaching a growth delay of 20–22 days compared to saline-treated control mice. Interestingly, two treatments with 2.5 mg/kg were more effective and resulted in a growth delay of 27 days [93]. A targeted ranpirnase was also effective in preclinical animal models (Figures 45.6 and 45.16) [30]. A multicenter phase II trial of ranpirnase as a single agent was conducted with patients suffering from unresectable and histologically confirmed malignant mesothelioma. Patients ($n = 105$) with Eastern Cooperative Oncology Group performance status 0–2 were enrolled onto the study [94]; 37% of patients had not responded to prior chemotherapy. Median survival times of 6 months for the intent-to-treat group and 8.3 months for the treatment target group populations were observed. The 1- and 2-year survival rates were 34 and 22% for the intent-to-treat group, respectively, and 42 and 27% for the treatment target group, respectively. Among the 81 patients assessable for tumor response, four had partial responses, two had minor regressions, and 35 experienced stabilization of previously progressive disease. Patients with responses and stable disease demonstrated markedly prolonged survival. Ranpirnase was well tolerated in the majority of patients and there were no drug-related deaths. Therefore, ranpirnase may be also developed to a promising toxin in targeted tumor therapies.

45.4 Conclusions and Perspectives

Forty years of targeted protein toxins have not yet brought about a masterstroke in tumor therapy and with the approval of only one product for cancer treatment thus far, the situation appears to be a gradual process. However, in the first two decades of development, the ideas were ahead of the technical capabilities of that time, and in the second two decades, a number of new challenges emerged from this utterly new approach, including production, immunogenicity, serious adverse events, and efficacy. During a lengthy learning process of alternating enthusiasm and disappointment, most of the teething troubles were successfully overcome. Even though a further decade may be required to round off half a century of research in targeted protein toxins before the final breakthrough will be declared, it can now be prognosticated with reasonable confidence that the pioneering work in the development of novel features including humanized molecules and strategies for efficient endosomal escape will result in emphatic success. It is expected that the new generations of targeted toxins will continue their way to potent anticancer drugs without considerable off-target effects. In the long term, even personalized fusion proteins may enter the market.

Acknowledgments

We acknowledge the financial support of our work on targeted tumor therapies by different foundations and organizations including the Deutsche Forschungsgemeinschaft, Deutsche Krebshilfe, Alexander von Humboldt-Stiftung, Sonnenfeldstiftung, and Berliner Krebsgesellschaft. We sincerely thank Suzanne Abdelazim for critically proofreading the manuscript.

References

1. Murphy, J.R., Williams, D.P., Bacha, P., Bishai, W., Waters, C., and Strom, T.B. (1988) Cell receptor specific targeted toxins: genetic construction and characterization of an interleukin 2 diphtheria toxin-related fusion protein. *J. Recept. Res.*, **8**, 467–480.
2. Platini, F., Perez-Tomas, R., Ambrosio, S., and Tessitore, L. (2010) Understanding autophagy in cell death control. *Curr. Pharm. Des.*, **16**, 101–113.
3. Fujisawa, T., Nakashima, H., Nakajima, A., Joshi, B.H., and Puri, R.K. (2011) Targeting IL-13Rα2 in human pancreatic ductal adenocarcinoma with combination therapy of IL-13–PE and gemcitabine. *Int. J. Cancer*, **128**, 1221–1223.
4. Hassan, R., Williams-Gould, J., Steinberg, S.M., Liewehr, D.J., Yokokawa, J., Tsang, K.Y., Surawski, R.J., Scott, T., and Camphausen, K. (2006) Tumor-directed radiation and the immunotoxin SS1P in the treatment of mesothelin-expressing tumor xenografts. *Clin. Cancer Res.*, **12**, 4983–4988.
5. Stewart, K.M., Horton, K.L., and Kelley, S.O. (2008) Cell-penetrating peptides as delivery vehicles for biology and medicine. *Org. Biomol. Chem.*, **6**, 2242–2255.
6. Vallera, D.A., Chen, H., Sicheneder, A.R., Panoskaltsis-Mortari, A., and Taras, E.P. (2009) Genetic alteration of a bispecific ligand-directed toxin targeting human CD19 and CD22 receptors resulting in improved efficacy against systemic B cell malignancy. *Leuk. Res.*, **33**, 1233–1242.
7. Vallera, D.A., Oh, S., Chen, H., Shu, Y., and Frankel, A.E. (2010) Bioengineering a unique deimmunized bispecific targeted toxin that simultaneously recognizes human CD22 and CD19 receptors in a mouse model of B-cell metastases. *Mol. Cancer Ther.*, **9**, 1872–1883.
8. Oh, S., Stish, B.J., Sachdev, D., Chen, H., Dudek, A.Z., and Vallera, D.A. (2009) A novel reduced immunogenicity bispecific targeted toxin simultaneously recognizing human epidermal

growth factor and interleukin-4 receptors in a mouse model of metastatic breast carcinoma. *Clin. Cancer Res.*, **15**, 6137–6147.

9. Moolten, F.L. and Cooperband, S.R. (1970) Selective destruction of target cells by diphtheria toxin conjugated to antibody directed against antigens on the cells. *Science*, **169**, 68–70.
10. Liu, S., Milne, G.T., Kuremsky, J.G., Fink, G.R., and Leppla, S.H. (2004) Identification of the proteins required for biosynthesis of diphthamide, the target of bacterial ADP-ribosylating toxins on translation elongation factor 2. *Mol. Cell. Biol.*, **24**, 9487–9497.
11. Jørgensen, R., Purdy, A.E., Fieldhouse, R.J., Kimber, M.S., Bartlett, D.H., and Merrill, A.R. (2008) Cholix toxin, a novel ADP-ribosylating factor from *Vibrio cholerae*. *J. Biol. Chem.*, **283**, 10671–10678.
12. Andersson, Y., Engebraaten, O., and Fodstad, O. (2009) Synergistic anti-cancer effects of immunotoxin and cyclosporin *in vitro* and *in vivo*. *Br. J. Cancer*, **101**, 1307–1315.
13. Blythman, H.E., Casellas, P., Gros, O., Gros, P., Jansen, F.K., Paolucci, F., Pau, B., and Vidal, H. (1981) Immunotoxins: hybrid molecules of monoclonal antibodies and a toxin subunit specifically kill tumour cells. *Nature*, **290** (5802), 145–146.
14. Mogridge, J., Cunningham, K., Lacy, D.B., Mourez, M., and Collier, R.J. (2002) The lethal and edema factors of anthrax toxin bind only to oligomeric forms of the protective antigen. *Proc. Natl. Acad. Sci. USA*, **99**, 7045–7048.
15. Kintzer, A.F., Thoren, K.L., Sterling, H.J., Dong, K.C., Feld, G.K., Tang, I.I., Zhang, T.T., Williams, E.R., Berger, J.M., and Krantz, B.A. (2009) The protective antigen component of anthrax toxin forms functional octameric complexes. *J. Mol. Biol.*, **392**, 614–629.
16. Liu, S., Redeye, V., Kuremsky, J.G., Kuhnen, M., Molinolo, A., Bugge, T.H., and Leppla, S.H. (2005) Intermolecular complementation achieves high-specificity tumor targeting by anthrax toxin. *Nat. Biotechnol.*, **23**, 725–730.
17. Liu, S., Netzel-Arnett, S., Birkedal-Hansen, H., and Leppla, S.H. (2000) Tumor cell-selective cytotoxicity of matrix metalloproteinase-activated anthrax toxin. *Cancer Res.*, **60**, 6061–6067.
18. Stirpe, F. (2004) Ribosome-inactivating proteins. *Toxicon*, **44**, 371–383.
19. Endo, Y., Mitsui, K., Motizuki, M., and Tsurugi, K. (1987) The mechanism of action of ricin and related toxic lectins on eukaryotic ribosomes. The site and the characteristics of the modification in 28 S ribosomal RNA caused by the toxins. *J. Biol. Chem.*, **262**, 5908–5912.
20. Citores, L., Ferreras, J.M., Munoz, R., Benitez, J., Jimenez, P., and Girbes, T. (2002) Targeting cancer cells with transferrin conjugates containing the non-toxic type 2 ribosome-inactivating proteins nigrin b or ebulin l. *Cancer Lett.*, **184**, 29–35.
21. Viel, T., Dransart, E., Nemati, F., Henry, E., Theze, B., Decaudin, D., Lewandowski, D., Boisgard, R., Johannes, L., and Tavitian, B. (2008) *In vivo* tumor targeting by the B-subunit of shiga toxin. *Mol. Imaging*, **7**, 239–247.
22. Endo, Y. and Wool, I.G. (1982) The site of action of alpha-sarcin on eukaryotic ribosomes. The sequence at the alpha-sarcin cleavage site in 28 S ribosomal ribonucleic acid. *J. Biol. Chem.*, **257**, 9054–9060.
23. D'Alatri, L., Di Massimo, A.M., Anastasi, A.M., Pacilli, A., Novelli, S., Saccinto, M.P., De Santis, R., Mele, A., and Parente, D. (1998) Production and characterisation of a recombinant single-chain anti ErbB2–clavin immunotoxin. *Anticancer Res.*, **18**, 3369–3373.
24. Wawrzynczak, E.J., Henry, R.V., Cumber, A.J., Parnell, G.D., Derbyshire, E.J., and Ulbrich, N. (1991) Biochemical, cytotoxic and pharmacokinetic properties of an immunotoxin composed of a mouse monoclonal antibody Fib75 and the ribosome-inactivating protein alpha-sarcin from *Aspergillus giganteus*. *Eur. J. Biochem.*, **196**, 203–209.

25. Rosenblum, M.G. and Barth, S. (2009) Development of novel, highly cytotoxic fusion constructs containing granzyme B: unique mechanisms and functions. *Curr. Pharm. Des.*, **15**, 2676–2692.
26. Gao, X. and Xu, Z. (2008) Mechanisms of action of angiogenin. *Acta Biochim. Biophys. Sin.*, **40**, 619–624.
27. Hetzel, C., Bachran, C., Fischer, R., Fuchs, H., Barth, S., and Stocker, M. (2008) Small cleavable adapters enhance the specific cytotoxicity of a humanized immunotoxin directed against CD64-positive cells. *J. Immunother.*, **31**, 370–376.
28. Russo, N., Shapiro, R., Acharya, K.R., Riordan, J.F., and Vallee, B.L. (1994) Role of glutamine-117 in the ribonucleolytic activity of human angiogenin. *Proc. Natl. Acad. Sci. USA*, **91**, 2920–2924.
29. Rybak, S.M. (2008) Antibody–onconase conjugates: cytotoxicity and intracellular routing. *Curr. Pharm. Biotechnol.*, **9**, 226–230.
30. Newton, D.L., Hansen, H.J., Mikulski, S.M., Goldenberg, D.M., and Rybak, S.M. (2001) Potent and specific antitumor effects of an anti-CD22-targeted cytotoxic ribonuclease: potential for the treatment of non-Hodgkin lymphoma. *Blood*, **97**, 528–535.
31. Mahmud, H., Dalken, B., and Wels, W.S. (2009) Induction of programmed cell death in ErbB2/HER2-expressing cancer cells by targeted delivery of apoptosis-inducing factor. *Mol. Cancer Ther.*, **8**, 1526–1535.
32. Tur, M.K., Neef, I., Jost, E., Galm, O., Jager, G., Stocker, M., Ribbert, M., Osieka, R., Klinge, U., and Barth, S. (2009) Targeted restoration of down-regulated DAPK2 tumor suppressor activity induces apoptosis in Hodgkin lymphoma cells. *J. Immunother.*, **32**, 431–441.
33. Li, H., Ray, G., Yoo, B.H., Erdogan, M., and Rosen, K.V. (2009) Down-regulation of death-associated protein kinase-2 is required for beta-catenin-induced anoikis resistance of malignant epithelial cells. *J. Biol. Chem.*, **284**, 2012–2022.
34. Pennarun, B., Meijer, A., de Vries, E.G., Kleibeuker, J.H., Kruyt, F., and de Jong, S. (2010) Playing the DISC: turning on TRAIL death receptor-mediated apoptosis in cancer. *Biochim. Biophys. Acta*, **1805**, 123–140.
35. Sawant, R. and Torchilin, V. (2010) Intracellular transduction using cell-penetrating peptides. *Mol. Biosyst.*, **6**, 628–640.
36. Snyder, E.L., Saenz, C.C., Denicourt, C., Meade, B.R., Cui, X.S., Kaplan, I.M., and Dowdy, S.F. (2005) Enhanced targeting and killing of tumor cells expressing the CXC chemokine receptor 4 by transducible anticancer peptides. *Cancer Res.*, **65**, 10646–10650.
37. Lorenzetti, I., Meneguzzi, A., Fracasso, G., Potrich, C., Costantini, L., Chiesa, E., Legname, G., Menestrina, G., Tridente, G., and Colombatti, M. (2000) Genetic grafting of membrane-acting peptides to the cytotoxin dianthin augments its ability to de-stabilize lipid bilayers and enhances its cytotoxic potential as the component of transferrin–toxin conjugates. *Int. J. Cancer*, **86**, 582–589.
38. Fuchs, H., Bachran, C., Li, T., Heisler, I., Durkop, H., and Sutherland, M. (2007) A cleavable molecular adapter reduces side effects and concomitantly enhances efficacy in tumor treatment by targeted toxins in mice. *J. Control. Release*, **117**, 342–350.
39. Olson, E.S., Aguilera, T.A., Jiang, T., Ellies, L.G., Nguyen, Q.T., Wong, E.H., Gross, L.A., and Tsien, R.Y. (2009) *In vivo* characterization of activatable cell penetrating peptides for targeting protease activity in cancer. *Integr. Biol.*, **1**, 382–393.
40. Fuchs, H., Bachran, C., Heisler, I., and Sutherland, M. (2005) A closer look at protein transduction domains as a tool in drug delivery. *Curr. Nanosci.*, **1**, 117–124.
41. Cizeau, J., Grenkow, D.M., Brown, J.G., Entwistle, J., and MacDonald, G.C. (2009) Engineering and biological characterization of VB6-845, an anti-EpCAM immunotoxin containing a T-cell epitope-depleted variant of the

plant toxin bouganin. *J. Immunother.*, **32**, 574–584.

42. Zhang, L., Zhao, J., Wang, T., Yu, C.J., Jia, L.T., Duan, Y.Y., Yao, L.B., Chen, S.Y., and Yang, A.G. (2008) HER2-targeting recombinant protein with truncated *Pseudomonas* exotoxin A translocation domain efficiently kills breast cancer cells. *Cancer Biol. Ther.*, **7**, 1226–1231.
43. Cao, Y., Marks, J.D., Marks, J.W., Cheung, L.H., Kim, S., and Rosenblum, M.G. (2009) Construction and characterization of novel, recombinant immunotoxins targeting the Her2/*neu* oncogene product: *in vitro* and *in vivo* studies. *Cancer Res.*, **69**, 8987–8995.
44. Hetzel, C., Bachran, C., Tur, M.K., Fuchs, H., and Stocker, M. (2009) Improved immunotoxins with novel functional elements. *Curr. Pharm. Des.*, **15**, 2700–2711.
45. Heisler, I., Keller, J., Tauber, R., Sutherland, M., and Fuchs, H. (2003) A cleavable adapter to reduce nonspecific cytotoxicity of recombinant immunotoxins. *Int. J. Cancer*, **103**, 277–282.
46. Del Gaizo, V. and Payne, R.M. (2003) A novel TAT-mitochondrial signal sequence fusion protein is processed, stays in mitochondria, and crosses the placenta. *Mol. Ther.*, **7**, 720–730.
47. Chen, X., Bai, Y., Zaro, J.L., and Shen, W.-C. (2010) Design of an *in vivo* cleavable disulfide linker in recombinant fusion proteins. *BioTechniques*, **49**, 513–518.
48. Wu, M. (1997) Enhancement of immunotoxin activity using chemical and biological reagents. *Br. J. Cancer*, **75**, 1347–1355.
49. Vago, R., Marsden, C.J., Lord, J.M., Ippoliti, R., Flavell, D.J., Flavell, S.U., Ceriotti, A., and Fabbrini, M.S. (2005) Saporin and ricin A chain follow different intracellular routes to enter the cytosol of intoxicated cells. *FEBS J.*, **272**, 4983–4995.
50. Davol, P.A., Bizuneh, A., and Frackelton, A.R. Jr. (1999) Wortmannin, a phosphoinositide 3-kinase inhibitor, selectively enhances cytotoxicity of receptor-directed-toxin chimeras *in vitro* and *in vivo*. *Anticancer Res.*, **19**, 1705–1713.
51. Bachran, C., Durkop, H., Sutherland, M., Bachran, D., Muller, C., Weng, A., Melzig, M.F., and Fuchs, H. (2009) Inhibition of tumor growth by targeted toxins in mice is dramatically improved by saponinum album in a synergistic way. *J. Immunother.*, **32**, 713–725.
52. Heisler, I., Sutherland, M., Bachran, C., Hebestreit, P., Schnitger, A., Melzig, M.F., and Fuchs, H. (2005) Combined application of saponin and chimeric toxins drastically enhances the targeted cytotoxicity on tumor cells. *J. Control. Release*, **106**, 123–137.
53. Berg, K., Folini, M., Prasmickaite, L., Selbo, P.K., Bonsted, A., Engesaeter, B.O., Zaffaroni, N., Weyergang, A., Dietze, A., Maelandsmo, G.M., Wagner, E., Norum, O.J., and Hogset, A. (2007) Photochemical internalization: a new tool for drug delivery. *Curr. Pharm. Biotechnol.*, **8**, 362–372.
54. Chen, Y.J. and Inouye, M. (2008) The intramolecular chaperone-mediated protein folding. *Curr. Opin. Struct. Biol.*, **18**, 765–770.
55. Borges, J.C. and Ramos, C.H. (2005) Protein folding assisted by chaperones. *Protein Pept. Lett.*, **12**, 257–261.
56. Shental-Bechor, D. and Levy, Y. (2009) Folding of glycoproteins: toward understanding the biophysics of the glycosylation code. *Curr. Opin. Struct. Biol.*, **19**, 524–533.
57. Fabbrini, M.S., Carpani, D., Soria, M.R., and Ceriotti, A. (2000) Cytosolic immunization allows the expression of preATF–saporin chimeric toxin in eukaryotic cells. *FASEB J.*, **14**, 391–398.
58. Giansanti, F., Di Leandro, L., Koutris, I., Pitari, G., Fabbrini, M.S., Lombardi, A., Flavell, D.J., Flavell, S.U., Gianni, S., and Ippoliti, R. (2010) Engineering a switchable toxin: the potential use of PDZ domains in the expression, targeting and activation of modified saporin variants. *Protein Eng. Des. Sel.*, **23**, 61–68.
59. Lombardi, A., Bursomanno, S., Lopardo, T., Traini, R., Colombatti, M.,

Ippoliti, R., Flavell, D.J., Flavell, S.U., Ceriotti, A., and Fabbrini, M.S. (2010) *Pichia pastoris* as a host for secretion of toxic saporin chimeras. *FASEB J.*, **24**, 253–265.

60. Weldon, J.E., Xiang, L., Chertov, O., Margulies, I., Kreitman, R.J., FitzGerald, D.J., and Pastan, I. (2009) A protease-resistant immunotoxin against CD22 with greatly increased activity against CLL and diminished animal toxicity. *Blood*, **113**, 3792–3800.
61. Veronese, F.M. and Mero, A. (2008) The impact of PEGylation on biological therapies. *BioDrugs*, **22**, 315–329.
62. Jevsevar, S., Kunstelj, M., and Porekar, V.G. (2010) PEGylation of therapeutic proteins. *Biotechnol. J.*, **5**, 113–128.
63. Su, D., Zhao, H., and Xia, H. (2010) Glycosylation-modified erythropoietin with improved half-life and biological activity. *Int. J. Hematol.*, **91**, 238–244.
64. An, Q., Lei, Y., Jia, N., Zhang, X., Bai, Y., Yi, J., Chen, R., Xia, A., Yang, J., Wei, S., Cheng, X., Fan, A., Mu, S., and Xu, Z. (2007) Effect of site-directed PEGylation of trichosanthin on its biological activity, immunogenicity, and pharmacokinetics. *Biomol. Eng.*, **24**, 643–649.
65. Tsutsumi, Y., Onda, M., Nagata, S., Lee, B., Kreitman, R.J., and Pastan, I. (2000) Site-specific chemical modification with polyethylene glycol of recombinant immunotoxin anti-Tac(Fv)–PE38 (LMB-2) improves antitumor activity and reduces animal toxicity and immunogenicity. *Proc. Natl. Acad. Sci. USA*, **97**, 8548–8553.
66. Onda, M., Beers, R., Xiang, L., Nagata, S., Wang, Q.C., and Pastan, I. (2008) An immunotoxin with greatly reduced immunogenicity by identification and removal of B cell epitopes. *Proc. Natl. Acad. Sci. USA*, **105**, 11311–11316.
67. Mathew, M. and Verma, R.S. (2009) Humanized immunotoxins: a new generation of immunotoxins for targeted cancer therapy. *Cancer Sci.*, **100**, 1359–1365.
68. Oldberg, A., Kalamajski, S., Salnikov, A.V., Stuhr, L., Morgelin, M., Reed, R.K., Heldin, N.E., and Rubin, K. (2007) Collagen-binding proteoglycan fibromodulin can determine stroma matrix structure and fluid balance in experimental carcinoma. *Proc. Natl. Acad. Sci. USA*, **104**, 13966–13971.
69. Baluna, R., Rizo, J., Gordon, B.E., Ghetie, V., and Vitetta, E.S. (1999) Evidence for a structural motif in toxins and interleukin-2 that may be responsible for binding to endothelial cells and initiating vascular leak syndrome. *Proc. Natl. Acad. Sci. USA*, **96**, 3957–3962.
70. Salvatore, G., Beers, R., Margulies, I., Kreitman, R.J., and Pastan, I. (2002) Improved cytotoxic activity toward cell lines and fresh leukemia cells of a mutant anti-CD22 immunotoxin obtained by antibody phage display. *Clin. Cancer Res.*, **8**, 995–1002.
71. Hansen, J.K., Weldon, J.E., Xiang, L., Beers, R., Onda, M., and Pastan, I. (2010) A recombinant immunotoxin targeting CD22 with low immunogenicity, low nonspecific toxicity, and high antitumor activity in mice. *J. Immunother.*, **33**, 297–304.
72. Yoon, D.J., Kwan, B.H., Chao, F.C., Nicolaides, T.P., Phillips, J.J., Lam, G.Y., Mason, A.B., Weiss, W.A., and Kamei, D.T. (2010) Intratumoral therapy of glioblastoma multiforme using genetically engineered transferrin for drug delivery. *Cancer Res.*, **70**, 4520–4527.
73. Liu, S., Bugge, T.H., and Leppla, S.H. (2001) Targeting of tumor cells by cell surface urokinase plasminogen activator-dependent anthrax toxin. *J. Biol. Chem.*, **276**, 17976–17984.
74. Liu, S., Aaronson, H., Mitola, D.J., Leppla, S.H., and Bugge, T.H. (2003) Potent antitumor activity of a urokinase-activated engineered anthrax toxin. *Proc. Natl. Acad. Sci. USA*, **100**, 657–662.
75. Su, Y., Ortiz, J., Liu, S., Bugge, T.H., Singh, R., Leppla, S.H., and Frankel, A.E. (2007) Systematic urokinase-activated anthrax toxin therapy produces regressions of subcutaneous human non-small cell lung tumor in athymic nude mice. *Cancer Res.*, **67**, 3329–3336.
76. Hoffmann, C., Bachran, C., Stanke, J., Elezkurtaj, S., Kaufmann, A.M.,

Fuchs, H., Loddenkemper, C., Schneider, A., and Cichon, G. (2010) Creation and characterization of a xenograft model for human cervical cancer. *Gynecol. Oncol.*, **118**, 76–80.
77. Benítez, J., Ferreras, J.M., Muñoz, R., Arias, Y., Iglesias, R., Córdoba-Díaz, M., del Villar, R., and Girbés, T. (2005) Cytotoxicity of an ebulin l–anti-human CD105 immunotoxin on mouse fibroblasts (L929) and rat myoblasts (L6E9) cells expressing human CD105. *Med. Chem.*, **1**, 65–70.
78. Stahnke, B., Thepen, T., Stocker, M., Rosinke, R., Jost, E., Fischer, R., Tur, M.K., and Barth, S. (2008) Granzyme B–H22(scFv), a human immunotoxin targeting CD64 in acute myeloid leukemia of monocytic subtypes. *Mol. Cancer Ther.*, **7**, 2924–2932.
79. Braschoss, S., Hirsch, B., Dubel, S., Stein, H., and Durkop, H. (2007) New anti-CD30 human pancreatic ribonuclease-based immunotoxin reveals strong and specific cytotoxicity *in vivo*. *Leuk. Lymphoma*, **48**, 1179–1186.
80. Tur, M.K., Neef, I., Jager, G., Teubner, A., Stocker, M., Melmer, G., and Barth, S. (2009) Immunokinases, a novel class of immunotherapeutics for targeted cancer therapy. *Curr. Pharm. Des.*, **15**, 2693–2699.
81. ten Cate, B., Bremer, E., de Bruyn, M., Bijma, T., Samplonius, D., Schwemmlein, M., Huls, G., Fey, G., and Helfrich, W. (2009) A novel AML-selective TRAIL fusion protein that is superior to gemtuzumab ozogamicin in terms of *in vitro* selectivity, activity and stability. *Leukemia*, **23**, 1389–1397.
82. Prince, H.M., Duvic, M., Martin, A., Sterry, W., Assaf, C., Sun, Y., Straus, D., Acosta, M., and Negro-Vilar, A. (2010) Phase III placebo-controlled trial of denileukin diftitox for patients with cutaneous T-cell lymphoma. *J. Clin. Oncol.*, **28**, 1870–1877.
83. Gerena-Lewis, M., Crawford, J., Bonomi, P., Maddox, A.M., Hainsworth, J., McCune, D.E., Shukla, R., Zeigler, H., Hurtubise, P., Chowdhury, T.R., Fletcher, B., Dyehouse, K., Ghalie, R., and Jazieh, A.R. (2009) A phase II trial of denileukin diftitox in patients with previously treated advanced non-small cell lung cancer. *Am. J. Clin. Oncol.*, **32**, 269–273.
84. Bacha, P.A., Forte, S.E., McCarthy, D.M., Estis, L., Yamada, G., and Nichols, J.C., (1991) Impact of interleukin-2-receptor-targeted cytotoxins on a unique model of murine interleukin-2-receptor-expressing malignancy. *Int. J. Cancer*, **49**, 96–101.
85. Huang, J., Fan, G., Zhong, Y., Gatter, K., Braziel, R., Gross, G., and Bakke, A. (2005) Diagnostic usefulness of aberrant CD22 expression in differentiating neoplastic cells of B-cell chronic lymphoproliferative disorders from admixed benign B cells in four-color multiparameter flow cytometry. *Am. J. Clin. Pathol.*, **123**, 826–832.
86. Kreitman, R.J., Stetler-Stevenson, M., Margulies, I., Noel, P., Fitzgerald, D.J., Wilson, W.H., and Pastan, I. (2009) Phase II trial of recombinant immunotoxin RFB4 (dsFv)–PE38 (BL22) in patients with hairy cell leukemia. *J. Clin. Oncol.*, **27**, 2983–2990.
87. Wayne, A.S., Kreitman, R.J., Findley, H.W., Lew, G., Delbrook, C., Steinberg, S.M., Stetler-Stevenson, M., Fitzgerald, D.J., and Pastan, I. (2010) Anti-CD22 immunotoxin RFB4 (dsFv)–PE38 (BL22) for CD22-positive hematologic malignancies of childhood: preclinical studies and phase I clinical trial. *Clin. Cancer Res.*, **16**, 1894–1903.
88. Kreitman, R.J., Tallman, M.S., Coutre, S., Robak, T., Wilson, W.H., Stetler-Stevenson, M., Noel, P., FitzGerald, D.J., Buzoianu, M., Lechleider, R., Kaucic, K., and Pastan, I. (2009) Phase I dose-escalation study of CAT-8015 (HA22), a CD22-specific targeted immunotoxin, in relapsed or refractory hairy cell leukemia. 51st ASH Annual Meeting and Exposition, New Orleans, LA, paper 22920.
89. Hassan, R. and Ho, M. (2008) Mesothelin targeted cancer immunotherapy. *Eur. J. Cancer*, **44**, 46–53.
90. Kreitman, R.J., Hassan, R., Fitzgerald, D.J., and Pastan, I. (2009) Phase I trial of continuous infusion anti-mesothelin recombinant immunotoxin SS1P. *Clin. Cancer Res.*, **15**, 5274–5279.

91. Kunwar, S., Chang, S., Westphal, M., Vogelbaum, M., Sampson, J., Barnett, G., Shaffrey, M., Ram, Z., Piepmeier, J., Prados, M., Croteau, D., Pedain, C., Leland, P., Husain, S.R., Joshi, B.H., and Puri, R.K. (2010) Phase III randomized trial of CED of IL13–PE38QQR vs Gliadel wafers for recurrent glioblastoma. *Neuro Oncol.*, **12**, 871–881.
92. Herrera, L., Bostrom, B., Gore, L., Sandler, E., Lew, G., Schlegel, P.G., Aquino, V., Ghetie, V., Vitetta, E.S., and Schindler, J. (2009) A phase 1 study of Combotox in pediatric patients with refractory B-lineage acute lymphoblastic leukemia. *J. Pediatr. Hematol. Oncol.*, **31**, 936–941.
93. Lee, I., Kalota, A., Gewirtz, A.M., and Shogen, K. (2007) Antitumor efficacy of the cytotoxic RNase, ranpirnase, on A549 human lung cancer xenografts of nude mice. *Anticancer Res.*, **27**, 299–307.
94. Mikulski, S.M., Costanzi, J.J., Vogelzang, N.J., McCachren, S., Taub, R.N., Chun, H., Mittelman, A., Panella, T., Puccio, C., Fine, R., and Shogen, K. (2002) Phase II trial of a single weekly intravenous dose of ranpirnase in patients with unresectable malignant mesothelioma. *J. Clin. Oncol.*, **20**, 274–281.

46
Drug Targeting to the Central Nervous System

Gert Fricker, Anne Mahringer, Melanie Ott, and Valeska Reichel

46.1
Introduction

Therapy of central nervous system (CNS) diseases is a continuing challenge in modern medicine, because most drugs are not able to enter the brain [1]. In particular, the treatment of brain tumors and brain metastases is a major problem. Despite advances in anticancer drug discovery and development, there has been little improvement in the prognosis of patients with brain cancer. Brain tumors are inherently serious and life-threatening because of their invasive and infiltrative character. As the brain is well protected by the skull, their detection mostly occurs at advanced stages when the presence of the tumor has side-effects that cause unexplained symptoms. In general, there are two types of brain tumors: (i) primary neoplasms that originate in the brain or the central spinal canal and (ii) secondary tumors or metastatic tumors that invade the brain from cancers that are primarily located somewhere else in the body. Glioblastoma multiforme – the most common and most aggressive type of primary brain tumor in humans – involves glial cells, and accounts for more than 50% of all parenchymal brain tumor cases and 20% of all intracranial tumors. Its treatment involves surgery, chemotherapy, radiation, antiangiogenic therapy, and corticosteroids. However, it is very difficult to treat due to several complicating factors: the brain is susceptible to damage, tumor cells are often resistant to conventional therapies, brain tissue has only a limited capacity for self-repair, and most drugs cannot cross the blood–brain barrier (BBB) to act on the tumor. Normally, the first stage of treatment of glioblastoma multiforme is surgery followed by radiotherapy. Further on, treatment includes chemotherapy during and after radiotherapy. The use of temozolomide (Temodal®) postradiotherapy results in a significant increase in median survival with minimal additional toxicity and is now standard for most cases of glioblastoma treatment. Recently, the US Food and Drug Administration has approved the antiangiogenetic Avastin® (bevacizumab) to treat patients with glioblastoma at progression after standard therapy. Boron neutron capture therapy (BNCT) has been tested as an alternative treatment for glioblastoma multiforme, but is not in common use.

Drug Delivery in Oncology: From Basic Research to Cancer Therapy, First Edition.
Edited by Felix Kratz, Peter Senter, and Henning Steinhagen.

However, despite all efforts of multimodality treatment, glioblastoma multiforme has a very poor prognosis, which is in fact the worst of any CNS malignancy. Often, promising agents for primary brain cancers *in vitro* show unsatisfying efficacy in clinical trials [2]. Patients with glioblastoma multiforme have to experience a very poor perspective of little more than 1-year mean survival time after surgical resection of the tumor, mainly because chemotherapy lacks long-term efficacy. In addition, most anticancer drugs tend to be highly cytotoxic and of limited specificity, and their prolonged use results in lethal damage to normal cells. Therefore, chemotherapeutic treatment of CNS tumors is associated with severe systemic toxic side-effects, thereby compromising the quality of life of the patient. With very few exceptions, anticancer drugs are not able to enter the brain at therapeutic concentrations. A dynamic interface between the CNS and the peripheral circulatory system – the brain microvessels forming the so-called BBB – functions as a regulator of ion homeostasis and nutrient transport, and as a barrier to potentially harmful molecules. Hence, the development of innovative drugs with reduced toxicity and targeted delivery methods is an urgent medical need, not only for brain tumors, but also for other CNS diseases.

46.2
Anatomy of the BBB

The BBB, which is formed by endothelial cells of brain capillaries, separates the bloodstream and brain parenchyma, and controls the passage of endogenous substances and xenobiotics into and out of the CNS (Figure 46.1).

Together with surrounding pericytes, foot processes of astrocytes, neurons, and the extracellular matrix, the microvessel endothelial cells constitute the so-called "neurovascular unit" that is essential for the health and function of the CNS.

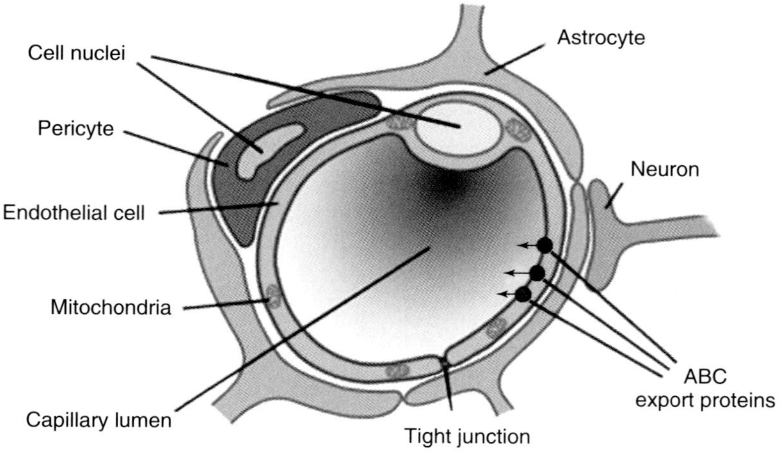

Figure 46.1 Schematic cross-section across the neurovascular unit.

Over a century ago scientists observed an uneven distribution of dyes in body and brain, which led to the conclusion of a separating wall between blood and brain [3]. In 1900, the German neurologist Max Lewandowsky was the first to use the term "Bluthirnschranke" when he studied the limited permeation of potassium ferrocyanate into the brain [4]. In 1921, the Russian physiologist Lina Stern described a "barrière hématoencéphalique." Both terms indicate the BBB. For several years the localization and function of this barrier was under debate until electron microscopy localized it within brain capillaries in brain slices. It was proposed that the endothelial cells were connected by tight junctions, thus forming a continuous membrane that constituted the BBB [5]. Further, it was suggested that astrocytes do not significantly contribute to the physical barrier [6].

The density of cerebral capillaries, especially in the cortical gray matter, is very high, with mean distances of approximately 40 μm. The capillary network has a total length of 600–650 km, the mean velocity of the blood flow is below 0.1 cm/s, and the luminal surface extends to approximately 15–30 m^2. Thus, the BBB represents an important surface for potential drug delivery. Brain microvessels significantly differ from peripheral capillaries – peripheral capillaries are fenestrated with openings up to 50 nm wide, whereas BBB endothelial cells are closely connected by tight junctions and zonulae occludentes, resulting in very high transendothelial resistances of up to 1500–2000 $\Omega \cdot cm^2$ in some species [7]. In fact, the BBB appears to be the tightest cell layer in the body. The capillaries are surrounded by a basal membrane enclosing pericytes. The function of these cells is not yet clear. It has been suggested that they are involved in blood flow regulation [8]. Other studies showed that pericyte-derived angiopoietin induces endothelial expression of occludin – an important tight junction protein [9]. In hypoxic states or traumatic brain injury, pericytes appear to move away from the BBB [10]. The outer surface of the basal membrane is covered by astrocytic foot processes. The exact role of astrocytes in BBB formation and maintenance of its integrity is also under debate. *In vitro*, coculture or culturing endothelial cells in astrocyte conditioned medium seems to improve BBB characteristics, such as tightness of cell monolayers or formation of adequate polarity [11, 12]. Several studies also suggest a regulation of BBB via dynamic Ca^{2+} signaling between astrocytes and the endothelium [13, 14].

Speaking of the "neurovascular unit" implies communication between neurons and the BBB, and there is indeed evidence that neurons are able to regulate several aspects of BBB function. There appears to be a direct innervation of the capillary endothelium and/or astrocytic foot processes by neurons [15, 16].

In addition to astrocytes, pericytes, and neurons, the extracellular matrix of the basal lamina interacts with the cerebral microvascular endothelium. Disruption of the extracellular matrix is strongly associated with increased BBB permeability in pathological states [17]. It has been shown that matrix proteins can influence the expression of endothelial tight junction proteins [18, 19], indicating that they are involved in tight junction maintenance.

A major characteristic of the BBB is the presence of junctional complexes, which include adherent junctions [20], tight junctions [21], and gap junctions [22]. The tight junctions mostly contribute to the high transendothelial electrical resistances. Important components are junctional adhesion molecule-1 [23], occludin [24], and claudins [25, 26]. In addition to the transmembrane proteins of the tight junctions, several accessory proteins are associated, such as ZO-1 (zonula occludens protein-1), ZO-2, ZO-3, and others. ZO-1 connects transmembrane proteins of the tight junctions to the acting cytoskeleton [27], and is therefore critical to the stability and function of the tight junctions. Dissociation of ZO-1 from the junctional complex is often connected with an increased permeability [28, 29]. For a more detailed description of BBB anatomy the reader is referred to a recent review [30].

In addition to these anatomical features, a second barrier element has been identified. It reflects the transport properties of multiple transport proteins, which are embedded in the luminal (blood-side) and abluminal (brain-side) plasma membranes of the endothelial cells (Figure 46.2).

First, carrier transport mechanisms are present at both luminal and abluminal plasma membranes to deliver nutrients, vitamins, or hormones to the brain and meet the extensive metabolic needs of brain cells. For example, glucose uptake is predominantly mediated by the glucose transporter (GLUT1), which is expressed at high levels at the BBB [31]. The transport of amino acids appears to be important for the control of the overall regulation of cerebral metabolism, including protein synthesis and neurotransmitter production [32, 33].

Second, efflux transport systems restrict the penetration of xenobiotics in the brain. At present, the mRNAs of several drug transporters have been detected in

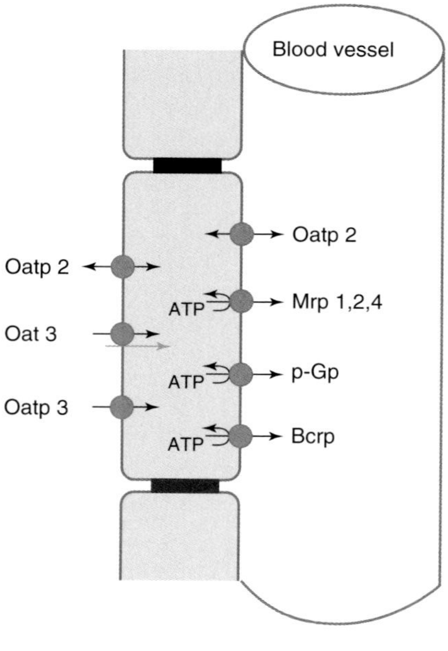

Figure 46.2 Drug transporters at the blood–brain barrier.

brain capillaries or brain capillary endothelial cell lines, including concentrative nucleoside transporters, organic cation transporters, organic anion transporting polypeptides (OATPs), organic anion transporters (OATs), equilibrative nucleoside transporters, and different members from the ATP-binding cassette (ABC) transporter superfamily, namely multidrug resistance protein (*mdr1* gene product, P-glycoprotein, ABCB1), multidrug resistance-associated proteins (ABCCs, MRPs), and breast cancer resistance protein (ABGG2, BCRP). Most likely, this list is incomplete and additional transport proteins remain to be detected.

Six ATP-driven drug export pumps (P-glycoprotein (ABCB1), BCRP (ABCG2), MRP1 (ABCC1), MRP2 (ABCC2), MRP4 (ABCC4), and MRP5 (ABCC5)) have been immunolocalized on the luminal plasma membrane, where they pump their substrates back into the blood circulation. Together these transporters handle a very wide range of anionic (MRPs), cationic (P-glycoprotein and BCRP), and uncharged (all six) xenobiotics. Additionally, several members of the SLCO/SLC22 and SLC22 family are expressed at the BBB. The organic anion transport protein OATP1a4, which handles the cardiac glycoside, digoxin [34], steroid, and drug conjugates as well as certain opioid peptides, is localized on both the luminal and abluminal membranes of the brain capillaries. Transport proteins in the basolateral plasma membrane (brain-side) include MRP1 [35], OATP1a5 [36, 37], and OAT3 [37]. When coupled to the appropriate ion gradients, both OAT3 and OATP1a5 are capable of driving organic anions into the endothelial cells. Thus, basolateral OAT1a5 and OAT3 may pair with luminal MRP2 and OATP1a5 to drive anionic xenobiotics out of the CNS.

Up until now, the primary active ATP-dependent export pump P-glycoprotein has received the most attention. This protein handles a remarkably large number of commonly prescribed drugs. This became particularly evident in dosing studies in P-glycoprotein knockout animals showing that brain/plasma ratios for a large number of P-glycoprotein substrates increased 5- to 50-fold [38]. In addition, treatment of the knockout animals with ivermectin, an anthelminthic drug, caused significantly elevated drug concentrations in the brain and dramatic neurotoxicity [39]. *Ex vivo* experiments with isolated brain capillaries using a fluorescent ivermectin derivative confirmed that the drug is indeed pumped back into the blood circulation [40] (Figure 46.3). For some other drugs the relevance of P-glycoprotein at the BBB has also been impressively demonstrated. A number of studies have shown that several HIV protease inhibitors including ritonavir and saquinavir are substrates of P-glycoprotein in brain capillary endothelial cells [41, 42]. Other clinically relevant drugs, which have been shown to be actively transported by P-glycoprotein and also other ABC transport proteins, include most small-molecule anticancer drugs, such as vinca alkaloids or doxorubicin (Table 46.1).

Similar observations have been made for the other export proteins in the BBB, and synergistic action has been discussed for BCRP and P-glycoprotein [43]. In addition, BCRP prevents brain entry of drugs like imatinib, prazosin, riluzole (which is used for amyotrophic lateral sclerosis treatment [44]), and others.

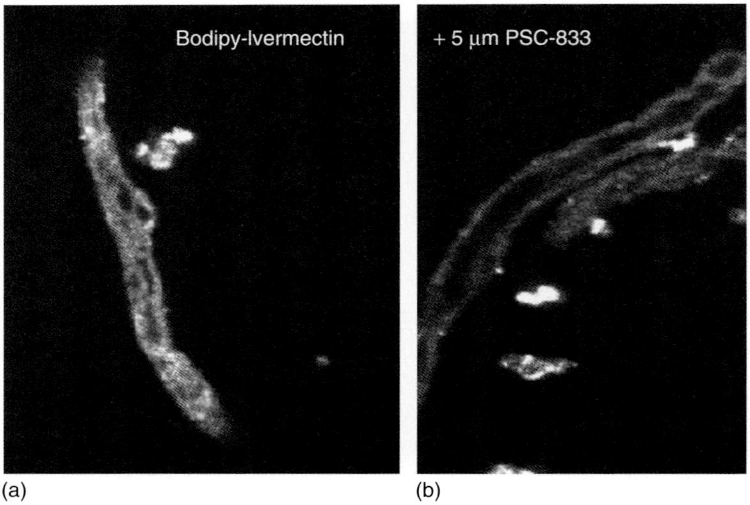

Figure 46.3 Confocal image of an isolated brain endothelial capillary incubated for 30 min with 1 µM BODIPY-ivermectin (a). The fluorescent compound is excreted into the capillary lumen. When the capillary is preincubated with the P-glycoprotein blocker PSC-833 (2 µM), BODIPY-ivermectin is taken up into the cells, but no longer secreted (b). (Reproduced with permission from [40].)

Table 46.1 Substrates and inhibitors of ABC transporters in the BBB (selected examples).

Export protein	Compound class	Drugs
P-glycoprotein (MDR1; ABCB1)	cytostatics	doxorubicin, paclitaxel, etoposide, idarubicin, vinblastine, mitoxantrone
	antiepileptics	carbamazepine, gabapentin, phenytoin, felbamate
	antidepressants	amitryptiline, dexepine, velafaxine, paroxetine
	antipsychotics	chlorpromazine, pimozide, fluphenazine, reserpine, triflupromazine
	anti-HIV	amprenavir, nelfinavir, saquinavir, ritonavir, lopinavir
MRP1 (ABCC1)	cytostatics	daunorubicin, doxorubicin, melphalan, methotrexate, teniposide, vincristine
	anti-HIV	saquinavir, ritonavir
MRP2 (ABCC2)	cytostatics	cisplatin, doxorubicin, epirubicin, vincristine, flavopiridol
	anti-HIV	saquinavir, ritonavir, indinavir
	antiepileptics	phenytoin
BCRP (ABCG2)	cytostatics	anthracycline, irinotecan, mitoxantrone, methotrexate, camptothecin, topotecan
	anti-HIV	AZT, lamivudine

46.3
Alterations of the BBB in Brain Tumors

It is presently under debate to what extent the BBB retains its integrity. Some important characteristics of the normal BBB are profoundly altered in brain tumors, which in turn might have a significant effect upon the disposition of anticancer drugs. Tight junctions may be altered (Figure 46.4) and several tight junction proteins may be downregulated (e.g., ZO-1, claudin-1, claudin-5, and occludin) [45, 46]. Thus, the vasculature appears to represent rather a "leaky" network than an intact BBB. However, particularly at the outer rim of the tumor the BBB may have conserved its integrity, making effective delivery a challenge [47]. Tumor uptake of drugs and macromolecules may also be influenced by interstitial fluid pressure, which could reduce penetration when it is elevated due to a leaky tumor vasculature. Concomitant administration of angiogenesis inhibitors may influence the structure and function of the tumor vasculature, and result in conditions that can be associated with improved BBB penetration [48].

The expression of the ABC transporters may also be altered in regions of brain tumors. For example, initial studies indicate upregulation of MRP1 and MRP3 in peritumor vascular endothelial cells [49] or downregulation of P-glycoprotein expression in the vasculature of gliomas [50]. However, more studies are necessary to clarify the role of drug pumps at the BBB or in the surroundings of intracerebral tumors.

46.4
Relevance of the BBB for Drug Delivery

The BBB constitutes the major hurdle in effective drug delivery to the CNS. Overcoming the barrier may be achieved by several approaches on a molecular/chemical level as well as on a physiological/pharmacological or a technological level, each of which will be discussed below.

46.4.1
Prodrug Approaches to Overcome the BBB

Drugs that exert their action in the CNS have to be either lipophilic enough to be able to permeate the BBB by passive diffusion or they need to be substrates of influx transporters being expressed in the BBB. In addition, they must not be substrates of efflux transporters. One type of chemical targeting where this goal has been achieved is the so-called retrometabolic drug design, which was introduced by the group of Bodor and which is applicable to a large variety of drugs, including steroids, antibiotics and antiviral drugs, neurotransmitters, antidementia and anticancer drugs as well as several peptides [51]. It uses a sequential metabolism approach. First, a precursor drug–conjugate moves freely into the brain before it is metabolically converted and trapped. The drug shuttle systems are based on the redox conversion of a lipophilic dihydropyridine into a positively charged, lipid-insoluble pyridinium salt. The dihydropyridinium-type

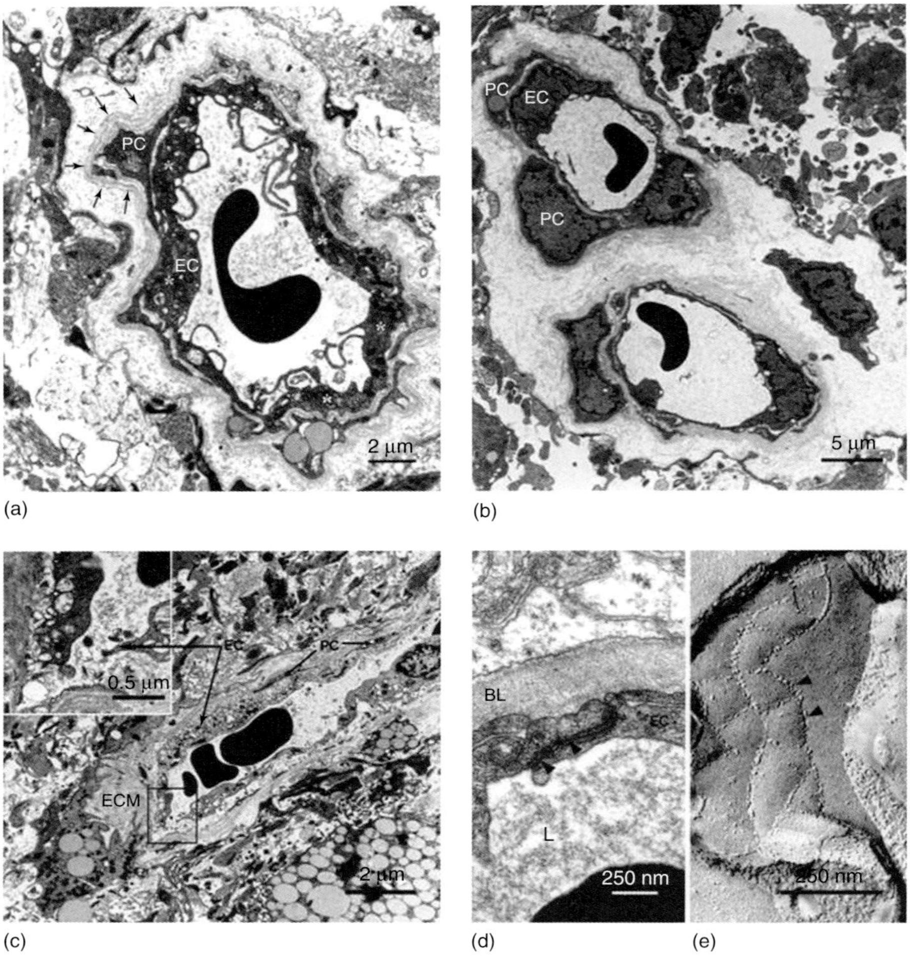

Figure 46.4 Electron microscopy of various microvessels in human glioblastoma multiforme. (a) Hyperplastic tumor microvessel. The circumference is formed by more than one endothelial cell. The luminal surface of endothelial cells is increased by numerous microfolds. Perivascular space is enlarged and the basal lamina is multilayered (arrows). (b) Microvessels from another tumor showing the variability of vascular alterations in different tumors concerning the endothelial surface, number of endothelial cells per circumference, and coverage by pericytes. Note the amount of extracellular matrix between the vessels. (c) Microvessel interrupted by a gap in the endothelial lining (see frame and insert). The endothelial cells are considerably vacuolized, but luminal microfolds are lacking. (d) High magnification of an interendothelial tight junction of a tumor microvessel. By this method, the morphology of the tight junction appears normal. Note tight junction "kisses" (arrowheads). (e) Freeze fracture replica of an endothelial cell tight junction of a tumor microvessel. The tight junction particles are predominantly associated with the E-face (arrowheads). EC, endothelial cell; PC, pericyte; ECM, perivascular extracellular matrix; BL, basal lamina; L, lumen. (Reproduced with permission from [46].)

carrier is sufficiently lipophilic to passively diffuse into the brain, where it undergoes enzymatic oxidation, forming the ionic pyridinium compound, which is then retained in the brain.

Targeting a transport system in the BBB by chemical modification of a drug was the approach chosen by Gynther *et al.* [52]: ketoprofen and indomethacin were conjugated with glucose, and the brain uptake mechanism of the prodrugs was determined with the *in situ* rat brain perfusion technique. The prodrugs were able to significantly inhibit the uptake of GLUT1-mediated uptake of glucose and to cross the BBB suggesting that the brain uptake of the prodrugs was carrier mediated. In a similar study ketoprofen was conjugated to L-tyrosine and concentration-dependent brain uptake could be observed that was significantly decreased by a specific inhibitor of the large amino acid transporter (LAT1) in the BBB. Thus, these results revealed that a drug–substrate conjugate is able to transport drugs into the brain via LAT1 [53].

46.4.2 Inhibition of ABC Export Proteins

Inhibition of ABC export proteins in the BBB offers an attractive approach to overcome the barrier. Thereby, the export of substrates will be suppressed, resulting in an accumulation of the drug of interest in the cerebral tissue. Recently, several relatively specific P-glycoprotein inhibitors have been developed and tested [54, 55]. The first generation of inhibitors are pharmacologically active drugs like verapamil or cyclosporine A, are rather unspecific inhibitors, and/or are highly susceptible to metabolism. The second generation of inhibitors includes valspodar (PSC-833), a nonimmunosuppressive cyclosporine analog, elacridar (GF 120918), biricodar (VX-710), and dexniguldipine (B8509-035). Unfortunately, the clinical outcome of these compounds as comedication in various cancer indications has not been convincing so far and most clinical studies have been terminated. The third generation of P-glycoprotein blockers (ONT-093; zosuquidar (LY335-979), tariquidar (XR9576), and laniquidar (R101-9333)) exhibits a more favorable transporter specificity as well as a better metabolic profile.

The inhibition of P-glycoprotein with orally administered valspodar led to significantly increased cerebral levels of intravenously administered paclitaxel (Taxol®), which under normal circumstances is not able to cross the BBB due to its interaction with the ABC transporter. As a consequence, a dramatic decrease of tumor size could be observed [56] in a mouse model of orthotopically implanted human glioblastoma (Figure 46.5).

This concept was confirmed in a recent study when coadministration of paclitaxel and HM30181A, a novel P-glycoprotein inhibitor, resulted in a significant therapeutic effect in a mouse brain tumor model [57]. Other studies with ABCG2-knockout mice and wild-type animals showed that BCRP in the BBB is one reason for the low permeability of the BCRP substrate imatinib (Gleevec®) [58]. The use of inhibitors and knowledge about the regulation of BCRP might be interesting for the application of BCRP substrates like gefitinib (Iressa®) [59], which showed interesting

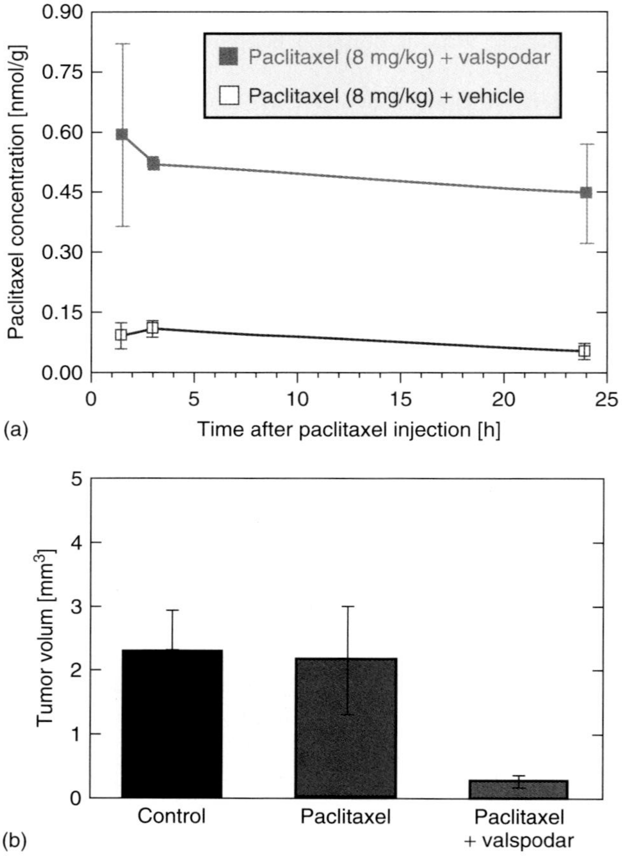

Figure 46.5 Effect of P-glycoprotein inhibition on efficacy of paclitaxel in a mouse brain tumor model (implanted intracerebral human U118 MG glioblastoma). (a) Cerebral concentration of paclitaxel in the absence of and after coadministration of the P-glycoprotein blocker valspodar to nude mice bearing a brain tumor. (b) Brain tumor size in control animals, in animals that had been treated with paclitaxel alone, and in animals that had been treated with paclitaxel and the P-glycoprotein blocker valspodar. (Reproduced with permission from [56].)

activity in a mouse model of brain tumors with expression of epidermal growth factor receptors, as well as in brain metastases in patients with a non-small-cell lung cancer [60, 61].

46.4.3 Intrathecal or Intraventricular Injection

This invasive method has been applied with some success for chemotherapy with methotrexate or cytarabine/cortisol in patients with aggressive lymphoma or acute lymphatic leukemia [62, 63].

46.4.4
Infusion of Hyperosmotic Solutions

The infusion of hyperosmotic solutions of, for example, mannitol or arabinose via the arteria carotis interna [64, 65] results in a shrinking of the endothelial cells with a concomitant opening of tight junctions. However, there is a relatively high risk of edema formation due to the very unselective opening of the BBB [66, 67]. Nevertheless, this approach has been clinically applied [68] when patients received intra-arterial chemotherapy combined with hyperosmotic perfusion. Survival and toxicity data appeared promising, and a plateau in survival curves suggested a cure for some patients. In addition, long-term survival may be achieved with focal or reduced-dose radiotherapy in some patients undergoing this treatment.

46.4.5
Focused Ultrasound Treatment

Ultrasound may be used for a focused opening of the BBB. Thereby, ultrasound is applied in the range of 0.5–2 MHz with pulse lengths in the millisecond range and repeating frequencies in the range of 1 Hz within a time interval of less than 1 min [69]. Most probably the opening of the BBB occurs by shear forces caused by microcurrents in the treated area. The opened areas can be identified by simultaneous magnetic resonance tomography. The method yields promising results, at least in animal studies [70]. Using magnetic resonance imaging (MRI)-guided focused ultrasound with preformed microbubbles to locally disrupt the BBB and systemic administration of doxorubicin, concentrations of 886 ± 327 ng/g tissue of the cytostatic drug could be achieved in the brain. In contrast, doxorubicin accumulation in nontargeted contralateral brain tissue remained significantly lower, suggesting that targeted delivery by focused ultrasound may render doxorubicin chemotherapy a viable treatment option against CNS tumors. In addition, MRI signal enhancement in the sonicated region correlated strongly with tissue doxorubicin concentration, suggesting that contrast-enhanced MRI could perhaps indicate drug penetration during image-guided interventions.

46.4.6
Vector-Coupled Drugs

An alternative to the direct manipulation of the BBB is the administration of targeted systems, which can be loaded with a drug of desire and which are modified at their surface in such a way that they recognize the BBB, are taken up into the endothelial cells, and are eventually released into the brain tissue. Targeting drugs to the CNS has successfully been applied by coupling substances to antibodies that recognize surface epitopes at the luminal side of the BBB.

A prime example is the use of transferrin or antibodies versus the transferrin receptor, which is expressed at high density at the luminal surface of microvessel endothelial cells [71, 72]. After binding to this receptor a ligand may undergo endocytosis and eventually transcytosis across the target cell [73, 74]. A drawback in using transferrin itself, however, is competitive inhibition by endogenous transferrin present in the blood. This disadvantage can be resolved using the antibody approach. Several studies demonstrated that drug–antibody conjugates are able to permeate the BBB. Coupled drugs include an 18mer antisense peptide nucleic acid specific for the *rev* gene of HIV-1 [75], glial cell line-derived neurotrophic factor [76], nerve growth factor [77, 78], azidothymidine [79], vasoactive intestinal peptide [80], and several others.

A similar strategy uses the iron-binding protein p97 (melanotransferrin (MTf)), which is able to cross the BBB [81]. One *in vivo* study in mice suggested that p97 has significant potential to be an effective vehicle for delivery of therapeutic drugs to the brain, demonstrating a 6- to 8-fold higher transport of adriamycin–p97 conjugates than transport of albumin or lactoferrin [82]. In recent experiments [83], Adenovirus serotype 5 (Ad5), which is widely used in the development of gene therapy protocols, was coupled to p97. It was found that this adaptor protein could redirect Ad5 to the p97 transcytosis pathway in an *in vitro* BBB model and the transcytosed Ad5 viral particles retained their native infectivity. Bispecific adaptor protein containing the extracellular domain of the coxsackie adenovirus receptor and the full-length p97 (sCAR-MTf)-mediated Ad5 transcytosis was temperature and dose dependent. In addition, the directionality of sCAR-MTf-mediated Ad5 transcytosis was examined, where the efficiency of apical-to-basal transcytosis was much higher than that of basal-to-apical direction, supporting a role of this strategy in transporting Ad5 vectors toward the brain. Thus, this approach might be interesting to facilitate gene delivery across the BBB. Similar observations were made when small-molecule anticancer drugs, such as paclitaxel or adriamycin, were coupled to p97 [84].

A similar brain drug delivery technology, designated 2B-Trans™, uses the membrane-bound precursor of heparin-binding epidermal growth factor, also known as diphtheria toxin receptor. Expression is amplified in disease conditions and therefore the receptor is suitable for site-specific disease targeting. Since there are no endogenous ligands present, competition appears to be unlikely. A nontoxic mutant of diphtheria toxin (CRM197 [85]), which has already been marketed for human use in vaccination programs with a proven safety profile, serves as a receptor specific carrier protein. *In vitro and in vivo* data demonstrated efficient diphtheria toxin receptor targeted delivery into the brain [86].

A further type of CNS-targeted delivery system are SynB™ vectors. They represent a small peptide vector that is able to enhance brain uptake of various anticancer drugs and others [87, 88]. Administration of these vectors with 10- to 27-amino-acid residues significantly enhanced brain uptake of molecules without opening BBB tight junctions. The mechanism of uptake for these vectors is not yet fully understood, but evidence was found for a receptor-independent entry into brain [89, 90].

Angiopep-2, a 19-amino-acid peptide, has been described as vector to target the low-density lipoprotein receptor-related protein. A conjugate of paclitaxel with Angiopep-2 was studied as a CNS drug delivery system [91] that showed therapeutic

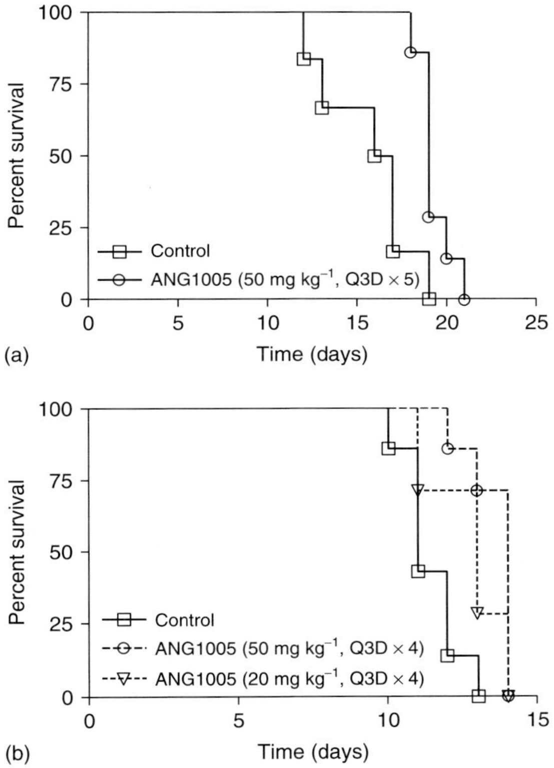

Figure 46.6 Percentage of survival (Kaplan–Meier plot) of mice with intracerebral U87 MG glioblastoma and NCI-H460 lung carcinoma tumors. (a) Nude mice received intracerebral implantation of U87 MG cells. At 3 days postimplantation, animals were treated by intravenous injection with vehicle only (control group) or ANG1005 (50 mg/kg, every third day, for five doses). (b) Nude mice received intracerebral implantation of NCI-H460 lung carcinoma cells. At 3 days postimplantation, animals were treated with vehicle only (control group) or ANG1005 (20 and 50 mg/kg, every third day, for four doses). The experiment was repeated separately at least 3 times. One representative experiment is shown ($n = 6$). (Reproduced with permission from [91].)

efficacy in preclinical models (Figure 46.6). It was shown that this construct possessed better brain permeability and *in vivo* antitumoral activity compared to paclitaxel in an orthotopic brain tumor model, partly due to its ability to bypass P-glycoprotein. Phase I clinical trials are ongoing to test its efficacy against recurrent primary or metastatic brain tumors.

Small single-domain antibodies with a size of approximately 14 kDa were able to transmigrate across cerebral endothelial cells *in vitro* and the BBB *in vivo* [92], with the ability to transport molecules up to 10 times their size into or across the target tissue. The efficacy of this antibody delivery system was improved by introducing avidity by multimerization. Cationized albumin or monoclonal antibodies against the insulin receptor were also tested as a chimeric peptide strategy to deliver drugs across the BBB [93].

One disadvantage of coupling a drug directly to the vector molecule is the limited loading capacity, allowing solely attachment of a few drug molecules to the carrier. Coupling a vector to a colloidal carrier (liposomes, nanoparticles), which can be loaded with a high number of drug molecules, certainly represents a significant improvement of this approach.

46.4.7
Liposomal Drug Delivery to the CNS

Targeted liposomes represent an advancement compared to direct linkage of a drug to a vector. However, a general problem with this approach is the exclusivity of targeting the BBB. All target-seeking vectors used so far are not specific for the BBB, but are also recognized at other parts of the body. In addition, colloidal carrier systems may be recognized by the reticuloendothelial system, which is built up by macrophages in blood, liver, spleen, lung, bone marrow, and other organs. A key element of this process is the so-called opsonization. Thereby, the surface of colloidal particles is covered by immunoglobulins and factors of the complement system (opsonins). As a consequence, the colloidal systems will be recognized and attacked by macrophages. One strategy to circumvent opsonization has successfully been applied in liposomes, when they have been coupled to poly(ethylene glycol) (PEG) chains, thus avoiding opsonization with the result of significantly prolonged circulation times in plasma. Additionally, PEGylation may decrease adverse effects caused by the large variations in peak-to-trough plasma drug concentrations associated with frequent administration and by the immunogenicity of unmodified proteins [94, 95].

An advantage of using colloidal carrier systems is their high loading capacity; recent calculations showed that up to 30 000 drug molecules may be loaded into a single liposome being targeted to the BBB [96].

Transferrin-conjugated PEGylated liposomes have been suggested as a colloidal carrier to achieve tumor-specific delivery of sodium borocaptate ($Na_2^{10}B_{12}H_{11}SH$) to malignant gliomas as BNCT [97]. This strategy is based on the nuclear reactions between ^{10}B and thermal neutrons resulting in high linear energy transfer α particles (^4He) and ^7Li nuclei that show a narrow distribution in tissue (5–9 mm), thus reducing nonspecific radiation damage. A key issue of this strategy is the selective delivery of a sufficient number of ^{10}B atoms to tumor cells [98].

The coupling of a transferrin antibody to the surface of PEGylated liposomes yielded interesting results. *In vitro* studies with capillary endothelial cells [99] demonstrated that such antibody-coupled liposomes are indeed able to permeate across the cells and release their content on the abluminal side. The permeation was temperature dependent and could be inhibited by the presence of free antibody, suggesting a specific mechanism. Transcytosis of these immunoliposomes was confirmed *in vivo* by the brain perfusion and capillary depletion technique, when the immunoliposomes were detected within the postvascular compartment of brain parenchyma and were not associated with the brain microvasculature.

In a rat study these antibody-directed liposomes were used for delivery of the antineoplastic agent daunomycin to the brain. The antibody was coupled to the terminal end of a PEG-conjugated linker lipid. Unconjugated liposomes did not permeate across the barrier, whereas coupling of 30 antibodies per liposome resulted in optimal brain delivery of the drug. Saturation of delivery was observed at higher antibody densities. Determination of brain levels over 24 h revealed that the immunoliposomes accumulated in brain tissue. The same kind of liposomes was also used for gene delivery to the brain [100]. After intravenous administration of a 6- to 7-kb expression plasmid encoding luciferase packaged in the interior of antitransferrin receptor immunoliposomes, luciferase gene expression in the brain peaked at 48 h after injection of 10 μg of plasmid DNA per rat – a dose that was 30- to 100-fold lower than that used for gene expression in rodents with cationic liposomes. The liposome formulation was stable in blood and was not entrapped in the lung. When a plasmid for β-galactosidase was loaded, β-galactosidase histochemistry demonstrated gene expression throughout the CNS, including neurons, choroid plexus epithelium, and the brain microvasculature. Thus, gene expression in the brain could be achieved by using a formulation that did not employ viruses or cationic liposomes.

Other researchers used liposomes coupled to antibodies versus the insulin receptor at the BBB [101, 102] or to fragments of apolipoprotein E, which is recognized by the low-density lipoprotein and similar receptors and undergoes endocytosis at the BBB [103]. When an apolipoprotein E-derived peptide, A2, was coupled to liposomes a nonselective internalization in an *in vitro* model of the BBB was observed via a clathrin- and caveolin-independent endocytosis [104]. Furthermore, covalent coupling of the highly cationic tandem dimer of apolipoprotein E residues onto PEG-derivatized liposomes resulted in an efficient, energy-dependent translocation of liposomes across the membrane of brain capillary endothelial cells. Liposomes without surface-located peptides displayed neither membrane accumulation nor cellular uptake. Enzymatic digestion of heparan sulfate proteoglycan (HSPG) with heparinase I and addition of heparin and poly(L-lysine) as competitors of HSPG and HSPG ligands, respectively, resulted in a significant loss in liposome internalization, suggesting that HSPG played a major role in the apolipoprotein E peptide-mediated uptake of liposomes into brain microvessel endothelial cells [105].

An increased liposomal uptake into cultured brain microvessel endothelial cells as well as in isolated functionally intact brain capillaries (Figure 46.7) suggests an improved liposomal brain uptake after coupling of cationized albumin to the surface of PEGylated liposomes [106].

Thereby, cellular uptake could be inhibited by free cationized albumin, phenylarsine oxide, nocodazole, and filipin, but not by dansylcadaverine, suggesting a caveolae-mediated cytotoxic process (Figure 46.8).

Recently, a new drug carrier for brain delivery, lactoferrin-modified procationic liposomes, was evaluated *in vitro* and *in vivo* [107]. So-called procationic liposomes, which were neutral or negatively charged at physiological pH, where changed into

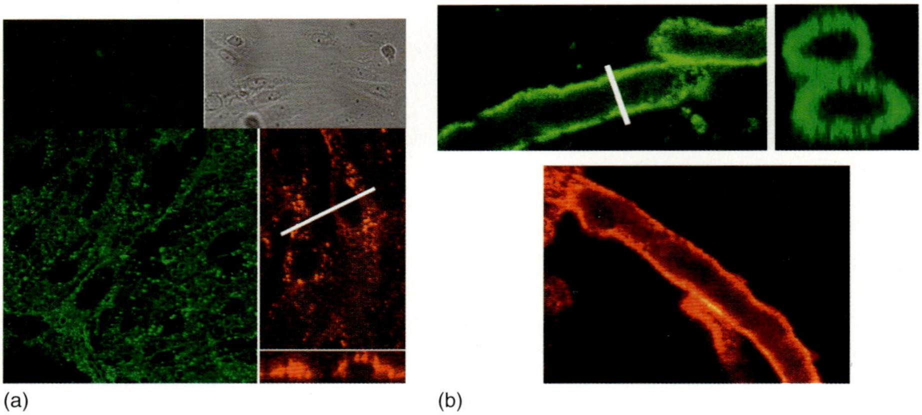

Figure 46.7 (a) Interaction of brain capillary endothelial cells with protein-coupled liposomes. (Top panel) Bovine serum albumin-coupled liposomes loaded with carboxyfluorescein (30 min incubation, lipid concentration 100 nmol/ml); left column, fluorescence imaging; right column, phase contrast imaging. (Bottom left panel) Cationized bovine serum albumin (CBSA)-coupled liposomes loaded with carboxyfluorescein (30 min incubation, lipid concentration 100 nmol/ml); image size: 140 × 75 μm. (Bottom right panel) CBSA-coupled liposomes loaded with Rh-DPPE as fluorescent marker (30 min incubation, lipid concentration 100 nmol/ml); image size 45 × 70 μm; white line: optical cross-section across the cells; lower image: three-dimensional reconstruction along the optical section. (b) Confocal laser scanning microscopy imaging of isolated brain capillaries incubated with CBSA-linked liposomes for 2 h. (Top panel) Rh-DPPE-containing liposomes, image size 75 × 55 μm; white line: optical cross-section across the capillary; right insert: three-dimensional reconstruction along the optical section. (Bottom panel) Carboxyfluorescein-containing liposomes, image size 65 × 30 μm; (Reproduced with permission from [106].)

cationic liposomes when they came in contact with brain capillary endothelial cells with the help of a brain-targeting ligand, lactoferrin. Compared with conventional liposomes these liposomes showed an improved performance in terms of uptake efficiency and cytotoxicity. The endocytosis involved in crossing the BBB was mediated by both receptor- and absorption-mediated transcytosis.

Several other vectors have been suggested for liposomal brain targeting, such as a leptin-derived peptide [108], cell-penetrating peptides [109] including TAT protein (86mer polypeptide) from HIV-1 [110], tamoxifen/wheat germ agglutinin [111], interleukin-13 [112], and others. Most of these systems showed efficacy in animal models; however, applicability after long-term administration including safety profile studies has still to be demonstrated for these systems.

Recently, liposomes have been introduced that are coated with the tripeptide glutathione at the tips of PEG to safely enhance the delivery of free drug to the brain. The therapeutic benefit of doxorubicin-loaded glutathione–PEG liposomes has been demonstrated. These liposomes resulted in a reduced brain tumor growth in proof-of-concept studies, which provides a strong basis for a further clinical development (*www.to-bbb.com*).

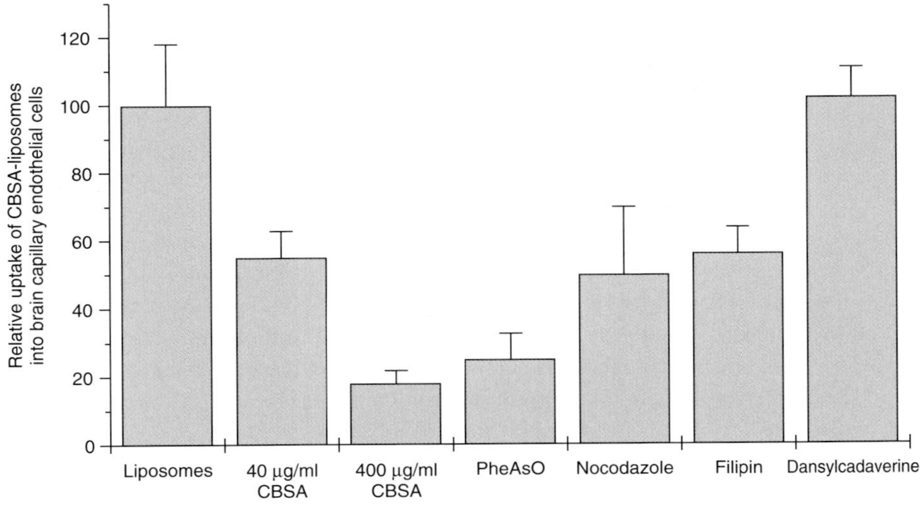

Figure 46.8 Inhibition of uptake of CBSA-linked liposomes by brain capillary endothelial cells. Incubation time 1 h; lipid concentration: 80 nmol/ml corresponding to around 4 μg/ml CBSA; concentrations of uptake modulators: 40 μg/ml CBSA; 400 μg/ml CBSA; PheAsO = phenylarsine oxide 20 μM; nocodazole = 4 μM; filipin = 3 μg/ml; dansylcadaverine = 100 μM. (Reproduced with permission from [106].)

Liposomes have also been used for a gene therapeutic approach to treat malignant glioblastoma. However, in these studies the liposomes were administered intracranially. Adenoviral vector containing herpes simplex virus thymidine kinase was administered followed by administration of ganciclovir. When the liposome–gene complex enters the tumor cell, the gene is incorporated into cellular chromosomes and cells begin to synthesize thymidine kinase, normally not produced by human cells. Thymidine kinase makes the tumor cells vulnerable for ganciclovir – a drug being registered for the treatment of certain viral diseases. Normal cells are not affected by ganciclovir, but only cells synthesizing the viral protein thymidine kinase are susceptible to treatment. Since the liposome–gene complex enters predominantly rapidly proliferating cells, it may be assumed that normal cells are not significantly affected [113, 114].

46.4.8
CNS Drug Delivery by Polymer Nanoparticles

An interesting alternative to liposomes are polymer nanoparticles, made from biocompatible and biodegradable materials, such as poly(lactic acid), poly(glycolic acid), copolymers thereof (poly(D,L-lactide-*co*-glycolide)), poly(butyl cyanoacrylate) (PBCA), or proteins such as albumin. An important aspect is that some of the materials have already been registered for parenteral use (e.g., poly(lactic acid) and poly(glycolic acid) copolymers are used for implants (Zoladex®), and PBCA is used as a tissue glue (Indermil®)).

The therapeutic efficacy of these colloidal carrier systems was shown in a rodent model of cerebral ischemia and reperfusion. The enzyme superoxide dismutase incorporated into poly(D,L-lactide-*co*-glycolide) nanoparticles yielded a 65% reduction of the infarct volume, whereas the enzyme alone in solution had no effect [115]. The efficacy of PBCA nanoparticles was demonstrated in several studies, where only drug, which was incorporated into nanoparticles, exhibited central activity [116]. Targeting of the BBB was achieved by surface modification of the nanoparticles with surfactants (e.g., Polysorbate-80 (Tween-80®) or Poloxamer 188 (Pluronic® F68). Apparently, after intravenous injection the surfactant-treated particles bind to apolipoproteins (A1, B, and E), and are subsequently recognized by low-density lipoprotein receptors and/or scavenger receptor class B type I within the BBB. A recent study using fluorescently labeled PBCA nanoparticles and confocal laser scanning microscopy showed that particles are able to cross the BBB and to distribute in brain tissue within 2–3 h after intravenous administration to rats [117] (Figure 46.9). PBCA nanoparticles may be loaded with diverse active ingredients, including doxorubicin [117, 118]. In particular, a major advantage of nanoparticle-embedded doxorubicin is its significantly reduced toxicity compared to toxicity of the drug administered in solution.

The nanoparticles may also serve as a controlled release system. A novel *N*-methyl-D-aspartic acid receptor antagonist showed a prolonged anticonvulsive action, suggesting that these particles act in the CNS via a controlled drug release [119].

Passage across the BBB was also confirmed for albumin nanoparticles, when electron microscopy was applied, indicating that a transcytosis occurred (Figure 46.10) [120].

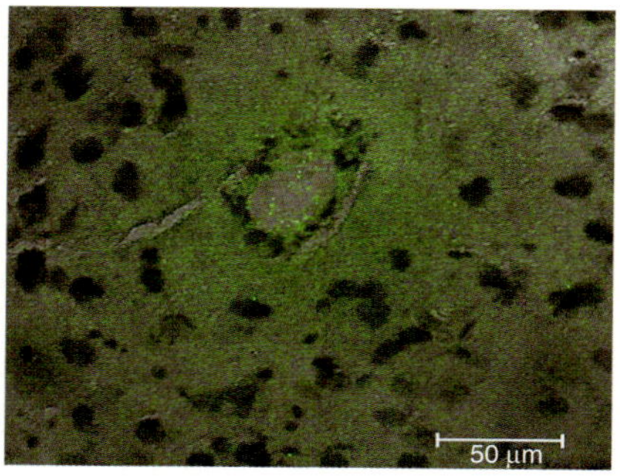

Figure 46.9 Cerebral distribution of rhodamine-123-labeled Polysorbate 80-coated nanoparticles in rat brain after administration via a tail vein. Sixty minutes after administration particle-associated fluorescence can be assigned to the brain capillary lumen, the endothelial cells, and the perivascular brain tissue. (Reproduced with permission from [117].)

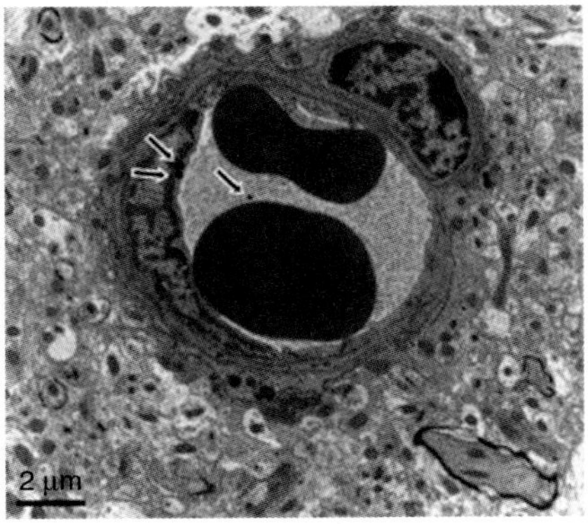

Figure 46.10 Electron microscopy of mouse brain tissue shows that nanoparticles with covalently bound apolipoprotein E are endocytosed after intravenous injection by brain endothelial cells and transported into the surrounding tissue by transcytosis. (Reproduced with permission from [120].)

46.4.9
Magnetically Controlled CNS Drug Delivery

Another technique to accumulate drugs is so-called magnetically controlled drug targeting. Thereby, drugs are reversibly bound to 50- to 500-nm magnetic particles (nanoparticles, liposomes) that may be concentrated in the area of interest by application of an external magnetic field [121].

Chertok *et al.* [122] studied nanoparticles composed of a magnetic (e.g., iron oxide/magnetite) core and a biocompatible polymeric shell (e.g., dextran, starch) to target brain tumors. Magnetic nanoparticles (12 mg Fe/kg) were injected in 9L gliosarcoma-bearing rats under a magnetic field. Magnetic resonance images were acquired before and immediately after administration of nanoparticles at 1-h intervals for 4 h. The magnetic targeting induced a 5-fold increase in the total glioma over nontargeted tumors and a 3.6-fold enhancement in the target selectivity index (e.g., nanoparticles accumulate in glioma over the normal brain). Thus, proof of principle has been demonstrated in mice, but for a substantial clinical application it has still to be demonstrated that magnetic delivery systems are really able to cross the BBB.

In a modified procedure – magnetic fluid hyperthermia – tumor cells may be destroyed in an alternating magnetic field after direct instillation of the magnetic fluid in the tumor, resulting in a subsequent heating [123, 124]. The efficacy of this approach is being evaluated in a phase II study. In brain autopsies the installed magnetic nanoparticles were dispersed or distributed as aggregates within geographic tumor necroses, restricted in distribution to the sites of instillation. Dispersed particles and particle aggregates were phagocytosed mainly by macrophages, whereas glioblastoma cells showed an uptake to a minor extent. Bystander effects such as sarcomatous tumor formation, formation of a sterile abscess, or foreign body giant cell reaction were not observed and the patients did not present any clinical symptoms related to possible adverse effects of this therapy.

46.4.10 Polymeric Micelles and Dendrimers

Apart from liposomes and nanoparticles, micelles or dendrimers have been employed for circumventing the BBB. Self-assembly of polymeric micelles with a size of 10–100 nm occurs in aqueous solutions of amphiphilic block copolymers when the copolymer concentration reaches the critical micelle concentration. The core of such micelles can be formed by hydrophobic polymer blocks, such as poly(propylene glycol), poly(D,L-lactide), poly(caprolactone), and others) and a shell of hydrophilic polymer (e.g., PEG). Pluronic/polyethylene block copolymers inhibit P-glycoprotein *in vitro* [125] and enhance transport of therapeutic agents across biological membranes, including the BBB.

Dendrimers are highly branched polymer molecules forming particles of small dimensions down to below 20 nm in size. A recent *in vitro* study [126] introduced polyether-*co*-polyester dendrimers loaded with methotrexate and conjugated to D-glucosamine. Glucose conjugation to the dendrimers conferred enhanced delivery across brain capillary endothelial cells as well as improved antitumor activity, which was evaluated against glioma cells and vascular human glioma tumor spheroids. More glucosylated dendrimers were found to be endocytosed than nonglucosylated dendrimers in both cell lines, suggesting a higher uptake after glucosamine coupling. Thus, these systems might also offer promising strategies for CNS delivery; however, proof of concept has still to be shown in *in vivo* studies.

46.4.11 Solid Lipid Nanoparticles

Solid lipid nanoparticles are dispersions of solid lipids stabilized with emulsifiers in aqueous solutions. In recent years, the potential use of solid lipid nanoparticles for brain drug delivery has been widely studied (for an overview, see [127, 128]), including anticancer drugs, such as camptothecin, paclitaxel, and doxorubicin, which all exhibit a very low cerebral availability. Drug concentrations in the brain were significantly increased by drug administration within solid lipid nanoparticles. Their low cytotoxicity and the biodegradability of the lipids used for manufacture make them very attractive candidates for brain delivery and tumor treatment. It was demonstrated that doxorubicin formulated in solid lipid nanoparticles achieved 12- to 50-fold higher intratumoral concentrations compared to free solutions within 24 h. In addition, in the contralateral healthy hemisphere in which BBB was not disrupted, doxorubicin–solid lipid nanoparticles reached only low subtherapeutic concentrations, whereas the free drug did not reach significant levels [128]. Intravenous administration of solid lipid nanoparticles loaded with paclitaxel to rabbits resulted in drug concentrations in brain tissue that were 10-fold higher than paclitaxel control solutions. These results clearly showed that solid lipid nanoparticles are able to increase cerebral availability of different antineoplastic agents usually ineffective against brain tumors. Subsequently, systemic toxicity was decreased by reducing the total amount of drug incorporated and maintaining an effective concentration in the tumor target. Therefore, solid lipid nanoparticles may be regarded as effective carriers for chemotherapeutic drugs, but also gene therapeutic agents or diagnostic tools in neuro-oncology. Nevertheless, further studies are needed to improve efficacy and develop optimized targeted therapies.

46.5
Intranasal Delivery to Bypass the BBB

Intranasal delivery provides an interesting noninvasive method of bypassing the BBB to deliver therapeutic agents to the CNS [129]. This technology allows drug delivery to the brain within minutes, thereby eliminating the need for systemic administration. Connections between the brain and external environment provided by olfactory and trigeminal nerves allow targeting of both small molecules and macromolecules to the olfactory system. Several *in vivo* studies showed the potential of this strategy for various drugs, including chemotherapeutics [130]. However, despite positive animal studies a debate is ongoing about whether this route of administration is feasible in humans considering the large anatomical differences between the olfactory areas of animals and humans. A careful analysis of the present literature [131] showed that only a few papers presented a sound experimental design to study direct nose–CNS transport of drugs. Of these, only two studies in rats were able to provide results that can be regarded as an indication for direct transport from the nose to the CNS. No pharmacokinetic evidence could be found to support a claim that nasal administration of drugs in humans will result in an enhanced delivery to their target sites in the brain compared with intravenous administration of the same drug under similar dosage conditions. Therefore, further studies are required to validate this approach.

46.6
Conclusion and Perspectives

Targeted drug delivery to the brain has been wishful thinking for decades. However, the development of CNS drug targeting has recently been experiencing a remarkable upswing. Good BBB permeability and hence accumulation in the CNS is a critical feature for the successful therapy of all CNS-related diseases. Recognition of underlying mechanisms of the BBB (identification of export proteins, their regulation and substrate selectivity, use of cytotic mechanisms, and others) and knowledge of the molecular biology of diseased CNS tissue offers a broad set of possibilities to overcome this obstacle and to deliver drugs into the brain. In recent years it has clearly been recognized that a shift is ongoing from traditional cytotoxic chemotherapy toward targeted approaches and, therefore, the development of new targeted chemical compounds as well as noninvasive targeting strategies are gaining more and more attention. The above discussed vector technology and/or surface modification of colloidal carrier systems offers promising tools for new therapeutic areas. Modified carriers loaded with vaccines, anti-inflammatory drugs, new antibiotics, and cytostatics or used as gene shuttles show first positive results in animal studies and in clinical applications. Even if many obstacles have to be conquered, the continuously ongoing optimization of carrier systems, such as by use of enzymatically cleavable bonds or improved signal structures, will lead to new biodegradable composites, offering new possibilities of drug delivery to the CNS.

References

1. Pardridge, W. (2003) Blood–brain barrier drug targeting: the future of brain drug development. *Mol. Interv.*, **3**, 90–105.
2. Omuro, A.M., Faivre, S., and Raymond, E. (2007) Lessons learned in the development of targeted therapy for malignant gliomas. *Mol. Cancer Ther.*, **6**, 1909–1919.
3. Ehrlich P. (1885) *Das Sauerstoff-bedürfniss des Organismus. Eine farbenanalytische Studie*, Hirschwald, Berlin.
4. Lewandowsky, M. (1900) Zur lehre von der cerebrospinalflussigkeit. *Z. Klein. Med.*, **40**, 480–494.
5. Reese, T.S. and Karnovsky, M.J. (1967) Fine structural localization of a blood–brain barrier to exogenous peroxidase. *J. Cell Biol.*, **34**, 207–217.
6. Brightman, M.W. and Reese, T.S. (1969) Junctions between intimately apposed cell membranes in the vertebrate brain. *J. Cell Biol.*, **40**, 648–677.
7. Crone, C. and Olesen, S.P. (1982) Electrical resistance of brain microvascular endothelium. *Brain Res.*, **241**, 49–55.
8. Bandopadhyay, R., Orte, C., Lawrenson, J.G., Reid, A.R., De Silva, S., and Allt, G. (2001) Contractile proteins in pericytes at the blood–brain and blood–retinal barriers. *J. Neurocytol.*, **30**, 35–44.
9. Hori, S., Ohtsuki, S., Hosoya, K., Nakashima, E., and Terasaki, T. (2004) A pericyte-derived angiopoietin-1 multimeric complex induces occludin gene expression in brain capillary endothelial cells through Tie-2 activation *in vitro*. *J. Neurochem.*, **89**, 503–513.
10. Dore-Duffy, P., Owen, C., Balabanov, R., Murphy, S., Beaumont, T., and Rafols, J.A. (2000) Pericyte migration from the vascular wall in response to traumatic brain injury. *Microvasc. Res.*, **60**, 55–69.
11. Tao-Cheng, J.H., Nagy, Z., and Brightman, M.W. (1987) Tight junctions of brain endothelium *in vitro* are enhanced by astroglia. *J. Neurosci.*, **7**, 3293–3299.
12. Neuhaus, J., Risau, W., and Wolburg, H. (1991) Induction of blood–brain barrier characteristics in bovine brain endothelial cells by rat astroglial cells in transfilter coculture. *Ann. NY Acad. Sci.*, **633**, 578–580.
13. Braet, K., Paemeleire, K., D'Herde, K., Sanderson, M.J., and Leybaert, L. (2001) Astrocyte–endothelial cell calcium signals conveyed by two signalling pathways. *Eur. J. Neurosci.*, **13**, 79–91.
14. Zonta, M., Angulo, M.C., Gobbo, S., Rosengarten, B., Hossmann, K.A., Pozzan, T., and Carmignoto, G. (2003) Neuron-to-astrocyte signaling is central to the dynamic control of brain microcirculation. *Nat. Neurosci.*, **6**, 43–50.
15. Cohen, Z., Molinatti, G., and Hamel, E. (1997) Astroglial and vascular interactions of noradrenaline terminals in the rat cerebral cortex. *J. Cereb. Blood Flow Metab.*, **17**, 894–904.

16. Kobayashi, H., Magnoni, M.S., Govoni, S., Izumi, F., Wada, A., and Trabucchi, M. (1985) Neuronal control of brain microvessel function. *Experientia*, **41**, 427–434.
17. Rosenberg, G.A., Estrada, E., Kelley, R.O., and Kornfeld, M. (1993) Bacterial collagenase disrupts extracellular matrix and opens blood–brain barrier in rat. *Neurosci. Lett.*, **160**, 117–119.
18. Tilling, T., Korte, D., Hoheisel, D., and Galla, H.J. (1998) Basement membrane proteins influence brain capillary endothelial barrier function *in vitro*. *J. Neurochem.*, **71**, 1151–1157.
19. Savettieri, G., Di Liegro, I., Catania, C., Licata, L., Pitarresi, G.L., D'Agostino, S., Schiera, G., De Caro, V., Giandalia, G., Giannola, L.I., and Cestelli, A. (2000) Neurons and ECM regulate occludin localization in brain endothelial cells. *Neuroreport*, **11**, 1081–1084.
20. Schulze, C. and Firth, J.A. (1993) Immunohistochemical localization of adherens junction components in blood–brain barrier microvessels of the rat. *J. Cell Sci.*, **104**, 773–782.
21. Kniesel U. and Wolburg H. (2000) Tight junctions of the blood–brain barrier. *Cell. Mol. Neurobiol.*, **20**, 57–76.
22. Dejana, E., Lampugnani, M.G., Martinez-Estrada, O., and Bazzoni, G. (2000) The molecular organization of endothelial junctions and their functional role in vascular morphogenesis and permeability. *Int. J. Dev. Biol.*, **44**, 743–748.
23. Lippoldt, A., Kniesel, U., Liebner, S., Kalbacher, H., Kirsch, T., Wolburg, H., and Haller, H. (2000) Structural alterations of tight junctions are associated with loss of polarity in stroke-prone spontaneously hypertensive rat blood–brain barrier endothelial cells. *Brain Res.*, **885**, 251–261.
24. Nitta, T., Hata, M., Gotoh, S., Seo, Y., Sasaki, H., Hashimoto, N., Furuse, M., and Tsukita, S. (2003) Size-selective loosening of the blood–brain barrier in claudin-5-deficient mice. *J. Cell Biol.*, **161**, 653–660.
25. Witt, K.A., Mark, K.S., Hom, S., and Davis, T.P. (2003) Effects of hypoxia–reoxygenation on rat blood–brain barrier permeability and tight junctional protein expression. *Am. J. Physiol.*, **285**, H2820–H2831.
26. Wolburg, H., Wolburg-Buchholz, K., Kraus, J., Rascher-Eggstein, G., Liebner, S., Hamm, S., Duffner, F., Grote, E.H., Risau, W., and Engelhardt, B. (2003) Localization of claudin-3 in tight junctions of the blood–brain barrier is selectively lost during experimental autoimmune encephalomyelitis and human glioblastoma multiforme. *Acta Neuropathol.*, **105**, 586–592.
27. Fanning, A.S., Jameson, B.J., Jesaitis, L.A., and Anderson, J.M. (1998) The tight junction protein ZO-1 establishes a link between the transmembrane protein occludin and the actin cytoskeleton. *J. Biol. Chem.*, **273**, 29745–29753.
28. Abbruscato, T.J., Lopez, S.P., Mark, K.S., Hawkins, B.T., and Davis, T.P. (2002) Nicotine and cotinine modulate cerebral microvascular permeability and protein expression of ZO-1 through nicotinic acetylcholine receptors expressed on brain endothelial cells. *J. Pharm. Sci.*, **91**, 2525–2538.
29. Mark, K.S. and Davis, T.P. (2002) Cerebral microvascular changes in permeability and tight junctions induced by hypoxia–reoxygenation. *Am. J. Physiol.*, **282**, H1485–H1494.
30. Hawkins, T. and Davis, T.P. (2005) The blood–brain barrier/neurovascular unit in health and disease. *Brian Pharm. Rev.*, **57**, 173–185.
31. Maher, F., Vannucci, S.J., and Simpson, I.A. (1994) Glucose transporter proteins in brain. *FASEB J.*, **8**, 1003–1011.
32. Pardridge, W. (1999) Blood–brain barrier biology and methodology. *J. Neurovirol.*, **5**, 556–569.
33. Smith, Q.R. (2000) Transport of glutamate and other amino acids at the blood–brain barrier. *J. Nutr.*, **130** (Suppl.), 1016S–1022S.
34. Meier, P.J. and Stieger, B. (2002) Bile salt transporters. *Annu. Rev. Physiol.*, **64**, 635–661.
35. Wijnholds, J., de Lange, E.C., Scheffer, G.L., van den Berg, D.J., Mol, C.A.,

van der Valk, M., Schinkel, A.H., Scheper, R.J., Breimer, D.D., and Borst, P. (2000) Multidrug resistance protein 1 protects the choroid plexus epithelium and contributes to the blood–cerebrospinal fluid barrier. *J. Clin. Invest.*, **105**, 279–285.

36. Gao, B., Stieger, B., Noe, B., Fritschy, J.M., and Meier, P.J. (1999) Localization of the organic anion transporting polypeptide 2 (OATP2) in capillary endothelium and choroid plexus epithelium of rat brain. *J. Histochem. Cytochem.*, **47**, 1255–1264.

37. Ohtsuki, S., Asaba, H., Takanaga, H., Deguchi, T., Hosoya, K., Otagiri, M., and Terasaki, T. (2002) Role of blood–brain barrier organic anion transporter 3 (OAT3) in the efflux of indoxyl sulfate, a uremic toxin: its involvement in neurotransmitter metabolite clearance from the brain. *J. Neurochem.*, **83**, 57–66.

38. Schinkel, A.H., Wagenaar, E., Mol, C.A., and van Deemter, L. (1996) P-glycoprotein in the blood–brain barrier of mice influences the brain penetration and pharmacological activity of many drugs. *J. Clin. Invest.*, **97**, 2517–2524.

39. Schinkel, A.H., Smit, J.J., van Tellingen, O., Beijnen, J.H., Wagenaar, E., van Deemter, L., Mol, C.A., van der Valk, M.A., Robanus-Maandag, E.C., te Riele, H.P., Berns, A.J.M., and Borst, P. (1994) Disruption of the mouse *mdr1a* P-glycoprotein gene leads to a deficiency in the blood–brain barrier and to increased sensitivity to drugs. *Cell*, **77**, 491–502.

40. Nobmann, S., Bauer, B., and Fricker, G. (2001) Ivermectin excretion by isolated functionally intact brain endothelial capillaries. *Br. J. Pharmacol.*, **132**, 722–728.

41. Kim, R.B., Fromm, M.F., Wandel, C., Leake, B., Wood, A.J., Roden, D.M., and Wilkinson, G.R. (1998) The drug transporter P-glycoprotein limits oral absorption and brain entry of HIV-1 protease inhibitors. *J. Clin. Invest.*, **101**, 289–294.

42. Drewe, J., Gutmann, H., Fricker, G., Török, M., Beglinger, C., and Huwyler, J. (1999) HIV protease inhibitor ritonavir: a more potent inhibitor of P-glycoprotein than the cyclosporine analog SDZ PSC 833. *Biochem. Pharmacol.*, **57**, 1147–1152.

43. Kodaira, H., Kusuhara, H., Ushiki, J., Fuse, E., and Sugiyama, Y. (2010) Kinetic analysis of the cooperation of P-glycoprotein (P-glycoprotein/Abcb1) and breast cancer resistance protein (Bcrp/Abcg2) in limiting the brain and testis penetration of erlotinib, flavopiridol, and mitoxantrone. *J. Pharmacol. Exp. Ther.*, **333**, 788–796.

44. Milane, A., Vautier, S., Chacun, H., Meininger, V., Bensimon, G., Farinotti, R., and Fernandez, C. (2009) Interactions between riluzole and ABCG2/BCRP transporter. *Neurosci. Lett.*, **452**, 12–16.

45. Sawada, T., Kato, Y., Kobayashi, M., and Takekekawa, Y. (2000) Immunohistochemical study of tight junction-related protein in neovasculature in astrocytic tumor. *Brain Tumor Pathol.*, **17**, 1–6.

46. Liebner, S., Fischmann, A., Rascher, G., Duffner, F., Grote, E.H., Kalbacher, H., and Wolburg, H. (2000) Claudin-1 and claudin-5 expression and tight junction morphology are altered in blood vessels of human glioblastoma multiforme. *Acta Neuropathol.*, **100**, 323–331.

47. de Vries, N.A., Beijnen, J.H., Boogerd, W., and van Tellingen, O. (2006) Blood–brain barrier and chemotherapeutic treatment of brain tumors. *Expert Rev. Neurother.*, **6**, 1199–1209.

48. Zhou, Q. and Gallo, J.M. (2009) Differential effect of sunitinib on the distribution of temozolomide in an orthotopic glioma model. *Neuro. Oncol.*, **11**, 301–310.

49. Haga, S., Hinoshita, E., Ikezaki, K., Fukui, M., Scheffer, G.L., Uchiumi, T., and Kuwano, M. (2001) Involvement of the multidrug resistance protein 3 in drug sensitivity and its expression in human glioma. *Jpn. J. Cancer Res.*, **92**, 211–219.

50. Becker, I., Becker, K.F., Meyermann, R., and Höllt, V. (1991) The multidrug-resistance gene MDR1 is expressed in human glial tumors. *Acta Neuropathol.*, **82**, 516–519.

51. Prokai, L., Prokai-Tatrai, K., and Bodor, N. (2000) Targeting drugs to the brain by redox chemical delivery systems. *Med. Res. Rev.*, **20**, 367–316.
52. Gynther, M., Ropponen, J., Laine, K., Leppänen, J., Haapakoski, P., Peura, L., Järvinen, T., and Rautio, J. (2009) Glucose promoiety enables glucose transporter mediated brain uptake of ketoprofen and indomethacin prodrugs in rats. *J. Med. Chem.*, **52**, 3348–3353.
53. Gynther, M., Laine, K., Ropponen, J., Leppänen, J., Mannila, A., Nevalainen, T., Savolainen, J., Järvinen, T., and Rautio, J. (2008) Large neutral amino acid transporter enables brain drug delivery via prodrugs. *J. Med. Chem.*, **51**, 932–936.
54. Kemper, E.M., van Zandbergen, A.E., Cleypool, C., Mos, H.A., Boogerd, W., Beijnen, J.H., and van Tellingen, O. (2003) Increased penetration of paclitaxel into the brain by inhibition of P-glycoprotein. *Clin. Cancer Res.*, **9**, 2849–2855.
55. Kemper, E.M., Cleypool, C., Boogerd, W., Beijnen, J.H., and van Tellingen, O. (2004) The influence of the P-glycoprotein inhibitor zosuquidar trihydrochloride (LY335979) on the brain penetration of paclitaxel in mice. *Cancer Chemother. Pharmacol.*, **53**, 173–178.
56. Fellner, S., Bauer, B., Miller, D.S., Schaffrik, M., Fankhänel, M., Spruss, T., Bernhardt, G., Graeff, C., Färber, L., Gschaidmeier, H., Buschauer, A., and Fricker, G. (2002) Transport of paclitaxel (Taxol) across the blood–brain barrier *in vitro* and *in vivo*. *J. Clin. Invest.*, **110**, 1309–1318.
57. Joo, K.M., Park, K., Kong, D.S., Song, S.Y., Kim, M.H., Lee, G.S., Kim, M.S., and Nam, D.H. (2008) Oral paclitaxel chemotherapy for brain tumors: ideal combination treatment of paclitaxel and P-glycoprotein inhibitor. *Oncol. Rep.*, **19**, 17–23.
58. Breedveld, P., Pluim, D., Cipriani, G., Wielinga, P., van Tellingen, O., Schinkel, A.H., and Schellens, J.H. (2005) The effect of Bcrp1 (Abcg2) on the *in vivo* pharmacokinetics and brain penetration of imatinib mesylate (Gleevec): implications for the use of breast cancer resistance protein and P-glycoprotein inhibitors to enable the brain penetration of imatinib in patients. *Cancer Res.*, **65**, 2577–2582.
59. Elkind, N.B., Szentpétery, Z., Apáti, A., Ozvegy-Laczka, C., Várady, G., Ujhelly, O., Szabó, K., Homolya, L., Váradi, A., Buday, L., Kéri, G., Németh, K., and Sarkadi, B. (2005) Multidrug transporter ABCG2 prevents tumor cell death induced by the epidermal growth factor receptor inhibitor Iressa (ZD1839, Gefitinib). *Cancer Res.*, **65**, 1770–1777.
60. Heimberger, A.B., Learn, C.A., Archer, G.E., McLendon, R.E., Chewning, T.A., Tuck, F.L., Pracyk, J.B., Friedman, A.H., Friedman, H.S., Bigner, D.D., and Sampson, J.H. (2002) Brain tumors in mice are susceptible to blockade of epidermal growth factor receptor (EGFR) with the oral, specific, EGFR-tyrosine kinase inhibitor ZD1839 (Iressa). *Clin. Cancer Res.*, **8**, 3496–3502.
61. Ceresoli, G.L., Cappuzzo, F., Gregorc, V., Bartolini, S., Crinò, L., and Villa, E. (2004) Gefitinib in patients with brain metastases from non-small-cell lung cancer: a prospective trial. *Ann. Oncol.*, **15**, 1042–1047.
62. Kwong, Y., Yeung, D.Y., and Chan, J.C. (2009) Intrathecal chemotherapy for hematologic malignancies: drugs and toxicities. *Ann. Hematol.*, **88**, 193–201.
63. Berg, S. and Chamberlain, M.C. (2005) Current treatment of leptomeningeal metastases: systemic chemotherapy, intrathecal chemotherapy and symptom management. *Cancer Treat Res.*, **125**, 121–146.
64. Rapaport, S.I., Hori, M., and Klatzo, I. (1971) Reversible osmotic opening of the blood–brain barrier. *Science*, **173**, 1026–1028.
65. Rapoport, S.I., Fredericks, W.R., Ohno, K., and Pettigrew, K.D. (1980) Quantitative aspects of reversible osmotic opening of the blood–brain barrier. *Am. J. Physiol.*, **238**, 421–431.

66. Neuwelt, E., Maravilla, K.R., Frenkel, E.P., Barnett, P., Hill, S., and Moore, R.J. (1980) Use of enhanced computerized tomography to evaluate osmotic blood–brain barrier disruption. *Neurosurgery*, **6**, 49–56.
67. Robinson, P.J. and Rapoport, S.I. (1990) Model for drug uptake by brain tumors: effects of osmotic treatment and of diffusion in brain. *J. Cereb. Blood Flow Metab.*, **10**, 153–161.
68. Jahnke, K., Kraemer, D.F., Knight, K.R., Fortin, D., Bell, S., Doolittle, N.D., Muldoon, L.L., and Neuwelt, E.A. (2008) Intraarterial chemotherapy and osmotic blood–brain barrier disruption for patients with embryonal and germ cell tumors of the central nervous system. *Cancer*, **112**, 581–588.
69. Liu, H.L., Hsu, P.H., Chu, P.C., Wai, Y.Y., Chen, J.C., Shen, C.R., Yen, T.C., and Wang, J.J. (2009) Magnetic resonance imaging enhanced by superparamagnetic iron oxide particles: usefulness for distinguishing between focused ultrasound-induced blood–brain barrier disruption and brain hemorrhage. *J. Magn. Reson. Imaging*, **29**, 31–38.
70. Treat, L.H., McDannold, N., Vykhodtseva, N., Zhang, Y., Tam, K., and Hynynen, K. (2007) Targeted delivery of doxorubicin to the rat brain at therapeutic levels using MRI-guided focused ultrasound. *Int. J. Cancer*, **121**, 901–907.
71. Moos, T. and Morgan, E.H. (2000) Transferrin and transferrin receptor function in brain barrier systems. *Cell. Mol. Neurobiol.*, **20**, 77–95.
72. Li, H. and Qian, Z.M. (2002) Transferrin/transferrin receptor-mediated drug delivery. *Med. Res. Rev.*, **22**, 225–250.
73. Friden, P.M., Walus, L.R., Musso, G.F., Taylor, M.A., Malfroy, B., and Starzyk, R.M. (1991) Anti-transferrin receptor antibody and antibody–drug conjugates cross the blood–brain barrier. *Proc. Natl. Acad. Sci. USA*, **88**, 4771–4775.
74. Pardridge, W.M., Buciak, J.L., and Friden, P.M. (1991) Selective transport of an anti-transferrin receptor antibody through the blood–brain barrier *in vivo*. *J. Pharmacol. Exp. Ther.*, **259**, 66–70.
75. Penichet, M.L., Kang, Y.S., Pardridge, W.M., Morrison, S.L., and Shin, S.U. (1999) An antibody–avidin fusion protein specific for the transferrin receptor serves as a delivery vehicle for effective brain targeting: initial applications in anti-HIV antisense drug delivery to the brain. *J. Immunol.*, **163**, 4421–4426.
76. Albeck, D.S., Hoffer, B.J., Quissell, D., Sanders, L.A., Zerbe, G., and Granholm, A.C. (1997) A non-invasive transport system for GDNF across the blood–brain barrier. *Neuroreport. J.*, **8**, 2293–2298.
77. Granholm, A.C., Bäckman, C., Bloom, F., Ebendal, T., Gerhardt, G.A., Hoffer, B., Mackerlova, L., Olson, L., Söderström, S., Walus, L.R. *et al.* (1994) NGF and anti-transferrin receptor antibody conjugate: short and long-term effects on survival of cholinergic neurons in intraocular septal transplants. *J. Pharmacol. Exp. Ther.*, **268**, 448–459.
78. Kordower, J.H., Charles, V., Bayer, R., Bartus, R.T., Putney, S., Walus, L.R., and Friden, P.M. (1994) Intravenous administration of a transferrin receptor antibody–nerve growth factor conjugate prevents the degeneration of cholinergic striatal neurons in a model of Huntington disease. *Proc. Natl. Acad. Sci. USA*, **91**, 9077–9080.
79. Tadayoni, B.M., Friden, P.M., Walus, L.R., and Musso, G.F. (1993) Synthesis, *in vitro* kinetics, and *in vivo* studies on protein conjugates of AZT: evaluation as a transport system to increase brain delivery. *Bioconjug. Chem.*, **4**, 139–145.
80. Bickel, U., Yoshikawa, T., Landaw, E.M., Faull, K.F., and Pardridge, W.M. (1993) Pharmacologic effects *in vivo* in brain by vector-mediated peptide drug delivery. *Proc. Natl. Acad. Sci. USA*, **90**, 2618–2622.
81. Moroo, I., Ujiie, M., Walker, B.L., Tiong, J.W., Vitalis, T.Z., Karkan, D., Gabathuler, R., Moise, A.R., and Jefferies, W.A. (2003) Identification of a novel route of iron transcytosis across the mammalian blood–brain barrier. *Microcirculation*, **10**, 457–462.

82. Demeule, M., Poirier, J., Jodoin, J., Bertrand, Y., Desrosiers, R.R., Dagenais, C., Nguyen, T., Lanthier, J., Gabathuler, R., Kennard, M., Jefferies, W.A., Karkan, D., Tsai, S., Fenart, L., Cecchelli, R., and Beliveau, R. (2002) High transcytosis of melanotransferrin (P97) across the blood–brain barrier. *J. Neurochem.*, **83**, 924–933.
83. Tang, Y., Han, T., Everts, M., Zhu, Z.B., Gillespie, G.Y., Curiel, D.T., and Wu, H. (2007) Directing adenovirus across the blood–brain barrier via melanotransferrin (P97) transcytosis pathway in an *in vitro* model. *Gene Ther.*, **14**, 523–532.
84. Karkan, D., Pfeifer, C., Vitalis, T.Z., Arthur, G., Ujiie, M., Chen, Q., Tsai, S., Koliatis, G., Gabathuler, R., and Jefferies, W.A. (2008) A unique carrier for delivery of therapeutic compounds beyond the blood–brain barrier. *PLoS ONE*, **3**, e2469.
85. Proia, R.L., Hart, D.A., Holmes, R.K., Holmes, K.V., and Eidels, L. (1979) Immunoprecipitation and partial characterization of diphtheria toxin-binding glycoproteins from surface of guinea pig cells. *Proc. Natl. Acad. Sci. USA*, **76**, 685–689.
86. Wang, P., Xue, Y., Shang, X., and Liu, Y. (2010) Diphtheria toxin mutant CRM197-mediated transcytosis across blood–brain barrier *In vitro*. *Cell. Mol. Neurobiol.*,**30**, 717–725.
87. Rousselle, C., Clair, P., Lefauconnier, J.M., Kaczorek, M., Scherrmann, J.M., and Temsamani, J. (2000) New advances in the transport of doxorubicin through the blood–brain barrier by a peptide vector-mediated strategy. *Mol. Pharmacol.*, **57**, 679–686.
88. Rousselle, C., Clair, P., Smirnova, M., Kolesnikov, Y., Pasternak, G.W., Gac-Breton, S., Rees, A.R., Scherrmann, J.M., and Temsamani, J. (2003) Improved brain uptake and pharmacological activity of dalargin using a peptide-vector-mediated strategy. *J. Pharmacol. Exp. Ther.*, **306**, 371–376.
89. Drin, G., Cottin, S., Blanc, E., Rees, A.R., and Temsamani, J. (2003) Studies on the internalization mechanism of cationic cell-penetrating peptides. *J. Biol. Chem.*, **278**, 31192–31201.
90. Dri, G., Rouselle, C., Scherrmann, J.M., Rees, A.R., and Temsamani, J. (2002) Peptide delivery to the brain via adsorptive-mediated endocytosis: advances with SynB vectors. *AAPS Pharm. Sci.*, **4**, E26.
91. Régina, A., Demeule, M., Ché, C., Lavallée, I., Poirier, J., Gabathuler, R., Béliveau, R., and Castaigne, J.P. (2008) Antitumour activity of ANG1005, a conjugate between paclitaxel and the new brain delivery vector Angiopep-2. *Br. J. Pharmacol.*, **155**, 185–197.
92. Abulrob, A., Sprong, H., Van Bergen en Henegouwen, P., and Stanimirovic, D. (2005) The blood–brain barrier transmigrating single domain antibody: mechanisms of transport and antigenic epitopes in human brain endothelial cells. *J Neurochem.*, **95**, 1201–1214.
93. Coloma, M.J., Lee, H.J., Kurihara, A., Landaw, E.M., Boado, R.J., Morrison, S.L., and Pardridge, W.M. (2000) Transport across the primate blood–brain barrier of a genetically engineered chimeric monoclonal antibody to the human insulin receptor. *Pharm. Res.*, **17**, 266–274.
94. Harris, J.M., Martin, N.E., and Modi, M. (2001) Pegylation: a novel process for modifying pharmacokinetics. *Clin. Pharmacokinet.*, **40**, 539–551.
95. Jain, N.K. and Nahar, M. (2010) PEGylated nanocarriers for systemic delivery. *Methods Mol. Biol.*, **624**, 221–234.
96. Huwyler, J., Wu, D., and Pardridge, W.M. (1996) Brain drug delivery of small molecules using immunoliposomes. *Proc. Natl. Acad. Sci. USA*, **93**, 14164–14169.
97. Doi, A., Kawabata, S., Iida, K., Yokoyama, K., Kajimoto, Y., Kuroiwa, T., Shirakawa, T., Kirihata, M., Kasaoka, S., Maruyama, K., Kumada, H., Sakurai, Y., Masunaga, S., Ono, K., and Miyatake, S. (2008) Tumor-specific targeting of sodium borocaptate (BSH) to malignant glioma by transferrin-PEG liposomes: a modality for boron neutron capture therapy. *J. Neurooncol.*, **87**, 287–294.

98. Yanagie, H., Ogata, A., Sugiyama, H., Eriguchi, M., Takamoto, S., and Takahashi, H. (2008) Application of drug delivery system to boron neutron capture therapy for cancer. *Expert Opin. Drug Deliv.*, **5**, 427–443.
99. Cerletti, A., Drewe, J., Fricker, G., Eberle, A.N., and Huwyler, J. (2000) Endocytosis and transcytosis of an immunoliposome-based brain drug delivery system. *J. Drug Target.*, **8**, 435–446.
100. Shi, N. and Pardridge, W.M. (2000) Noninvasive gene targeting to the brain. *Proc. Natl. Acad. Sci. USA*, **97**, 7567–7572.
101. Boado, R.J. (2007) Blood–brain barrier transport of non-viral gene and RNAi therapeutics. *Pharm Res.*, **24**, 1772–1787.
102. Pardridge, W.M. (2010) Preparation of Trojan horse liposomes (THLs) for gene transfer across the blood–brain barrier. *Cold Spring Harb. Protoc.*, **2010** (4), pdb.prot5407.
103. Hülsermann, U., Massing, U., Hoffmann, M., and Fricker, G. (2009) Uptake of apolipoprotein E fragment coupled liposomes by cultured brain microvessel endothelial cells and intact brain capillaries. *J. Drug Target.*, **17**, 610–618.
104. Leupold, E., Nikolenko, H., and Dathe, M. (2009) Apolipoprotein E peptide-modified colloidal carriers: the design determines the mechanism of uptake in vascular endothelial cells. *Biochim. Biophys. Acta*, **1788**, 442–449.
105. Sauer, I., Dunay, I.R., Weisgraber, K., Bienert, M., and Dathe, M. (2005) An apolipoprotein E-derived peptide mediates uptake of sterically stabilized liposomes into brain capillary endothelial cells. *Biochemistry*, **44**, 2021–2029.
106. Thöle, M., Nobmann, S., Huwyler, J., Bartmann, A., and Fricker, G. (2002) Uptake of cationizied albumin coupled liposomes by cultured porcine brain microvessel endothelial cells and intact brain capillaries. *J. Drug Target.*, **10**, 337–344.
107. Chen, H., Tang, L., Qin, Y., Yin, Y., Tang, J., Tang, W., Sun, X., Zhang, Z., Liu, J., and He, Q. (2010) Lactoferrin-modified procationic liposomes as a novel drug carrier for brain delivery. *Eur. J. Pharm. Sci.*, **40**, 94–102.
108. Tamaru, M., Akita, H., Fujiwara, T., Kajimoto, K., and Harashima, H. (2010) Leptin-derived peptide, a targeting ligand for mouse brain-derived endothelial cells via macropinocytosis. *Biochem. Biophys. Res. Commun.*, **394**, 587–592.
109. Hervé, F., Ghinea, N., and Scherrmann, J.M. (2008) CNS delivery via adsorptive transcytosis. *AAPS J.*, **10**, 455–472.
110. Rapoport, M. and Lorberboum-Galski, H. (2009) TAT-based drug delivery system – new directions in protein delivery for new hopes? *Expert Opin. Drug Deliv.*, **6**, 453–463.
111. Du, J., Lu, W.L., Ying, X., Liu, Y., Du, P., Tian, W., Men, Y., Guo, J., Zhang, Y., Li, R.J., Zhou, J., Lou, J.N., Wang, J.C., Zhang, X., and Zhang, Q. (2009) Dual-targeting topotecan liposomes modified with tamoxifen and wheat germ agglutinin significantly improve drug transport across the blood–brain barrier and survival of brain tumor-bearing animals. *Mol. Pharm.*, **6**, 905–917.
112. Madhankumar, A.B., Slagle-Webb, B., Wang, X., Yang, Q.X., Antonetti, D.A., Miller, P.A., Sheehan, J.M., and Connor, J.R. (2009) Efficacy of interleukin-13 receptor-targeted liposomal doxorubicin in the intracranial brain tumor model. *Mol. Cancer Ther.*, **8**, 648–654.
113. Ryuke, Y., Mizuno, M., Natsume, A., and Yoshida, J. (2000) Transduction efficiency of adenoviral vectors into human glioma cells increased by association with cationic liposomes. *Neurol. Med. Chir.*, **40**, 256–260.
114. von Eckardstein, K.L., Patt, S., Zhu, J., Zhang, L., Cervós-Navarro, J., and Reszka, R. (2001) Short-term neuropathological aspects of *in vivo* suicide gene transfer to the F98 rat glioblastoma using liposomal and viral vectors. *Histol. Histopathol.*, **16**, 735–744.

115. Reddy, M.K. and Labhasetwar, V. (2009) Nanoparticle-mediated delivery of superoxide dismutase to the brain: an effective strategy to reduce ischemia-reperfusion injury. *FASEB J.*, **23**, 1384–1395.

116. Kreuter, J. (2004) Influence of the surface properties on nanoparticle-mediated transport of drugs to the brain. *J. Nanosci. Nanotechnol.*, **4**, 484–488.

117. Reimold, I., Domke, D., Bender, J., Seyfried, C.A., Radunz, H.E., and Fricker, G. (2008) Delivery of nanoparticles to the brain detected by fluorescence microscopy. *Eur. J. Pharm. Biopharm.*, **70**, 627–632.

118. Steiniger, S.C., Kreuter, J., Khalansky, A.S., Skidan, I.N., Bobruskin, A.I., Smirnova, Z.S., Severin, S.E., Uhl, R., Kock, M., Geiger, K.D., and Gelperina, S.E. (2004) Chemotherapy of glioblastoma in rats using doxorubicin-loaded nanoparticles. *Int. J. Cancer*, **109**, 759–767.

119. Friese, A., Seiller, E., Quack, G., Lorenz, B., and Kreuter, J. (2000) Increase of the duration of the anticonvulsive activity of a novel NMDA receptor antagonist using poly(butylcyanoacrylate) nanoparticles as a parenteral controlled release system. *Eur. J. Pharm. Biopharm.*, **49**, 103–109.

120. Zensi, A., Begley, D., Pontikis, C., Legros, C., Mihoreanu, L., Wagner, S., Büchel, C., von Briesen, H., and Kreuter, J. (2009) Albumin nanoparticles targeted with Apo E enter the CNS by transcytosis and are delivered to neurones. *J. Control. Release*, **137**, 78–86.

121. Rivière, C., Martina, M.S., Tomita, Y., Wilhelm, C., Tran Dinh, A., Ménager, C., Pinard, E., Lesieur, S., Gazeau, F., and Seylaz, J. (2007) Magnetic targeting of nanometric magnetic fluid loaded liposomes to specific brain intravascular areas: a dynamic imaging study in mice. *Radiology*, **244**, 439–448.

122. Chertok, B., Moffat, B.A., David, A.E., Yu, F., Bergemann, C., Ross, B.D., and Yang, V.C. (2008) Iron oxide nanoparticles as a drug delivery vehicle for MRI monitored magnetic targeting of brain tumors. *Biomaterials*, **29**, 487–496.

123. Jordan, A. and Maier-Hauff, K. (2007) Magnetic nanoparticles for intracranial thermotherapy. *J. Nanosci. Nanotechnol.*, **7**, 4604–4606.

124. van Landeghem, F.K., Maier-Hauff, K., Jordan, A., Hoffmann, K.T., Gneveckow, U., Scholz, R., Thiesen, B., Brück, W., and von Deimling, A. (2009) Post-mortem studies in glioblastoma patients treated with thermotherapy using magnetic nanoparticles. *Biomaterials*, **30**, 52–57.

125. Batrakova, E.V. and Kabanov, A.V. (2008) Pluronic block copolymers: evolution of drug delivery concept from inert nanocarriers to biological response modifiers. *J. Control. Release*, **130**, 98–106.

126. Dhanikula, R.S., Argaw, A., Bouchard, J.-F., and Hildgen, P. (2008) Methotrexate loaded polyether-copolyester dendrimers for the treatment of gliomas: enhanced efficacy and intratumoral transport capability. *Mol. Pharm.*, **5**, 105–116.

127. Blasi, P., Giovagnoli, S., Schoubben, A., Ricci, M., and Rossi, C. (2007) Solid lipid nanoparticles for targeted brain drug delivery. *Adv. Drug Deliv. Rev.*, **59**, 454–477.

128. Brioschi, A., Zenga, F., Zara, G.P., Gasco, M.R., Ducati, A., Mauro, A. (2007) Solid lipid nanoparticles: could they help to improve the efficiacy of pharmacological treatments of brain tumors. *Neurol. Res.*, **29**, 324–330.

129. Frey, W.H. II (2002) Bypassing the blood–brain barrier to delivery therapeutic agents to the brain and spinal cord. *Drug Deliv. Technol.*, **5**, 46–49.

130. Wang, D., Gao, Y., and Yun, L. (2005) Study on brain targeting of raltitrexed following intranasal administration in rats. *Cancer Chemother. Pharmacol.*, **57**, 97–104.

131. Merkus, F.W. and van den Berg, M.P. (2007) Can nasal drug delivery bypass the blood–brain barrier?: questioning the direct transport theory. *Drugs R D*, **8**, 133–144.

47
Liver Tumor Targeting

Katrin Hochdörffer, Giuseppina Di Stefano, Hiroshi Maeda, and Felix Kratz

47.1
Introduction

Liver cancers or hepatic cancers develop from liver tissue (primary liver cancer), in contrast to liver metastases that are formed by cancer cells migrating from other organs to the liver (secondary liver cancer). There are three types of primary liver cancer: cholangiocarcinoma, hepatoblastoma (which occurs predominantly in childhood), and hepatocellular carcinoma (HCC), which all differ regarding their cause, symptoms, diagnosis, and treatment. Due to the frequency of HCC (approximately 80%), this malignant disease will be discussed in detail in this chapter [1].

47.1.1
Epidemiology and Incidence of HCC

Currently, HCC is the fifth most common malignant tumor in the world. The geographic distribution of the incidence of HCC as shown in Figure 47.1 is variable and increases in developed countries [2]. The HCC incidence varies from less than 10 cases per 100 000 persons per year in Western countries to 50–150 cases per 100 000 people per year in parts of Africa and Asia [3, 4]. The American Cancer Society expected that in the United States the number of new cases of liver cancer would reach around 24 120 and predictable mortalities for liver cancer around 18 910 for both sexes in the year 2010 [5].

Apart from chronic hepatitis B, C, and D virus infections, the highest HCC risk factor in Western countries is alcohol-induced liver disease. Other risk factors include diabetes mellitus, nonalcoholic steatohepatitis, and obesity for males. HCC prevalence is more than twice as high in men as in women. Patients with chronic liver disease, in particular liver cirrhosis, have an increased risk of developing HCC. The HCC risk also correlates with the etiology, duration, and activity of the underlying liver disease. In general, the highest HCC risks pertain to patients with chronic hepatitis B or C virus with hereditary hemochromatosis or alcoholic toxic liver cirrhosis [6]. Patients with liver cirrhosis caused by a primary biliary

Drug Delivery in Oncology: From Basic Research to Cancer Therapy, First Edition.
Edited by Felix Kratz, Peter Senter, and Henning Steinhagen.

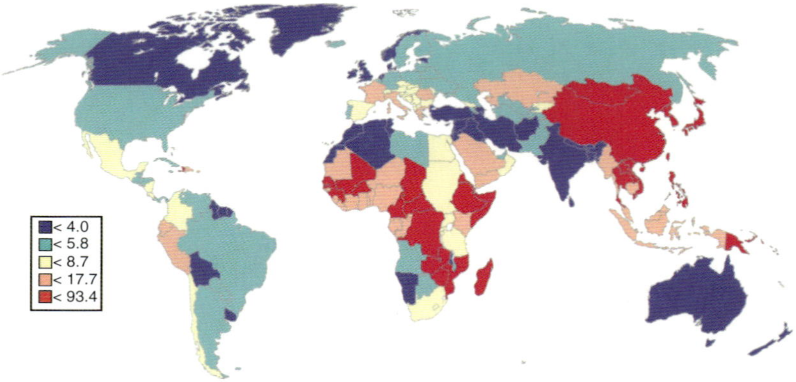

Figure 47.1 Worldwide incidence of HCC. The age-adjusted incidence rates are reported per 100 000 inhabitants [2].

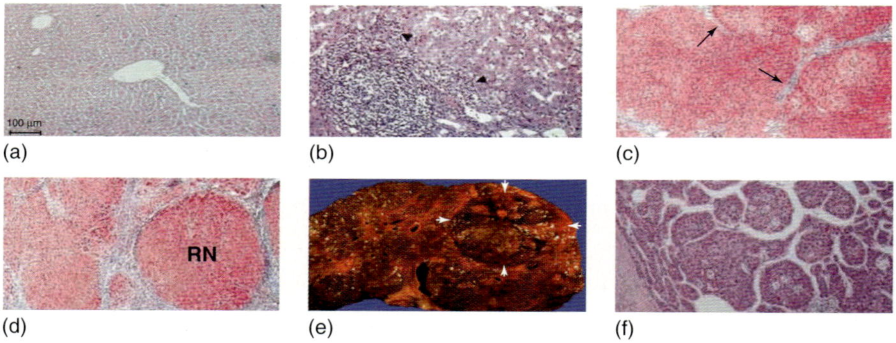

Figure 47.2 Clinical development of HCC. (a) healthy liver, (b) inflammation, (c) fibroses, (d) cirrhosis (RN are pseudolobuli), and (e) and (f) HCC [7].

cirrhosis, classified as Wilson's disease or autoimmune hepatitis, have a lower risk of developing HCC. Usually, HCC arises after years or even decades of a chronic, progressive hepatopathy, which subsequently leads to liver fibrosis and progresses to liver cirrhosis (Figure 47.2). The latency period between hepatitis B and C infection and HCC development is 30–60 and 20–30 years, respectively. HCC is a very malignant tumor and without any treatment the prognosis is poor [7].

47.1.2
Therapeutic Options for Treating Liver Cancer

The choice of a suitable treatment depends on the tumor stage, the localization of the tumor in the liver, the liver function as well as the age and state of health of the patient. The therapeutic modalities, such as HCC resection, liver transplantation, and local ablative strategies (e.g., percutaneous ethanol injection (PEI) or radiofrequency ablation (RFA)) are considered potentially curative approaches, and a 5-year survival rate between 50 and 70% can be reached. When these options are not possible, radio- or chemotherapy is used, but is mostly ineffective.

47.1.2.1 Liver Resection

At an early stage, surgical resection is the treatment of choice for HCC in noncirrhotic liver [8, 9]. The resection of 70–80% of functional liver tissues can be achieved in patients without liver cirrhosis. After successful resection, recurrence of HCC occurs in over 70% of patients during the first 5 years. The major cause for these relapses is the formation of intrahepatic metastases, which often appear in an advanced primary tumor with low grading and vascular invasion [9].

When dealing with an advanced tumor stage at the time of diagnosis, and often simultaneous presence of liver cirrhosis as well as comorbidity, old age, and other factors, surgical interventions are possible in about 20% of patients with HCC [10]. Liver resection actually represents a curative treatment as it simultaneously removes the underlying cirrhosis disease. If strict selection criteria are observed, such as the number and the size of nodules (one nodule below 5 cm or three nodules below 3 cm diameter per nodule), a 5-year survival rate of 70% with a relapse rate of lower than 15% can be achieved [10].

47.1.2.2 Local Ablative Therapy

Local ablative strategies include the process of injecting a chemical substance such as alcohol or acetic acid, or the process of inserting a hand-held probe (a so-called transducer) into the tumor, which then uses radiofrequency, microwaves, or laser light to destroy the tumor tissue. These strategies are the best curative treatment options for patients with small tumors who are not candidates for surgical resection or liver transplantation [11]. PEI and RFA are effective for patients with maximally three tumor foci and a diameter of 3 cm or less for each tumor. In this tumor stage a complete ablation is expected for 80% of the patients with a 5-year survival rate between 40 and 70%. A complete remission is achieved in 50% of the patients where the HCC tumor size is between 3 and 5 cm. The indication for PEI or RFA is not safe for tumors larger than 5 cm.

47.1.2.3 Transarterial Chemoembolization

At an intermediate stage of HCC, transarterial chemoembolization (TACE) is a further therapeutic option for patients with inoperable liver cancer or metastases and for patients with large or multifocal tumors (intermediate stage B [12]) that cannot be treated with RFA or PEI [13, 14]. TACE is a minimal invasive method in which an anticancer agent is simultaneously applied regionally with an emulsion such as Lipiodol® to shut off arteries, thus prolonging the activity of the anticancer agent. The main effect of TACE is most likely based on receptacle occlusion; the choice of the chemotherapeutic agent (e.g., doxorubicin (DOX), epirubicin, cisplatin, or mitomycin) and the choice of the occlusion materials are less decisive for the therapeutic success. Other special transarterial interventions include intra-arterial ^{131}I-Lipiodol therapy as well as intra-arterial injection of ^{90}Y-microspheres, which act as selective radiotherapy *in situ* [8, 9].

A response rate between 15 and 55% can be reached. Recently, in a number of randomized trials, a significant survival rate could be achieved for patients, above all in those with a good liver function [15, 16].

47.1.2.4 **Chemotherapy/Targeted Therapy**

The use of cytotoxic agents in advanced HCC has been unsatisfactory because HCC is a relatively chemoresistant tumor and is highly refractory to conventional chemotherapy. DOX, the agent that is most often employed and given as systemic chemotherapy, was shown to produce a limited response rate in HCC patients [17]. In addition, other chemotherapeutic agents, such as cisplatin, epirubicin, 5-fluorouracil (5-FU), and their combinations, have been investigated, but showed minimal antitumor response against advanced HCC [8, 18, 19]. Similarly, clinical studies with the newer generation of chemotherapeutic agents, such as gemcitabine, irinotecan, and PEGylated liposomal DOX, have shown no survival benefit [20, 21].

Recently, a modest survival improvement was reported after the introduction of the multikinase inhibitor sorafenib (Nexavar®): median survival and time to radiologic progression were nearly 3 months longer for patients treated with this drug than for those given a placebo [22–24]. A number of review articles have been published that discuss molecular-targeted therapies in HCC [25–27].

In summary, the therapeutic options for treating inoperable HCC and liver metastases are unsatisfactory. Anticancer agents lack selectivity for liver tumors so that chemotherapy is insufficient and associated with numerous systemic side-effects. Therefore, there is an urgent need to develop therapeutic concepts that increase the cytotoxic potential of anticancer drugs by selectively delivering the drug to liver tumors and specifically releasing it inside the tumor and tumor cells.

47.2 Rationale for Drug Delivery Concepts for Treating Liver Cancer

Efficient drug delivery systems are characterized by selectively transporting an encapsulated or carrier-linked drug to the tumor tissue, and specifically releasing the drug extra- or intracellularly in the tumor due to biochemical or physiological features unique for the tumor and tumor cells. Basic approaches of targeted drug delivery involve active and passive targeting or a combination of both.

A passive targeting strategy is based on the hypervasculature, defective vascular architecture, and ineffective lymphatic drainage of the malignant tissue. The accumulation of drugs in tumor tissue is obtained by using macromolecules (e.g., synthetic polymers or serum proteins) or nanocarriers (liposomes, micelles, nanoparticles) as carriers that do not primarily interact with tumor cells, but influence the drug's biodistribution and tumor uptake. This phenomenon has been termed the enhanced permeability and retention (EPR) effect and was elucidated by Matsumura and Maeda [28, 29] as well as Jain [30, 31] in the mid-1980s (see Chapter 3 for a detailed description).

Uptake of macromolecules and nanoparticles in the liver and in liver tumors is further mediated by the reticuloendothelial system (RES). The term "RES" was coined by L. Aschoff in 1924 and describes a number of cells of the mesenchyme that are capable of phagocytosis (i.e., they are able to take up and store foreign particles). A major function of the RES is the production of antibodies that subsequently elicit cellular immune reactions. The RES includes the stellate cells/Kupffer cells of the liver, the sinus cells of the spleen as well as the cells of the reticular connective tissue. When nanosized carriers are present, they can be opsonized by plasma proteins that are quickly recognized as foreign particles and are removed by the RES [32–34]. Depending on the size and composition of the drug carriers, they can be taken up by the RES within minutes after administration and are removed from the circulation [32].

In contrast, active targeting uses carriers that specifically recognize receptors or antigens expressed on the surface of tumor cells. As carriers for liver tumor targeting, low-molecular-weight ligands or antibodies are mostly used that can optionally be attached onto the surface of nanoparticles, such as synthetic polymers, serum proteins, carbon nanotubes, liposomes, and micelles. Typical examples are shown in Figure 47.3 [35].

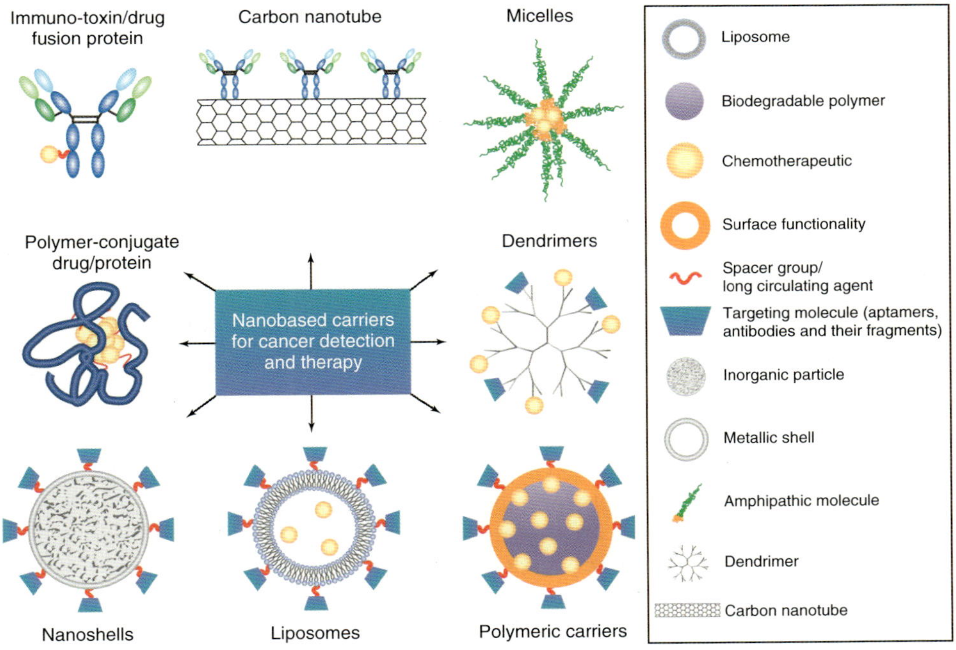

Figure 47.3 Types of nanosized carriers for targeting solid tumors [35].

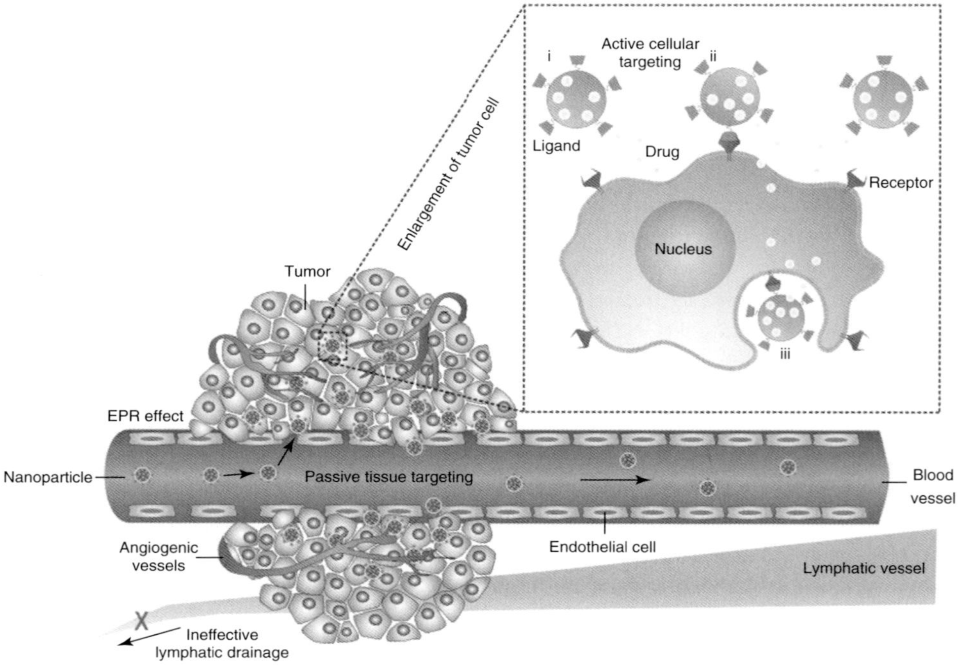

Figure 47.4 Schematic illustration of ligand-based nanocarriers that act by passive and active targeting. Passive tissue targeting is achieved by extravasation and retention of nanoparticles through anomalies in the vascular network of malignant tissue. Active targeting can be achieved by modifying the surface of nanoparticles with ligands that can interact specifically with their cellular target [35].

When elucidating the mode of action of ligand-based nanocarriers, it is important to realize that in most cases passive as well as active targeting play a role in delivering the drug to the tumor and tumor cells as illustrated in Figure 47.4 [35].

The best-studied example of a receptor that is expressed on liver and liver tumor cells is the Ashwell receptor that is specific for asialoglycoprotein (ASGP) and is described in the following section.

47.2.1
Receptor for ASGPs: A Target for Delivering Drugs to Hepatocytes

In 1968, Ashwell and Morell [36] observed that serum glycoproteins bearing *N*-linked oligosaccharides are rapidly removed from the bloodstream by hepatic parenchymal liver cells after losing their terminal sialic acid residues. The binding of ASGPs on hepatocytes is mediated by a C-type lectin recognizing galactose moieties, which is exposed after the removal of sialic acid residues. This lectin, which is involved in binding and endocytosis of a wide range of macromolecules exposing galactose or *N*-acetylgalactosamine, was named Ashwell's receptor or the receptor for ASGPs (ASGPR).

The first studies that characterized ASGPR (for a review, see [37]) indicated that the ASGPR is composed of subunits (two or three different peptides depending on the animal species) that are expressed on the hepatocyte membrane in an oligomerized state. The most frequently observed form is the heterotrimer, which was also found in human cells.

It is known that ASGPR is an oligomeric and integral membrane protein, and is composed of two homologous proteins – the human lectins (HL-1 and -2) [38]. HL-1 and -2 are glycoproteins that have 55% identical amino acids in their structures. These glycoproteins consist of a cytoplasmic N-terminal domain, built up of 40 amino acids, a short transmembrane domain, and a long C-terminal exoplasmic domain with 230 amino acids. On the C-terminal end of the exoplasmic domain are binding sites for calcium ions [39]. It is also probable that the ASGPR preferentially forms a heterotetramer containing two molecules of HL-1 and -2 at a time [40].

The functional binding activity of the receptor requires the presence of all subunits. The sugar-binding site appears to be relatively small and involves only terminal sugars bearing an axial hydroxy group on carbon-4. A cluster of three to five close sugar residues is enough to obtain an optimal binding strength with a dissociation constant in the nanomolar range. The tetra-antennary oligosaccharides of asialoorosomucoid have the highest dissociation constants of all carbohydrate structures; oligosaccharides lacking the third branch (e.g., those of asialotransferrin) show a significantly reduced binding affinity. A high affinity between ASGPR and desialyted glycoprotein terminal residues of β-D-galactopyranosyl-(galactose-, Gal-) or 2-acetamido-2-deoxy-β-D-galactopyranosyl-(*N*-acetylgalactosamine-, GalNAc-) has been observed. In the presence of several neighboring saccharide groups (multivalent ligands or so-called glycoside clusters) the binding constant is extremely high. In binding studies it was observed that dissociation constants of di- and trivalent galactose ligands were in the range of around 10^{-6} to even 5×10^{-9} M, whereas monovalent galactose ligands showed binding constants in a millimolar range. This phenomena is called the cluster glycoside effect and is predominantly due to thermodynamic features of multivalent ligands (e.g., chelate effects) [41]. Several synthetic ligands take advantage of the cluster glycoside effect. The majority of these ligands consist of dendritic molecules often based on glutamic acid containing terminal galactose or *N*-acetylgalactosamine groups (Figure 47.5).

To the best of our knowledge, the dendritic compound YEE(GalNAcAH)$_3$ (Figure 47.5) is the most effective synthetic ligand for the ASGPR. The dissociation constant is in the subnanomolar range due to the use of *N*-acetylgalactosamine, which showed a high binding affinity [42, 43]. Apart from the nature of the monosaccharide ligand, the geometry has an strong influence on the binding constant of synthetic glycoside clusters [44]. Upon binding to the receptor, the ASGPR–ligand complex associates with clathrin within coated pits and is internalized. The endocytosed vesicle forms endosomes, where due to the increasing acidity of the environment the receptor–ligand complex dissociates. The receptor is recycled back to the cell surface to be reutilized, while the ligand is carried to the lysosomal compartment for degradation.

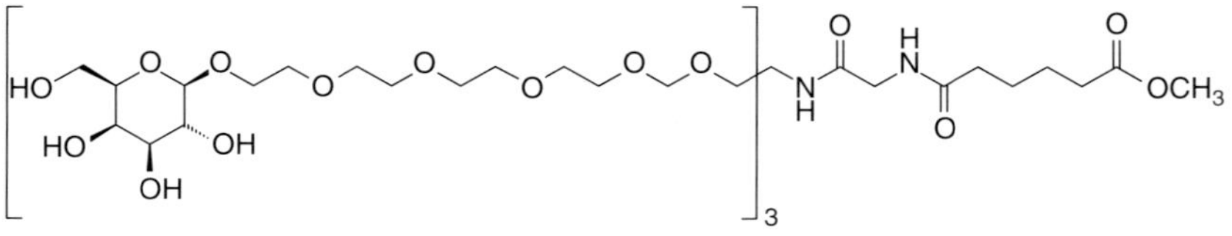

TG(20 Å), $K_d = 2\times10^{-7}$ M

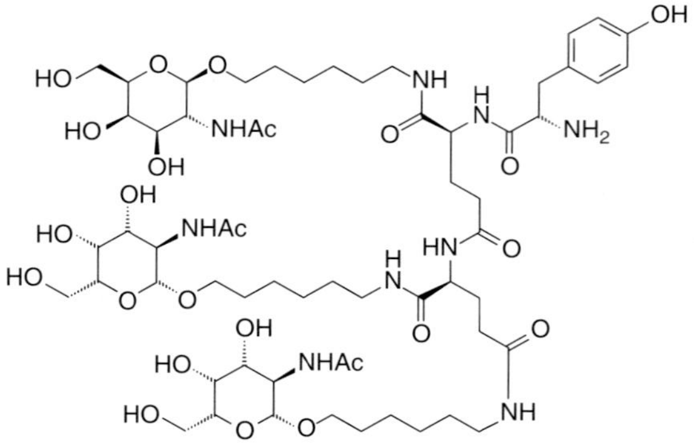

YEE(GalNAcAH)$_3$, $K_d < 10^{-9}$ M

Figure 47.5 Structures of synthetic ligands with high affinity for ASGPR [42, 43].

The ASGPR is expressed at high levels only on the surface of parenchymal liver cells, where it is mainly located at the basolateral surface. Very reduced levels of ASGPR have also been documented in other organs of the digestive system, in the kidneys, and in the spleen. In these extrahepatic tissues, however, the binding capacity of the receptor is merely 1–5% compared to that of the liver, and no evidence of endocytosis and subsequent ligand degradation has been observed.

When the discovery of ASGPRs was reported, it soon became evident that due to their high binding selectivity for sugar-bearing ligands and the fact that their localization is restricted to a single cell type, these low-molecular-weight ligands can be exploited to deliver ligand-bound drugs to hepatocytes. These compounds are useful to treat liver pathologies, but also cause unwanted side-effects in other organs. To circumvent this drawback, drugs were covalently linked with galactosylated macromolecules. ASGPR-mediated endocytosis of such designed drug conjugates should depend only on the binding of galactose residues and not be affected by other characteristics of the molecule; this allows for the synthesis of hepatotropic conjugates of drugs suitable for the potential clinical treatment of HCC. Moreover, the internalization of macromolecular conjugates in liver cells via the ASGPR is facilitated by the structure of hepatic sinusoids, which have highly fenestrated capillaries and do not form a barrier for circulating macromolecules.

The best-studied carriers for developing hepatotropic drug conjugates with glycosides are fetuin, human serum albumin (HSA), and the synthetic polymer *N*-(2-hydroxypropyl)methacrylamide (HPMA). Examples of DOX with these carriers will be described in Section 47.3.2.

It is worth mentioning that a number of polysaccharides interact with the ASGPR and hepatocytes, such as pullulan, arabinogalactan, xyloglucan, and polygalactosamine, and a few drug conjugates have been developed and studied primarily in *in vitro* studies (see Chapter 23).

47.2.2
Designing Drug-Encapsulated Nanoparticles for Liver Tumor Uptake by the RES

Polyacrylcyanoacrylate (PACA) nanoparticles were already investigated in *in vivo* studies 30 years ago. It was shown that they are potential drug carriers for passive targeting [45]. As a result, the colloidal particles are taken up by the RES. Some advantages of such nanoparticles, which ideally are biodegradable and bioavailable polymers, include sustained drug action on the liver tumor lesions, reduced systemic side-effects, facilitated extravasation into the tumor, high capability to cross various physiological barriers as well as controlled and targeted delivery of the drug [46].

Polybutylcyanoacrylate (PBCA) and polyisohexylcyanoacrylate (PIHCA) belong to the class of PACA nanoparticles. PBCA and PIHCA nanoparticles were loaded with several anticancer agents, and examined in detail in *in vitro* and *in vivo* studies [45, 47]. Two DOX-loaded PIHCA nanoparticles [48, 49] and a PBCA nanoparticle loaded with mitoxantrone have been or are being evaluated in clinical trials. Details will be described in Sections 47.3 and 47.4.

47.2.3
Liver Tumor Targeting Using HepDirect Prodrugs

Substances that specifically inhibit the activity of viral enzymes prevent viral replication. Usually, these substances are nucleoside analogs and are incorporated in the viral DNA. Nucleosides are effective against many viral infections and cancers, and are phosphorylated via nucleoside kinase to nucleoside 5′-monophosphate (NMP) and consequently to nucleoside triphosphate (NTP) [50, 51]. These NTPs can inhibit the viral and cellular DNA and RNA polymerases, or they can cause a chain termination and then be incorporated with a growing DNA or RNA strand [50]. A promising approach for targeting liver tumors is the development of cell-permeable prodrugs of antitumor NMPs that bypass the nucleoside kinase, thus increasing the NTP production (Figure 47.6). This new class of phosphate and phosphonate prodrugs that incorporate a cyclic 1,3-propanyl ester **1** is shown in Figure 47.6.

Erion *et al.* [50, 52] nicknamed this approach HepDirect™ (a registered trademark of Metabasis Therapeutics). Apart from the ester bond, these prodrugs contain a ring substituent that additionally allows the prodrugs to be oxidized. This oxidative cleavage reaction is catalyzed by a cytochrome P450. Prodrugs that have an aryl

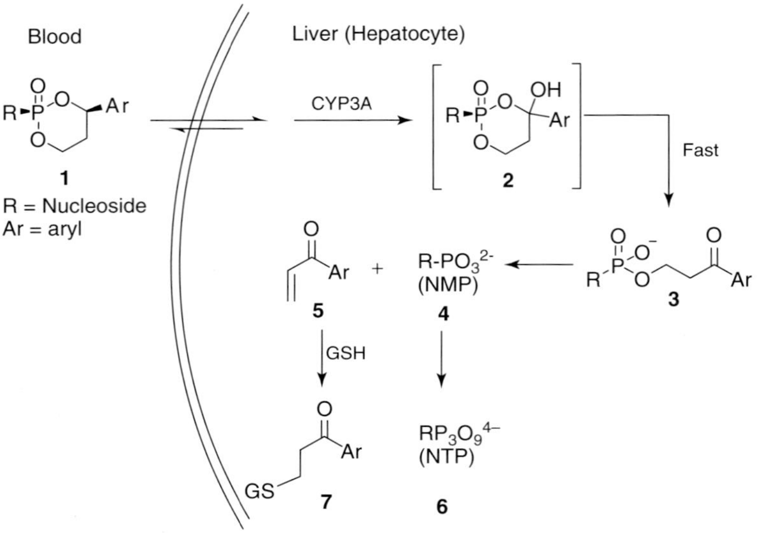

Figure 47.6 HepDirect: schematic presentation of a new class of phosphate and phosphonate prodrugs and their cleavage mechanism [52].

substituent in position 4 are specifically oxidized by the cytochrome P450 isoenzyme family CYP3A. The latter is expressed mainly in the parenchymal cells of the liver and not significantly in the enterocytes of the small intestine [53].

The mechanism, shown in Figure 47.6, begins with an oxidation, which causes a ring opening and generates a short-lived negatively charged intermediate (**3**). This intermediate is retained inside the cell. The next step is a β-elimination reaction, which produces the phosphate or phosphonate prodrug and the byproduct, which undergoes rapid conjugation with glutathione (GSH). The latter exists at millimolar levels in the liver [54]. The NMP **4** is converted to the biologically active NTP analog **6** by an intracellular nucleotide kinase. The *in vitro* and *in vivo* results of these HepDirect prodrugs are described in Section 47.3.

47.3
Preclinical Development of Hepatotropic Drug Delivery Systems

During the past 30 years drug delivery systems and new strategies have been developed to combat primary and secondary liver cancers. In particular, two drug delivery approaches have been investigated in detail: (i) exploiting the ASGPR, which is expressed in around 80% of patients with HCC, and (ii) the development of high-molecular weight drug delivery systems where uptake by the liver and liver tumors is mediated by the RES and the EPR effect. Furthermore, a new approach was developed using phosphate or phosphonate prodrugs, which represent a potential strategy for targeting drugs to the liver. A number of drug delivery systems are listed in Table 47.1, including the corresponding anticancer agents and development status.

Selected drug delivery systems showing promising results in *in vitro* and *in vivo* studies such as the HepDirect prodrugs, the drug–polymer conjugates PK2, L-HSA–DOX, and SMANCS, and the nanoparticles Doxorubicin Transdrug, YCC-DOX, and mitoxantrone-loaded nanoparticles are described in detail in the following subsections.

47.3.1 HepDirect Prodrugs

As mentioned in Section 47.2, phosphate and phosphonate prodrugs, named HepDirect, are suitable for potentially treating HCC. In a study, the activity of HepDirect prodrugs of two structurally different NMP analogs, MB06866 [(2*R*,4*S*)-9-[2-[4-(3-chlorophenyl)-2-oxo-1,3,2-dioxaphosphorian-2-yl]methoxyethyl] adenine (remofovir)], an analog of adefovir (PMEA), and MB07133 [(2*R*,4*S*)-4-amino-1-[5-*O*-[2-oxo-4-(4-pyridyl)-1,3,2-dioxaphosphorian-2-yl]-β-D-arabinofuranosyl]-2(1*H*)-pyrimidinone], a cytarabine (ara-C) 5′-monophosphate, was assessed in an *in vivo* model using overnight-fasted male Simonsen albino rats or *ad libitium*-fed male NIH Swiss mice. MB06866 showed a 12-fold increase in liver uptake relative to bis-POM PMEA (adefovir dipivoxil), which failed in clinical trials due to renal toxicity [52, 74]. The second HepDirect prodrug MB07133, a prodrug of ara-C 5′-monophosphate, indicated a greater potential for targeting drugs to the liver (Figure 47.7). ara-C is an inactive agent against solid tumors probably due to deactivation by cytidine deaminase or due to its low conversion to ara-CTP (cytarabine triphosphate) [75]. Proof of concept for the HepDirect prodrug MB07133 has been performed in non-tumor-bearing mice (Figure 47.7). In these experiments a considerably enhanced ara-CTP production in the liver could be shown compared to the bone marrow and in plasma. Furthermore, MB07133 was less toxic than ara-C against bone marrow cells and produced significantly less body weight loss [52].

Owing to the high levels of CYP3A activity in primary liver tumors [76], MB07133 should be converted to ara-CTP in hepatocarcinoma cells. ara-CTP is expected to inhibit DNA polymerase activity, and consequently inhibit DNA synthesis and tumor cell growth.

47.3.2 Drug–Polymer Conjugates

In the following subsections we describe selected drug–polymer conjugates for which *in vivo* proof of concepts were obtained.

47.3.2.1 PK2: A HPMA-Based Copolymer with *N*-Galactosamine

Water-soluble polymers based on HPMA are nontoxic and nonimmunogenic, have a manifold/versatile chemistry, and have good biocompatibility – properties that make them particularly suitable for targeted drug carriers. Originally, the

Table 47.1 Overview of the different drug delivery systems that have been developed with the aim of targeting primary and secondary liver tumors.

Drug delivery system	Description	Development status	References
Apolipoprotein A-I	apolipoprotein A-I-mediated small interfering RNA	*in vitro/in vivo*	[55]
PLA-PLL-EGFR mAb	epidermal growth factor receptor monoclonal antibody	*in vitro/in vivo*	[56]
YCC-DOX	multifunctional DOX-loaded SPIO nanoparticles	*in vitro/in vivo*	[57]
SMANCS	poly(styrene-*co*-maleic acid) and neocarzinostatin	market approval	[58]
HepDirect prodrugs	phosphate or phosphonate prodrugs combined with antitumor nucleoside analogs	*In vitro/in vivo*	[52]
Doxorubicin Transdrug	DOX-loaded PIHCA nanoparticle	phase II	*www.bioalliancepharma.com*
PK2	HPMA-based copolymer with *N*-galactosamine and DOX	phase I	[59]
Mitoxantrone-loaded nanoparticles	mitoxantrone-loaded PBCA nanoparticle	phase II	[46]
tSLN	docetaxel-loaded lipid nanoparticles	*in vitro/in vivo*	[60]
CTS/PEG-GA	glycyrrhetinic acid-modified chitosan/poly(ethylene glycol) nanoparticles	*in vitro/in vivo*	[61]
Direct-nano	apotransferrin-loaded nanoparticles	*in vitro/in vivo*	[62]
HAPN	hydroxyapatite nanoparticles	*in vitro*	[63]
A54-nanoshells	gold nanoshells	*in vitro*	[64]
L-BNC	bionanocapsule composed of large (L) proteins	*in vitro*	[65]
PE-sub	phycoerythrin subunit liposome	*in vitro*	[66]
QD-Ls	quantum dot liposome	*in vitro*	[67]
Plasmid DNA liposomes	encapsulation of plasmid DNA into negatively charged liposomes	*in vitro*	[68]
PMBN-preS1	phosphorylcholine-based amphiphilic block copolymer micelles	*in vitro*	[69]
LA-P105	lactobionic acid-conjugated Pluronic® P105 micelles	*in vitro*	[70]
Lac-PIC micelles	lactose-modified poly(ethylene glycol)	*in vitro/in vivo*	[71]
PEG-*b*-PPA/DNA micelles	poly(ethylene glycol)/ polyphosphoramidate micelles	*in vitro/in vivo?*	[72]
LNP01	lipidoid small interfering RNA	*in vivo*	[73]
L-HSA-DOXO	acid-sensitive doxorubicin conjugate of lactosaminated human serum albumin	*in vivo*	[141]

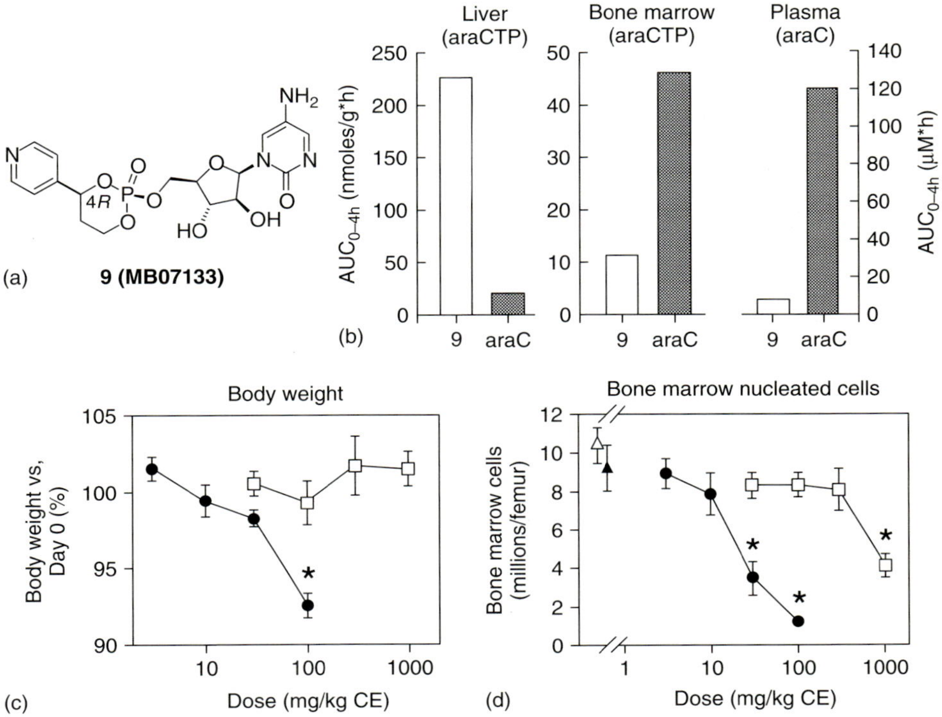

Figure 47.7 (a) Structure of MB07133 (**9**). (b) Mean liver and bone marrow ara-CTP AUC_{0-4h} and plasma ara-C AUC_{0-4h} determined from samples collected at 0.5, 1, 2, and 4 h after intraperitoneal injection of a 100 mg/kg ara-C-equivalents (CE) dose of MB07133 or ara-C to normal mice. Ara-CTP was not detected in the bone marrow in MB07133-treated mice or in liver samples of ara-C-treated mice more than 2 h after dosing. (c) Body weight change (%) of **9A**: 1:1 mixture of *R*- and *S*-isomers of MB07133, and ara-C (circles) in male mice. (d) Cytotoxicity of **9A** (squares) and ara-C (circles) on bone marrow nucleated cells measured on day 5 following intraperitoneal injection on five consecutive days compared with vehicle-treated (open triangle); solid triangle = untreated mice; $^*P < 0.05$ [52].

development of a HPMA copolymer containing the topoisomerase II inhibitor DOX that is taken up by the EPR effect by solid tumors was pursued. DOX was linked to the polymer backbone through a tetrapeptide spacer (Gly–Phe–Leu–Gly), known as PK1, that is cleaved by lysosomal enzymes such as cathepsin B and releases native DOX. In preclinical studies it was found that the *in vivo* activity of PK1 correlated with the level of lysosomal cathepsins in solid tumors. On the basis of these promising data, PK1 was the first HPMA-based macromolecular prodrug to enter clinical trials (for further information, see [77, 78] and Chapter 26).

When additionally conjugated with antibodies, proteins, or sugars, such polymer therapeutics showed good results in animals [79–84]. With respect to liver tumor targeting, PK2 is a sister compound of PK1, but additionally incorporates

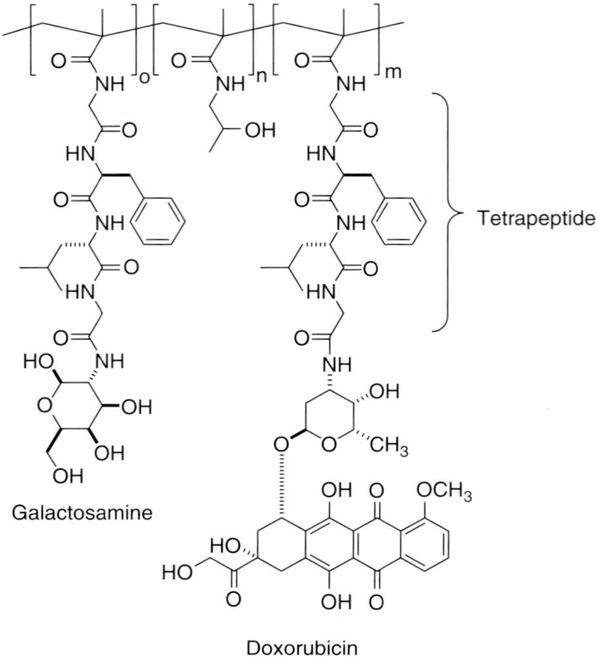

Figure 47.8 Structure of PK2 – a HPMA-based copolymer with galactosamine as the ASGPR-affine ligand and in which DOX is bound through a cathepsin B-cleavable tetrapeptide (Gly–Phe–Leu–Gly).

galactosamine as a targeting ligand that was designed to be taken up by the ASGPR of liver tumor cells [85]. The conjugate PK2 contains 7.5 wt% DOX as well as 2.0 wt% galactosamine bound to the polymer backbone via the same peptide linker as in PK1 (Figure 47.8) wherein the galactosamine moiety binds to the ASGPR [86, 87].

Several pharmacokinetic studies in animals have revealed that intravenous administration of PK2 delivers DOX preferentially to the liver [82, 88, 89], which was shown in an early individual treatment attempt in one patient [90]. Furthermore, clinical signs of cardiotoxicity were not seen in any animals treated intravenously with PK2 [86]. Due to the promising results, the conjugate has been studied in a phase I clinical trial (see below).

47.3.2.2 **Lactosaminated Albumin: A Safe and Efficient Hepatotropic Carrier for Treating Liver Tumors**

One of the first glycoproteins that was considered for selective hepatocyte delivery of drugs via the ASGPR was desialylated fetuin. Fetuin is a glycoprotein from fetal calf serum that in its desialylated form displays high binding affinity for the ASGPR. Drug conjugates with desialylated fetuin are efficiently internalized by hepatocytes via the ASGPR. However, a drawback that should be taken seriously is that they are prone to induce antibodies that could both inactivate the conjugates and produce allergic reactions [91]. This problem can be overcome by using as the hepatotropic drug carrier lactosaminated homologous albumin (L-SA) (i.e., albumin derived from the same animal species to which the drug conjugate is administered and derivatized with lactose residues) [92, 93]. L-SA was proposed for the first time as a hepatotropic carrier of drugs by Luigi Fiume. Several years ago, he suggested that a protein can be made to be selectively targeted to liver cells by conjugating it with smaller molecules for which a specific binding site exists on the cell membrane [94, 95]. According to this hypothesis, it was established that proteins after conjugation with small molecules exposing galactosyl residues [96–98] bind to ASGPR and are internalized by hepatocytes. A very simple way of attaching galactosyl residues was developed by Wilson [98], who used α-lactose and applied the procedure of Gray [99] and Schwartz and Gray [100]. These authors coupled reducing carbohydrates to proteins in a single step in aqueous solution at neutral pH value. The method relies on the ability of a cyanoborohydride anion to selectively reduce the Schiff bases without reacting with the free aldehyde groups [101]. The reaction scheme is depicted in Figure 47.9 for HSA.

According to this procedure, the glucose moiety of lactose is bound to the ε-amino groups of the lysine residues of HSA through its aldehyde group, while the galactose moiety remains unchanged and can interact with the ASGPR. When 20–30 lactose residues are attached to one albumin molecule, the neoglycoprotein L-HSA is selectively taken up by the liver parenchymal cells [102]. Drug conjugates prepared with lactosaminated homologous albumin do not induce antibodies in mice [91, 103] and in humans [104]. L-HSA has another advantage over asialofetuin and

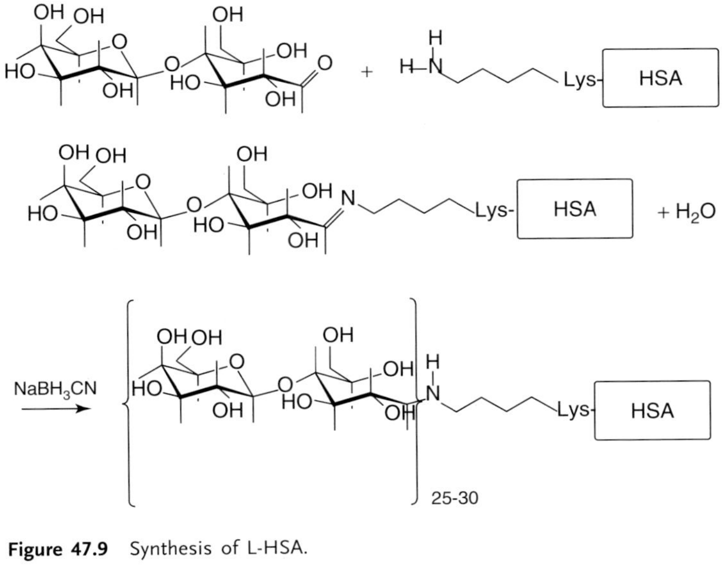

Figure 47.9 Synthesis of L-HSA.

other naturally occurring desialylated glycoproteins since it can easily be obtained in the amounts required for clinical purposes. The safety and efficacy of L-HSA as a hepatotropic carrier of drugs was demonstrated in patients with chronic type B hepatitis using a conjugate of the antiviral nucleoside analog adenine arabinoside (ara-A) [104–107]. These studies proved the validity of a targeted chemotherapeutic approach based on drug conjugation to hepatotropic carriers for the treatment of liver pathologies.

In subsequent experiments L-HSA was tested as a potential carrier of antineoplastic drugs to primary and secondary liver tumors.

47.3.2.2.1 L-HSA Conjugate of 5-Fluoro-2′-Deoxyuridine to Increase the Drug Concentrations in Hepatic Micrometastases During the studies of L-HSA conjugated to ara-A in laboratory animals, it was observed that after the uptake of the conjugate in hepatocytes and the intracellular release of the drug from L-HSA, araA was partly released in the bloodstream [108]. Although this release reduces the efficacy of hepatocyte targeting, it has a useful consequence since it can result in higher drug concentrations in hepatic blood than in the systemic circulation. Therefore, administration of anticancer nucleoside analogs bound to L-HSA can be a way to expose neoplastic cells fed by liver sinusoids to enhanced drug levels, thus accomplishing a locoregional noninvasive treatment of hepatic micrometastases. This possibility was investigated with the goal of improving the adjuvant chemotherapy of colon cancer. After surgical resection of this tumor, about 50% of patients develop hepatic metastases, presumably due to undetectable, microscopic foci of neoplastic cells located in liver sinusoids already present at the time of surgery. Due to this high frequency of disease recurrence, an adjuvant chemotherapy is usually recommended. The adjuvant chemotherapy administered to patients with colon cancer is almost universally based on administration of 5-FU – a fluoropyrimidine that is given alone or in combination [109]. 5-FU is a prodrug which mainly acts after conversion to 5-fluoro-2′-deoxyuridine (FUdR)and in its phosphorylated form inhibits thymidylate synthase [110]. Although effective in the treatment of colon cancer, fluoropyrimidines have a drawback, since they are characterized by high hepatic extraction [111, 112] and as a consequence during systemic chemotherapy with fluoropyrimidines, the cells of liver micrometastases are exposed to drug concentrations lower than those achievable in systemic circulation. This is a serious disadvantage, since micrometastases should be the major targets of adjuvant chemotherapy. Attempts have been made to enhance the efficacy of fluoropyrimidines against liver micrometastases with locoregional treatments, performed by infusing 5-FU into the portal vein [113–115] or administering FUdR via the hepatic artery [116]. However, portal vein infusions of 5-FU often result in catheter complications and only permit a single cycle every 7 days. In addition, administration of FUdR via the hepatic artery is often followed by the appearance of biliary sclerosis [116, 117], which is a consequence of the drug delivered in high concentrations to bile duct cells through the hepatic artery.

Following the observations with L-HSA–ara-A, it was hypothesized that the systemic administration of FUdR bound to L-HSA, by producing a local release of the drug in liver blood, could be a way to expose neoplastic cells infiltrating hepatic sinusoids to higher and hence more effective concentrations of FUdR [118, 119].

To obtain the conjugate L-HSA–FUdR, FUdR was first phosphorylated at the 5′-OH group according to Yoshikawa *et al.* [120]. The 5′-phosphoric ester of FUdR was then converted into its imidazolide, which was subsequently allowed to react with L-HSA at alkaline pH value (Figure 47.10) [121].

^{31}P-nuclear magnetic resonance (NMR) spectroscopy of this conjugate showed that the FUdR monophosphate (FUdRMP) was linked to L-HSA by two phosphoamide bonds: one, which was predominant (80% of total bonds), formed with the ε-amino group of lysine residues and the other with one of the imidazole nitrogens of histidine [122]. Conjugates with a molar ratio FUdRMP/L-HSA ranging from 13 to 16 were used in biological studies. In animals that were intravenously injected with L-HSA–FUdRMP, the drug that released from hepatocytes back into the bloodstream after liver uptake of the conjugate was the dephosphorylated nucleoside (i.e., FUdR). In parallel experiments, free FUdR and the conjugate were given to rats by bolus or by slow infusion, and the concentrations of FUdR in hepatic veins and in the infrahepatic vena cava were determined [118, 119]. These concentrations are a measure of the drug level in the liver blood and in the systemic circulation, respectively. The ratio between the levels of FUdR in hepatic veins and those in the infrahepatic vena cava was 5–7 times higher in rats injected with the conjugate than in animals administered with the free drug. The anticancer activities of free and L-HSA-conjugated FUdR were compared in mice with liver micrometastases induced by intrasplenic injection of cells from a murine colon carcinoma [118]. Coupling to L-HSA substantially enhanced the anticancer activity of FUdR: the dose inhibiting tumor growth was several times lower when the drug was injected in the conjugated form. The release of the drug locally in hepatic blood can account for this dose reduction. Since FUdR administered in its conjugated form is concentrated in liver cells, a possible hepatotoxicity of the conjugate must be taken into consideration. However, clinical data indicate a resistance of hepatocytes to FUdR [116, 117]. The release of FUdR in hepatic sinusoids should not be harmful even for bile duct cells since the biliary tree is exclusively fed by the hepatic artery and not by sinusoidal blood [123–125]. Moreover, bile excretion of FUdR has not been reported [126].

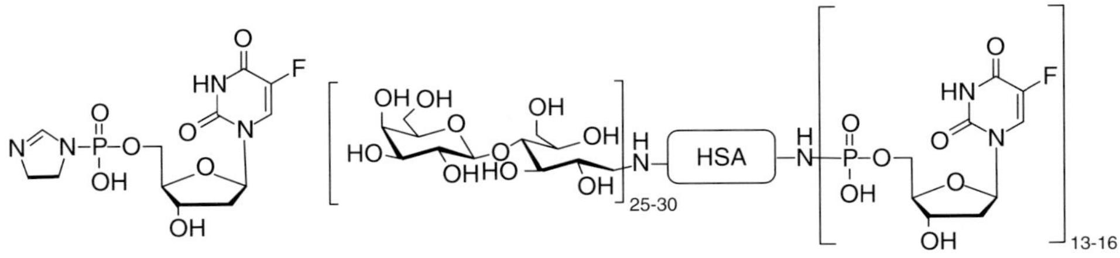

Figure 47.10 Imidazolide of FUdRMP and the conjugate L-HSA–FUdR (80% of FUdRMP is bound to the ε-amino groups of lysines on the surface of albumin).

In conclusion, L-HSA–FUdRMP, by causing a local release of drug in hepatic sinusoids, has the potential to accomplish a regional chemotherapy of liver micrometastases of colon carcinoma similar to that performed by the portal vein infusion of FU. Compared to portal vein infusion, administration of L-HSA–FUdRMP by the peripheral venous route would have the important advantage of being a noninvasive procedure, thus avoiding the risks of catheter complications and allowing repeated cycles of treatment starting prior to surgery.

47.3.2.2.2 Development of an Acid-Sensitive Drug Conjugate L-HSA–DOX for Treating HCC In a study on needle biopsies from 60 consecutive cases of human HCCs, ASGPR was histochemically detected on all the cells in 28 out of 35 (80%) well-differentiated (WD) and in five out of 25 (25%) poorly differentiated (PD) forms of the tumor [127]. This result justified the attempts to develop a therapeutic strategy of exploiting the ASGPR expressed in HCC [128–130]. To this aim, DOX was conjugated to L-HSA.

DOX was coupled to L-HSA using the 6-maleimidocaproyl hydrazone derivative of the drug (DOXO-EMCH), first synthesized to conjugate DOX with a monoclonal antibody recognizing a tumor-associated antigen (Figure 47.11) [131]. DOXO-EMCH is also the first albumin-binding prodrug under clinical development (see Chapter 26).

During synthesis, the maleimide moiety of DOXO-EMCH rapidly reacts with the HS groups of reduced cysteines of HSA that were made available by prior reduction of disulfides with tris(2-carboxyethyl) phosphine in a one-pot reaction. The maleimide moiety of DOXO-EMCH forms a thioether bond with HS groups that is stable under physiological conditions [132]. Cysteine was the only amino acid residue of L-HSA that reacted with DOXO-EMCH as demonstrated by ^{13}C-NMR spectroscopy of a conjugate synthesized using a DOXO-EMCH in which the carbon atoms of the double bond of the maleimide group were enriched with the ^{13}C isotope [133]. The L-HSA–DOX used in the experiments reported below had a molar ratio DOX/L-HSA ranging from 5 to 7 in the different conjugate preparations (1 mg conjugate contained 36–50 μg DOX) [134].

For a conjugate to be pharmacologically active, the bond linking the drug to the carrier must be stable in the bloodstream, but it needs to be rapidly cleaved after entering the cells. The hydrazone bond of DOXO-EMCH fulfills this property because it is sufficiently stable at the neutral pH value of plasma, yet is rapidly hydrolyzed at the acidic pH value of endosomal and lysosomal compartments (pH 4–6) inside the cells [135] (Figure 47.12). This was demonstrated in rats with HCCs (see below) that were intravenously injected with L-HSA–DOX at the pharmacologically active dose of 1 mg/kg. At 2–3 h after administration, when the conjugate was essentially cleared from the bloodstream, the amounts of conjugated DOX taken up by the tumors and the surrounding liver were completely set free from the carrier [134]. After release from L-HSA, DOX remains confined in the cells to which it was transported by the carrier for a relatively long time [136].

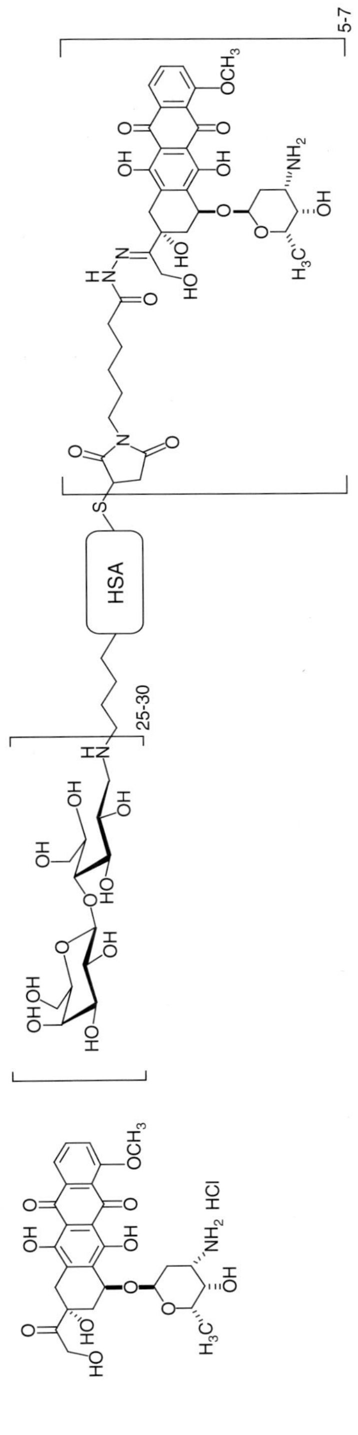

Figure 47.11 DOX and its conjugate with L-HSA (L-HSA–DOX).

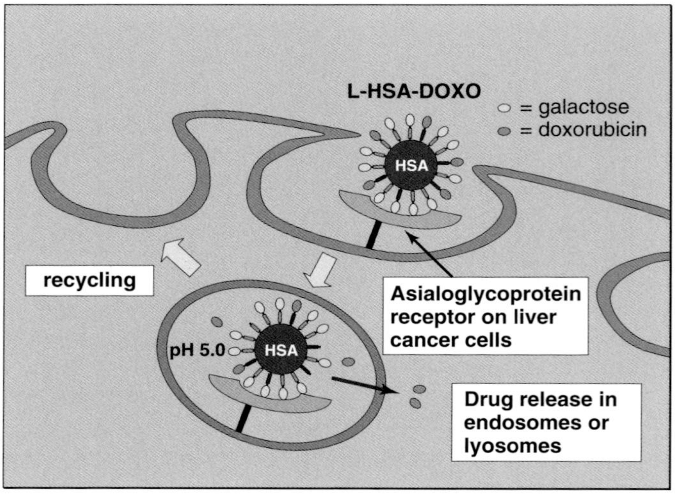

Figure 47.12 Uptake of L-HSA–DOX by liver tumor cells through endocytosis and release of DOX in the acidic environment of endosomes or lysosomes.

Anticancer Activity of L-HSA–DOX in Rats Bearing HCCs The anticancer activity of L-HSA–DOX was studied in rats with HCCs induced by diethylnitrosamine (DENA), which was administered in the rats' drinking water (100 mg/l) for 2 months [137]. One month after the last day of DENA administration, multiple nodules with sizes ranging from 2 to 10 mm in diameter could be observed spread over the liver surface. All histologically examined nodules were classified as HCCs, with either a trabecular (WD = well differentiated), solid (PD = poorly differntiated), or intermediate (MD = moderately differntiated) pattern (Figure 47.13).

As first proof of concepts, the anticancer effect of L-HSA–DOX on rat HCCs was studied in two experiments. In a first study, L-HSA–DOX was given intravenously to rats (1 mg/kg once a week for 4 weeks) starting 1 week after the last day of DENA administration when established tumors had not yet been formed. This dose is twice that administered weekly to humans (20 mg/m^2, corresponding to approximately 0.5 mg/kg). In this experiment, L-HSA–DOX significantly reduced the number of HCCs developed from preneoplastic lesions [138]; in contrast, the free drug, administered at the same dose and schedule, was completely ineffective (Figure 47.14).

In addition, therapy with DOX was associated with a body weight change of −10%, whereas therapy with the conjugate produced no body weight change (+1%). Biodistribution studies in healthy rats showed a strongly increased area under the curve (AUC) of DOX concentration in the livers of animals administered with the L-HSA conjugated drug. In contrast, in rats injected with the free drug comparable levels of DOX were measured in the liver, heart, intestine, spleen, and kidneys (Figure 47.14b and Table 47.2) [138].

These results clearly suggested that treatment with L-HSA–DOX could be useful to prevent recurrences due to metachronous HCCs, but gave no information about

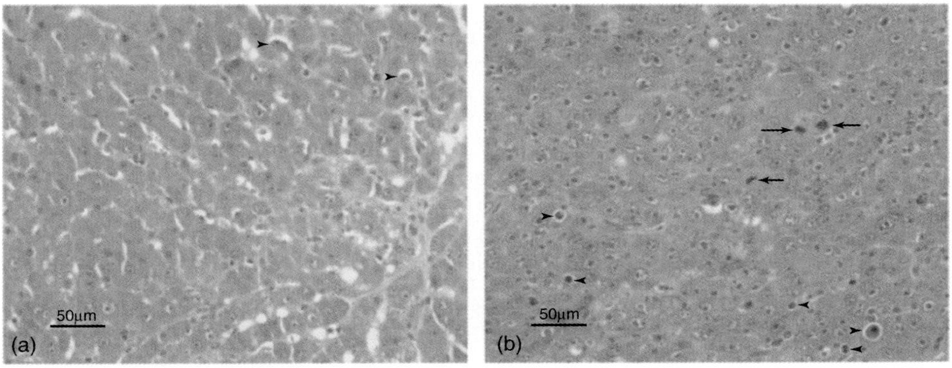

Figure 47.13 WD (a) and PD (b) rat HCCs. (a) Isomorphic hepatocytes with eosinophilic cytoplasm and prominent nucleoli are arranged in trabeculae separated by vascular channels; low atypias. A few apoptotic bodies are present (arrowheads). (b) Hepatocytes with polymorphic nuclei, enlarged nucleoli, and basophilic cytoplasm are arranged in a solid pattern. Several mitotic cell structures (arrows) and apoptotic bodies (arrowheads) are present.

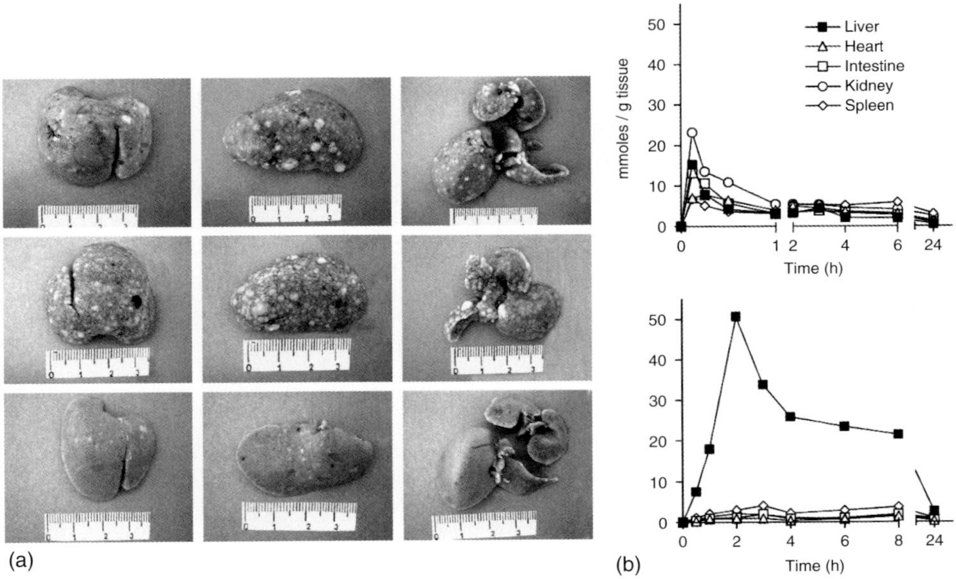

Figure 47.14 (a) Macroscopic views of formalin-fixed liver lobes from three representative rats in the saline-, free-DOX- (4 × 1 mg/kg), and L-HSA–DOX-treated groups (4 × 1 mg/kg DOX-equivalents) (upper, medium, and lower set of photos, respectively). (b) Concentrations of DOX in healthy liver, heart, intestine, spleen, and kidney for DOX (A) and L-HSA–DOX (B).

Table 47.2 AUC_{0-24h} of DOX concentrations in rat organs after administration of the same dose (1 μg/g) of free or L-HSA coupled DOX (L-HSA–DOX).

Compound	AUC_{0-24h} (nmol·h/g tissue)				
	Liver	Heart	Intestine	Kidney	Spleen
DOX	60.5	100.0	109.0	145.6	169.4
L-HSA–DOX	360.0	28.8	33.2	48.3	119.6

The values reported for conjugate-injected animals refer to DOX that has been set free from the carrier inside the cells.

its potential to reduce the growth of already established tumors. Hence, the effect of L-HSA–DOX on HCCs was studied by tracking the tumors over time by means of high-frequency ultrasound [139]. Rats with HCCs detected by ultrasound received saline, free, or conjugated DOX (1 mg/kg), intravenously injected twice a week for 4 weeks. During the period of drug administration, the growth of HCCs was observed in three imaging sessions. In this study, L-HSA–DOX not only prevented the development of new tumors from preneoplastic lesions, as previously found, but also significantly inhibited the growth of established HCCs. In contrast, free-DOX exerted an effect on tumor growth only during the first period of administration (Figure 47.15) and did not impair the appearance of new HCCs.

Further biodistribution experiments were performed in rats bearing DENA-induced HCCs in order to evaluate the DOX levels in tumor nodules after administration of the drug given in the free or L-HSA conjugated form. In these experiments it was unexpectedly observed that administration of L-HSA–DOX can increase DOX concentrations also in PD HCCs, which lack the ASGPR. This is illustrated by the results reported in Table 47.3, which lists the AUC_{0-24h} of DOX levels in the three forms of HCCs.

Contrary to L-HSA–DOX, L-^{14}C-HSA, the albumin carrier without conjugated DOX, was taken up by WD HCCs, but not by PD HCCs, as previously reported [137].

The mechanism by which L-HSA–DOX is actively taken up by neoplastic hepatocytes, which do not express ASGPR, is not precisely known, but preliminary data suggests that uptake of L-HSA–DOX by the cells of these tumors is mediated by the DOX residues themselves since DOX molecules bear a positive charge that allow them to adhere to the cell surface and induce adsorptive endocytosis [140].

To verify whether lactose residues play a role in the cellular uptake of LHSA–DOX by PD HCCs, tumor-bearing rats were administered with a conjugate prepared with nonlactosaminated albumin (HSA–DOX) and the DOX concentrations were determined in HCCs [141]. L-HSA–DOX and HSA–DOX (intravenously injected at 1 mg DOX/kg), both loaded with five to seven molecules of DOX, produced similar levels of the drug in the different grades of the liver tumor nodules; therefore an

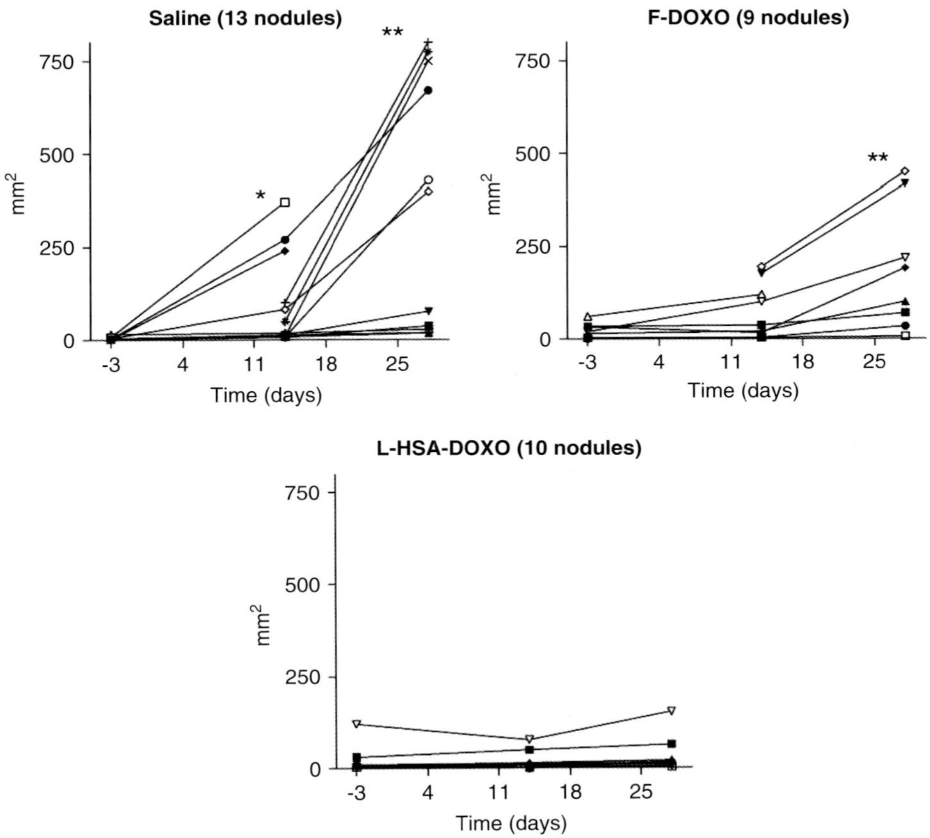

Figure 47.15 Growth of individual HCCs tracked on successive imaging sessions using ultrasound. Data were evaluated by a paired *t*-test. Statistically significant differences $^{*}P < 0.05$ and $^{**}P < 0.01$, respectively, using the values of the previous imaging session. F-DOXO = free-DOX; L-HSA–DOXO = L-HSA–DOX.

Table 47.3 AUC_{0-24h} of DOX concentrations in WD, MD, and PD HCCs in rats injected with the same dose (1 μg/g) of free or L-HSA-coupled DOX (L-HSA–DOX).

Compound	AUC_{0-24h} (nmol·h/g tissue)		
	WD HCCs	MD HCCs	PD HCCs
DOX	42.2	52.9	43.9
L-HSA–DOX	132.6	98.5	84.7

exclusive role of lactose for the uptake of L-HSA–DOX by PD HCCs could be ruled out. On the other hand, contrary to L-HSA–DOX, the nonlactosaminated DOX conjugate was shown to accumulate in spleen and bone marrow, and induced a leukopenia that was not produced by the lactosaminated conjugate [141, 142]. Considerable DOX accumulation in bone marrow (a target organ of the drugs toxicity) caused by five to seven molecules of DOX bound to HSA discouraged from pursuing further anticancer studies with this conjugate. Experimental evidence suggested that the lower drug concentrations in spleen and bone marrow in mice and rats injected with L-HSA–DOX could be caused by a more rapid uptake in the liver and liver tumors after systemic administration or cellular uptake of the conjugate by these organs is hindered due to the lactose residues bound to HSA [142]. If this were true, lactose might be replaced by other molecules producing the same effect. However, lactose has the clear advantage of enhancing conjugate penetration through the ASGPR in WD HCCs and also in preneoplastic liver lesions, which express the receptor [143] (see above). Moreover, L-HSA has already been shown to be a safe and efficient carrier in humans.

Tolerability in Animals The high drug concentrations produced in the liver by L-HSA–DOX raises the possibility of hepatic damage in a clinical use of the conjugate, particularly considering that the majority of HCCs in Western countries arise in cirrhotic livers. This issue was addressed by studying the effect of the conjugate, given at the same doses and with the same schedule as in the experiments evaluating anticancer activity (see above), on serum parameters of liver function and viability in normal rats, in rats with regenerating liver after partial hepatectomy, and in rats with fibrosis/cirrhosis induced by carbon tetrachloride (CCl_4) or DENA. In normal rats, L-HSA–DOX did not modify any clinically relevant serum liver parameter [144]. Administered to partially hepatectomized rats, it neither impaired the viability of regenerating hepatocytes nor produced changes in their ultrastructure and caused only a small delay of hepatic DNA recovery [145]. In rats with fibrosis/cirrhosis induced by CCl_4, it only caused moderate increases of aspartate transaminase and alanine transaminase serum levels, not statistically different from those produced by the free drug [144]. In these animals, free-DOX produced a decrease in albumin concentration, which was probably due to kidney damage and proteinuria caused by the drug in rats. The only effect observed in conjugate treated rats was an increase in alkaline phosphatase [139]. This effect was not due to cholestasis, as indicated by the levels of γ-glutamyltransferase, which were not modified, but was probably caused by the carrier L-HSA, since it was also observed in patients with chronic type B hepatitis who received the conjugate L-HSA–ara-AMP as well as in cynomolgus monkeys treated with nonconjugated L-HSA [104]. The excellent tolerability of L-HSA–DOX was also confirmed in HCC-bearing rats. In these animals the free drug caused a marked decrease in body weight, but systemic toxicity was not observed in rats administered with the conjugate [138, 139]. These reduced side-effects can be easily explained by the lower drug concentrations caused by the conjugate in the extrahepatic tissues [141].

In summary, L-HSA–DOX is a promising lactosaminated albumin conjugate of DOX that has pronounced antitumor activity in an autochthonous liver tumor model, is effective against all forms of HCCs, and has a very favorable toxicity profile due to low levels in extrahepatic tissues.

47.3.2.3 SMANCS: A Conjugate of Poly(Styrene-*co*-Maleic Acid) and the Antitumor Agent Neocarzinostatin

Neocarzinostatin (NCS) is a macromolecular chromoprotein of a highly potent bicyclic dienediyne antibiotic (as shown in Figure 47.16) bound tightly and non-covalently with high affinity ($K_d \sim 10^{-10}$ M) to a 113-amino-acid apoprotein. The chromophore is a very potent and labile DNA-damaging agent, and is protected and released from the apoprotein to interact with its target DNA. Opening of the epoxide under reductive conditions present in cancer cells leads to a diradical intermediate through a Bergman cyclization and eventually double-strand DNA cleavage [148].

The major limitations of NCS are its great toxicity (primarily bone marrow suppression) and its very fast clearance rate. Thus, in order to improve the pharmacokinetic profile, to reduce the systemic toxicity as well as the tumor targeting properties, poly(styrene-*co*-maleic acid) (SMA) was conjugated to NCS by coupling amino groups of the apoprotein to the maleic anhydride groups of the alternating copolymer of SMA (Figure 47.17) [146, 147].

Due to a considerably increased lipophilicity, SMANCS exhibits high affinity to a lipid contrast agent (Lipiodol), and thus a lipid formulation, SMANCS/Lipiodol, was used in clinical practice where an intra-arterial route of administration gave the best preclinical and clinical results [146–153].

In preclinical models by infusing a lipid contrast agent, such as Lipiodol, with/without the polymeric anticancer drug SMANCS via the tumor-feeding arterial route, Lipiodol is very effectively taken up by the tumor [149]. As an example, the results of treatment with SMANCS in a liver tumor model in rabbits are shown in

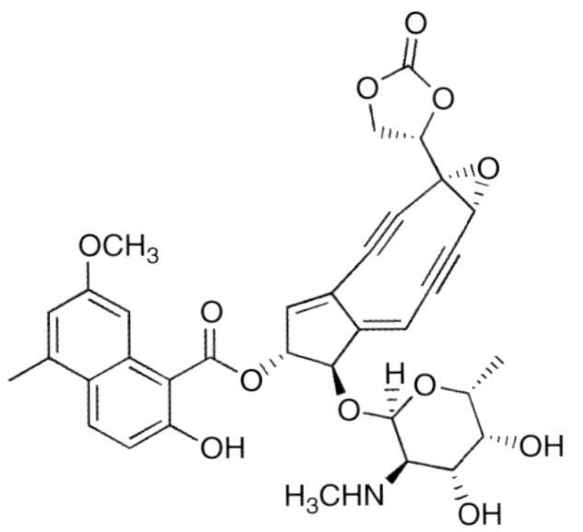

Figure 47.16 Chemical structure of the highly toxic chromophore dienediyne antibiotic of NCS (see ref. 148).

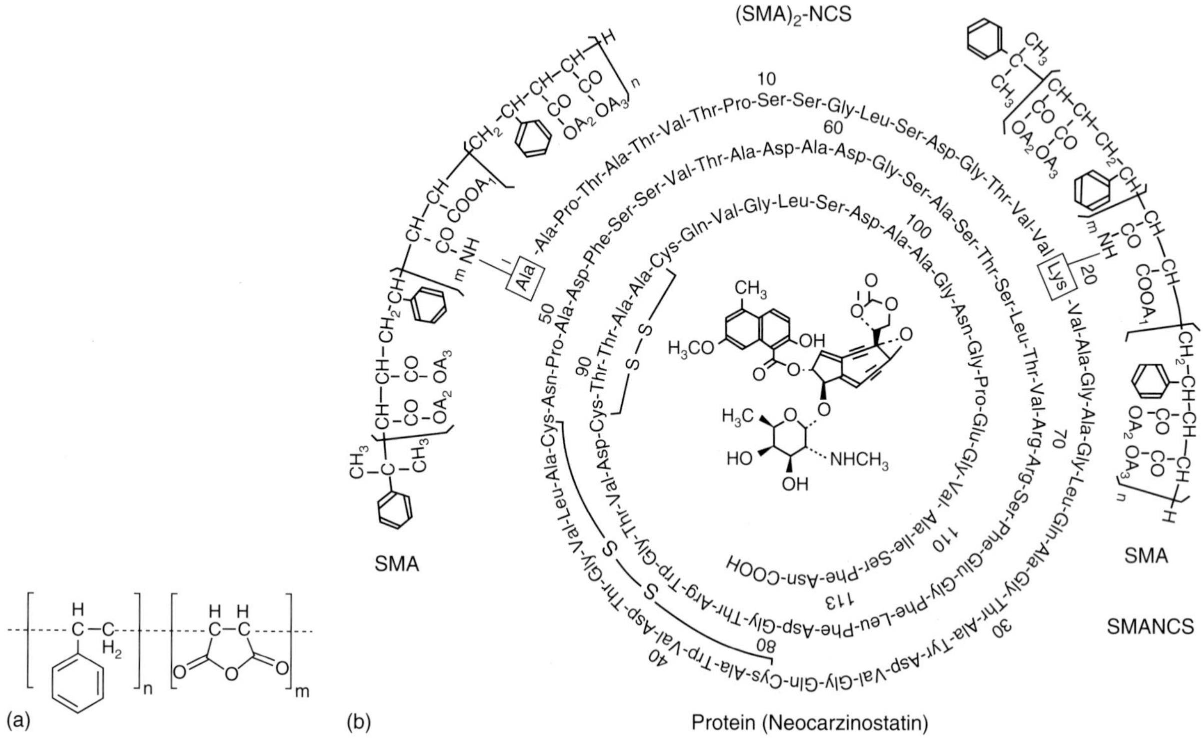

Figure 47.17 (a) Schematic structure of SMA. (b) Structure of SMANCS, which consists of the NCS (protein + chromophore) and SMA.

Figure 47.18a–d, in which VX-2 papilloma cells (around 2×10^6) were implanted in subcapsular parenchyma of the left anterior lobe of the rabbit liver [151]. In Figure 47.18a–d, soft X-rays of the liver with large size tumors are shown after SMANCS/Lipiodol (0.1 mg/0.1 ml) was injected into the proper hepatic artery. All liver tumors show significant tumor selective uptake of Lipiodol as white stains that were retained for more than 7 days, whereas no clear uptake in the normal liver parenchyma was noted after day 3 [151]. Quantitation of radioactive Lipiodol indicated that tumor selectivity over other normal organs or tissues was more than 100-fold [149], and the ratio of tissue drug concentration of the tumor/blood was

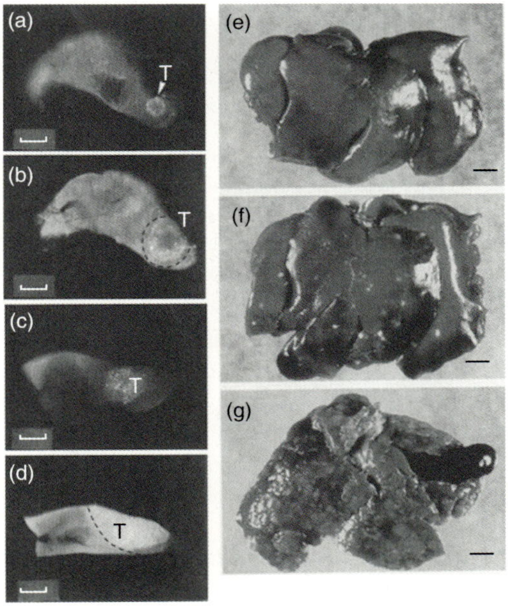

Figure 47.18 (a)–(d) Soft X-ray film images of sliced liver with experimentally implanted VX-2 tumor obtained after arterial injection of SMANCS/Lipiodol(0.1 mg/0.1 ml): (a) 15 min after injection, (b) after 1 day, (c) after 3 days, and (d) after 7 days. Note: at 15 min in (a) and day 1 in (b), Lipiodol is still retained in the vascular bed, which gradually disappeared after a few days, as shown in (c), day 3. One day after the intra-arterial injection, Lipiodol is still retained in normal parenchyma although Lipiodol is more clearly seen in the tumor nodules. By days 3 and 7, tumor staining became more distinct as Lipiodol was cleared by the lymphatic system in the normal tissue in contrast to tumor. (e)–(g) Suppression of metastatic liver tumor (VX-2) by SMANCS/Lipiodol in rabbit. Tumor cells (VX-2) were inoculated via the portal vein of rabbits ($n = 12$ per group) and SMANCS was injected on the same day via the same route. (e) SMANCS/Lipiodol(0.4 mg/0.4 ml/kg), (f) SMANCS in 5% glucose (0.4 mg/0.4 ml/kg), and (g) control, with vehicle 0.4 ml saline only. Bar = 1 cm. All livers were removed 12 days after drug injection. The SMANCS/Lipiodol group showed no tumor nodules in 44% of tested rabbits. In contrast, the majority of the livers of the control group (no drug) showed more than 500 tumor nodules/rabbit in 58%, > 100 nodules in 90% of the rabbits ($n = 12$) [151].

about 2000. When such rabbit livers were examined at later timepoints, remarkable differences of tumor growth compared to the control group without drug were seen (Figure 47.18e–g), where SMANCS/Lipiodol given via the proper hepatic artery resulted in remarkable suppression of tumor growth. Even SMANCS alone in 5% glucose (Figure 47.18f) showed significant effects when compared with the untreated control group (Figure 47.18g).

Due to these promising results and subsequent toxicological studies, SMANCS was investigated in clinical trials for treating patients with HCC [152, 153] (see Section 47.4). SMANCS/Lipiodol was approved in 1993 for the treatment of HCC and marketed by Yamauchi Pharmaceutical (now Astellas Pharma).

47.3.3 Development of Nanoparticles for Treating Liver Tumors

Prominent examples of drug-encapsulated nanoparticles are Doxorubicin Transdrug and a PBCA–mitoxantrone nanoparticle. A DOX-loaded PIHCA nanoparticle, also known as Doxorubicin Transdrug, was determined in *in vitro* and *in vivo* studies, and later in clinical trials. The results of the *in vitro* data were promising due to the high antitumor efficacy on HCC of PIHCA–DOX versus free-DOX as control. These nanoparticles can bypass the multidrug resistance (MDR) phenotype, which is responsible for the chemoresistance of HCC [154]. They showed promising antitumor efficacy in preclinical tumor models and Doxorubicin Transdrug was subsequently studied in clinical trials for regional therapy of liver tumors (see Section 47.4).

A further nanoparticle – a PBCA nanoparticle loaded with mitoxantrone (dihydroxyanthracenedione (DHAD)), an antineoplastic agent used in the treatment of various forms of cancer – showed promising results in a phase II clinical trial in the treatment of patients with unresected HCC (see below).

In contrast, in a phase I clinical trial in patients with refractory solid tumor a nanoparticle with the same polymer (i.e., a DOX-loaded PIHCA nanoparticle) was unsuccessful due to side-effects such as allergic reactions, fever, and bone pain [48].

47.3.3.1 Doxorubicin Transdrug

PIHCA nanoparticles, which are known to bypass MDR, were loaded with DOX (PIHCA–DOX) and tested in *in vitro* and *in vivo* studies. The 50% inhibitory concentration (IC_{50}) of PIHCA–DOX and DOX was determined in different human hepatoma cell lines, and the results showed higher cytotoxicity of PIHCA–DOX versus DOX. Conversely, unloaded PIHCA nanoparticles and DOX that were administered together did not increase the chemosensitivity/antitumor property of free-DOX. Consequently, the antitumor efficacy of PIHCA–DOX was due to the encapsulation of DOX into PIHCA nanoparticles [49].

The antitumor efficacy was determined *in vivo* in a transgenic murine model. In a first study the maximum tolerated dose (MTD) was found to be 9 mg/kg and this value was used for administration to transgenic mice. Four groups of transgenic mice were intravenously administered with one injection of PIHCA–DOX

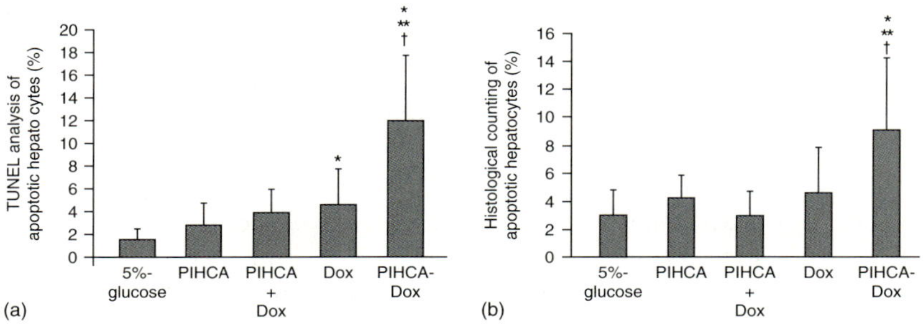

Figure 47.19 *In vivo* antitumor cytotoxicity of PIHCA–DOX versus DOX on HCC. (a) TUNEL analysis and (b) histological counting of apoptotic hepatocytes ($^*P < 0.01$ versus 5% glucose or PIHCA + DOX, $^{**}P < 0.05$ versus PIHCA, and $^\dagger P < 0.01$ versus DOX injected mice) [49].

(9 mg/kg DOX–120 mg/kg PIHCA; $n = 15$), DOX (9 mg/kg; $n = 13$), PIHCA (120 mg/kg; $n = 6$), PIHCA + DOX (120 + 9 mg/kg; $n = 3$), or 5% glucose. After 10 days, the mice were sacrificed and the antitumor effect of PIHCA–DOX and DOX in HCC tumors was assessed by using two different methods: the first being nuclear fragmented DNA staining using the terminal deoxynucleotidyl transferase dUTP nick-end-labeling (TUNEL) technique [155] and the second being histological counting of apoptotic bodies (Figure 47.19) [49, 156]. Both methods showed a significant increase of apoptosis after injecting PIHCA–DOX (9.0 ± 5.0%; Figure 47.19b) in comparison to DOX (4.6 ± 3.3%; Figure 47.19b).

Since antitumor benefits of chemotherapy are closely linked to tumor cell apoptosis induced by antineoplastic drugs, one can expect that a higher apoptosis rate induced by PIHCA–DOX will induce a better antitumor effect and result in an improved overall survival rate of tumor-bearing mice.

The histological examination indicates the presence of large areas of tumor necrosis in some animals treated with PIHCA–DOX, while this could not be seen in any of the animals treated with DOX (Figure 47.20) [49].

In conclusion, the *in vitro* and *in vivo* studies showed a significantly improved antitumor activity against HCC using PIHCA–DOX versus DOX that encouraged BioAlliance Pharma to initiate clinical trials (see below).

47.3.3.2 **Mitoxantrone-Loaded Nanoparticles**

PBCA nanoparticles loaded with mitoxantrone (DHAD) were evaluated for tumor-inhibiting effects and acute toxicity. Both orthotopic and heterotopic transplantation models of HCC were used in an *in vivo* study with nude mice using DOX and DHAD as controls. DHAD-PBCA-NPs were intravenously administered to four groups of five mice each: physiological saline group (0.1 ml/10 g), DOX group (20 μg/10 g), DHAD group (20 μg/10 g), and DHAD-PBCA-NP group (15 μg/10 g) 36 h after the transplantation of HCC. After the last injection on day 14, the animals were sacrificed and their livers and tumors were removed and examined [47].

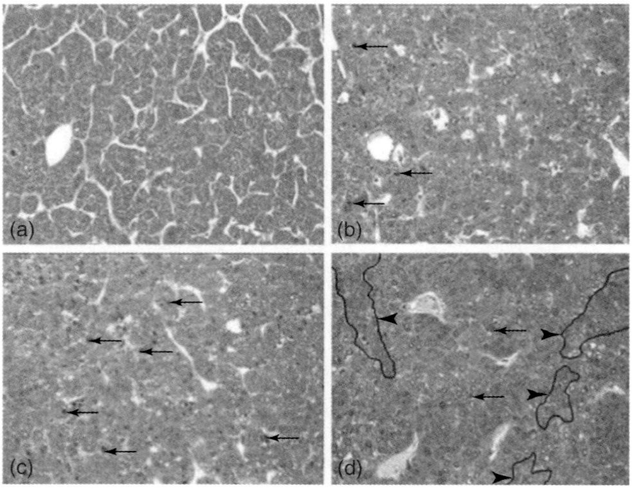

Figure 47.20 Histological examination in X/myc transgenic livers that were injected with PIHCA–DOX or DOX. WD HCC of trabecular type seen in glucose-treated animals (a). Arrows show apoptotic bodies in HCC tumors that were treated with one intravenous injection of DOX (b) or PIHCA–DOX (c). In some animals treated with PIHCA–DOX necrotic tumor areas were observed that are highlighted with arrowheads in (d). Hematoxylin & eosin stain, original magnification ×25 [49].

In contrast, the antitumor effects of all mice treated with DOX (20 μg/10 g), DHAD (20 μg/10 g), or DHAD-PBCA-NP in the heterotopic model were similar. The MTD of DHAD-PBCA-NP was 4.5 mg/kg, and the intravenous administration of DHAD-PBCA-NP to mice showed no obvious local irritation and no significant side-effects on heart, spleen, lung, and liver cells [47]. In summary, the antitumor effect of DHAD-PBCA-NP was considerably higher in comparison to DHAD and DOX in the orthotopically transplanted HCC, and systemic toxicity was low at the doses that were used in these experiments.

Phase I and II trials were subsequently performed in China with DHAD-PBCA-NP in patients with unresected HCC (see below).

47.3.3.3 **YCC-DOX: A Multifunctional DOX-Loaded Superparamagnetic Iron Oxide Nanoparticle**

Maeng *et al.* [57] have developed a novel polymeric nanoparticle system (YCC-DOX, Figure 47.21a) composed of poly(ethylene oxide)–trimellitic anhydride chloride–folate (PEO–TMA–FA, Figure 47.21b), DOX, and superparamagnetic iron oxide (SPIO; Fe_3O_4).

SPIO is a magnetic resonance imaging (MRI) agent that is taken up by Kupffer cells (part of the RES). Due to its degradation into nontoxic iron ions in the body, it is used for liver diagnosis [157]. The targeted delivery of diagnostic or therapeutic agents to the folate receptor which is overexpressed in various human cancers such as breast, lung, kidney, and ovarian cancer was established in HCC cell lines and in

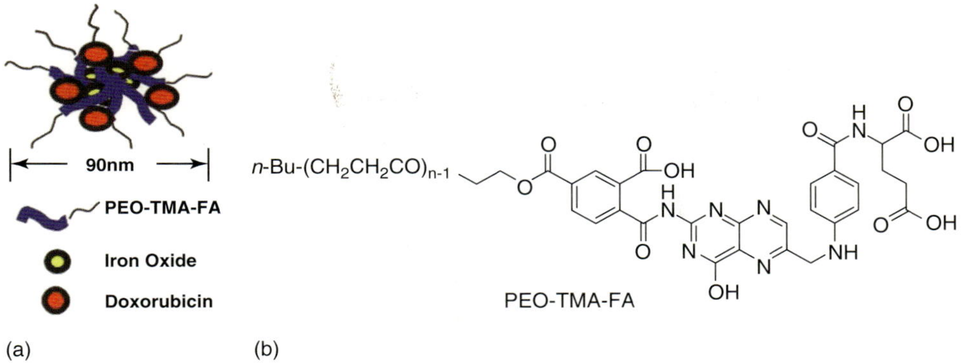

Figure 47.21 (a) PEO–TMA–FA polymer loaded with DOX and iron oxide. (b) Structure of PEO–TMA–FA [57].

liver cancer *in vivo* models. In an *in vitro* study using Hep3B and KB cell lines it was shown that the folate receptor was overexpressed in liver cancer and subsequently the cellular uptake of YCC-DOX was determined in these cell lines. As shown in Figure 47.22, the fluorescent intensity of DOX in YCC-DOX-treated Hep3B and KB cells was strong, whereas the cells that were additionally treated with FA showed a lower intensity. This observation indicates that FA inhibits binding of YCC-DOX to the folate receptor in a competitive manner [57].

The antitumor activity of YCC-DOX nanoparticles was evaluated in *in vitro* and *in vivo* models in comparison with free-DOX and Doxil® (a PEGylated liposomal formulation with DOX). In the animals treated with YCC-DOX, the tumor growth was significantly suppressed compared with free-DOX and Doxil. Furthermore, the MRI contrast effect of YCC-DOX nanoparticles was assessed using the conventional MRI contrast agent Resovist® as control. Both *in vitro* and *in vivo*, YCC-DOX showed higher MRI sensitivity in comparison to Resovist.

The anticancer effect of YCC-DOX is shown in Figure 47.23 for the autochthonous rat liver tumor model. In this rat model the substances containing DOX suppress tumor growth in comparison to the control group treated with

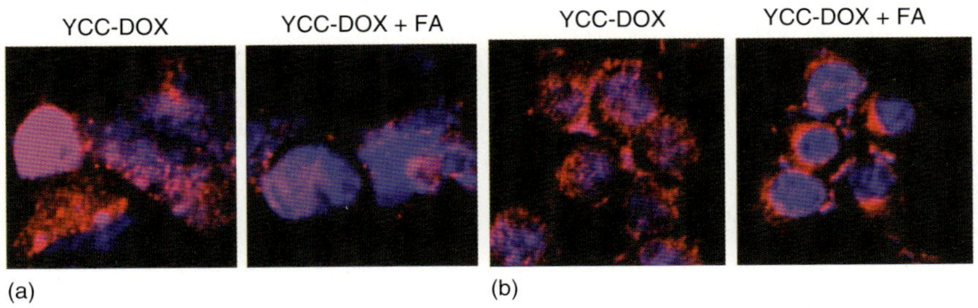

Figure 47.22 Fluorescence imaging of DOX (red) and nucleus (blue) in YCC-DOX-treated (a) Hep3B and (b) KB cell lines with and without FA [57].

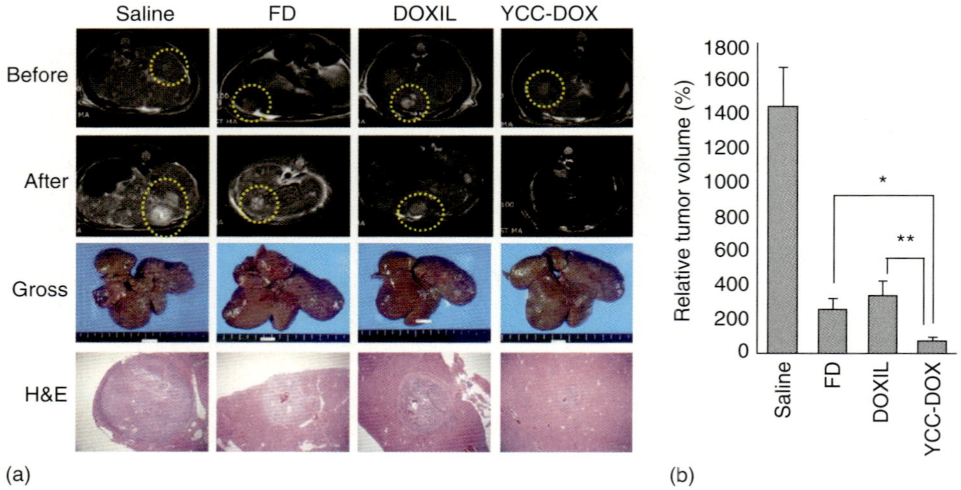

Figure 47.23 Anticancer effects in the rat liver tumor model. (a) Representative magnetic resonance images, gross images, and hematoxylin & eosin images. (b) Relative tumor volumes in the liver of rats treated with saline, free-DOX (FD), Doxil, and YCC-DOX ($^*P < 0.05$;$^{**} P < 0.002$). H&E, hematoxylin & eosin.

saline. As seen in Figure 47.23b, the relative tumor volume of YCC-DOX-treated animals is decreased 19.3-, 3.5-, and 4.5-fold compared to the saline-, free-DOX-, and Doxil-treated groups. The magnetic resonance images and the relative tumor volume values demonstrate that YCC-DOX significantly inhibits tumor growth and accumulates in liver cancer cells.

Additionally, the antiproliferation, antiangiogenesis, and apoptosis effects of YCC-DOX nanoparticles were studied with the aid of Ki-67 and CD34 antibodies, which are direct markers of angiogenesis and cell proliferation of cancer cells. The immunohistochemical analysis showed a lower fluorescent density of the YCC-DOX group in contrast to the other groups and in the TUNEL assay a higher number of apoptotic cells were observed in the YCC-DOX-treated rat tumors than in the saline-, free-DOX-, or Doxil-treated groups (Figure 47.24) [57].

In summary, the YCC-DOX nanoparticle is a promising substance that can act as a drug delivery system of antitumor agents as well as a MRI contrast agent for the therapy and diagnosis of primary liver cancer.

47.4 Clinical Development

Clinical trials with drug delivery systems for treating primary and/or secondary liver cancer have been performed with two drug–polymer conjugates: PK2

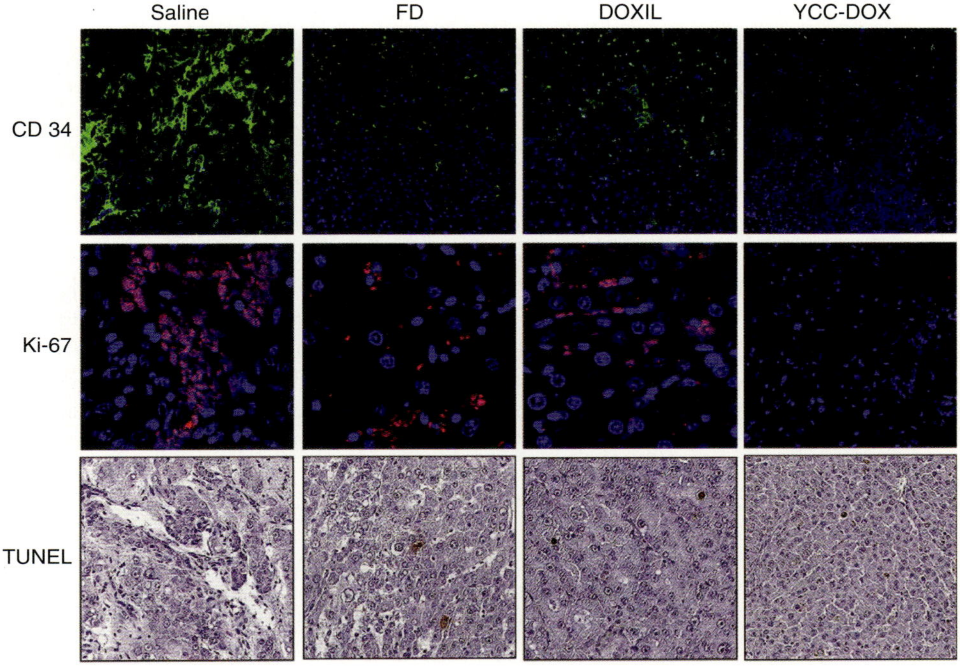

Figure 47.24 Effects on the proliferation, angiogenesis, and apoptosis of liver cancer. The images show liver cancer cells of rats treated with saline, free-DOX (FD), Doxil, or YCC-DOX; the pink and green coloration indicates positive anti-Ki-67 (original magnification ×400) and anti-CD34 (original magnification ×200) staining, respectively. In TUNEL images, the brown coloration is indicates the presence of apoptotic cells (original magnification ×400).

(a DOX–HPMA copolymer conjugated with *N*-galactosamine) and SMANCS (a conjugate of SMA and the highly cytotoxic agent NCS dissolved in SMANCS/Lipiodol, a lipid contrast agent).

In addition, two nanoparticles with DOX (Doxorubicin Transdrug) and mitoxantrone (DHAD-PBCA-NP) have been evaluated in phase II trials.

SMANCS/Lipiodol is the only polymer therapeutic that has been approved for treating HCC. The pivotal results of the clinical trials with the above-mentioned drug delivery systems are described below.

47.4.1
Phase I Study with PK2: A HPMA-Based Copolymer with *N*-Galactosamine

PK2, a DOX–HPMA copolymer conjugated with *N*-galactosamine as a ligand targeting the ASGPR, was determined in a phase I study with 31 patients with primary or metastatic liver cancer. The aim of this study was to determine the following parameters:

- Identification of side-effects and determination of the MTD after intravenous infusion of PK2
- Analysis of the efficiency of hepatic targeting by radioimaging with ^{123}I-PK2
- Assessment of the antineoplastic efficacy of PK2 [59].

The administration of PK2 was administered intravenously over 1 h and was repeated every 3 weeks. The MTD was a dose of 160 mg/m^2 of DOX-equivalents, which is approximately 2.5-fold higher that the standard dose for DOX (60–75 mg/m^2). Dose-limiting toxicities (DLTs) were associated with severe fatigue, neutropenia, and mucositis above the MTD. An imaging study in one patient with primary hepatoma showed increased uptake of radiolabeled ^{123}I-PK2 over time (Figure 47.25). Targeting of ^{123}I-labeled PK2 to peripheral metastases was also investigated. A selective and increased uptake was observed in disseminated metastases in comparison to healthy tissue. Two partial responses in patients with advanced liver cancer and one minor remission 47 months after treatment were achieved in this study.

In conclusion, it was established that the galactosamine targeted polymer is mainly delivered to the liver and potentially opens an avenue for using similarly designed HPMA drug conjugates with tethered galactosamine for treating diseases such as cirrhosis, hepatic malarial infection, HCC, and viral hepatitis. To date, no further clinical studies have been performed with PK2.

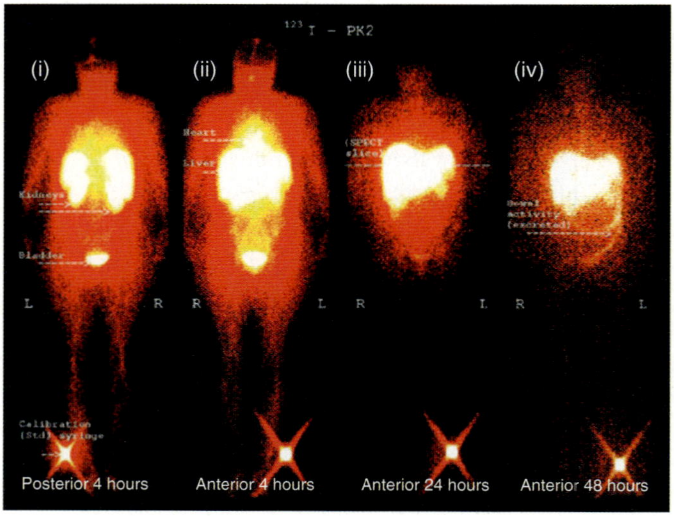

Figure 47.25 Planar γ-camera imaging of a patient at 4, 24, and 48 h after administration of PK2 (120 mg DOX-equivalents/m^2) [59].

47.4.2
Doxorubicin Transdrug: A DOX Nanoparticle with PIHCA that Advanced to Phase II/III Trials

In 2006, BioAlliance Pharma received orphan drug status by the European Medicines Agency and the US Food and Drug Administration for the treatment of HCC with Doxorubicin Transdrug. Doxorubicin Transdrug was developed by BioAlliance Pharma and is a product of a proprietary nanotechnology using PIHCA to encapsulate drugs. In a phase I/II clinical trial, Doxorubicin Transdrug loaded with DOX was evaluated in 20 patients with advanced primary liver cancer. During this study, at least one single injection of Doxorubicin Transdrug was administered into the hepatic artery of the patients. The MTD was $30\,mg/m^2$ and an objective response in three patients (16.67%) was achieved after one injection. During the same year, BioAlliance Pharma received approval by the Agence Francaise de Securite Sanitaire des Produits de Sante, the French medical regulatory agency, to start randomized phase II/III clinical trials. The main objective of these studies was to further determine the efficacy and tolerance of Doxorubicin Transdrug and to compare it with the current standard of care (frequently TACE). Even though the initial data displayed promising results, the phase II/III was prematurely interrupted due to frequent and severe pulmonary damage. In the phase II study, patients received three intra-arterial injections of Doxorubicin Transdrug and a survival rate of 88.9% was observed after 18 months compared to a 54.5% survival rate observed in patients who were treated with TACE with a cytotoxic drug. The increased survival rate was considered to be statistically significant. Based on this data, BioAlliance Pharma will investigate new application and dosing strategies for Doxorubicin Transdrug in order to reduce pulmonary adverse events that led to discontinuation of the trial (*www.bioalliancepharma.com*)

47.4.3
Phase I/II Trials of Mitoxantrone-Loaded PBCA Nanoparticles

The toxicity and antitumor activity of mitoxantrone-loaded PBCA nanoparticles (DHAD-PBCA-NPs) were determined in a randomized multicenter phase II study with 108 patients with unresected HCC. The DHAD-PBCA-NPs had a mean diameter of around 55.8 nm and were loaded with around 47% of mitoxantrone (DHAD). In this clinical trial, free DHAD was administered in the control arm. Both DHAD and DHAD-PBCA-NPs were injected intravenously within at least 15 min, a dose of $12\ mg/m^2$ mitoxantrone-equivalents being administered every 3 weeks, and each patient in the study underwent at least two treatment cycles. The response rates to the treatment are summarized in Table 47.4.

As apparent in Table 47.4, six patients (10.5%) treated with DHAD-PBCA-NPs had a partial response and 35 (61.4%) had stable disease. In contrast, patients who received a DHAD injection showed no objective responses and stable disease was achieved in 23 patients (45.1%). In the group treated with DHAD-PBCA-NPs, the

Table 47.4 Response rates of patients with HCC after treatment with DHAD or DHAD-PBCA-NPs [46].

Treatment group	Number of cases	CR (*n* (%))	PR (*n* (%))	SD (*n* (%))	PD (*n* (%))	OR (*n* (%))
DHAD-PBCA-NPs	57	0 (0.0)	6 (10.5)	35 (61.4)	16 (28.1)	6 (10.5)
DHAD	51	0 (0.0)	0 (0.0)	23 (45.1)	28 (54.9)	0 (0.0)

CR, complete response (complete disappearance of the tumor lesions for at least 4 weeks); PR, partial response, (more than 50% reduction of the tumor size for at least 4 weeks); SD, stable disease (a decrease of less than 50% or an increase of less than 25% of the tumor volume for at least 4 weeks); PD, progressive disease (25% or greater increase of the tumor size or any appearance of new lesions at any time during the study); OR, objective response (CR or PR).

survival rate after 1 year was 13.6% (eight patients). In the control group, however, none of the patients were alive after 1 year.

Several toxic side-effects occurred, such as leukopenia (47.4% in the DHAD-PBCA-NP arm and 74.5% in the DHAD arm) and anemia (65% with DHAD-PBCA-NP and 37.3% with DHAD).

In summary, intravenous administration of DHAD-PBCA-NPs showed improved antitumor activity against hepatic tumors and the median survival was extended to 5.46 months in comparison to 3.23 months in patients treated with free DHAD. Consequently, therapy with DHAD-PBCA-NPs seems to be a promising therapeutic option for patients with unresected HCC that should be further confirmed in phase III trials.

47.4.4
ThermoDox®: A Heat-Sensitive Liposomal Formulation of DOX in Phase II Trials

ThermoDox is a thermosensitive liposome encapsulating the active ingredient DOX that is given intravenously and in combination with hyperthermia or ablation for treating liver cancers. The thermally responsive nature of ThermoDox is due to the lipid molecules rapidly changing their structures by increasing the temperature to 39 °C or above that create defects in the bilayer of the liposomes so that DOX is released and can diffuse into the surrounding tissue (Figure 47.26). The released anticancer agent DOX is stable up to 73 °C [158].

Due to the promising results in preclinical studies, ThermoDox was investigated in a phase I study to determine the MTD and DLTs. In this clinical trial ThermoDox was intravenously administered to 24 patients with HCC or metastatic liver cancer during a period of 30 and 15 min before starting RFA. The patients, who had up to four lesions in a range of 3–7 cm in diameter, were treated with 20, 30, 40, 50, or 60 mg/m^2 of ThermoDox. The MTD was 50 mg/m^2 DOX with the most common side-effect being myelosuppression. Time to treatment failure for five patients receiving greater than 50 mg/m^2 DOX was 374 days on average, whereas

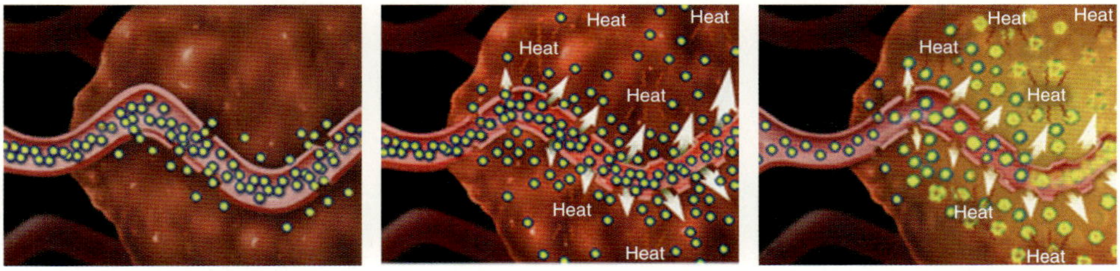

Figure 47.26 (a) Leaky tumor vessels (37 °C), (b) heat adds permeability (39 < T < 42 °C), and (c) mechanical release at 39–42 °C. (Reproduced courtesy of Celsion.)

15 patients receiving less than 50 mg/m^2 DOX had an average time to treatment failure of 80 days. Based on this data, Celsion has initiated a global phase III HEAT study with ThermoDox that is being conducting under a Special Protocol Assessment with the FDA. Six hundred patients are being assessed in this clinical trial in sites in the United States, Hong Kong, Canada, Taiwan, South Korea, China, and Italy. The antitumor efficacy is determined in patients receiving ThermoDox in combination with RFA compared to patients who receive RFA as control. The primary endpoint of this global trial is progression-free survival with a secondary confirmative endpoint of overall survival. Celsion expects an end of the clinical study by the middle of 2011 (for further information, see *www.celsion.com*).

47.4.5
SMANCS: A Conjugate of SMA and the Antitumor Agent NCS

As early as 1982, Maeda *et al.* reported on the remarkable therapeutic effect of SMANCS on primary hepatoma (HCC), in which SMANCS dissolved at a concentration of 1 mg/ml in the lipid contrast agent Lipiodol was infused via the hepatic artery [152, 153, 159]. The dose with respect to the volume of the SMANCS/Lipiodol solution that is applied may vary depending on the size of the tumor [58, 160, 161]. Usually, for small size tumors with maximum cross-sections less than 2 cm, the administered volume may be about 1–1.5 ml, for those with a diameter of 2–3 cm, the administered volume can be increased to about 1.5–3 ml, and for those with a tumor diameter of 4–6 cm, the administered volume can be increased to 4–5 ml. As stated below for larger tumors (greater than 6 cm), the infusion volume should be divided into multiple doses with intervals of about 4 weeks be repeated 2–3 times. Most HCC patients need subsequent treatment after 4 months. As described Chapter 3 in this volume, arterial administration of SMANCS/Lipiodol, results in selective drug delivery to cancer tissue with great efficiency (i.e., the tumor/blood plasma ratio of the drug is greater than 2000) [149]. The EPR effect is clearly observed in computed tomography (CT) scan images taken 2–3 days after infusion of SMANCS/Lipiodol, and one can follow the tumor-selective targeting as well as response using this method. This pronounced

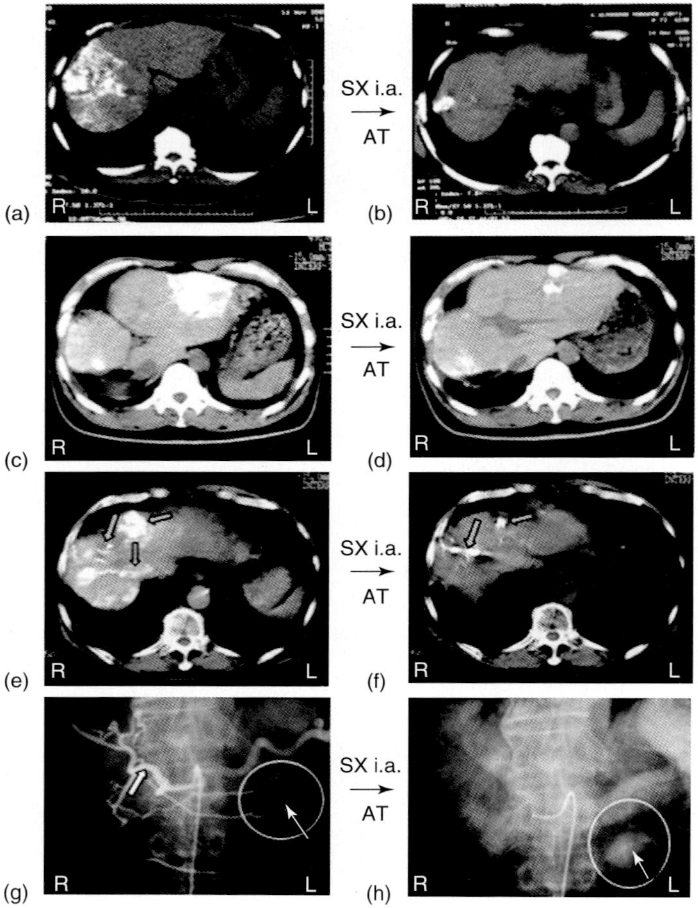

Figure 47.27 X-ray CT scan images of HCC either solitary/massive type (a and c) or recurrent case (e) with arterio-portal shunt. The figures show CT scan images of the malignant liver of the patients before and after arterial infusion of SMANCS/Lipiodol (SX i.a.) with concomitant angiotensin II (AT)-induced hypertension. In (a)–(f), white areas indicate tumors with SMANCS/Lipiodol retention as well as the spinal and costal bones [162]. All three cases showed rapid tumor regression within 1 month (see text). In (g) metastatic tumor nodule is invisible in the angiography under the normotension. However, it becomes visible under the angiotensin II induced hypertensive state in the angiogram (h) (see arrow in the circle) indicating enhanced drug delivery effect under hypertensive state.

targeting effect may be due to the EPR effect as well as the first-pass effect (see Figure 3.1, 3.5, 3.8 and others in Chapter 3, and Figures 47.27 and 47.28).

In patients with HCC, the response rate with SMANCS/Lipiodol, when properly infused into the hepatic artery, is more than 90% for Child A and B cirrhotic stage of the liver. White areas demonstrate tumors that have accumulated

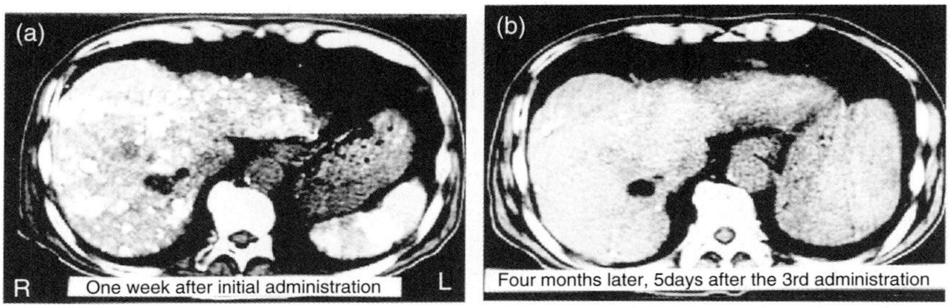

Figure 47.28 X-ray CT scan images of multinodular HCC after arterial infusion of SMANCS/Lipiodol. (a) One week after the infusion under normotensive states. Note: numerous tumor nodules in the entire liver have taken up SMANCS/Lipiodol. (b) The same image after 4 months. The patient was treated with three infusions of the drug under normotension over 4 months. Please note disappearance of numerous nodules.

SMANCS/Lipiodol as illustrated in Figure 47.27a and b, which demonstrates the response to treatment with SMANCS/Lipiodol under angiotensin II-induced hypertension after 1 month (see Chapter 3 for this therapeutic method).

Figure 47.27c and d demonstrates the case of a massive HCC treated with SMANCS/Lipiodol similar to Figure 47.27a and b; under angiotensin II induced hypertension a remarkable regression of the tumor was obtained during the follow-up period of 1 month. Another case report of recurrent HCC, 2.5 years after tumor resection that was treated similarly as above, is depicted in Figure 47.27e and f. Antitumor activity against HCC with an arterio-portal shunt administration of SMANCS/Lipiodol resulted in a formidable outcome with significant regression of the hepatoma (Figure 47.27e and f), which is usually uncontrollable by conventional treatments including surgical resection. In the angiograms (Figure 47.27g and h), a unique branching off from the right proper hepatic artery is seen that extends to the left lower part (arrow in the circle). Only under hypertension induced by angiotensin II did the metastatic tumor become diagnostically visible (see arrow in Figure 47.27g).

The arterial infusion of the normotensive state is also effective but takes a longer time to achieve 50% tumor reduction (see Chapter 3). The tumor-selective delivery of SMANCS in Lipiodol is not only observed in highly vascularized solitary HCC, but also in multinodular type HCC as seen in Figure 47.28a, in which SMANCS/Lipiodol is taken up effectively into the small micronodules of sizes less than 5 mm. The majority of small nodules disappeared in 4 months (Figure 47.28b).

We have observed this prominent drug uptake in HCC even under normotensive blood pressure. However, when the Seldinger arterial infusion is performed under angiotensin II-induced hypertensive conditions (the Seldinger technique is a well-established procedure in clinical practice used to introduce catheters by puncturing the vessel with a needle, inserting the Seldinger or plastic probe into the vessel thus ensuring a permanent access to the artery), the time that is required for the tumor to decrease to less than 50% of its original size (cross-section) will be much shorter (less than 1 month) due to a higher and more selective drug accumulation (see Section 3.4. Figure 3.11 and 3.12, and Figure 47.27a, c and e).

A postmarketing survey of SMANCS therapy for HCC in about 4000 cases was published as summarized in Table 47.5 [163]. It is seen that the drug caused very few serious adverse effects even in the advanced stages of HCC and yet a good therapeutic response was documented.

The effect on metastatic liver cancer is also encouraging when SMANCS/Lipiodol is infused into the tumor-feeding artery under angiotensin II-induced high blood pressure (e.g., 110 → 150 mmHg) [162]. The therapeutic efficacy of SMANCS/Lipiodol injected similarly into the tumor-feeding artery is also promising for cancers of the lung and other difficult-to-treat abdominal tumors, such as cancers of the kidney and pancreas [152, 160, 161], bile duct, and gallbladder [162].

Table 47.5 Adverse effects of intra-arterial SMANCS/Lipiodol therapy in hepatoma patients [163].

Symptoms	Parameter	Change (%)
Dermatological (exanthema)	–	0.36
Nausea	–	5.35[a]
Vomiting	–	4.06[a]
Anorexia	–	3.63[a]
Abdominal pain(transitory)	–	5.53
Liver function		
glutamyl oxaloacetic transaminase	increased	2.16[a]
glutamyl pyruvic transaminase	increased	2.12[a]
bilirubin	(> 1.5 mg/dl)	3.45[a]
Hypotension	–	2.22
Blood counts		
white blood cells	decreased	0.38
	increased	0.83[a]
polymorphonuclear leukocytes	decreased	0.04
	increased	0.28
Platelets	decreased	0.83
Renal function	impaired	0.71
blood urea nitrogen	increased	0.41
Anaphylaxis/shock	–	0.14
Rigor (transitory)	–	4.88
Chest pain (transitory)	–	0.20
Fever (low grade, 2–7 days)	–	27.80
C-reactive protein	increased	0.67
Ascites formation	–	1.35[a]

Based on 3956 patients (by Yamauchi Pharmaceutical, PMS, 2003).
[a]These issues are potentially associated with liver disease such as liver cirrhosis per se, not necessary induced by the drug, SMANCS.

Additional comments and precautions for arterial infusion of SMANCS/Lipiodol in the arterial infusion into hepatic artery include:

- Excessive and rapid infusion of SMANCS/Lipiodol will result in backlash flow of injected drug into the gastroduodenal artery, which may cause gastric or duodenal ulcer.
- The feeding artery of a individual tumor may be different from normal feeding artery (e.g., the normal feeding artery for hepatoma is the hepatic artery; for lung cancer, the bronchial artery, etc.); however, frequently there are anomalous vascular-feeding routes that may occur, from, such as, the costal, or even from the renal arteries, or other branching in hepatoma.
- A continuous flow (push) using a syringe connected to the catheter should be avoided; on the contrary, an intermittent push to avoid homeostasis, thrombus formation, or shock should be applied that maintains normal blood flow after the procedure. This method is not the embolization method.
- Do not try to fill a large tumor completely at once, since a large tumor may collapse under this treatment and extensive bleeding may result with a risk of causing complications.
- Angiotensin II-induced hypertension (e.g., $100 \rightarrow 150$ mmHg) will generally result in an improved delivery of SMANCS/Lipiodol and other polymeric drugs in general [162].
- Most adverse side-effects such as shock, which occurs every once in a while in angiography, can be avoided by appropriate use of glucocorticoids (such as betamethasone) and/or antihistamines. Patients with iodine allergy should be desensitized similarly by injection of a glucocorticoid 1 day before the procedure. The prick test using microgram quantity of SMANCS/Lipiodol may be helpful to predict allergic reaction.

47.5 Conclusions and Perspectives

Liver cancer, especially HCC, has become a major global health problem and is the fifth most common cancer worldwide. Since surgical or regional therapy with anticancer agents is restricted to patients at an early tumor stage, there is an urgent need to develop new therapeutic strategies for treating patients with advanced stages of HCC and also multiple liver metastases, which are typically a result of breast, esophageal, lung, stomach, or colorectal cancer. Since the RES, the EPR effect of liver metastases as well as the expression of certain liver-associated receptors, such as ASGPR, are prominent in the liver and liver tumors, tailor-made drug delivery systems relying on passive as well as active targeting can be considered ideal for improving the palliative and curative therapy of primary liver tumors and liver metastases.

Examples of drug–polymer conjugates with HPMA or serum albumin bearing galactose molecules and DOX bound though a cathepsin B-cleavable or acid-sensitive linker have shown impressive preclinical results. In addition, two drug nanoparticles that are taken up by the RES of the liver have advanced to the clinic: Doxorubicin Transdrug, a nanoparticle comprising PIHCA and DOX, reached phase II studies, but further development is on hold due to lung toxicity. A second nanoparticle with mitoxantrone encapsulated in PBCA showed promising activity in a phase II trial in the treatment of patients with unresected HCC with an overall increase in survival of around 2.2 months compared to the mitoxantrone control arm.

The most successful drug–polymer conjugate for treating HCC to date is SMANCS – a conjugate of two synthetic copolymers of SMA and the highly potent chromoprotein NCS that has been approved for the treatment of HCC in Japan since 1993. SMANCS is administered via the hepatic artery dissolved in Lipiodol, a lipid contrast agent, and has meanwhile demonstrated convincing antitumor activity in thousands of patients. Indeed, because a drug–polymer conjugate is applied combined with a contrast agent Lipiodol, an ethyl ester of iodinated poppy seed oil that allows X-ray detection of liver tumor nodules, SMANCS/Lipiodol can be viewed as a first successful clinical application of a theranostic approach.

For the future, in the era of nanomedicine it can be expected that the development of numerous polymer- or lipid-based nanoparticles with or without targeting ligands will be intensively pursued that target liver tumors with the aim of improving the therapeutic options for treating patients with primary and secondary liver tumors.

In addition, a global phase III HEAT study with ThermoDox, a heat-sensitive liposomal formulation of DOX, is being conducting under a Special Protocol Assessment with the FDA. Six hundred patients will be assessed in this clinical trial worldwide. The antitumor efficacy of ThermoDox in combination with RFA will be compared to patients who receive RFA as a control.

References

1. Schmitz, V. and Sauerbruch, T. (2007) Früherkennung des hepatozelluären Karzinoms. *Gastroenterologie*, **2**, 356–364.
2. El-Serag, H.B. and Rudolph, K.L. (2007) Hepatocellular carcinoma: epidemiology and molecular carcinogenesis. *Gastroenterology*, **132**, 2557–2576.
3. Lok, A.S., Seeff, L.B., Morgan, T.R. *et al.* (2009) Incidence of hepatocellular carcinoma and associated risk factors in hepatitis C-related advanced liver disease. *Gastroenterology*, **136**, 138–148.
4. Lawson, A., Hagan, S., Rye, K. *et al.* (2007) The natural history of hepatitis C with severe hepatic fibrosis. *J. Hepatol.*, **47**, 37–45.
5. American Cancer Society (2010) *Cancer Facts and Figures 2010*, American Cancer Society, Washington, DC, pp. 1–66.
6. Schütte, K., Bornschein, J., and Malfertheiner, P. (2009) Hepatocellular carcinoma – epidemiological trends and risk factors. *Digest. Dis.*, **27**, 80–92.
7. Blum, H.E. (2007) Epidemiologie, Diagnostik und Prävention. *Gastroenterologe*, **2**, 6–11.
8. Giuliani, F. and Colucci, G. (2009) Treatment of hepatocellular carcinoma. *Oncology*, **77** (Suppl. 1), 43–49.
9. Kubicka, S. and Manns, M.P. (2008) Hepatozelluläres Karzinom. *Gastroenterologe*, **3**, 147–157.
10. Spangenberg, H.C., Thimme, R., von Weizsäcker, F. *et al.* (2004) Hepatozelluläres Karzinom. *Internist*, **45**, 777–785.
11. Cabrera, R. and Nelson, D.R. (2010) Review article: the management of

hepatocellular carcinoma. *Aliment. Pharmacol. Ther.*, **31**, 461–476.

12. Boucher, W.E., Forner, A., Reig, M. *et al.* (2009) New drugs for the treatment of hepatocellular carcinoma. *Liver Int.*, **29**, 148–158.
13. Kuhl, C. (2009) Transarterielle Chemoembolisation bei hepatozellulärem Karzinom-neue Entwicklungen. *Gastroenterologe*, **4**, 330–339.
14. Shin, S.W. (2009) The current practice of transarterial chemoembolization for the treatment of hepatocellular carcinoma. *Korean J. Radiol.*, **10**, 425–434.
15. Llovet, J.M., Real, M.I., Montaña, X. *et al.* (2002) Arterial embolisation or chemoembolisation versus symptomatic treatment in patients with unresectable hepatocellular carcinoma: a randomised controlled trial. *Lancet*, **359**, 1734–1739.
16. Lo, C.M., Ngan, H., Tso, W.K. *et al.* (2002) Randomized controlled trial of transarterial lipiodol chemoembolization for unresectable hepatocellular carcinoma. *Hepatology*, **35**, 1164–1171.
17. Yeo, W., Mok, T.S., Zee, B. *et al.* (2005) A randomized phase III study of doxorubicin versus cisplatin/interferon-2b/doxorubicin/fluorouracil (PIAF) combination chemotherapy for unresectable hepatocellular carcinoma. *J. Natl. Cancer Inst.*, **97**, 1532–1538.
18. Chaparro, M., Moreno, L.G., Trapero-Marugan, M. *et al.* (2008) Review article: pharmacological therapy for hepatocellular carcinoma with sorafenib and other oral agents. *Aliment. Pharmacol. Ther.*, **28**, 1269–1277.
19. Yau, T., Chan, P., Epstein, R. *et al.* (2009) Management of advanced hepatocellular carcinoma in the era of targeted therapy. *Liver Int.*, **29**, 10–17.
20. O'Reilly, E.M., Stuart, K.E., Sanz-Altamira, P.M. *et al.* (2001) A phase II study of irinotecan in patients with advanced hepatocellular carcinoma. *Cancer*, **91**, 101–105.
21. Halm, U., Etzrodt, G., Schiefke, I. *et al.* (2000) A phase II study of pegylated liposomal doxorubicin for treatment of advanced hepatocellular carcinoma. *Ann. Oncol.*, **11**, 113–114.
22. Llovet, J.M., Ricci, S., Mazzaferro, V. *et al.* (2008) Sorafenib in advanced hepatocellular carcinoma. *N. Engl. J. Med.*, **359**, 378–390.
23. Greten, T.F., Manns, M.P., and Malek, N. (2009) Sorafenib for the treatment of HCC – the beginning of a new era in the treatment of HCC. *Z. Gastroenterol.*, **47**, 55–60.
24. Keating, G.M. and Santoro, A. (2009) Sorafenib: a review of its use in advanced hepatocellular carcinoma. *Drugs*, **69**, 223–240.
25. Greten, T.F., Korangy, F., Manns, M.P. *et al.* (2009) Molecular therapy for the treatment of hepatocellular carcinoma. *Br. J. Cancer*, **100**, 19–23.
26. Tanaka, S. and Arii, S. (2009) Molecularly targeted therapy for hepatocellular carcinoma. *Cancer Sci.*, **100**, 1–8.
27. Thomas, M. (2009) Molecular targeted therapy for hepatocellular carcinoma. *J. Gastroenterol.*, **44** (Suppl. XIX), 136–141.
28. Matsumura, Y. and Maeda, H. (1986) A new concept for macromolecular therapeutics in cancer chemotherapy: mechanism of tumoritropic accumulation of proteins and the antitumor agent SMANCS. *Cancer Res.*, **46**, 6387–6392.
29. Maeda, H., Wu, J., Sawa, T. *et al.* (2000) Tumor vascular permeability and the EPR effect in macromolecular therapeutics: a review. *J. Control. Release*, **65**, 271–284.
30. Jain, R.K. (1987) Transport of molecules in the tumor interstitium: a review. *Cancer Res.*, **6**, 3039–3051.
31. Jain, R.K. (1987) Transport of molecules across tumor vasculature. *Cancer Metastasis Rev.*, **6**, 559–593.
32. Zamboni, W.C. (2008) Concept and clinical evaluation of carrier-mediated anticancer agents. *Oncologist*, **13**, 248–260.
33. Allen, T.M. and Hansen, C. (1991) Pharmacokinetics of stealth versus conventional liposomes: effect of dose. *Biochim. Biophys. Acta*, **1068**, 133–141.
34. Drummond, D.C., Meyer, O., Hong, K. *et al.* (1999) Optimizing liposomes for delivery of chemotherapeutic agents

to solid tumors. *Pharmacol. Rev.*, **51**, 691–743.
35. Peer, D., Karp, J.M., Hong, S. *et al.* (2007) Nanocarriers as an emerging platform for cancer therapy. *Nanotechnology*, **2**, 751–760.
36. Morell, A.G., Irvine, R.A., Sternlieb, I. *et al.* (1968) Physical and chemical studies on ceruloplasmin. V. Metabolic studies on sialic acid-free ceruplasmin *in vivo*. *J. Biol. Chem.*, **243**, 155–159.
37. Stockert, R.J. (1995) The asialoglycoprotein receptor: relationship between structure, function and expression. *Physiol. Rev.*, **75**, 591–609.
38. Geffen, I. and Spiess, M. (1992) Asiaglycoprotein receptor. *Int. Rev. Cytol.*, **173B**, 181–219.
39. Meier, M., Bider, M.D., Malashkevich, V.N. *et al.* (2000) Crystal structure of the carbohydrate recognition domain of the H1 subunit of the asialoglycoprotein receptor. *J. Mol. Biol.*, **300**, 857–865.
40. Bider, M.D., Wahlberg, J.M., Kammerer, R.A. *et al.* (1996) The oligomerization domain of the asialoglycoprotein receptor preferentially forms 2:2 heterotetramers *in vitro*. *J. Biol. Chem.*, **271**, 31996–32001.
41. Lundquist, J.J. and Toone, E.J. (2002) The cluster glycoside effect. *Chem. Rev.*, **102**, 555–578.
42. Lee, T.R. and Lee, Y.C. (1987) Preparation of cluster glycosides of *N*-acetylgalactosamine that have subnanomolar binding constants towards the mammalian hepatic Gal/Gal-NAc-specific receptor. *Glycoconj. J.*, **4**, 317–328.
43. Lee, R.T. (1991) Ligand structural requirements for recognition and binding by the hepatic asialoglycoprotein receptor. *Targeted Diagn. Ther. Ser.*, **4**, 65–86.
44. Biessen, E.A.L., Beuting, D.M., Roelen, H.C.P.F. *et al.* (1995) Synthesis of cluster galactosides with high affinity for the hepatic asialoglycoprotein receptor. *J. Med. Chem.*, **38**, 1538–1546.
45. Zhang, Z., Liao, G., Nagai, T. *et al.* (1996) Mitoxantrone polybutyl cyanoacrylate nanoparticles as an anti-neoplastic targeting drug delivery system. *Int. J. Pharm.*, **139**, 1–8.
46. Zhou, Q., Sun, X., Zeng, L. *et al.* (2009) A randomized multicenter phase II clinical trial of mitoxantrone-loaded nanoparticles in the treatment of 108 patients with unresected hepatocellular carcinoma. *Nanomedicine*, **5**, 419–423.
47. Zhang, Z., He, Q., Liao, G.-T. *et al.* (1999) Study on the anticarcinogenic effect and acute toxicity of liver-targeting mitoxantrone nanoparticles. *World J. Gastroenterol.*, **5**, 511–514.
48. Kattan, J., Droz, J., Couvreur, P. *et al.* (1992) Phase I clinical trial and pharmacokinetic evaluation of doxorubicin carried by polyisohexylcyanoacrylate nanoparticles. *Invest. New Drugs*, **10**, 191–199.
49. Barraud, L., Merle, P., Soma, E. *et al.* (2005) Increase of doxorubicin sensitivity by doxorubicin-loading into nanoparticles for hepatocellular carcinoma cells *in vitro* and *in vivo*. *J. Hepatol.*, **42**, 736–743.
50. Erion, M.D., Reddy, K.R., Boyer, S.H. *et al.* (2004) Design, synthesis, and characterization of a series of cytochrome P450 3A-activated prodrugs (HepDirect prodrugs) useful for targeting phosph(on)ate-based drugs to the liver. *J. Am. Chem. Soc.*, **126**, 5154–5163.
51. Arner, E.S. and Eriksson, S. (1995) Mammalian deoxyribonucleoside kinases. *Pharmacol. Ther.*, **67**, 155–186.
52. Erion, M.D., van Poelje, P.D., MacKenna, D.A. *et al.* (2005) Liver-targeted drug delivery using HepDirect prodrugs. *J. Pharmacol. Exp. Ther.*, **312**, 554–560.
53. de Waziers, I., Cugnenc, P.H., Yang, C.S. *et al.* (1990) Cytochrome P450 isoenzymes, epoxide hydrolase and glutathione transferases in rat and human hepatic and extrahepatic tissues. *J. Pharmacol. Exp. Ther.*, **253**, 387–394.
54. Meister, A. (1983) Metabolism and transport of glutathione and other gamma-glutamyl compounds in *Functions of Glutathione: Biochemical, Physiological, Toxicological and Clinical Aspects*

(ed. A. Larson), Raven Press, New York, pp. 1–22.

55. Kim, S.I., Shin, D., Choi, T.H. *et al.* (2007) Systemic and specific delivery of small interfering RNAs to the liver mediated by apolipoprotein A-I. *Mol. Ther.*, **5**, 1145–1152.

56. Liu, P., Li, Z., Zhu, M. *et al.* (2010) Preparation of EGFR monoclonal antibody conjugated nanoparticles and targeting to hepatocellular carcinoma. *J. Mater. Sci. Mater. Med.*, **21**, 551–556.

57. Maeng, J.H., Lee, D.-H., Jung, K.H. *et al.* (2010) Multifunctional doxorubicin loaded superparamagnetic iron oxide nanoparticles for chemotherapy and magnetic resonance imaging in liver cancer. *Biomaterials*, **31**, 4995–5006.

58. Maeda, H., Sawa, T., and Konno, T. (2001) Mechanism of tumor-targeted delivery of macromolecular drugs, including the EPR effect in solid tumor and clinical overview of the prototype polymeric drug SMANCS. *J. Control. Release*, **74**, 47–61.

59. Seymour, L.W., Ferry, D.R., Anderson, D. *et al.* (2002) Hepatic drug targeting: phase I evaluation of polymer-bound doxorubicin. *J. Clin. Oncol.*, **20**, 1668–1676.

60. Xu, Z., Chen, L., Gu, W. *et al.* (2009) The performance of docetaxel-loaded solid lipid nanoparticles targeted to hepatocellular carcinoma. *Biomaterials*, **30**, 226–232.

61. Tian, Q., Zhang, C.-N., Wang, X.-H. *et al.* (2010) Glycyrrhetinic acid-modified chitosan/poly(ethylene glycol) nanoparticles for liver-targeted delivery. *Biomaterials*, **31**, 4748–4756.

62. Krishna, A.D.S., Mandraju, R.K., Kishore, G. *et al.* (2009) An efficient targeted drug delivery through apotransferrin loaded nanoparticles. *PloS ONE*, **4**, e7240.

63. Yuan, Y., Liu, C., Qian, J. *et al.* (2010) Size-mediated cytotoxicity and apoptosis of hydroxyapatite nanoparticles in human hepatoma HepG2 cells. *Biomaterials*, **31**, 730–740.

64. Liu, S.-Y., Liang, Z.-S., Gao, F. *et al.* (2010) *In vitro* photothermal study of gold nanoshells functionalized with small targeting peptides to liver cancer cells. *J. Mater. Sci. Mater. Med.*, **21**, 665–674.

65. Nagaoka, T., Fukuda, T., Yoshida, S. *et al.* (2007) Characterization of bio-nanocapsule as a transfer vector targeting human hepatocyte carcinoma by disulfide linkage modification. *J. Control. Release*, **118**, 348–356.

66. Hu, L., Huang, B., Zou, M. *et al.* (2008) Preparation of the phycoerythrin subunit liposome in a photodynamic experiment on liver cancer cells. *Acta Pharmacol. Sin.*, **29**, 1539–1546.

67. Bothun, G.D., Rabideau, A.E., and Stoner, M.A. (2009) Hepatoma cell uptake of cationic multifluorescent quantum dot liposomes. *J. Phys. Chem. B*, **113**, 7725–7728.

68. Zhang, H.-W., Zhang, L., Sun, X. *et al.* (2007) Successful transfection of hepatoma cells after encapsulation of plasmid DNA into negatively charged liposomes. *Biotechnol. Bioeng.*, **96**, 118–124.

69. Miyata, R., Ueda, M., Jinno, H. *et al.* (2009) Selective targeting by preS1 domain of hepatitis B surface antigen conjugated with phosphorylcholine-based amphilic block copolymer micelles as a biocompatible, drug delivery carrier for treatment of human hepatocellular carcinoma with paclitaxel. *Int. J. Cancer*, **124**, 2460–2467.

70. Li, X., Huang, Y., Chen, X. *et al.* (2009) Self-assembly and characterization of Pluronic P105 micelles for liver-targeted delivery of silybin. *J. Drug Target.*, **17**, 739–750.

71. Yang, K.W., Li, X.R., Yang, Z.L. *et al.* (2007) Novel polyion complex micelles for liver-targeted delivery of diammonium glycyrrhizinate: *in vitro* and *in vivo* characterization. *J. Biomed. Mater. Res. A*, **88**, 140–148.

72. Jiang, X., Dai, H., Ke, C.-Y. *et al.* (2007) PEG-*b*-PPA/DNA micelles improve transgene expression in rat liver through intrabiliary infusion. *J. Control. Release*, **122**, 297–304.

73. Akinc, A., Goldberg, M., Qin, J. *et al.* (2009) Development of lipidoid-siRNA

formulations for systemic delivery to the liver. *Mol. Ther.*, **17**, 872–879.

74. Marcellin, P., Chang, T.-T., Lim, S.G. *et al.* (2003) Adefovir dipivoxil for the treatment of hepatitis B e antigen-positive chronic hepatitis B. *N. Engl. J. Med.*, **348**, 808–816.
75. Heinemann, V., Hertel, L.W., Grindey, G.B. *et al.* (1988) Comparison of the cellular pharmacokinetics and toxicity of 2′,2′-diflurodeoxycytidine and 1-β-D-arabinofuranosylcytosine. *Cancer Res.*, **48**, 4024–4031.
76. Zhang, Y.J., Chen, S., Tsai, W.Y. *et al.* (2000) Expression of cytochrome P450 1A1/2 and 3A4 in liver tissues of hepatocellular carcinoma cases and controls from Taiwan and their relationship to hepatitis B virus and aflatoxin B_1- and 4-aminobiphenyl-DNA adducts. *Biomarkers*, **5**, 295–306.
77. Vasey, P.A., Kaye, S.B., Morrison, R. *et al.* (1999) Phase I clinical and pharmacokinetic study of PK1 [*N*-(2-hydroxypropyl)methacrylamide copolymer doxorubicin]: first member of a new class of chemotherapeutic agents – drug–polymer conjugates. *Clin. Cancer Res.*, **5**, 83–94.
78. Bilim, V. (2003) Technology evaluation: PK1, Pfizer/Cancer Research UK. *Curr. Opin. Mol. Ther.*, **5**, 326–330.
79. Ulbrich, K., Strohalm, J., Subr, V. *et al.* (1996) Polymeric conjugates of drugs and antibodies for site-specific drug delivery. *Macromol. Symp.*, **103**, 177–192.
80. Flanagan, P.A., Duncan, R., Subr, V. *et al.* (1992) Evaluation of protein–*N*-(2-hydroxypropyl)-methacrylamide copolymer conjugates as targetable drug-carriers: 2. Body distribution of conjugates containing transferrin, antitransferrin receptor antibody or anti-Thy 1.2 antibody and effectiveness of transferrin-containing daunomycin conjugates against mouse L1210 leukemia *in vivo*. *J. Control. Release*, **18**, 25–37.
81. Rihova, B. (1995) Antibody-targeted polymer-bound drugs. *Folia Microbiol.*, **40**, 367–384.
82. Seymour, L.W., Ulbrich, K., Wedge, S.R. *et al.* (1991) *N*-(2-Hydroxypropyl)methacrylamide copolymers targeted to the hepatocyte galactose receptor: Pharmacokinetics in DBA2 mice. *Br. J. Cancer*, **63**, 859–866.
83. Duncan, R., Seymour, L.C.W., Scarlett, L. *et al.* (1986) Fate of *N*-(2-hydroxypropyl)methacrylamide copolymers with pendent galactosamine residues after intravenous administration to rats. *Biochim. Biophys. Acta*, **880**, 62–71.
84. Seymour, L.W. (1994) Soluble polymers for lectin-mediated drug targeting. *Adv. Drug Deliv. Rev.*, **14**, 89–111.
85. Duncan, R., Kopecek, J., Rejmanova, P. *et al.* (1983) Targeting of *N*-(2-hydroxypropyl)methacrylamide copolymers to liver by incorporation of galactose residues. *Biochim. Biophys. Acta*, **755**, 518–521.
86. Hopewell, J.W., Duncan, R., Wilding, D. *et al.* (2001) Preclinical evaluation of the cardiotoxicity of PK2: a novel HPMA copolymer–doxorubicin–galactosamine conjugate antitumor agent. *Hum. Exp. Toxicol.*, **20**, 461–470.
87. Seymour, L.W., Ulbrich, K., Strohalm, J. *et al.* (1991) Pharmacokinetics of a polymeric drug carrier targeted to the hepatocyte galactose receptor. *Br. J. Cancer*, **63**, 859–866.
88. Pimm, M.V., Perkins, A.C., Strohalm, J. *et al.* (1996) Gamma scintigraphy of a ^{123}I-labelled *N*-(2-hydroxypropyl)methacrylamide copolymer–doxorubicin conjugate containing galactosamine following intravenous administration to nude mice bearing hepatic human colon carcinoma. *J. Drug Target.*, **3**, 385–390.
89. Pimm, M.V., Perkins, A.C., Duncan, R. *et al.* (1993) Targeting of *N*-(2-hydroxypropyl)methacrylamide copolymer–doxorubicin conjugate to the hepatocyte galactose-receptor in mice: visualisation and quantification by gamma scintigraphy as a basis for clinical targeting studies. *J. Drug Target.*, **1**, 125–131.
90. Julyan, P.J., Seymour, L.W., Ferry, D.R. *et al.* (1999) Preliminary clinical study of the distribution of HPMA

copolymers bearing doxorubicin and galactosamine. *J. Control. Release*, **57**, 281–290.

91. Fiume, L., Mattioli, A., Busi, C. *et al.* (1982) Conjugates of adenine-9-β-D-arabinofuranoside monophosphate (ara-AMP) with lactosaminated homologous albumin are not immunogenic in the mouse. *Experientia*, **38**, 1087–1089.
92. Fiume, L., Busi, C., Mattioli, A. *et al.* (1981) Hepatocyte targeting of adenine-9-β-D-arabinofuranoside 5′-monophosphate (ara-AMP) coupled to lactosaminated albumin. *FEBS Lett.*, **129**, 261–264.
93. Fiume, L., Bassi, B., Busi, C. *et al.* (1986) A chemically stable conjugate of 9-β-D-arabinofuranosyladenine 5′-monophosphate with lactosaminated albumin accomplishes a selective delivery of the drug to liver cells. *Biochem. Pharmacol.*, **35**, 967–972.
94. Fiume, L. (1969) Penetration of β-amanitin–rabbit-albumin conjugate into hepatic parenchymal cells. *Lancet*, **2**, 853–854.
95. Fiume, L., Campadelli, G., and Wieland, T. (1971) Facilitated penetration of amanitin–albumin conjugates into hepatocytes after coupling with fluorescein. *Nat. New Biol.*, **230**, 219–220.
96. Rogers, J.C. and Kornfeld, S. (1971) Hepatic uptake of proteins coupled to fetuin glycopeptide. *Biochem. Biophys. Res. Commun.*, **45**, 622–629.
97. Krantz, M.J., Holtzman, N.A., Stowell, C.P. *et al.* (1976) Attachment of thioglycoside to proteins: enhancement of liver membrane binding. *Biochemistry*, **15**, 3963–3968.
98. Wilson, G. (1978) Effect of reductive lactosamination on the hepatic uptake of bovine pancreatic ribonuclease A dimer. *J. Biol. Chem.*, **235**, 2070–2072.
99. Gray, G.R. (1974) The direct coupling of oligosaccharides to proteins and derivatized gels. *Arch. Biochem. Biophys.*, **163**, 426–428.
100. Schwartz, B.A. and Gray, G.R. (1977) Proteins containing reductively aminated disaccharides. Synthesis and chemical characterization. *Arch. Biochem. Biophys.*, **181**, 542–549.
101. Borch, R.F., Bernstein, M.D., and Durst, H.D. (1971) The cyanohydroborate anion as a selective reducing agent. *J. Am. Chem. Soc.*, **93**, 2897–2904.
102. Fiume, L., Busi, C., and Mattioli, A. (1982) Lactosaminated human serum albumin as hepatotropic drug carrier. Rate of uptake by mouse liver. *FEBS Lett.*, **146**, 42–46.
103. Fiume, L., Busi, C., Preti, P. *et al.* (1987) Conjugates of ara-AMP with lactosaminated albumin: a study on their immunogenicity in mouse and rat. *Cancer Drug Deliv.*, **4**, 145–150.
104. Cerenzia, M., Fiume, L., De Bernardi Venon, W. *et al.* (1996) Adenine arabinoside monophosphate coupled to lactosaminated human albumin administered for 4 weeks in patients with chronic type B hepatitis decreased viremia without producing significant side effects. *Hepatology*, **23**, 657–661.
105. Fiume, L., Torrani Cerenzia, M.R., Bonino, F. *et al.* (1988) Inhibition of hepatitis B virus replication by vidarabine monophosphate conjugated with lactosaminated serum albumin. *Lancet*, **2**, 13–15.
106. Torrani Cerenzia, M.R., Fiume, L., Busi, C. *et al.* (1994) Inhibition of hepatitis B virus replication by adenine arabinoside monophosphate coupled to lactosaminated albumin. Efficacy and minimal active dose. *J. Hepatol.*, **20**, 307–309.
107. Zarski, J.P., Barange, K., Souvignet, C. *et al.* (2001) Efficacy and safety of lactosaminated human serum albumin–adenine arabinoside monophosphate in chronic hepatitis B patients non-responders to interferon therapy: a randomised clinical trial. *J. Hepatol.*, **34**, 487–488.
108. Fiume, L., Busi, C., Corzani, S. *et al.* (1994) Organ distribution of a conjugate of adenine arabinoside monophosphate with lactosaminated albumin in the rat. *J. Hepatol.*, **20**, 681–682.
109. MacDonald, J.S. and Astrow, A.B. (2001) Adjuvant therapy of colon cancer. *Semin. Oncol.*, **28**, 30–40.

110. van Laar, J.A.M., Rustum, Y.M., Ackland, S.P. *et al.* (1998) Comparison of 5-fluoro-2′-deoxyuridine with 5-fluorouracil and their role in the treatment of colorectal cancer. *Eur. J. Cancer*, **34**, 296–306.
111. Ensminger, W.D., Rosowsky, A., Raso, V. *et al.* (1978) A clinical-pharmacological evaluation of hepatic arterial infusions of 5-fluoro-2′-deoxyuridine and 5-fluorouracil. *Cancer Res.*, **38**, 3784–3792.
112. Wagner, J.G., Gyves, J.W., Stetson, P.L. *et al.* (1986) Steady-state nonlinear pharmacokinetics of 5-fluorouracil during hepatic arterial and intravenous infusions in cancer patients. *Cancer Res.*, **46**, 1499–1506.
113. Taylor, I., Machin, D., Mullee, M. *et al.* (1985) A randomised controlled trial of adjuvant portal vein cytotoxic perfusion in colorectal cancer. *Br. J. Surg.*, **72**, 359–363.
114. Fielding, L.P., Hittinger, R., Grace, R.H. *et al.* (1992) Randomised controlled trial of adjuvant chemotherapy by portal-vein perfusion after curative resection for colorectal adenocarcinoma. *Lancet*, **340**, 502–506.
115. Rougier, P., Sahmoud, T., Nitti, D. *et al.* (1998) Adjuvant portal-vein infusion of fluorouracil and heparin in colorectal cancer: a randomised trial. *Lancet*, **351**, 1677–1681.
116. Kemeny, N., Seiter, K., Niedzwiecki, D. *et al.* (1992) A randomized trial of intrahepatic infusion of fluorodeoxyuridine with dexamethasone versus fluorodeoxyuridine alone in the treatment of metastatic colorectal cancer. *Cancer*, **69**, 327–334.
117. Hohn, D.C., Melnick, J., Stagg, R. *et al.* (1985) Biliary sclerosis in patients receiving hepatic arterial infusion of floxuridine. *J. Clin. Oncol.*, **3**, 98–102.
118. Di Stefano, G., Busi, C., and Fiume, L. (2002) Floxuridine coupling with lactosaminated human albumin to increase the drug efficacy on liver micrometastases. *Dig. Liver Dis.*, **34**, 439–446.
119. Di Stefano, G., Lanza, M., Busi, C. *et al.* (2002) Conjugates of nucleoside analogs with lactosaminated human albumin to selectively increase the drug levels in liver blood: requirements for a regional chemotherapy. *J. Pharmacol. Exp. Ther.*, **301**, 638–642.
120. Yoshikawa, M., Kato, T., and Takeshini, T. (1967) A novel method for phosphorylation of nucleosides to 5′-nucleotides. *Tetrahedron Lett.*, **50**, 5065–5068.
121. Fiume, L., Busi, C., Di Stefano, G. *et al.* (1993) Coupling of antiviral nucleoside analogs to lactosaminated human albumin by using the imidazolides of their phosphoric esters. *Anal. Biochem.*, **212**, 407–411.
122. Di Stefano, G., Tubaro, M., Lanza, M. *et al.* (2003) Synthesis and physicochemical characteristics of a liver-targeted conjugate of fluorodeoxyuridine monophosphate with lactosaminated human albumin. *Rapid Commun. Mass Spectrom.*, **17**, 2503–2507.
123. Mitra, S.K. (1966) The terminal distribution of hepatic artery with special reference to arterio-portal anastomosis. *J. Anat.*, **100**, 651–663.
124. Rappaport, A.M. (1973) The microcirculatory hepatic unit. *Microvasc. Res.*, **6**, 212–228.
125. Cho, K.J. and Lundequist, A. (1983) The peribiliary vascular plexus: the microvascular architecture of the bile duct in the rabbit and in clinical cases. *Radiology*, **147**, 357–364.
126. Andrews, J.C., Kunsten, C., Terio, P. *et al.* (1991) Hepatobiliary toxicity of 5-fluoro-2′-deoxyuridine. Intra-arterial versus portal venous routes of infusion. *Invest. Radiol.*, **26**, 461–464.
127. Trerè, D., Fiume, L., Badiali De Giorgi, L. *et al.* (1999) The asialoglycoprotein receptor in human hepatocellular carcinomas: its expression on the proliferating cells. *Br. J. Cancer*, **81**, 404–408.
128. Schneider, Y., Abarca, J., Aboud-Pirak, E. *et al.* (1984) Drug targeting in human cancer chemotherapy in *Receptor-Mediated Targeting of Drugs*, NATO ASI Series A: Life Sciences, vol. 82 (eds G. Gregoriadis, G. Poste, J. Senior, and

A. Trouet), Plenum Press, New York, pp. 1–25.

129. O'Hare, K.B., Hume, I.C., Scarlett, L. *et al.* (1989) Effect of galactose on interaction of *N*-(2-hydroxypropyl) methacrylamide copolymers with hepatoma cells in culture: preliminary applications to an anticancer agents, daunomycin. *Hepatology*, **10**, 207–214.

130. Di Stefano, G., Busi, C., Mattioli, A. *et al.* (1999) Inhibition of [^{3}H]thymidine incorporation into DNA of rat regenerating liver by 2′,2′-difluorodeoxycytidine coupled to lactosaminated poly-L -lysine. *Biochem. Pharmacol.*, **57**, 793–799.

131. Willner, D., Trail, P.A., Hofstead, S.J. *et al.* (1993) (6-Maleimidocaproyl)hydrazone derivative of doxorubicin – a new derivative for the preparation of immunoconjugates of doxorubicin. *Bioconjugate Chem.*, **4**, 521–527.

132. Di Stefano, G., Lanza, M., Kratz, F. *et al.* (2004) A novel method for coupling doxorubicin to lactosaminated human albumin by an acid sensitive hydrazone bond: synthesis, characterization and preliminary biological properties of the conjugate. *Eur. J. Pharm. Sci.*, **23**, 393–397.

133. Boga, C., Fiume, L., Baglioni, M. *et al.* (2009) Characterisation of the conjugate of the (6-maleimidocaproyl) hydrazone derivative of doxorubicin with lactosaminated human albumin by ^{13}C NMR spectroscopy. *Eur. J. Pharm. Sci.*, **38**, 262–269.

134. Di Stefano, G., Fiume, L., Baglioni, M. *et al.* (2008) Doxorubicin coupled to lactosaminated albumin: effect of heterogeneity in drug load on conjugate disposition and hepatocellular carcinoma uptake in rats. *Eur. J. Pharm. Sci.*, **33**, 191–198.

135. Greenfield, R.S., Kaneko, T., Daues, A. *et al.* (1990) Evaluation *in vitro* of adriamycin immunoconjugates synthesized using an acid-sensitive hydrazone linker. *Cancer Res.*, **50**, 6600–6607.

136. Di Stefano, G., Kratz, F., Lanza, M. *et al.* (2003) Doxorubicin coupled to lactosaminated human albumin remains confined within mouse liver cells after the intracellular release from the carrier. *Dig. Liver Dis.*, **35**, 428–433.

137. Di Stefano, G., Fiume, L., Bolondi, L. *et al.* (2005) Enhanced uptake of lactosaminated human albumin by rat hepatocarcinomas: implications for an improved chemotherapy of primary liver tumors. *Liver Int.*, **25**, 854–860.

138. Fiume, L., Bolondi, L., Busi, C. *et al.* (2005) Doxorubicin coupled to lactosaminated albumin inhibits the growth of hepatocellular carcinomas induced in rats by diethylnitrosamine. *J. Hepatol.*, **43**, 645–652.

139. Di Stefano, G., Fiume, L., Baglioni, M. *et al.* (2008) Efficacy of doxorubicin coupled to lactosaminated albumin on rat HCCs evaluated by ultrasound imaging. *Dig. Liver Dis.*, **40**, 278–284.

140. Goormaghtigh, E., Chatelain, P., Caspers, J. *et al.* (1980) Evidence of a specific complex between adriamycin and negatively-charged phospholipids. *Biochim. Biophys. Acta*, **597**, 1–14.

141. Di Stefano, G., Fiume, L., Baglioni, M. *et al.* (2006) A conjugate of doxorubicin with lactosaminated albumin enhances the drug concentrations in all the forms of rat hepatocellular carcinomas independently of their differentiation grade. *Liver Int.*, **26**, 726–733.

142. Di Stefano, G., Fiume, L., Baglioni, M. *et al.* (2007) Coupling of lactose molecules to the carrier protein hinders the spleen and bone marrow uptake of doxorubicin conjugated with human albumin. *Eur. J. Pharm. Sci.*, **30**, 136–142.

143. Harris, L., Preat, V., and Farber, E. (1987) Patterns of ligand binding to normal, regenerating, preneoplastic, and neoplastic rat hepatocytes. *Cancer Res.*, **47**, 3954–3958.

144. Di Stefano, G., Fiume, L., Domenicali, M. *et al.* (2006) Doxorubicin coupled to lactosaminated albumin: effects on rats with liver fibrosis and cirrhosis. *Dig. Liver Dis.*, **38**, 404–408.

145. Di Stefano, G., Derenzini, M., Kratz, F. *et al.* (2004) Liver targeted doxorubicin: effects on regenerating rat hepatocytes. *Liver Int.*, **24**, 246–252.

146. Maeda, H., Ueda, M., Morinaga, T. *et al.* (1985) Conjugation of poly(styrene-*co*-maleic acid) derivatives to the antitumor protein neocarzinostatin: pronounced improvements in pharmacological properties. *J. Med. Chem.*, **28**, 455–461.
147. Maeda, H., Takeshita, J., and Kanamaru, R. (1979) A lipophilic derivative of neocarzinostatin: a polymer conjugation of an antitumor protein antibiotic. *Int. J. Pept. Protein Res.*, **14**, 81–87.
148. Maeda, H., Edo, K., and Ishida, N. (1997) *Neocarzinostatin: The Past, Present, and Future on an Anticancer Drug*, Springer, Tokyo, pp. 227–267.
149. Iwai, K., Maeda, H., and Konno, T. (1984) Use of oily contrast medium for selective drug targeting to tumor: enhanced therapeutic effect and X-ray image. *Cancer Res.*, **44**, 2115–2121.
150. Maeda, H., Takeshita, J., Kanamaru, R. *et al.* (1979) Antimetastatic and antitumor activity of a derivative of neocarzinostatin: an organic solvent- and water-soluble polymer-conjugated protein. *Gann*, **70**, 601–606.
151. Yamasaki, K., Konno, T., Miyauch, Y. *et al.* (1987) Reduction of hepatic metastases in rabbits by administration of an oily anticancer agent into the portal vein. *Cancer Res.*, **47**, 852–855.
152. Konno, T., Maeda, H., Iwai, K. *et al.* (1983) Effect of arterial administration of high-molecular-weight anticancer agent SMANCS with lipid lymphographic agent on hepatoma: a preliminary report. *Eur. J. Cancer Clin. Oncol.*, **19**, 1053–1065.
153. Konno, T., Maeda, H., Iwai, K. *et al.* (1984) Selective targeting of anticancer drug and simultaneous image enhancement in solid tumors by arterially administered lipid contrast medium. *Cancer*, **54**, 2367–2374.
154. Cuvier, C., Roblot-Treupel, L., Millot, J.M. *et al.* (1992) Doxorubicin-loaded nanospheres bypass tumor cell multidrug resistance. *Biochem. Pharmacol.*, **44**, 509–517.
155. Merle, P., Barraud, L., Lefrancois, L. *et al.* (2003) Long-term high-dose interferon-alpha therapy delays Hepadnavirus-related hepatocarcinogenesis in X/myc transgenic mice. *Oncogene*, **22**, 2762–2771.
156. Lowe, S.W., Bodis, S., McClatchey, A. *et al.* (1994) p53 Status and the efficacy of cancer therapy *in vivo*. *Science*, **266**, 807–810.
157. Yu, M.K., Jeong, Y.Y., Park, J. *et al.* (2008) Drug-loaded superparamagnetic iron oxide nanoparticles for combined cancer imaging and therapy *in vivo*. *Angew. Chem. Int. Ed.*, **47**, 5362–5365.
158. Poon, R.T.P. and Borys, N. (2009) Lyso-thermosensitive liposomal doxorubicin: a novel approach to enhance efficacy of themal ablation of liver cancer. *Expert Opin. thermal Pharmacother.*, **10**, 333–343.
159. Konno, T., Maeda, H., Yokoyama, I. *et al.* (1982) Use of a lipid lymphographic agent, lipiodol, as a carrier of high molecular weight antitumor agent, SMANCS, for hepatocellular carcinoma. *Jpn. J. Cancer Chemother.*, **9**, 2005–2015.
160. Seymour, L.W., Olliff, S.P., Poole, C.J. *et al.* (1998) A novel dosage approach for evaluation of SMANCS [poly-(styrene-*co*-maleyl-half-*n*-butylate)–neocarzinostatin] in the treatment of primary hepatocellular carcinoma. *Int. J. Oncol.*, **12**, 1217–1223.
161. Maki, S., Konno, T., and Maeda, H. (1985) Image enhancement in computerized tomography for sensitive diagnosis of liver cancer and semiquantitation of tumor selective drug targeting with oily contrast medium. *Cancer*, **56**, 751–757.
162. Nagamitsu, A., Greish, K., and Maeda, H. (2009) Elevating blood pressure as a strategy to increase tumor targeted delivery of macromolecular drug SMANCS: cases of advanced solid tumors. *Jpn. J. Clin. Oncol.*, **39**, 756–766.
163. Greish, K., Fang, J., Inuzuka, T. *et al.* (2003) Macromolecular anticancer therapeutics for effective solid tumor targeting: advantages and prospects. *Clin. Pharmacokinet.*, **42**, 1089–1105.

48
Photodynamic Therapy: Photosensitizer Targeting and Delivery

Pawel Mroz, Sulbha K. Sharma, Timur Zhiyentayev, Ying-Ying Huang, and Michael R.Hamblin

48.1
Introduction

Photodynamic therapy (PDT) is a promising new therapeutic procedure for the management of a variety of solid tumors. It is a two-step procedure that involves administration of a nontoxic dye, or photosensitizer, followed by activation of the drug with nonthermal light of a specific wavelength [1–3]. PDT generates singlet oxygen and other reactive oxygen species(ROS) that cause an oxidative stress and membrane damage in the treated cells, and eventual cell death. The process usually involved injection of the photosensitizer into the bloodstream followed by a waiting period to allow the photosensitizer to accumulate in the malignant lesion followed by illumination of the tumor with red or near-IR that is able to penetrate the tissue. The selectivity of PDT is a consequence of a low-to-moderate degree of selective photosensitizer uptake caused by proliferating malignant cells and abnormal tumor vasculature combined with spatial confinement of the illumination. Tumor destruction is caused by a combination of direct tumor cell cytotoxicity, a dramatic antivascular effect that impairs blood supply to the irradiated area, and an activation of the systemic antitumor immune response [4–6] (Figure 48.1).

48.2
Photochemistry and Photophysics

The two most important processes that define PDT are the light absorption and energy transfer from the ground singlet state to the triplet excited state photosensitizer [7]. The Jablonski diagram (Figure 48.2) graphically illustrates the processes of light absorption and energy transfer that are at the heart of PDT. The ground singlet photosensitizer state (PS^0) has two electrons with opposite spins in the lowest energy molecular orbital. Following the absorption of photons, one of the electrons is boosted into a high-energy orbital, but keeps its spin to form the short-lived first excited singlet state ($^1PS^*$). The $^1PS^*$ can lose its energy by emitting fluorescent photons (light) or by internal conversion into heat. It may

Drug Delivery in Oncology: From Basic Research to Cancer Therapy, First Edition.
Edited by Felix Kratz, Peter Senter, and Henning Steinhagen.

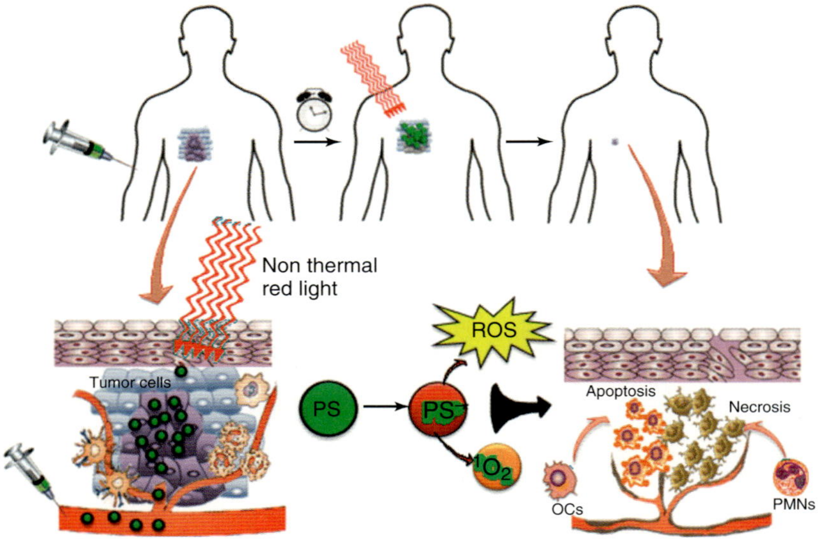

Figure 48.1 Schematic illustration of the mechanism of PDT. The photosensitizer is injected systemically and after sufficient time to allow its accumulation in the tumor light is delivered to produce ROS. The tumor cells are killed by a mixture of necrosis and apoptosis, the blood supply is damaged, and the host immune system is activated. PS, photosensitizer; DCs, dendritic cells; PMNs, polymorphoneutrophils.

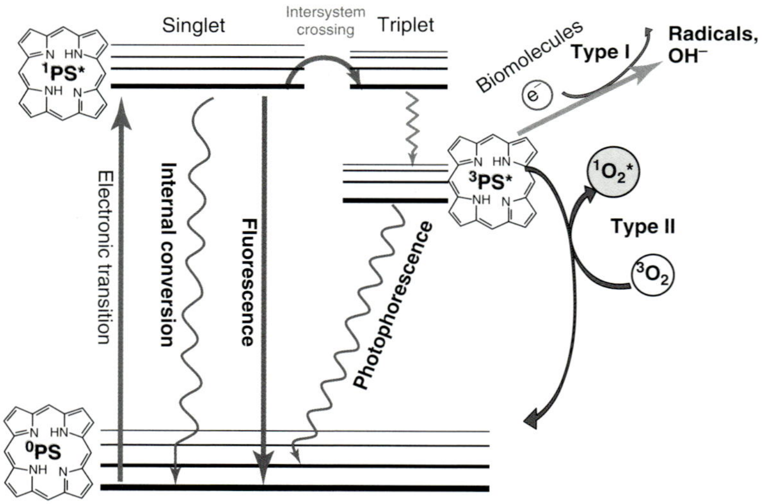

Figure 48.2 Jablonski diagram. The ground state photosensitizer absorbs a photon of the correct wavelength to excite its electron to the first excited singlet state that may (in addition to losing energy by heat or fluorescence emission) undergo intersystem crossing to the long-lived triplet state. This can undergo photochemistry by either electron transfer (Type I) or by energy transfer (Type II) to molecular oxygen to produce ROS.

also convert to a long-lived excited triplet state ($^3PS^*$) with the electron spins now being parallel via the process known as intersystem crossing. This excited triplet state is the photoactive state, which may generate ROS by undergoing two main reactions. (i) In the Type 1 reaction, $^3PS^*$ can react directly with a substrate (electron donor) to form the radical anion $PS^{\bullet-}$ that can further react with oxygen to produce superoxide radical anion $O_2^{\bullet-}$. The $O_2^{\bullet-}$ can further react to produce more ROS such as hydroxyl radicals. (ii) In the Type 2 reaction, $^3PS^*$ can transfer its energy directly to molecular oxygen (itself a triplet in the ground state) to form excited state singlet oxygen $^1O_2$. The ROS generated in the Type 1 pathway, together with singlet oxygen produced via the Type 2 pathway, are oxidizing agents that can directly react with many biological molecules [8]. However, due to the short lifetime of ROS, the initial extent of the damage is limited to the localization site of the photosensitizer, which may include the mitochondria, plasma membrane, Golgi apparatus, lysosomes, endosomes, and endoplasmic reticulum (ER) [9], as well as to amino acid residues in proteins [10] and DNA in nuclei [11].

48.3 Photosensitizers

The prerequisites for an ideal photosensitizer have been defined several times [12, 13], and they include high chemical purity, selectivity for cancer cells, chemical and physical stability, pharmacokinetics that allow the use of a short drug–light interval, increased accumulation within tumor tissues, activation at red/near-IR wavelengths with deep tissue penetration, and rapid clearance [14].

The majority of photosensitizers, used both clinically and experimentally, are derived from the tetrapyrrole aromatic nucleus found in many naturally occurring pigments such as heme chlorophyll and bacteriochlorophyll. Tetrapyrroles usually have a relatively large absorption band in the region of 400 nm, known as the Soret band, and a set of progressively smaller absorption bands as the spectrum moves into the red wavelengths, known as the Q-bands. Another set of classical chemical derivatives generally obtained from naturally occurring porphyrins and chlorins includes such structures like purpurins, pheophorbides, pyropheophorbides, pheophytins, and phorbins.

A second widely studied structural group of photosensitizers is the phthalocyanines and, to a lesser extent, their related cousins, the naphthalocyanines. However, the presence of four phenyl groups (or even worse four naphthyl groups) causes significant solubility and aggregation problems, and therefore phthalocyanines are frequently prepared with sulfonic acid groups to provide water solubility or with centrally coordinated metal atoms [15, 16].

Another broad class of potential photosensitizers includes completely synthetic, non-naturally occurring, conjugated pyrrolic ring systems. These comprise such structures such as texaphyrins [17], porphycenes [18], and sapphyrins [19].

The last class of compounds that have been studied as photosensitizers are non-tetrapyrrole-derived naturally occurring or synthetic dyes. Examples include hypericin (from the plant known as St. John's wort, *Hypericum perforatum*) [20], toluidine blue O [21], Rose Bengal [22], and functionalized fullerenes [23]. Quantitative structure–activity relationship experiments with several series of structurally related analogs [24, 25] revealed that photosensitizer structure, charge, and hydrophobicity may determine how the photosensitizer molecule interacts with its surroundings and provide additional information for future rational design [26].

Figure 48.3 shows the chemical structures of selected photosensitizers, particularly those that have been employed in the drug delivery strategies that are covered in this chapter.

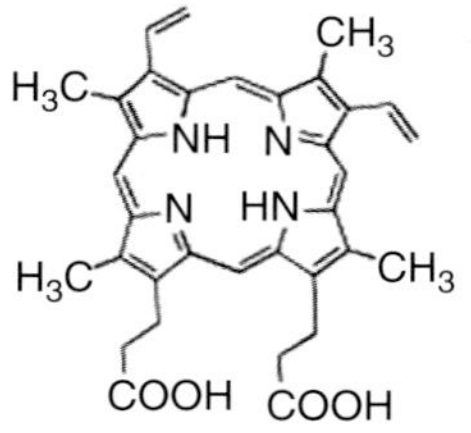

Protoporphyrin IX

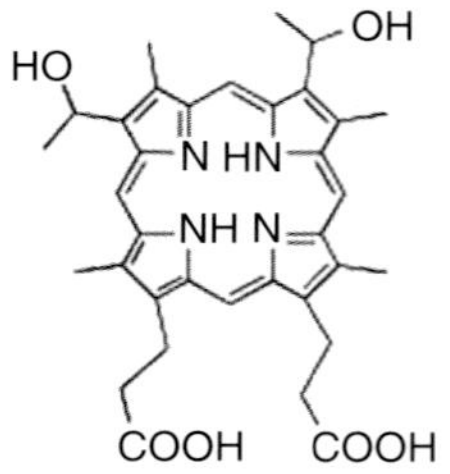

Hematoporphyrin

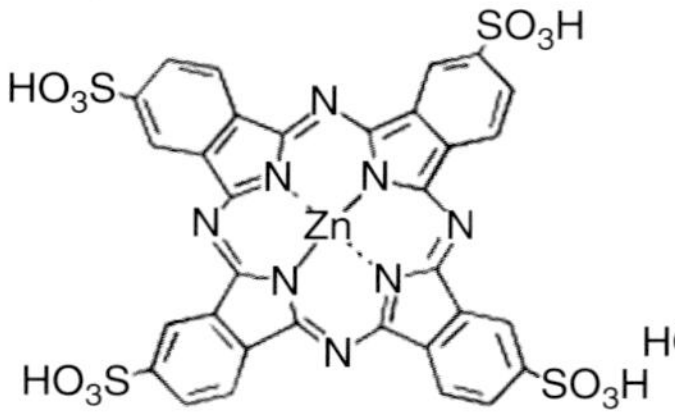

Zinc phthalocyanine tetrasulfonate

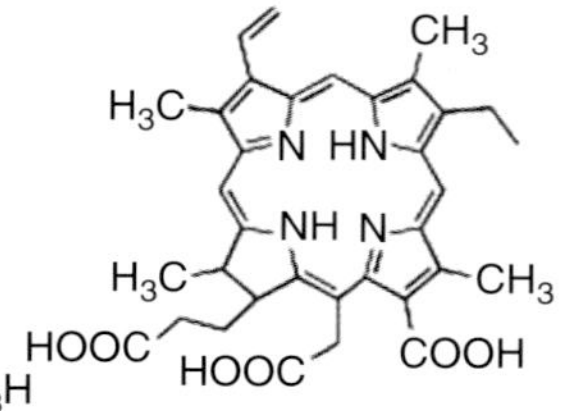

Chlorin(e6)

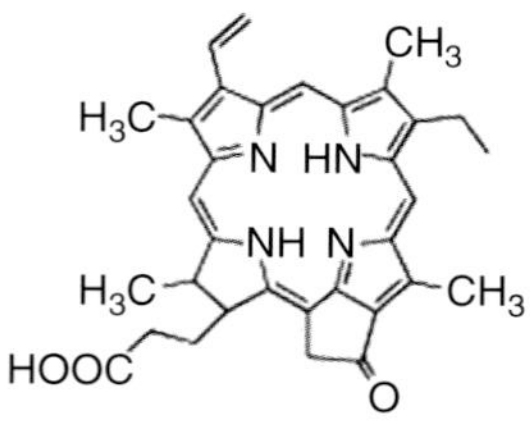

Pyropheophorbide-a

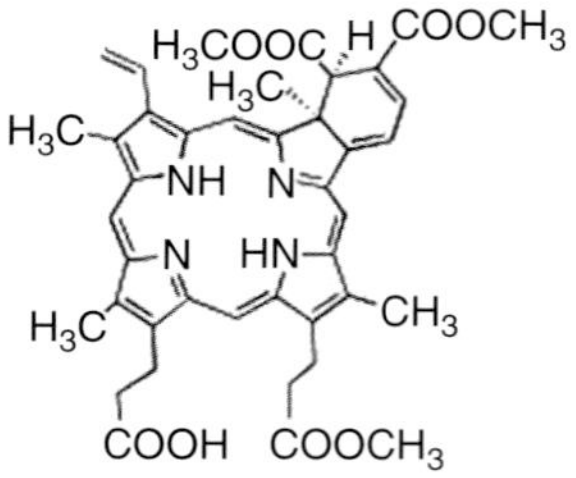

Benzoporphyrin derivative

Figure 48.3 Structures of photosensitizers that have been used in drug delivery strategies: protoporphyrin IX, hematoporphyrin, zinc phthalocyanine tetrasulfonate, chlorin e6, pyropheophorbide-a, and benzoporphyrin derivative mono acid ring A.

48.4
Subcellular Localization

Among the important factors determining the effectiveness of PDT is where the photosensitizer localizes within the tumor cells [27]. Particular photosensitizers have been reported to localize in intracellular organelles, such as the mitochondria, ER, Golgi apparatus, and lysosomes. Less commonly reported localizations are the plasma membrane and the nucleus. Subcellular localization may change with incubation time and the photosensitizer may relocate to other organelles after illumination has started. The particular cell death pathways that are activated after PDT have been reported to include apoptosis, necrosis, autophagy, and mitotic catastrophe ref. [28], and photosensitizer localization is perhaps the most important determinant of which of these mechanisms is predominant. It is generally considered that photosensitizer localization in the mitochondria or the ER is the most effective at inducing apoptosis and can therefore kill tumor cells at the lowest PDT dose (combination of photosensitizer concentration and light fluence).

48.5
Targeting in PDT

Due to the suboptimal nature of tumor targeting obtained by most commonly used free photosensitizers, and taking into consideration their generally hydrophobic nature and pronounced tendency to aggregate, considerable efforts have been made to improve photosensitizer performance by employing the strategies used in drug delivery and targeting. The most important targeting strategies will be covered in the rest of the chapter.

48.6
Preclinical Developments

48.6.1
Drug Delivery Vehicles: Liposomes Micelles and Nanoparticles

The spontaneous ability of block copolymer molecules to assemble in aqueous solution is widely utilized for delivery of antitumor drugs both in preclinical and clinical trials [29]. Often the polymeric molecule used is a diblock copolymer with one hydrophobic and one hydrophilic block (usually poly(ethylene glycol) (PEG)). This molecule forms a hydrophobic core–hydrophilic shell particle in aqueous solution, which is called a polymeric micelle (or simply, a micelle). The amphiphilic nature of the polymer micelle allows loading of the hydrophobic core with a hydrophobic anticancer drug. Additionally, the hydrophobic core facilitates disaggregation of the drug's molecular aggregates and the hydrophilic shell sterically protects the drug from interaction with unwanted particles. Often the hydrophobic drug molecules are noncovalently loaded into the micelle core and

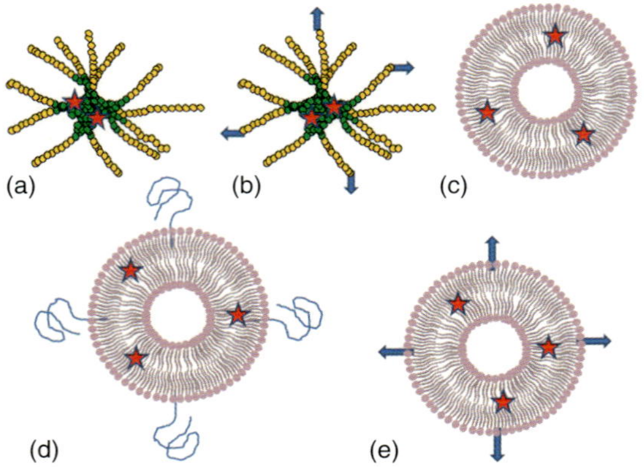

Figure 48.4 Nanoparticle delivery vehicles used in PDT: (a) polymer micelle, (b) polymer micelle with targeting ligands attached, (c) unilamellar liposome, (d) sterically stabilized liposome (PEGylated), and (e) liposome with targeting ligands attached.

the hydrophilic shell of the micelle is not designed to target cancer cells specifically (Figure 48.4a). The hydrophilic molecular "tails" of the shell can be tagged with a tumor-specific ligand (folate, peptide, antibody) to enhance selectivity of the vehicle (Figure 48.4b). The nature of the drug–micelle interaction is not always based on hydrophobic forces, but alternatively the ionic and covalent bonds can be used to load/attach the desired drug to the micelle. Two relevant reviews have covered various strategies to apply polymer micelles for drug and gene delivery [29], and for PDT treatment of eye neovascular disorders [30].

Some lipids under certain conditions are able to form unilamellar spherical lipid bilayers in aqueous solution, called liposomes (Figure 48.4c). The inner space of liposomes is filled with water or buffer. The potential ability of liposomes to assist in drug delivery and targeting depend on many factors: lipid composition of the liposome, liposome stabilization by polymers, bound or attached tags, structure and lipophilicity of drug, nature of target, and finally ionic strength, pH, and temperature. Here, we review various liposomes used as photosensitizer delivery vehicles to enhance PDT outcome: conventional (Figure 48.4c), cationic, sterically stabilized (Figure 48.4d), and actively targeted liposomes (Figure 48.4e).

Conventional liposomes consist of one lipid; in many cases dipalmitoylphosphatidylcholine (DPPC) is used due to its availability. Alternatively the liposome as a delivery vehicle may consist of mixture of two and more lipids, and sometimes cholesterol. By varying the lipid content one can modulate stability, microviscosity, overall charge, and pH- and thermosensitivity of the delivery vehicle. The correlation between lipid composition of a liposome and its pharmacological properties is not very well understood.

Cationic charge can determine two important features of the delivery vehicle. (i) Charge on liposomes prevents both liposome aggregation with serum proteins and detachment of hydrophobic photosensitizers from the liposome to serum proteins. (ii) The positive charge facilitates the accumulation in the anionic plasma membrane. The stabilization of liposomes is usually achieved by incorporation of PEG lipid molecules into liposomal membrane. The PEG hydrophilic chains buried at the outer lipid layer of the liposome interact with water, creating a water shell that prevents interaction of the membrane with serum proteins and helps the liposome to escape from the reticuloendothelial system [31]. Liposomes can be modified to target cancer cells actively owing to the fact that some types of cancer cells are known to overexpress certain receptors (e.g., folate receptors). By attaching folate molecules to the liposomes one can effectively target those cancer cells [32].

Nanoparticles aim to enhance both selectivity and activity of photosensitizer delivery. While these strategies are not able to offer Ehrlich's "magic bullet" they perform considerably better than free photosensitizer. A recent review published by Chatterjee *et al.* [33] suggested the following classification of nanoparticles for photoactive drugs employed by PDT: if the vehicle participates in photosensitizer excitation then it is termed "active," otherwise it is called "passive". Passive carriers include polymers [34, 35], lipid emulsions, gold [36], iron oxide [37], silica, and ormosil (amino-functionalized organically modified silica) nanoparticles; active carriers include quantum dots (QDs), and upconverting and self-illuminating nanoparticles [38].

The utilization of QDs in PDT has attracted attention since recent studies [39] showed that QDs possess both a decent ability to generate ROS and high photostability. The enhanced photostability has made QDs a very powerful imaging tool in biology. However, QD utilization in PDT is limited because direct photoactivation of QDs leads to a poor rate of ROS production. This limitation explains why most of the studies performed in recent years are devoted to QD–photosensitizer hybrids such as QD–phthalocyanines, QD–porphines, and others. The mechanism of ROS generation by these hybrids is known as Förster resonance energy transfer (FRET). There are two major types of such QD–photosensitizer hybrids. In the first type of QD–photosensitizer hybrid, called upconverting QDs, the near-IR electromagnetic radiation is absorbed by a QD in a process called two-photon excitation, and then the QD emits higher-energy photons that in turn are absorbed by photosensitizers [40]. In the second type of QD–photosensitizer hybrid, called X-ray-induced PDT nanoparticles, the QD absorbs X-ray radiation and in a process termed scintillation emits visible photons that can be absorbed by organic molecule photosensitizers [39]. It is important to mention that excitation of both types of hybrids described above does not actually require visible light, and that both near-IR, and X-ray radiation have considerably greater tissue penetration ability than visible light (Table 48.1).

48.6.2 Photosensitizer Targeting via Antibodies

Antibodies were one of the first targeting vehicles tested for photosensitizer delivery. The development of a number of monoclonal antibodies (mAbs) that

Table 48.1 Drug delivery vehicles for PDT.

Delivery vehicle	Target	Photosensitizer	References
Micelles from (PEG2000)–(PCL2600) polymer	human breast cancer MCF-7 cells	pheophorbide-a	[41]
(Me-PEG5000)–(PCL4100) micelles	murine RIF-1 cells	protoporphyrin IX	[42]
PEG–PCL copolymer	MCF-7c3 human breast cancer cells	silicon phthalocyanine	[43]
Poly(2-aminoethyl methacrylate)–PCL	HepG2 cells	aminoporphyrin	[44]
PEG–diacyl lipid micelles	HeLa cells	pyropheophorbide-a derivative	[45]
PEG–diacyl lipid micelles	melanoma-bearing C57BL/6 mice	5,10,15,20-tetraphenyl-21H, 23H-porphine	[46]
PEG-*b*-poly(L-lysine)	mouse neovascularization model	dendrimer porphyrin	[47]
DPPC liposomes	male C57/Black mice bearing a transplanted Lewis lung carcinoma	Zn(II)-2, 3-naphthalocyanines	[48]
DPPC liposomes	mice bearing Ehrlich carcinomas and B16 melanomas	Zn(II)-phthalocyanine	[49]
DPPC liposomes	MDCK cells and chorioallantoic membrane of chick embryo	tetrakis (methoxyethyl) porphycene	[50]
DPPC liposomes	human colon (colo-205) cells	purpurin-18	[51]
DPPC liposomes and cholesterol	MCF-7c3 human breast cancer cells implanted in BALB/c mice	Zn(II)-phthalocyanine	[52]
DMPC liposomes	MCF-7c3 human breast cancer cells and the LM2 adenocarcinoma	Zn(II)-phthalocyanine derivative	[53]
DPPC/DMPC liposomes	EMT6 xenografted nude mice	*m*-tetrahydroxyphenylchlorin	[54]
DPPC/DPPG/ cholesterol liposomes and acetylated PEI	human vascular endothelial ECV304 cell line	benzoporphyrin derivative	[55]
DMPC liposomes and cationic gemini surfactant	glioblastoma cell lines	*m*-tetrahydroxyphenylchlorin	[56]
PEG2000–DSPE liposomes	gastric cancer cell lines and tumor-bearing nude mice	chlorin e6 sodium salt	[57]

Table 48.1 (*continued*)

Delivery vehicle	Target	Photosensitizer	References
Monomethoxy-PEG−2, 3-dimyristoyl glycerol-stabilized liposomes	M5076 ovarian sarcoma	photofrin	[58]
PEG liposomes	Meth-A sarcoma bearing mice	benzoporphyrin derivative	[59]
Folate–diplasmenylcholine liposomes	human nasopharyngeal cancer KB cells	chloroaluminum phthalocyanine tetrasulfonate	[60]
APRPG pentapeptide-modified liposomes	Meth-A sarcoma-bearing mice	benzoporphyrin derivative	[61]
polylactic acid (PLA), PEG-coated PLA and Cremophor EL oil/water emulsion	EMT-6 mammary tumor in mice	hexadecafluoro Zn(II)-phthalocyanine	[62]
Gold nanoparticles	HeLa cells	Zn(II)-phthalocyanine	[63]
Iron oxide nucleus/chitosan	SW40 carcinoma both *in vitro* and *in vivo* (mice)	porphyrin derivative	[64]
ORMOSIL particles	colon 26 and RIF-1 cells, A375 and B16-F10 melanoma cells	iodobenzylpyropheophorbide	[65]
Polymer and silica-based particles	C6 glioma tumors in rat	methylene blue	[66]

PLA, polylactic acid; PEG, polyethylene glycol; ORMOSIL, organically modified silicate

recognized human tumor-associated antigens led to investigators covalently attaching photosensitizers to the IgG molecule in the expectation that the resulting photoimmunoconjugate (PIC) would preferentially deliver the photosensitizer to the tumor. The advantages claimed for this approach include those advantages specific to mAbs (high specificity and affinity for their target antigens) and those advantages specific for photosensitizers (generally nontoxic to normal tissues that do not receive light). A disadvantage of using other possible cytotoxic payloads such as toxins, cytotoxic drugs, and radioisotopes for conjugation to mAbs is that these payloads have nonspecific toxicity to organs such as the liver that tend to accumulate mAb conjugates. It was thought that internalization of the PIC into target tumor cells would not be necessary for the mAb–photosensitizer since the ROS generated upon illumination could diffuse into the cells from the membrane and produce fatal damage. However, it is now thought that PICs would kill cells more efficiently if they are internalized. Since it is necessary to have a relatively large number (at least 1 million) of photosensitizer molecules per single cancer cell to produce efficient light-mediated killing, the mAb–photosensitizer conjugates required high photosensitizer/mAb ratios, which made the synthesis

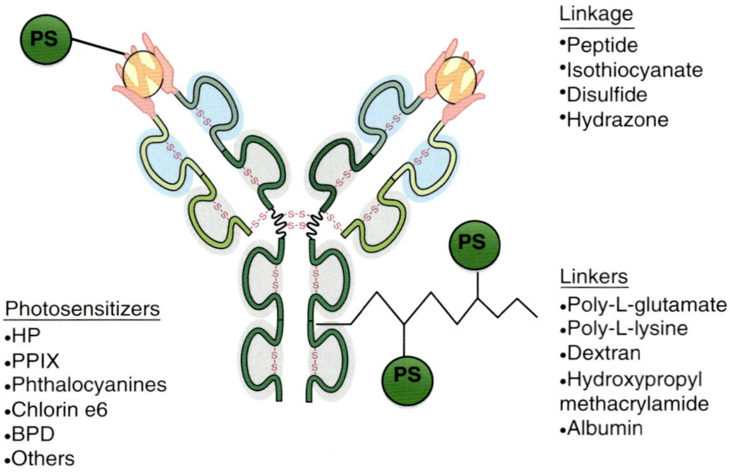

Figure 48.5 Strategies for conjugation of photosensitizers to mAbs. Photosensitizers can be directly attached to the antibody (usually via lysine amino groups) or indirectly attached by first conjugating them to a linker that is subsequently attached to the antibody via carbohydrate or disulfide linkages. PS, photosensitizer; HP, hematoporphyrin; PPIX, protoporphyrin IX; BPD, benzoporphyrin derivative.

and purification complicated. The goal of any such synthesis should be to retain features essential for both photosensitizer and antibody activities, and at the same time allow maximal photosensitizer incorporation.

The following two basic approaches have been used for the synthesis of PICs (Figure 48.5).

48.6.2.1 **Direct Photosensitizer–mAab Conjugates**

These have usually been prepared by reaction between primary amino groups present on the mAb and a reactive group (frequently an activated ester of a carboxyl group) on the photosensitizer (Table 48.2).

48.6.2.2 **Photosensitizer Linked to mAab via Polymers or Other Macromolecular Linkers**

In these conjugates photosensitizers are attached to a linker in the first step and the linker–photosensitizer conjugate is then attached to the antibody in a second step. This indirect linkage method has certain advantages over the direct linkage procedure. (i) The number of photosensitizers attached per single mAb can be much higher, thereby increasing the likelihood of a sufficiently large number of photosensitizer molecules being delivered to kill each cell with achievable light fluences. (ii) It is possible to prepare and characterize the linker–photosensitizer conjugate first before attaching to the antibody, thus increasing the chances of having a well-characterized final conjugate. (iii) The macromolecular linker is often a hydrophilic water-soluble polymer, and can play a role in improving water

Table 48.2 Direct photosensitizer–mAb conjugates.

mAb	Target	Photosensitizer	Linkage	References
Anti-M-1	DBA/2 myosarcoma M-1	hematoporphyrin	direct	[67]
B16G	suppressor T-cells	hematoporphyrin	direct	[2]
UCD/AB 6.01	52-kDa protein like keratin 8	hematoporphyrin derivative	direct	[68]
a-PNAr-I	gastric cancer cells	hematoporphyrin	direct	[69]
U36	CD44 variant, head and neck squamous cancer	*m*-tetrahydroxyphenylchlorin	direct	[70]
425	EGFR	TrisMPyP-PhiCO_2H	direct	[71]
E48	16- to 22-kDa glycosylphosphatidy-linositol-anchored surface antigen	AlPc$(SO_2Ngly)_4$	direct	[72]
C225	EGFR	chlorin e6	direct	[73]
C225	EGFR	benzoporphyrin derivative	direct/PEG	[74]
HER50, HER66	HER2/*neu* oncogene	pyropheophorbide-a	direct/PEG	[75]
C6.5 scFv	HER2/*neu* oncogene	benzoporphyrin derivative	direct	[76]
FSP 77 17.1A	internalizing antigens	tris-phenolic, tris-pyridinium porphyrins	direct	[77]
scFv	phage-display derived	porphyrins	direct	[78]

solubility and reducing the tendency to aggregate of the final mAb–photosensitizer conjugate. (iv) The attachment point to the mAb may not necessarily be the primary amino groups used in direct conjugation that are frequently located on the variable region that is involved in target-specific recognition. Attachment of linker–photosensitizer conjugates has been reported to the periodate-oxidized carbohydrate groups in the hinge region by hydrazide reaction [79] and to the sulfhydryl groups obtained by reduction of disulfide bonds in the middle of the molecule [80]. In principle, these attachment sites allow for minimal losses in the immunoreactivity of the mAb (Table 48.3).

48.6.3
Peptide or Growth Factor Conjugates

Peptides have been used as delivery vehicles to target specific receptors that in some conditions may be expressed or overexpressed on tumor cells. These peptides have been targeted to some of the receptors expressed on cancer cells, such as epidermal growth factor receptor (EGFR), neuropilin-1 (NRP-1), or the integrins (overexpressed on tumor microvascular endothelial cells). Some peptides have been used to direct the photosensitizer to specific cellular organelles, such as the

Table 48.3 Indirect photosensitizer-linker-mAb conjugates.

mAb	Target	Photosensitizer	Linkage	References
Anti-Leu-1	T-cells	chlorin e6	dextran linker	[81]
OC125	human ovarian cancer	chlorin e6-monoethylene-diamine monoamide	polyglutamic acid linker	[82]
5E8	human squamous lung cancer	cenzoporphyrin derivative	polyvinyl alcohol linker	[83]
2.1	human melanoma	Sn(IV) chlorin e6	hydrazide-linked dextran	[84]
OV-TL 16	human ovarian cancer	mesochlorin e6	*N*-(2-hydroxypropyl) methacrylamide linker	[85]
Rituximab	CD20	pyropheophorbide-a	fullerene-malonate linker	[86]
OC125F(ab′)$_2$	CA125 on human ovarian cancer	chlorin e6	poly(L-lysine) linker	[87]
17.1A	human colorectal cancer	chlorin e6	poly(L-lysine) linker	[88]
2C5	mouse cancer cells	meso-tetraphenyl-porphine	PEG/phosphatidy-lethanola-mine micelles	[89]

mitochondria or the nucleus. Another approach is to increase the cellular uptake of photosensitizers by conjugation to cell-penetrating peptides (CPPs). Overall efforts have been made to use much smaller peptides as targeting vehicles to overcome the difficulties found in delivering large molecules such as large proteins and antibodies through the blood vessels and allowing them to extravasate and penetrate the tumor.

There have been many reports regarding the use of these peptides as delivery vehicles in PDT that are summarized in Table 48.4.

48.6.4
Conjugates between Photosensitizer and Nonantibody Proteins

The lipophilic nature and relatively high hydrophobicity of photosensitizers are the reasons why photosensitizers interact with different types of serum proteins, including lipoproteins. In addition, hydrophobic interactions between combinations of the ionic pairs, hydrogen bonds and aromatic stacking interactions play an important role in the formation of photosensitizer–protein complexes.

Lipoproteins function as carriers of cholesterol and tri- and diacyl lipids. The most important type of lipoproteins is called low-density lipoprotein (LDL). The molecular weight of LDL is around 3×10^6 Da. LDL consists of a cholesterol ester core and

Table 48.4 Peptide and growth factor-photosensitizer conjugates.

Peptide	Target	Photosensitizer	Linkage	References
EGF	EGFRs highly overexpressed on some tumor cells such as squamous cell carcinoma human A431	Sn(IV) chlorin e6	dextran or polyvinylalcohol	[90]
EGF	EGFRs	Sn(IV) chlorin e6	serum albumin (human) or dextran	[91]
$\alpha_v\beta_3$ integrin-specific peptide RGD (H-Arg-Gly-Asp-OH)	$\alpha_v\beta_3$ integrins present on tumor microvascular endothelial cells	5-(4-carboxyphenyl)-10,15,20-triphenylchlorin or porphyrin	direct	[92]
Heptapeptide [H-Ala-Thr-Trp-Leu-Pro-Pro-Arg-OH (ATWLPPR)	NRP-1	5-(4-carboxyphenyl)-10,15,20-triphenylchlorin	spacer (6-aminohexanoic acid)	[93]
cRGDfK (Arg-Gly-Asp-Phe-Lys)	integrins (heterodimeric glycoproteins upregulated on the surface of proliferating endothelial cells)	protoporphyrin IX	direct	[94]
ATWLPPR	NRP-1 recombinant chimeric protein	5-(4-carboxyphenyl)-10,15,20-triphenylchlorin	spacer (6-aminohexanoic acid)	[95]
Peptide	NRP-1	chlorin-type photosensitizer	direct	[96]
Bombesin	gastrin-releasing peptide receptor	tetrasulfonated aluminum phthalocyanines ($AlPcS_4$)	C-14 spacer chain	[97]

(continued overleaf)

Table 48.4 (*continued*)

Peptide	Target	Photosensitizer	Linkage	References
Agonist, [D-Lys6]GnRH, or to a GnRH antagonist, [D-pGlu1, D-Phe2, D-Trp3, D-Lys6]GnRH	GnRH receptor	protoporphyrin IX	–	[98]
Bovine serum albumin and the 51-amino-acid peptide hormone, insulin	–	chlorin e6	–	[99–103]
CPP, NLS, or bifunctional CPP–NLS or NLS–CPP sequences	human prostate cancer cells	hematoporphyrin derivative (porfimer sodium) and *m*-tetrahydroxy-phenylchlorin	direct	[104]
CPP and NLS	human HEp2 cells	porphyrins	direct	[105]
Membrane-penetrating arginine oligopeptide (R7)	tumor cells	5-(4-carboxyphenyl)-10,15,20-triphenylchlorin	direct	[106]
Poly(L-lysine)	HeLa cells	chlorin e6	direct	[107]
Poly(*S*-lysine)	proliferating keratinocyte NCTC 2544 cells	tricationic porphyrins	direct	[108]
Three new amphiphilic guanidines, a biguanidine, or a MLS peptide	cell mitochondria	three new amphiphilic porphyrin derivatives	direct	[109]
Nucleus-directed linear peptide or a branched peptide (loligomer)	nucleus of CHO and RIF-1 cells	chlorin e6	–	[110]

GnRh, gonadotropin-releasing hormone; NLS, nuclear localization signal; mitochondrial localization sequence (MLS).

Table 48.5 Protein–photosensitizer conjugates.

Protein	Tumor model	Photosensitizer	Linkage	References
LDL	Greene amelanotic melanoma in rabbits	benzoporphyrin derivative	noncovalent complex	[112]
LDL	human skin fibroblasts and human retinoblastoma cells	chlorin e6	covalent	[113]
LDL	human fibrosarcoma cells	hematoporphyrin IX and Zn(II)-phthalocyanine	noncovalent complex	[114]
Human serum albumin	C3H mice with radiation-induced fibrosarcoma tumors	pyropheophorbide-a analogs and bacteriopurpurinimides	noncovalent complex	[115]
Bovine serum albumin	EMT-6 tumor in BALB/c mice and human colon T380 carcinoma in nude mice	Zn(II)-phthalocyanine	noncovalent complex	[116]
Transferrin-conjugated liposome	AY-27 rat bladder carcinoma cells and corresponding tumor in rats	tetrasulfonated aluminum phthalocyanine ($AlPcS_4$)	complex between photosensitizer and liposome, covalent between transferrin and liposome	[117]
Transferrin	human MCF-7 and rat MTLn3 mammary adenocarcinoma cells	chlorin e6	covalent	[118]
Transferrin	U7.6 murine hybridoma and Friend's leukemia cells	hematoporphyrin	covalent	[91]
EGF	MDA-MB-468 (human breast adenocarcinoma) and A431 (human skin carcinoma) cells	Sn(IV) chlorin e6 monoethylenediamine	covalent	[119]

cholesterol/phospholipid shell; the shell contains a large protein called apoprotein B-100 (512 kDa). Since lipids and cholesterol are the main components of the cell lipid membranes then one can predict that tumor proliferating cells consume higher amounts of LDL. Indeed, it was shown that some tumor cells express higher levels of LDL receptors than normal cells [111]. Furthermore incorporation of photosensitizers into LDL generally increases drug accumulation and photodynamic yield (see Table 48.5). It is important to mention that the photosensitizer–LDL interaction may perturb the apoprotein structure and therefore the apoprotein binding to the LDL receptor may be reduced or eliminated.

Another important protein component of serum is albumin. It is the most abundant protein and is able to bind to a number of compounds. This soluble protein is known to be an important carrier for some hormones, hemin, and fatty acids. Albumin is also responsible for maintaining optimal osmotic pressure. Finally, albumin is an important source of amino acids and as a result this protein has a higher turnover rate in some tumors. Additionally, it was demonstrated that albumin–photosensitizer conjugates are targets for scavenger receptors on tumor-associated macrophages [120]. Table 48.5 lists a few examples of albumin–photosensitizer complexes and conjugates.

Transferrin is an iron-chelating protein and a major source of iron. Again, dividing cells need a constant iron supply and some types of tumors overexpress transferrin receptors. It was reported [120] that transferrin–photosensitizer conjugates are accumulated in cells through receptor-mediated transport and that accumulation can be significantly increased by upregulation of transferrin receptors with desferrioxamine.

EGF is responsible for binding to a specific receptor (EGFR), and facilitates growth of epidermal and epithelial cells. EGFRs are overexpressed in many cancer types; it was estimated that around 30% of ovarian tumors overexpress EGFRs. EGF protein was coupled with different photosensitizers and, in general, the phototoxicity of conjugates was found to be 7–100 times greater than free photosensitizer phototoxicity.

Two relevant reviews [121, 122] are recommended for further familiarization with delivery strategies in PDT.

48.6.5
Polymer–Photosensitizer Conjugates

In recent years much progress has been made in the use of conjugates between cytotoxic drugs and polymeric carriers to increase the therapeutic ratio of tumor treatment (i.e., to increase tumor selectivity while simultaneously reducing toxicity to normal organs) [123]. The theory and application of the enhanced permeability and retention (EPR) effect has been reviewed [124]. The leaky blood vessels that are characteristic to the neovasculature found in tumors combined with an absence of lymphatic drainage, also characteristic of tumors, encourages a time-dependent accumulation of macromolecules that are at the same time small enough to leak out of the blood vessels, but are also big enough to not diffuse away. Similar arguments have been made in favor of the use of polymer–photosensitizer conjugates to increase the targeting ability of photosensitizers in PDT. Another highly important consideration that is peculiar to PDT drug delivery depends on the hydrophobic nature of most photosensitizer molecules, and their high tendency to aggregate in aqueous and biological environments. By covalently attaching the photosensitizer to water-soluble polymers with hydrophilic functional groups it may be possible to solve both problems (insolubility and aggregation) at the same time. Many of the synthetic schemes for preparing polymer–photosensitizer conjugates have arisen from work on conjugates between mAbs and photosensitizers (as described above). The preparation of conjugates between tetrapyrrole photosensitizer and polymers poses special challenges. The constructs may aggregate to a greater or lesser extent due to the amphiphilic nature of hydrophobic tetrapyrroles joined to hydrophilic polymer chains. Water-soluble photosensitizer–polymer conjugates must be relatively hydrophilic, but may bear net cationic, anionic, or neutral charges. Many reports are concerned with covalent attachment of PEG to photosensitizers to increase solubility and reduce aggregation. For conjugates based on poly(L-lysine) that are naturally positively charged, it was possible to make the overall conjugate neutral by acetylating all the free amino groups or alternatively by succinylating the amino groups it is possible to make the conjugate have an overall negative charge [125–128]. Figure 48.6 shows the structures of the polymers that have been used to prepare covalent photosensitizer conjugates. Table 48.6 lists published studies concerned with polymer–photosensitizer conjugates.

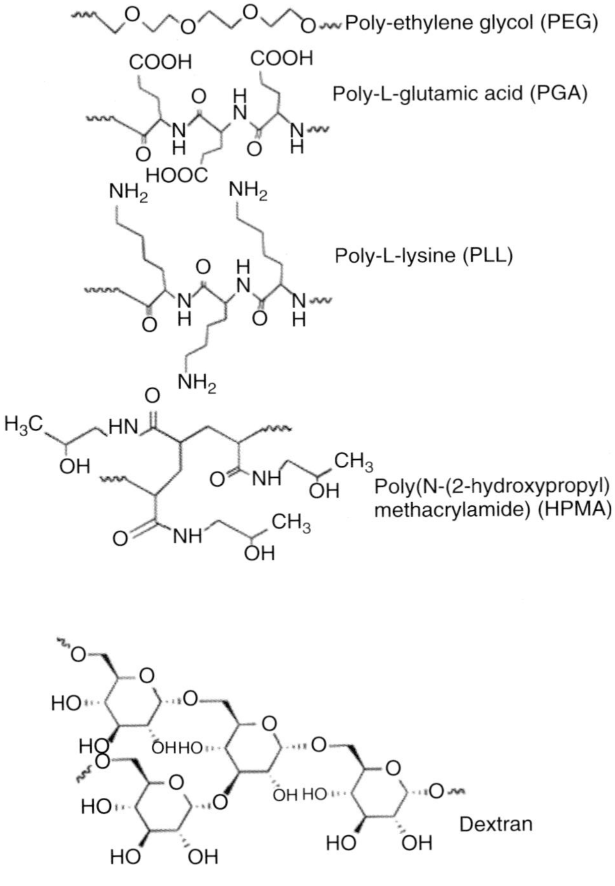

Figure 48.6 Structures of polymers used in photosensitizer–polymer conjugates. Structures of some of the polymers that have been attached to photosensitizers and either used as macromolecular photosensitizers or used to prepare indirect antibody conjugates.

Table 48.6 Conjugates between polymers and photosensitizer.

Polymer	Molecular weight (Da)	Photosensitizer	References
Polyvinyl alcohol	10000	benzoporphyrin derivative	[129]
N-(2-hydroxypropyl) methacrylamide copolymer	19000	chlorin e6	[130]
PEG	5000	*m*-tetrahydroxyphenylchlorin	[131]
PEG	500–750	metalated porphyrins	[132]
PEG	5000	Zn(II)-protoporphyrin	[133]
PEG	2000	chloroaluminum-phthalocyanine	[134]
Polyvinyl alcohol	18000		
Poly(L-lysine)	5000–55000	chlorin e6	[127]
PEG–poly(L-lysine) block copolymer	5000–40000	chlorin e6	[126]
PEG–poly(L-lysine) block copolymer	350000	chlorin e6	[135]

48.6.6
Enzyme-Cleavable Photosensitizer Conjugates

One of the proposed methods of photosensitizer targeting to tumor lesions that is characterized by increased specificity is the use of a photosensitizer conjugate that contains a covalently attached quencher and can target specific enzymes overexpressed in tumors (Figure 48.7). There are several factors that may influence the selection of photosensitizer for conjugation, including compatibility and yield, quencher compatibility, photosensitizer hydrophobicity, excitation profile, singlet oxygen quantum yield, fluorescence quantum yields, and photosensitizer dark toxicity. Additionally, the selection of photosensitizer is influenced by product

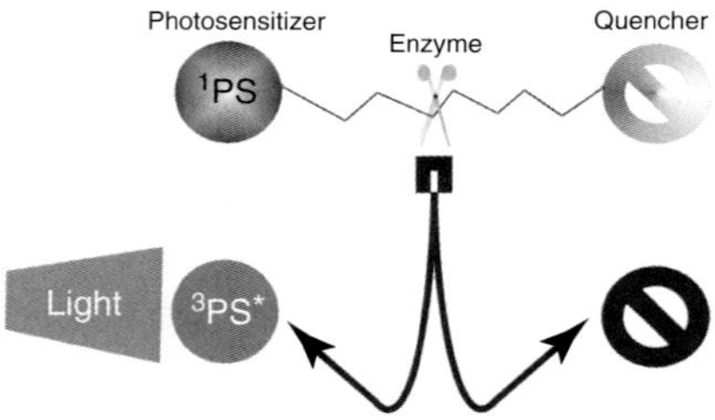

Figure 48.7 Enzyme-cleavable photosensitizer conjugates. The photosensitizer is attached to a quencher by a cleavable linker (often a specific peptide) that is recognized by a protease enzyme overexpressed in tumors. Upon cleavage the photosensitizer is released and becomes photoactive.

availability, cost, and required yield. Porphyrin-based photosensitizers have been often selected due to their strong singlet oxygen quantum yields and well-known chemistries [136]. The photosensitizer conjugate needs to remain photochemically inactive until the construct reaches its destination and photosensitizer is released by the targeted enzyme that cleaves the photosensitizer from the quencher. This assures the activation of the photosensitizer and subsequent PDT effect is limited to the treated lesion and that the surrounding tissues are spared.

There are many possible approaches to maintaining continued photosensitizer deactivation outside the targeted lesion. Contact quenching brings another molecule in close contact with the photosensitizer to alter the excitation properties of the photosensitizer. This interaction often results in a wavelength absorption shift [137]. Other methods include quenching through FRET, photoinduced electron transfer, self-quenching, dynamic quenching, and the heavy metal effect [138, 139].

There are several enzymes that may be specifically overexpressed in targeted tissue and this specific enzymatic activity became the basis behind the development of enzyme-activated photosensitizers. The advantages of this approach include photosensitizer activation confined to the location of the active enzyme and enzyme activation of numerous photosensitizer molecules, resulting in high signal amplification. Out of many candidate enzymes, the proteases have been reported as particularly good targets for this approach, mainly due to their well-characterized catalytic activity [140]. The main target for proteases is a peptide bond and photosensitizer conjugation has been dominated by standard *N*-hydroxysuccinimide active ester, resulting in stable amide couplings. However, other diverse conjugation strategies have been demonstrated, including thiol [141], isothiocyanate [142], and enyne metathesis [143] to conjugate photosensitizers.

To date, peptide-based photosensitizer conjugates have generally been based on either a polymer or short peptide sequence backbone. The polymeric polylysine backbone can contain hundreds of repeating lysine residues and holds potential to accommodate a high number of conjugated photosensitizers, while the interspersed PEG moieties can help to improve solubility. The short peptide linker-based photosensitizer conjugates comprise an amino acid sequence that binds a single photosensitizer and a quencher, and as a small molecule can enter target cells through the plasma membrane [144, 145].

The polymeric photosensitizer conjugate approach was tested by Campo *et al.* [146]. The polymeric photosensitizer prodrugs (PPPs) in which multiple photosensitizer units were covalently coupled to a polymeric backbone via protease-cleavable peptide linkers were tested *in vitro* using the T-24 bladder carcinoma cell line and *ex vivo* using mouse intestines. Both experiments illustrated the ability of these PPPs to fluoresce and induce phototoxicity upon enzymatic activation. Gabriel *et al.* further developed this approach [147]. Different pheophorbide-a peptide loading ratios and backbone net charges were evaluated with respect to their solubility, "self-quenching" capacity of fluorescence emission, and ROS generation. In addition, linker-sequence-impaired selectivity toward enzymatic cleavage was demonstrated. *In vitro* cell culture tests confirmed dose-dependent higher phototoxicity of enzymatically activated PPPs compared to the nonactivated conjugate after irradiation with white light. Another approach involved designing chlorin e6-containing macromolecules, which are sensitive to tumor-associated proteases [148]. The agents were nontoxic in their native state, but became fluorescent and produced singlet oxygen on protease conversion.

The short peptide technique was first reported in 2004 by Chen *et al.* [141] who constructed a caspase-3 cleavable construct consisting of GDEVDGSGK peptide, pyropheophorbide as the photosensitizer, and a carotenoid as the quencher moiety [149]. Another manifestation of this approach was the construction [144] of a matrix metalloproteinase (MMP)-7-triggered photodynamic molecular beacon (PMB) and achieving not only MMP-7-triggered production of singlet oxygen in solution, but also MMP-7-mediated photodynamic cytotoxicity in cancer cells. Preliminary *in vivo* studies also revealed the MMP-7-activated PDT efficacy of this PMB. Another recently developed approach explored the overexpression of β-lactamase in several drug-resistant bacteria. Specific photodynamic toxicity was detected toward β-lactamase-expressing methicillin-resistant *Staphylococcus aureus*. In this approach the usual mechanism for antibiotic resistance (cleavage of the β-lactam ring) was used to release the phototoxic component from the prodrug, leading to increased phototoxicity [150].

Provided that the photosensitizer conjugates are coupled with optimized delivery systems, they have been shown to (i) efficiently accumulate in tumors, (ii) be locally activated by targeted enzymes, (iii) locally accumulate in concentrations that could be measured by quantitative fluorescence assays, and (iv) effectively kill enzyme-positive cancer cells and tumors upon light illumination.

48.6.7
Small-Molecule–Photosensitizer Conjugates

Several small molecules, such as folic acid, steroid hormones, and sugars, have been conjugated with photosensitizers to increase tumor targeting of photosensitizers or to modify their tissue biodistribution. Cancer cells tend to overexpress estrogen or androgen receptors, therefore the covalent attachment of photosensitizers to steroid hormone receptor ligands can be used to target tumors such as breast, prostate, endometrial, and testicular cancer for PDT. This approach could potentially deliver drugs more selectively to specific target tissues, but they could also be used to target different subcellular locations inside a cell. Even though the targets of these conjugates are believed to be intracellular receptors, conjugates can still enter cells and elicit cellular responses.

Folic acid is important for cells and tissues that rapidly divide, and therefore rapidly dividing cancer cells tend to overexpress folate receptors to ensure that they obtain a sufficient supply. Folate is involved in the synthesis, repair, and functioning of DNA, and a deficiency of folate may result in damage to DNA that may lead to cancer. This overexpression combined with the high-affinity recognition displayed by the receptor–ligand binding has meant that folate receptors have become a popular tumor target by conjugating folic acid to anticancer molecules, including photosensitizers.

Table 48.7 Small molecule–photosensitizer conjugates.

Small molecule	Target	Photosensitizer	Linkage	References
β-Estradiol	MCF-7	tetraphenylporphyrin-C11	–	[151]
C17-α-alkynylestradiol	ER-positive MCF-7 and ER-negative HS578t human breast cancer cells	chlorin e6-dimethyl ester	–	[152]
Neurosteroid analogs	$GABA_A$ receptor	7-nitro-2,1,3-benzoxadiazol-4-yl amino or porphyrin	–	[153]
Folic acid	nasopharyngeal cell line expressing folate receptors	hexane-1,6-diamine	–	[154]
Folate	KB cancer cells (FR^+) compared to HT 1080 cancer cells (FR–)	pyropheophorbide-a	peptide sequence as a stable linker	[153]
Folate	nude mice	*m*-tetrahydroxyphenyl-chlorin	–	[155]
Mono- and diglucose	HT29 human adenocarcinoma cells	porphyrins chlorin	–	[156]
β-Galactose	–	purpurinimides	–	
Nonhydrolyzable saccharide	different malignant cell	porphyrin	–	[157]
Lactose	–	*N*-hexyl-mesopurpurinimide	–	[158]
Pullulan (water-soluble polysaccharide)	asialoglycoprotein receptors	fullerene (C_{60})	–	[159]

The rationale for conjugating sugar residues or saccharides to photosensitizers is to take advantage of the avid recognition and binding of various sugar residues by lectins. Lectins bind carbohydrate moieties either as free moieties in solution or as part of a protein/particle body. They agglutinate cells and/or precipitate glycoconjugates. Lectins have been reported to be overexpressed in many types of cancer cells, including liver, breast, prostate, lung, and bile duct cell types, and have therefore become a popular target for glycoconjugated anticancer molecules. Furthermore, sugars tend to be hydrophilic molecules with a high degree of water solubility, and can play a major role in solubilizing and disaggregating hydrophobic photosensitizer molecules (Table 48.7).

48.6.8 Photochemical Internalization

Photochemical internalization (PCI) is based on the photochemical damage of endocytic membranes and subsequent release of drugs trapped inside the vesicles.

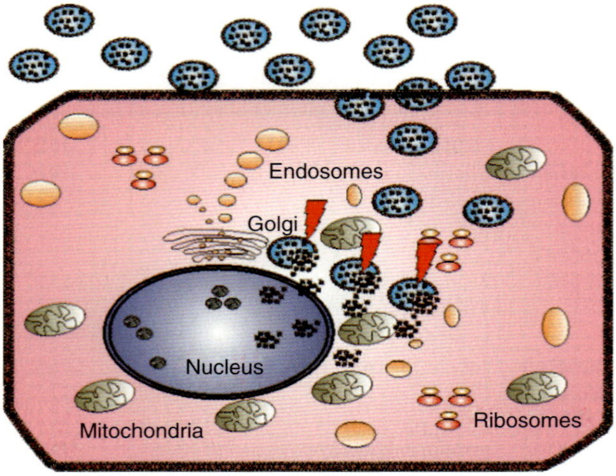

Figure 48.8 PCI. The photosensitizer is administered together with a cytotoxic macromolecule, which is difficult to get into cells. Both species are taken up into endosomes, where upon illumination the macromolecule is released to kill the cell.

It has been developed as an alternative technique to advance specificity and efficacy of delivering macromolecules and therapeutic agents to target tissue. PCI utilizes photosensitizing agents in the same manner as PDT, which upon exposure to light leads to the production of ROS, local cytotoxic effects, and shutdown of tumor vessels [160]. Additionally, during PCI the activation of the photosensitizer leads to destruction of the delivery vesicles, resulting in local release of carried agents. The advantages of PCI include improved selectivity of the therapeutic agents due to their local release in the light-illuminated regions and therefore reduced adverse effects (Figure 48.8) [161].

In order for PCI technology to induce increased translocation of therapeutic macromolecules to the cytosol the macromolecules need to be located in endocytic vesicles at some stage of the process. The two most popular photosensitizers used in the PCI approach are disulfonated meso-tetraphenylporphine ($TPPS_{2a}$) and disulfonated aluminum phthalocyanine ($AlPcS_{2a}$) due to the fact that the amphiphilic disulfonated compounds are mainly located in the vesicular membranes [162].

PCI effectiveness in therapeutic efficacy and specificity have been tested in several systems, including delivering protein toxins, DNA for gene therapy, oligonucleotides for post-transcriptional gene silencing, peptides and mRNA for cancer vaccination, and other molecules that do not readily penetrate through the cellular membranes [160, 163]. PCI has been shown to improve transgene delivery of plasmid/polyethylenimine (PEI) polyplexes *in vitro* [164], while *in vivo* it has been shown that $AlPcS_{2a}$-based PCI effectively delivered plasmids expressing p53 complexed to a glycosylated PEI, leading to a complete regression of squamous cell carcinomas deficient in active p53 [165].

PCI was also able to increase the number of adenoviral-transduced cells by up to 30-fold [166]. In another set of experiments Folini *et al.* [167] demonstrated PCI-mediated targeting of a naked peptide nucleic acid (PNA) to a catalytic component of human telomerase reverse transcriptase (hTERT-PNA). After photochemical treatment, cells treated with the hTERT-PNA showed a marked inhibition of telomerase activity and a reduced cell survival, which was not observed after treatment with hTERT-PNA alone. PCI also augmented the antisense effects (cytosolic/nuclear) of different PNA–peptide conjugates (Tat, Arg7, KLA) up to two orders of magnitude [168]. In addition, efficient gene silencing of the S100A4 gene by PNA delivered by PCI has also been demonstrated [169]. PCI has been used to aid the delivery of siRNA molecules complexed with lipofectamine from the endocytic vesicles [170] and combining anti-EGFR small interfering RNA (siRNA) treatment with PCI resulted in a 10-fold increased efficiency in knockdown of EGFR compared to siRNA treatment alone.

PCI has also been shown to increase the cytotoxic effect of the immunotoxin MOC31-gelonin that binds to the EGP-2 antigen that is found on most carcinomas [171], cetuximab-saporin [172], and the affinity toxin EGF-saporin [173].

The most remarkable application of PCI, however, is its ability to deliver and locally release chemotherapeutic agents inside the cancer cells. A study by Lou *et al.* [174] evaluated the effectiveness of PCI mediated by $TPPS_{2a}$ with doxorubicin in two breast cancer cell lines, MCF-7 and MCF-7/ADR (the latter being resistant to doxorubicin). They found out that for doxorubicin alone, the IC_{50} was 0.1 μM for MCF-7 and 1 μM for MCF-7/ADR. After PCI, the IC_{50} concentration decreased to 0.1 μM for both cell lines and doxorubicin released into the cytosol was able to enter cell nuclei. PCI was therefore able to reverse the doxorubicin phenotype of resistant breast cancer cells. Based on the current evidence is seems that the PCI may be a promising and novel treatment modality to locally deliver therapeutic agents, and selected examples may help to successfully overcome the resistance mechanism employed by tumor cells.

48.7
Clinical Developments

There have only been a limited number of reports concerning the clinical applications of PDT mediated by the various drug delivery techniques described in Section 48.6. Liposomes have been used to deliver photosensitizers clinically, including the successful Visudyne® (also known as verteporfin or liposomal benzoporphyrin derivative) that was used in many applications in ophthalmology [175]. Liposomal delivery of 5-aminolevulinic acid to the skin improved the effectiveness of PDT for acne [176] and for nonmelanoma skin cancer [177]. Zinc phthalocyanine formulated in liposomes prepared from phospholipids l-palmitoyl-2-oleoyl-*sn*-glycero-3-phosphocholine and 1,2-dioleoyl-*sn*-glycero-3-phospho-L-serine in a ratio of 9 : 1 was tested in phase I clinical trials for squamous cell carcinomas of the upper aerodigestive tract [178, 179].

The bacteriochlorin photosensitizer known as TOOKAD is in clinical trials for prostate cancer and is delivered in a micelle formulation formed from Cremophor EL® [180]. SnEt2 (purlytin) was also delivered in Cremophor micelles for mediating PDT of chest wall recurrence of breast cancer [181].

A group in Germany has described the clinical application of antibody targeted PDT [182]. Schmidt *et al.* demonstrated selectivity of a conjugate between phthalocyanine and antiovarian cancer mAb in photokilling of ovarian cancers cells *in vitro* [183]. Next they treated three women with advanced ovarian carcinoma (FIGO III) [184]. They showed some evidence of response after PDT by means of an ultramicroscopical analysis demonstrating a selective devitalization of tumor cells.

PCI has been recently tested in a phase I clinical trial for cancer. A study spearheaded by Dr. Colin Hopper at University College London Hospital is currently examining the safety of the PCI mediated by $TPCS_{2a}$ in combination with bleomycin in patients presenting with head and neck as well as skin neoplasms (*http://clinicaltrials.gov/ct2/show/NCT00993512*). The reported preliminary results show considerable promise.

48.8 Conclusions and Perspectives

The design and testing of new strategies to increase the selectivity and effectiveness of PDT has been a growth area in recent years, and continued progress is expected to be made in the foreseeable future. New drug delivery vehicles are a large part of the nanotechnology revolution, and nanoparticle formulations for photosensitizers are expected to play an increasing role in preclinical work and eventually in clinical applications. mAb therapy is becoming widespread in all of medicine and antibodies are expected to play a role in targeting photosensitizers to specific tumor antigens or receptors. Small peptides that have the same ability to recognize their receptors as large antibodies or proteins are also becoming more studied and will play a role in photosensitizer targeting. Enzyme-cleavable photosensitizer conjugates and PCI are drug delivery strategies that are unique to PDT.

Acknowledgments

Research in the Hamblin laboratory is supported by the National Institutes of Health, (grant **RO1AI050875**), US Air Force MFEL program (contract **FA9550-04-1-0079**), Center for Integration of Medicine and Innovative Technology (**DAMD17-02-2-0006**), and the Congressionally Directed Medical Research Program (**W81XWH-09-1-0514**). P.M. was partly supported by a Genzyme-Partners Translational Research Grant.

References

1. Henderson, B.W. and Dougherty, T.J. (1992) How does photodynamic therapy work? *Photochem. Photobiol.*, **55**, 145–157.
2. Steele, J.K., Liu, D., Stammers, A.T., Whitney, S., and Levy, J.G. (1988) Suppressor deletion therapy: selective elimination of T suppressor cells *in vivo* using a hematoporphyrin conjugated monoclonal antibody permits animals to reject syngeneic tumor cells. *Cancer Immunol. Immunother.*, **26**, 125–131.
3. Vrouenraets, M.B., Visser, G.W., Snow, G.B., and van Dongen, G.A. (2003) Basic principles, applications in oncology and improved selectivity of photodynamic therapy. *Anticancer Res.*, **23**, 505–522.
4. Dougherty, T.J., Gomer, C.J., Henderson, B.W., Jori, G., Kessel, D., Korbelik, M., Moan, J., and Peng, Q. (1998) Photodynamic therapy. *J. Natl. Cancer Inst.*, **90**, 889–905.
5. Engbreht, B.W., Menon, C., Kahur, A.V., Hahn, S.M., and Fraker, D.L. (1999) Photofrin-mediated photodynamic therapy induces vascular occlusion and apoptosis in a human sarcoma xenograft model. *Cancer Res.*, **59**, 4334–4342.
6. Castano, A.P., Mroz, P., and Hamblin, M.R. (2006) Photodynamic therapy and anti-tumour immunity. *Nat. Rev. Cancer*, **6**, 535–545.
7. Plaetzer, K., Krammer, B., Berlanda, J., Berr, F., and Kiesslich, T. (2009) Photophysics and photochemistry of photodynamic therapy: fundamental aspects. *Lasers Med. Sci.*, **24**, 259–268.
8. Hatz, S., Lambert, J.D., and Ogilby, P.R. (2007) Measuring the lifetime of singlet oxygen in a single cell: addressing the issue of cell viability. *Photochem. Photobiol. Sci.*, **6**, 1106–1116.
9. Buytaert, E., Dewaele, M., and Agostinis, P. (2007) Molecular effectors of multiple cell death pathways initiated by photodynamic therapy. *Biochim. Biophys. Acta*, **1776**, 86–107.
10. Grune, T., Klotz, L.O., Gieche, J., Rudeck, M., and Sies, H. (2001) Protein oxidation and proteolysis by the nonradical oxidants singlet oxygen or peroxynitrite. *Free Radic. Biol. Med.*, **30**, 1243–1253.
11. Ravanat, J.L. and Cadet, J. (1995) Reaction of singlet oxygen with 2′-deoxyguanosine and DNA. Isolation and characterization of the main oxidation products. *Chem. Res. Toxicol.*, **8**, 379–388.
12. O'Connor, A.E., Gallagher, W.M., and Byrne, A.T. (2009) Porphyrin and nonporphyrin photosensitizers in oncology: preclinical and clinical advances in photodynamic therapy. *Photochem. Photobiol.*, **85**, 1053–1074.
13. Dai, T., Huang, Y.Y., and Hamblin, M.R. (2009) Photodynamic therapy for localized infections – state of the art. *Photodiagn. Photodyn. Ther.*, **6**, 170–188.
14. Castano, A.P., Demidova, T.N., and Hamblin, M.R. (2004) Mechanisms in photodynamic therapy: part one – photosensitizers, photochemistry and cellular localization. *Photodiagn. Photodyn. Ther.*, **1**, 279–293.
15. Fingar, V.H., Wieman, T.J., Karavolos, P.S., Doak, K.W., Ouellet, R., and van Lier, J.E. (1993) The effects of photodynamic therapy using differently substituted zinc phthalocyanines on vessel constriction, vessel leakage and tumor response. *Photochem. Photobiol.*, **58**, 251–258.
16. Peng, Q., Moan, J., Nesland, J.M., and Rimington, C. (1990) Aluminum phthalocyanines with asymmetrical lower sulfonation and with symmetrical higher sulfonation: a comparison of localizing and photosensitizing mechanism in human tumor LOX xenografts. *Int. J. Cancer*, **46**, 719–726.
17. Detty, M.R., Gibson, S.L., and Wagner, S.J. (2004) Current clinical and preclinical photosensitizers for use in photodynamic therapy. *J. Med. Chem.*, **47**, 3897–3915.
18. Szeimies, R.M., Karrer, S., Abels, C., Steinbach, P., Fickweiler, S.,

Messmann, H. *et al.* (1996) 9-Acetoxy-2,7,12,17-tetrakis-(beta-methoxyethyl)-porphycene (ATMPn), a novel photosensitizer for photodynamic therapy: uptake kinetics and intracellular localization. *J. Photochem. Photobiol. B*, **34**, 67–72.

19. Kral, V., Davis, J., Andrievsky, A., Kralova, J., Synytsya, A., Pouckova, P. *et al.* (2002) Synthesis and biolocalization of water-soluble sapphyrins. *J. Med. Chem.*, **45**, 1073–1078.
20. Agostinis, P., Vantieghem, A., Merlevede, W., and de Witte, P.A. (2002) Hypericin in cancer treatment: more light on the way. *Int. J. Biochem. Cell Biol.*, **34**, 221–241.
21. Stockert, J.C., Juarranz, A., Villanueva, A., and Canete, M. (1996) Photodynamic damage to HeLa cell microtubules induced by thiazine dyes. *Cancer Chemother. Pharmacol.*, **39**, 167–169.
22. Bottiroli, G., Croce, A.C., Balzarini, P., Locatelli, D., Baglioni, P., Lo Nostro, P. *et al.* (1997) Enzyme-assisted cell photosensitization: a proposal for an efficient approach to tumor therapy and diagnosis. The rose bengal fluorogenic substrate. *Photochem. Photobiol.*, **66**, 374–383.
23. Mroz, P., Tegos, G.P., Gali, H., Wharton, T., Sarna, T., and Hamblin, M.R. (2007) Photodynamic therapy with fullerenes. *Photochem. Photobiol. Sci.*, **6**, 1139–1149.
24. Margaron, P., Gregoire, M.J., Scasnar, V., Ali, H., and van Lier, J.E. (1996) Structure–photodynamic activity relationships of a series of 4-substituted zinc phthalocyanines. *Photochem. Photobiol.*, **63**, 217–223.
25. Huang, Y.Y., Mroz, P., Zhiyentayev, T., Sharma, S.K., Balasubramanian, T., Ruzie, C. *et al.* (2010) *In vitro* photodynamic therapy and quantitative structure-activity relationship studies with stable synthetic near-infrared-absorbing bacteriochlorin photosensitizers. *J. Med. Chem.*, **53**, 4018–4027.
26. Vrouenraets, M.B., Visser, G.W., Snow, G.B., and van Dongen, G.A. (2003) Basic principles, applications in oncology and improved selectivity of photodynamic therapy. *Anticancer Res.*, **23**, 505–522.
27. Pazos, M.C. and Nader, H.B. (2007) Effect of photodynamic therapy on the extracellular matrix and associated components. *Braz. J. Med. Biol. Res.*, **40**, 1025–1035.
28. Mroz, P., Yaroskavsky, A., Kharkwal, G., and Hamblin, M.R. (2011) Cell death pathways in photodynamic therapy for cancer. *Cancers*, **3**, 2516–2539.
29. Nishiyama, N. and Kataoka, K. (2006) Current state, achievements, and future prospects of polymeric micelles as nanocarriers for drug and gene delivery. *Pharmacol. Ther.*, **112**, 630–648.
30. Christie, J.G. and Kompella, U.B. (2008) Ophthalmic light sensitive nanocarrier systems. *Drug Discov. Today*, **13**, 124–134.
31. Woodle, M.C. (1995) Sterically stabilized liposome therapeutics. *Adv. Drug Deliv. Rev.*, **16**, 249–265.
32. Oku, N. and Ishii, T. (2009) Antiangiogenic photodynamic therapy with targeted liposomes. *Methods Enzymol.*, **465**, 313–330.
33. Chatterjee, D.K., Fong, L.S., and Zhang, Y. (2008) Nanoparticles in photodynamic therapy: an emerging paradigm. *Adv. Drug Deliv. Rev.*, **60**, 1627–1637.
34. Konan, Y.N., Berton, M., Gurny, R., and Allemann, E. (2003) Enhanced photodynamic activity of meso-tetra(4-hydroxyphenyl)porphyrin by incorporation into sub-200 nm nanoparticles. *Eur. J. Pharm. Sci.*, **18**, 241–249.
35. Khdair, A., Gerard, B., Handa, H., Mao, G., Shekhar, M.P., and Panyam, J. (2008) Surfactant-polymer nanoparticles enhance the effectiveness of anticancer photodynamic therapy. *Mol. Pharm.*, **5**, 795–807.
36. Cheng, Y.A.C.S., Meyers, J.D., Panagopoulos, I., Fei, B., and Burda, C. (2008) Highly efficient drug delivery with gold nanoparticle vectors for *in vivo* photodynamic therapy of cancer. *J. Am. Chem. Soc.*, **130**, 10643–10647.
37. Reddy, G.R., Bhojani, M.S., McConville, P., Moody, J., Moffat, B.A.,

Hall, D.E. *et al.* (2006) Vascular targeted nanoparticles for imaging and treatment of brain tumors. *Clin. Cancer Res.*, **12**, 6677–6686.

38. Bechet, D., Couleaud, P., Frochot, C., Viriot, M.L., Guillemin, F., and Barberi-Heyob, M. (2008) Nanoparticles as vehicles for delivery of photodynamic therapy agents. *Trends Biotechnol.*, **26**, 612–621.
39. Juzenas, P., Chen, W., Sun, Y.P., Coelho, M.A., Generalov, R., Generalova, N. *et al.* (2008) Quantum dots and nanoparticles for photodynamic and radiation therapies of cancer. *Adv. Drug Deliv. Rev.*, **60**, 1600–1614.
40. Chatterjee, D.K. (2006) Upconveriting nanoparticles as nanotransducers for photodynamic therapy in cancer cells. *Nanomedicine*, **3**, 73–78.
41. Knop, K., Mingotaud, A.F., El-Akra, N., Violleau, F., and Souchard, J.P. (2009) Monomeric pheophorbide(a)-containing poly(ethyleneglycol-*b*-epsilon-caprolactone) micelles for photodynamic therapy. *Photochem. Photobiol. Sci.*, **8**, 396–404.
42. Li, B., Moriyama, E.H., Li, F., Jarvi, M.T., Allen, C., and Wilson, B.C. (2007) Diblock copolymer micelles deliver hydrophobic protoporphyrin IX for photodynamic therapy. *Photochem. Photobiol.*, **83**, 1505–1512.
43. Master, A.M., Rodriguez, M.E., Kenney, M.E., Oleinick, N.L., and Gupta, A.S. (2010) Delivery of the photosensitizer Pc 4 in PEG–PCL micelles for *in vitro* PDT studies. *J. Pharm. Sci.*, **99**, 2386–2398.
44. Wu, D.Q., Li, Z.Y., Li, C., Fan, J.J., Lu, B., Chang, C. *et al.* (2010) Porphyrin and galactosyl conjugated micelles for targeting photodynamic therapy. *Pharm. Res.*, **27**, 187–199.
45. Cinteza, L.O., Ohulchanskyy, T.Y., Sahoo, Y., Bergey, E.J., Pandey, R.K., and Prasad, P.N. (2006) Diacyllipid micelle-based nanocarrier for magnetically guided delivery of drugs in photodynamic therapy. *Mol. Pharm.*, **3**, 415–423.
46. Skidan, I., Dholakia, P., and Torchilin, V. (2008) Photodynamic therapy of experimental B-16 melanoma in mice with tumor-targeted 5,10,15,20-tetraphenylporphin-loaded PEG–PE micelles. *J. Drug Target.*, **16**, 486–493.
47. Sugisaki, K., Usui, T., Nishiyama, N., Jang, W.D., Yanagi, Y., Yamagami, S. *et al.* (2008) Photodynamic therapy for corneal neovascularization using polymeric micelles encapsulating dendrimer porphyrins. *Invest. Ophthalmol. Vis. Sci.*, **49**, 894–899.
48. Shopova, M., Wohrle, D., Stoichkova, N., Milev, A., Mantareva, V., Muller, S. *et al.* (1994) Hydrophobic Zn(II)-naphthalocyanines as photodynamic therapy agents for Lewis lung carcinoma. *J. Photochem. Photobiol. B*, **23**, 35–42.
49. Love, W.G., Duk, S., Biolo, R., Jori, G., and Taylor, P.W. (1996) Liposome-mediated delivery of photosensitizers: localization of zinc (II)-phthalocyanine within implanted tumors after intravenous administration. *Photochem. Photobiol.*, **63**, 656–661.
50. Toledano, H., Edrei, R., and Kimel, S. (1998) Photodynamic damage by liposome-bound porphycenes: comparison between *in vitro* and *in vivo* models. *J. Photochem. Photobiol. B*, **42**, 20–27.
51. Sharma, S., Dube, A., Bose, B., and Gupta, P.K. (2006) Pharmacokinetics and phototoxicity of purpurin-18 in human colon carcinoma cells using liposomes as delivery vehicles. *Cancer Chemother. Pharmacol.*, **57**, 500–506.
52. Oliveira, C.A., Machado, A.E., and Pessine, F.B. (2005) Preparation of 100 nm diameter unilamellar vesicles containing zinc phthalocyanine and cholesterol for use in photodynamic therapy. *Chem. Phys. Lipids*, **133**, 69–78.
53. Vittar, N.B., Prucca, C.G., Strassert, C., Awruch, J., and Rivarola, V.A. (2008) Cellular inactivation and antitumor efficacy of a new zinc phthalocyanine with potential use in photodynamic therapy. *Int. J. Biochem. Cell Biol.*, **40**, 2192–2205.

54. Lassalle, H.P., Dumas, D., Grafe, S., D'Hallewin, M.A., Guillemin, F., and Bezdetnaya, L. (2009) Correlation between *in vivo* pharmacokinetics, intratumoral distribution and photodynamic efficiency of liposomal mTHPC. *J. Control. Release*, **134**, 118–124.
55. Takeuchi, Y., Kurohane, K., Ichikawa, K., Yonezawa, S., Ori, H., Koishi, T. *et al.* (2003) Polycation liposome enhances the endocytic uptake of photosensitizer into cells in the presence of serum. *Bioconjug. Chem.*, **14**, 790–796.
56. Bombelli, C., Bordi, F., Ferro, S., Giansanti, L., Jori, G., Mancini, G. *et al.* (2008) New cationic liposomes as vehicles of *m*-tetrahydroxyphenylchlorin in photodynamic therapy of infectious diseases. *Mol. Pharm.*, **5**, 672–679.
57. Namiki, Y., Namiki, T., Date, M., Yanagihara, K., Yashiro, M., and Takahashi, H. (2004) Enhanced photodynamic antitumor effect on gastric cancer by a novel photosensitive stealth liposome. *Pharmacol. Res.*, **50**, 65–76.
58. Sadzuka, Y., Tokutomi, K., Iwasaki, F., Sugiyama, I., Hirano, T., Konno, H. *et al.* (2006) The phototoxicity of photofrin was enhanced by PEGylated liposome *in vitro*. *Cancer Lett.*, **241**, 42–48.
59. Ichikawa, K., Hikita, T., Maeda, N., Takeuchi, Y., Namba, Y., and Oku, N. (2004) PEGylation of liposome decreases the susceptibility of liposomal drug in cancer photodynamic therapy. *Biol. Pharm. Bull.*, **27**, 443–444.
60. Qualls, M.M. and Thompson, D.H. (2001) Chloroaluminum phthalocyanine tetrasulfonate delivered via acid-labile diplasmenylcholine–folate liposomes: intracellular localization and synergistic phototoxicity. *Int. J. Cancer*, **93**, 384–392.
61. Ichikawa, K., Hikita, T., Maeda, N., Yonezawa, S., Takeuchi, Y., Asai, T. *et al.* (2005) Antiangiogenic photodynamic therapy (PDT) by using long-circulating liposomes modified with peptide specific to angiogenic vessels. *Biochim. Biophys. Acta*, **1669**, 69–74.
62. Allemann, E., Brasseur, N., Benrezzak, O., Rousseau, J., Kudrevich, S.V., Boyle, R.W. *et al.* (1995) PEG-coated poly(lactic acid) nanoparticles for the delivery of hexadecafluoro zinc phthalocyanine to EMT-6 mouse mammary tumours. *J. Pharm. Pharmacol.*, **47**, 382–387.
63. Wieder, M.E., Hone, D.C., Cook, M.J., Handsley, M.M., Gavrilovic, J., and Russell, D.A. (2006) Intracellular photodynamic therapy with photosensitizer–nanoparticle conjugates: cancer therapy using a "Trojan horse". *Photochem. Photobiol. Sci.*, **5**, 727–734.
64. Sun, Y., Chen, Z.L., Yang, X.X., Huang, P., Zhou, X.P., and Du, X.X. (2009) Magnetic chitosan nanoparticles as a drug delivery system for targeting photodynamic therapy. *Nanotechnology*, **20**, 135102.
65. Ohulchanskyy, T.Y., Roy, I., Goswami, L.N., Chen, Y., Bergey, E.J., Pandey, R.K. *et al.* (2007) Organically modified silica nanoparticles with covalently incorporated photosensitizer for photodynamic therapy of cancer. *Nano Lett.*, **7**, 2835–2842.
66. Tang, W., Xu, H., Kopelman, R., and Philbert, M.A. (2005) Photodynamic characterization and *in vitro* application of methylene blue-containing nanoparticle platforms. *Photochem. Photobiol.*, **81**, 242–249.
67. Mew, D., Wat, C.K., Towers, G.H., and Levy, J.G. (1983) Photoimmunotherapy: treatment of animal tumors with tumor-specific monoclonal antibody–hematoporphyrin conjugates. *J. Immunol.*, **130**, 1473–1477.
68. Donald, P.J., Cardiff, R.D., He, D.E., and Kendall, K. (1991) Monoclonal antibody–porphyrin conjugate for head and neck cancer: the possible magic bullet. *Otolaryngol. Head Neck Surg.*, **105**, 781–787.
69. Berki, T. and Nemeth, P. (1992) Photo-immunotargeting with haematoporphyrin conjugates activated by a low-power He-Ne laser. *Cancer Immunol. Immunother.*, **35**, 69–74.
70. Vrouenraets, M.B., Visser, G.W., Stewart, F.A., Stigter, M.,

Oppelaar, H., Postmus, P.E. *et al.* (1999) Development of *meta*-tetrahydroxyphenylchlorin–monoclonal antibody conjugates for photoimmunotherapy. *Cancer Res.*, **59**, 1505–1513.

71. Vrouenraets, M.B., Visser, G.W., Loup, C., Meunier, B., Stigter, M., Oppelaar, H. *et al.* (2000) Targeting of a hydrophilic photosensitizer by use of internalizing monoclonal antibodies: a new possibility for use in photodynamic therapy. *Int. J. Cancer*, **88**, 108–114.
72. Vrouenraets, M.B., Visser, G.W., Stigter, M., Oppelaar, H., Snow, G.B., and van Dongen, G.A. (2001) Targeting of aluminum (III) phthalocyanine tetrasulfonate by use of internalizing monoclonal antibodies: improved efficacy in photodynamic therapy. *Cancer Res.*, **61**, 1970–1975.
73. Soukos, N.S., Hamblin, M.R., Keel, S., Fabian, R.L., Deutsch, T.F., and Hasan, T. (2001) Epidermal growth factor receptor-targeted immunophotodiagnosis and photoimmunotherapy of oral precancer *in vivo*. *Cancer Res.*, **61**, 4490–4496.
74. Savellano, M.D. and Hasan, T. (2003) Targeting cells that overexpress the epidermal growth factor receptor with polyethylene glycolated BPD verteporfin photosensitizer immunoconjugates. *Photochem. Photobiol.*, **77**, 431–439.
75. Savellano, M.D., Pogue, B.W., Hoopes, P.J., Vitetta, E.S., and Paulsen, K.D. (2005) Multiepitope HER2 targeting enhances photoimmunotherapy of HER2-overexpressing cancer cells with pyropheophorbide-a immunoconjugates. *Cancer Res.*, **65**, 6371–6379.
76. Kuimova, M.K., Bhatti, M., Deonarain, M., Yahioglu, G., Levitt, J.A., Stamati, I. *et al.* (2007) Fluorescence characterisation of multiply-loaded anti-HER2 single chain Fv–photosensitizer conjugates suitable for photodynamic therapy. *Photochem. Photobiol. Sci.*, **6**, 933–939.
77. Hudson, R., Carcenac, M., Smith, K., Madden, L., Clarke, O.J., Pelegrin, A. *et al.* (2005) The development and characterisation of porphyrin isothiocyanate–monoclonal antibody conjugates for photoimmunotherapy. *Br. J. Cancer*, **92**, 1442–1449.
78. Staneloudi, C., Smith, K.A., Hudson, R., Malatesti, N., Savoie, H., Boyle, R.W. *et al.* (2007) Development and characterization of novel photosensitizer: scFv conjugates for use in photodynamic therapy of cancer. *Immunology*, **120**, 512–517.
79. Goff, B.A., Bamberg, M., and Hasan, T. (1991) Photoimmunotherapy of human ovarian carcinoma cells *ex vivo*. *Cancer Res.*, **51**, 4762–4767.
80. Hamblin, M.R., Miller, J.L., and Hasan, T. (1996) Effect of charge on the interaction of site-specific photoimmunoconjugates with human ovarian cancer cells. *Cancer Res.*, **56**, 5205–5210.
81. Oseroff, A.R., Ohuoha, D., Hasan, T., Bommer, J.C., and Yarmush, M.L. (1986) Antibody-targeted photolysis: selective photodestruction of human T-cell leukemia cells using monoclonal antibody–chlorin e6 conjugates. *Proc. Natl. Acad. Sci. USA*, **83**, 8744–8748.
82. Hasan, T., Lin, C.W., and Lin, A. (1989) Laser-induced selective cytotoxicity using monoclonal antibody–chromophore conjugates. *Prog. Clin. Biol. Res.*, **288**, 471–477.
83. Jiang, F.N., Jiang, S., Liu, D., Richter, A., and Levy, J.G. (1990) Development of technology for linking photosensitizers to a model monoclonal antibody. *J. Immunol. Methods*, **134**, 139–149.
84. Rakestraw, S.L., Tompkins, R.G., and Yarmush, M.L. (1990) Preparation and characterization of immunoconjugates for antibody-targeted photolysis. *Bioconjug. Chem.*, **1**, 212–221.
85. Shiah, J.G., Sun, Y., Kopeckova, P., Peterson, C.M., Straight, R.C., and Kopecek, J. (2001) Combination chemotherapy and photodynamic therapy of targetable *N*-(2-hydroxypropyl)methacrylamide copolymer–doxorubicin/mesochlorin e(6)–OV-TL 16 antibody immunoconjugates. *J. Control. Release*, **74**, 249–253.
86. Rancan, F., Helmreich, M., Molich, A., Ermilov, E.A., Jux, N., Roder, B. *et al.*

(2007) Synthesis and *in vitro* testing of a pyropheophorbide-a–fullerene hexakis adduct immunoconjugate for photodynamic therapy. *Bioconjug. Chem.*, **18**, 1078–1086.

87. Hamblin, M.R. (2002) Covalent photosensitizer conjugates for targeted photodynamic therapy. *Trends Photochem. Photobiol.*, **9**, 1–24.

88. Del Governatore, M., Hamblin, M.R., Piccinini, E.E., Ugolini, G., and Hasan, T. (2000) Targeted photodestruction of human colon cancer cells using charged 17.1A chlorin e6 immunoconjugates. *Br. J. Cancer*, **82**, 56–64.

89. Roby, A., Erdogan, S., and Torchilin, V.P. (2006) Solubilization of poorly soluble PDT agent, meso-tetraphenylporphin, in plain or immunotargeted PEG–PE micelles results in dramatically improved cancer cell killing *in vitro*. *Eur. J. Pharm. Biopharm.*, **62**, 235–240.

90. Gijsens, A. and De Witte, P. (1998) Photocytotoxic action of EGF–PVA–Sn(IV)chlorin e6 and EGF–dextran–Sn(IV)chlorin e6 internalizable conjugates on A431 cells. *Int. J. Oncol.*, **13**, 1171–1177.

91. Gijsens, A., Missiaen, L., Merlevede, W., and de Witte, P. (2000) Epidermal growth factor-mediated targeting of chlorin e6 selectively potentiates its photodynamic activity. *Cancer Res.*, **60**, 2197–2202.

92. Frochot, C., Di Stasio, B., Vanderesse, R., Belgy, M.J., Dodeller, M., Guillemin, F. *et al.* (2007) Interest of RGD-containing linear or cyclic peptide targeted tetraphenylchlorin as novel photosensitizers for selective photodynamic activity. *Bioorg. Chem.*, **35**, 205–220.

93. Tirand, L., Thomas, N., Dodeller, M., Dumas, D., Frochot, C., Maunit, B. *et al.* (2007) Metabolic profile of a peptide-conjugated chlorin-type photosensitizer targeting neuropilin-1: an *in vivo* and *in vitro* study. *Drug Metab. Dispos.*, **35**, 806–813.

94. Conway, C.L., Walker, I., Bell, A., Roberts, D.J., Brown, S.B., and Vernon, D.I. (2008) *In vivo* and *in vitro* characterisation of a protoporphyrin IX–cyclic RGD peptide conjugate for use in photodynamic therapy. *Photochem. Photobiol. Sci.*, **7**, 290–298.

95. Tirand, L., Frochot, C., Vanderesse, R., Thomas, N., Trinquet, E., Pinel, S. *et al.* (2006) A peptide competing with VEGF165 binding on neuropilin-1 mediates targeting of a chlorin-type photosensitizer and potentiates its photodynamic activity in human endothelial cells. *J. Control. Release*, **111**, 153–164.

96. Thomas, N., Bechet, D., Becuwe, P., Tirand, L., Vanderesse, R., Frochot, C. *et al.* (2009) Peptide-conjugated chlorin-type photosensitizer binds neuropilin-1 *in vitro* and *in vivo*. *J. Photochem. Photobiol. B*, **96**, 101–108.

97. Dubuc, C., Langlois, R., Benard, F., Cauchon, N., Klarskov, K., Tone, P. *et al.* (2008) Targeting gastrin-releasing peptide receptors of prostate cancer cells for photodynamic therapy with a phthalocyanine–bombesin conjugate. *Bioorg. Med. Chem. Lett.*, **18**, 2424–2427.

98. Rahimipour, S., Ben-Aroya, N., Ziv, K., Chen, A., Fridkin, M., and Koch, Y. (2003) Receptor-mediated targeting of a photosensitizer by its conjugation to gonadotropin-releasing hormone analogues. *J. Med. Chem.*, **46**, 3965–3974.

99. Akhlynina, T.V., Jans, D.A., Rosenkranz, A.A., Statsyuk, N.V., Balashova, I.Y., Toth, G. *et al.* (1997) Nuclear targeting of chlorin e6 enhances its photosensitizing activity. *J. Biol. Chem.*, **272**, 20328–20331.

100. Akhlynina, T.V., Rosenkranz, A.A., Jans, D.A., Gulak, P.V., Serebryakova, N.V., and Sobolev, A.S. (1993) The use of internalizable derivatives of chlorin e6 for increasing its photosensitizing activity. *Photochem. Photobiol.*, **58**, 45–48.

101. Akhlynina, T.V., Rosenkranz, A.A., Jans, D.A., and Sobolev, A.S. (1995) Insulin-mediated intracellular targeting enhances the photodynamic activity of chlorin e6. *Cancer Res.*, **55**, 1014–1019.

102. Sobolev, A.S., Akhlynina, T.V., Yachmenev, S.V., Rosenkranz, A.A., and Severin, E.S. (1992) Internalizable insulin–BSA–chlorin E6 conjugate is a more effective photosensitizer than chlorin E6 alone. *Biochem. Int.*, **26**, 445–450.

103. Akhlynina, T.V., Jans, D.A., Statsyuk, N.V., Balashova, I.Y., Toth, G., Pavo, I. *et al.* (1999) Adenoviruses synergize with nuclear localization signals to enhance nuclear delivery and photodynamic action of internalizable conjugates containing chlorin e6. *Int. J. Cancer*, **81**, 734–740.

104. Sehgal, I., Sibrian-Vazquez, M., and Graca, H.V.M. (2008) Photoinduced cytotoxicity and biodistribution of prostate cancer cell-targeted porphyrins. *J. Med. Chem.*, **51**, 6014–6020.

105. Sibrian-Vazquez, M., Jensen, T.J., and Vicente, M.G. (2008) Synthesis, characterization, and metabolic stability of porphyrin–peptide conjugates bearing bifunctional signaling sequences. *J. Med. Chem.*, **51**, 2915–2923.

106. Choi, Y., McCarthy, J.R., Weissleder, R., and Tung, C.H. (2006) Conjugation of a photosensitizer to an oligoarginine-based cell-penetrating peptide increases the efficacy of photodynamic therapy. *ChemMedChem*, **1**, 458–463.

107. Ogura, S., Yazaki, K., Yamaguchi, K., Kamachi, T., and Okura, I. (2005) Localization of poly-L -lysine–photosensitizer conjugate in nucleus. *J. Control. Release*, **103**, 1–6.

108. Nuno Silva, J., Haigle, J., Tome, J.P., Neves, M.G., Tome, A.C., Maziere, J.C. *et al.* (2006) Enhancement of the photodynamic activity of tri-cationic porphyrins towards proliferating keratinocytes by conjugation to poly-*S*-lysine. *Photochem. Photobiol. Sci.*, **5**, 126–133.

109. Sibrian-Vazquez, M., Nesterova, I.V., Jensen, T.J., and Vicente, M.G. (2008) Mitochondria targeting by guanidine- and biguanidine-porphyrin photosensitizers. *Bioconjug. Chem.*, **19**, 705–713.

110. Bisland, S.K., Singh, D., and Gariepy, J. (1999) Potentiation of chlorin e6 photodynamic activity *in vitro* with peptide-based intracellular vehicles. *Bioconjug. Chem.*, **10**, 982–992.

111. Gueddari, N., Favre, G., Hachem, H., Marek, E., Le Gaillard, F., and Soula, G. (1993) Evidence for up-regulated low density lipoprotein receptor in human lung adenocarcinoma cell line A549. *Biochimie*, **75**, 811–819.

112. Schmidt-Erfurth, U., Flotte, T.J., Gragoudas, E.S., Schomacker, K., Birngruber, R., and Hasan, T. (1996) Benzoporphyrin-lipoprotein-mediated photodestruction of intraocular tumors. *Exp. Eye Res.*, **62**, 1–10.

113. Schmidt-Erfurth, U., Diddens, H., Birngruber, R., and Hasan, T. (1997) Photodynamic targeting of human retinoblastoma cells using covalent low-density lipoprotein conjugates. *Br. J. Cancer*, **75**, 54–61.

114. Polo, L., Valduga, G., Jori, G., and Reddi, E. (2002) Low-density lipoprotein receptors in the uptake of tumour photosensitizers by human and rat transformed fibroblasts. *Int. J. Biochem. Cell Biol.*, **34**, 10–23.

115. Chen, Y., Miclea, R., Srikrishnan, T., Balasubramanian, S., Dougherty, T.J., and Pandey, R.K. (2005) Investigation of human serum albumin (HSA) binding specificity of certain photosensitizers related to pyropheophorbide-a and bacteriopurpurinimide by circular dichroism spectroscopy and its correlation with *in vivo* photosensitizing efficacy. *Bioorg. Med. Chem. Lett.*, **15**, 3189–3192.

116. Larroque, C., Pelegrin, A., and Van Lier, J.E. (1996) Serum albumin as a vehicle for zinc phthalocyanine: photodynamic activities in solid tumour models. *Br. J. Cancer*, **74**, 1886–1890.

117. Derycke, A.S., Kamuhabwa, A., Gijsens, A., Roskams, T., De Vos, D., Kasran, A. *et al.* (2004) Transferrin-conjugated liposome targeting of photosensitizer AlPcS4 to rat bladder carcinoma cells. *J. Natl. Cancer Inst.*, **96**, 1620–1630.

118. Cavanaugh, P.G. (2002) Synthesis of chlorin e6–transferrin and demonstration of its light-dependent *in vitro* breast cancer cell killing ability. *Breast Cancer Res. Treat.*, **72**, 117–130.

119. Laptev, R., Nisnevitch, M., Siboni, G., Malik, Z., and Firer, M.A. (2006) Intracellular chemiluminescence activates targeted photodynamic destruction of leukaemic cells. *Br. J. Cancer*, **95**, 189–196.

120. Hamblin, M.R. and Newman, E.L. (1994) Photosensitizer targeting in photodynamic therapy. I. Conjugates of haematoporphyrin with albumin and transferrin. *J. Photochem. Photobiol. B*, **26**, 45–56.

121. Sharman, W.M., van Lier, J.E., and Allen, C.M. (2004) Targeted photodynamic therapy via receptor mediated delivery systems. *Adv. Drug Deliv. Rev.*, **56**, 53–76.

122. Konan, Y.N., Gurny, R., and Allemann, E. (2002) State of the art in the delivery of photosensitizers for photodynamic therapy. *J. Photochem. Photobiol. B*, **66**, 89–106.

123. Luo, Y. and Prestwich, G.D. (2002) Cancer-targeted polymeric drugs. *Curr. Cancer Drug Targets*, **2**, 209–226.

124. Maeda, H., Wu, J., Sawa, T., Matsumura, Y., and Hori, K. (2000) Tumor vascular permeability and the EPR effect in macromolecular therapeutics: a review. *J. Control. Release*, **65**, 271–284.

125. Hamblin, M.R., Miller, J.L., Rizvi, I., Loew, H.G., and Hasan, T. (2003) Pegylation of charged polymer–photosensitiser conjugates: effects on photodynamic efficacy. *Br. J. Cancer*, **89**, 937–943.

126. Hamblin, M.R., Miller, J.L., Rizvi, I., Ortel, B., Maytin, E.V., and Hasan, T. (2001) Pegylation of a chlorin$_{e6}$ polymer conjugate increases tumor targeting of photosensitizer. *Cancer Res.*, **61**, 7155–7162.

127. Hamblin, M.R., Rajadhyaksha, M., Momma, T., Soukos, N.S., and Hasan, T. (1999) *In vivo* fluorescence imaging of the transport of charged chlorin e6 conjugates in a rat orthotopic prostate tumour. *Br. J. Cancer*, **81**, 261–268.

128. Soukos, N.S., Hamblin, M.R., and Hasan, T. (1997) The effect of charge on cellular uptake and phototoxicity of polylysine chlorin$_{e6}$ conjugates. *Photochem. Photobiol.*, **65**, 723–729.

129. Davis, N., Liu, D., Jain, A.K., Jiang, S.Y., Jiang, F., Richter, A. *et al.* (1993) Modified polyvinyl alcohol-benzoporphyrin derivative conjugates as phototoxic agents. *Photochem. Photobiol.*, **57**, 641–647.

130. Peterson, C.M., Lu, J.M., Sun, Y., Peterson, C.A., Shiah, J.G., Straight, R.C. *et al.* (1996) Combination chemotherapy and photodynamic therapy with *N*-(2-hydroxypropyl) methacrylamide copolymer-bound anticancer drugs inhibit human ovarian carcinoma heterotransplanted in nude mice. *Cancer Res.*, **56**, 3980–3985.

131. Rovers, J.P., Saarnak, A.E., de Jode, M., Sterenborg, H.J., Terpstra, O.T., and Grahn, M.F. (2000) Biodistribution and bioactivity of tetra-pegylated *meta*-tetra(hydroxyphenyl)chlorin compared to native *meta*-tetra(hydroxyphenyl)chlorin in a rat liver tumor model. *Photochem. Photobiol.*, **71**, 211–217.

132. Mewis, R.E., Savoie, H., Archibald, S.J., and Boyle, R.W. (2009) Synthesis and phototoxicity of polyethylene glycol (PEG) substituted metal-free and metallo-porphyrins: effect of PEG chain length, coordinated metal, and axial ligand. *Photodiagn. Photodyn. Ther.*, **6**, 200–206.

133. Regehly, M., Greish, K., Rancan, F., Maeda, H., Bohm, F., and Roder, B. (2007) Water-soluble polymer conjugates of ZnPP for photodynamic tumor therapy. *Bioconjug. Chem.*, **18**, 494–499.

134. Brasseur, N., Ouellet, R., La Madeleine, C., and van Lier, J.E. (1999) Water-soluble aluminium phthalocyanine–polymer conjugates for PDT: photodynamic activities and pharmacokinetics in tumour-bearing mice. *Br. J. Cancer*, **80**, 1533–1541.

135. Choi, Y., Weissleder, R., and Tung, C.H. (2006) Selective antitumor effect of novel protease-mediated photodynamic agent. *Cancer Res.*, **66**, 7225–7229.

136. Kim, W.J., Kang, M.S., Kim, H.K., Kim, Y., Chang, T., Ohulchanskyy, T. *et al.* (2009) Water-soluble porphyrin–polyethylene glycol conjugates with enhanced cellular uptake for photodynamic therapy. *J. Nanosci. Nanotechnol.*, **9**, 7130–7135.

137. Marras, S.A., Kramer, F.R., and Tyagi, S. (2002) Efficiencies of fluorescence resonance energy transfer and contact-mediated quenching in oligonucleotide probes. *Nucleic Acids Res.*, **30**, e122.

138. Yogo, T., Urano, Y., Ishitsuka, Y., Maniwa, F., and Nagano, T. (2005) Highly efficient and photostable photosensitizer based on BODIPY chromophore. *J. Am. Chem. Soc.*, **127**, 12162–12163.

139. McCarthy, J.R. and Weissleder, R. (2007) Model systems for fluorescence and singlet oxygen quenching by metalloporphyrins. *ChemMedChem*, **2**, 360–365.

140. Turk, B. (2006) Targeting proteases: successes, failures and future prospects. *Nat. Rev. Drug Discov.*, **5**, 785–799.

141. Chen, J., Stefflova, K., Niedre, M.J., Wilson, B.C., Chance, B., Glickson, J.D. *et al.* (2004) Protease-triggered photosensitizing beacon based on singlet oxygen quenching and activation. *J. Am. Chem. Soc.*, **126**, 11450–11451.

142. Hammer, R.P., Owens, C.V., Hwang, S.H., Sayes, C.M., and Soper, S.A. (2002) Asymmetrical, water-soluble phthalocyanine dyes for covalent labeling of oligonucleotides. *Bioconjug. Chem.*, **13**, 1244–1252.

143. Zheng, G., Graham, A., Shibata, M., Missert, J.R., Oseroff, A.R., Dougherty, T.J. *et al.* (2001) Synthesis of beta-galactose-conjugated chlorins derived by enyne metathesis as galectin-specific photosensitizers for photodynamic therapy. *J. Org. Chem.*, **66**, 8709–8716.

144. Zheng, G., Chen, J., Stefflova, K., Jarvi, M., Li, H., and Wilson, B.C. (2007) Photodynamic molecular beacon as an activatable photosensitizer based on protease-controlled singlet oxygen quenching and activation. *Proc. Natl. Acad. Sci. USA*, **104**, 8989–8994.

145. Chen, J., Lovell, J.F., Lo, P.C., Stefflova, K., Niedre, M., Wilson, B.C. *et al.* (2008) A tumor mRNA-triggered photodynamic molecular beacon based on oligonucleotide hairpin control of singlet oxygen production. *Photochem. Photobiol. Sci.*, **7**, 775–781.

146. Campo, M.A., Gabriel, D., Kucera, P., Gurny, R., and Lange, N. (2007) Polymeric photosensitizer prodrugs for photodynamic therapy. *Photochem. Photobiol.*, **83**, 958–965.

147. Gabriel, D., Campo, M.A., Gurny, R., and Lange, N. (2007) Tailoring protease-sensitive photodynamic agents to specific disease-associated enzymes. *Bioconjug. Chem.*, **18** (4), 1070–1077.

148. Choi, Y., Weissleder, R., and Tung, C.H. (2006) Protease-mediated phototoxicity of a polylysine-chlorin$_{E6}$ conjugate. *ChemMedChem*, **1**, 698–701.

149. Stefflova, K., Chen, J., Marotta, D., Li, H., and Zheng, G. (2006) Photodynamic therapy agent with a built-in apoptosis sensor for evaluating its own therapeutic outcome *in situ*. *J. Med. Chem.*, **49**, 3850–3856.

150. Zheng, X., Sallum, U.W., Verma, S., Athar, H., Evans, C.L., and Hasan, T. (2009) Exploiting a bacterial drug-resistance mechanism: a light-activated construct for the destruction of MRSA. *Angew. Chem. Int. Ed.*, **48**, 2148–2151.

151. James, D.A., Swamy, N., Paz, N., Hanson, R.N., and Ray, R. (1999) Synthesis and estrogen receptor binding affinity of a porphyrin–estradiol conjugate for targeted photodynamic therapy of cancer. *Bioorg. Med. Chem. Lett.*, **9**, 2379–2384.

152. Swamy, N., James, D.A., Mohr, S.C., Hanson, R.N., and Ray, R. (2002) An estradiol–porphyrin conjugate selectively localizes into estrogen receptor-positive breast cancer cells. *Bioorg. Med. Chem.*, **10**, 3237–3243.

153. Shu, H.J., Eisenman, L.N., Wang, C., Bandyopadhyaya, A.K., Krishnan, K., Taylor, A. *et al.* (2009) Photodynamic effects of steroid-conjugated fluorophores on GABAA receptors. *Mol. Pharmacol.*, **76**, 754–765.

154. El-Akra, N., Noirot, A., Faye, J.C., and Souchard, J.P. (2006) Synthesis of estradiol–pheophorbide a conjugates:

evidence of nuclear targeting, DNA damage and improved photodynamic activity in human breast cancer and vascular endothelial cells. *Photochem. Photobiol. Sci.*, **5**, 996–999.

155. Schneider, R., Schmitt, F., Frochot, C., Fort, Y., Lourette, N., Guillemin, F. *et al.* (2005) Design, synthesis, and biological evaluation of folic acid targeted tetraphenylporphyrin as novel photosensitizers for selective photodynamic therapy. *Bioorg. Med. Chem.*, **13**, 2799–2808.

156. Di Stasio, B., Frochot, C., Dumas, D., Even, P., Zwier, J., Muller, A. *et al.* (2005) The 2-aminoglucosamide motif improves cellular uptake and photodynamic activity of tetraphenylporphyrin. *Eur. J. Med. Chem.*, **40**, 1111–1122.

157. Chen, X., Hui, L., Foster, D.A., and Drain, C.M. (2004) Efficient synthesis and photodynamic activity of porphyrin–saccharide conjugates: targeting and incapacitating cancer cells. *Biochemistry*, **43**, 10918–10929.

158. Pandey, S.K., Zheng, X., Morgan, J., Missert, J.R., Liu, T.H., Shibata, M. *et al.* (2007) Purpurinimide carbohydrate conjugates: effect of the position of the carbohydrate moiety in photosensitizing efficacy. *Mol. Pharm.*, **4**, 448–464.

159. Liu, J. and Tabata, Y. (2010) Photodynamic therapy of fullerene modified with pullulan on hepatoma cells. *J. Drug Target.*, **18**, 602–610.

160. Norum, O.J., Selbo, P.K., Weyergang, A., Giercksky, K.E., and Berg, K. (2009) Photochemical internalization (PCI) in cancer therapy: from bench towards bedside medicine. *J. Photochem. Photobiol. B*, **96**, 83–92.

161. Shum, P., Kim, J.M., and Thompson, D.H. (2001) Phototriggering of liposomal drug delivery systems. *Adv. Drug Deliv. Rev.*, **53**, 273–284.

162. Prasmickaite, L., Hogset, A., and Berg, K. (2001) Evaluation of different photosensitizers for use in photochemical gene transfection. *Photochem. Photobiol.*, **73**, 388–395.

163. Berg, K., Selbo, P.K., Prasmickaite, L., and Hogset, A. (2004) Photochemical drug and gene delivery. *Curr. Opin. Mol. Ther.*, **6**, 279–287.

164. Prasmickaite, L., Hogset, A., Engesaeter, B.B., Bonsted, A., and Berg, K. (2004) Light-directed gene delivery by photochemical internalisation. *Expert Opin. Biol. Ther.*, **4**, 1403–1412.

165. Ndoye, A., Merlin, J.L., Leroux, A., Dolivet, G., Erbacher, P., Behr, J.P. *et al.* (2004) Enhanced gene transfer and cell death following p53 gene transfer using photochemical internalisation of glucosylated PEI–DNA complexes. *J. Gene Med.*, **6**, 884–894.

166. Engesaeter, B.O., Bonsted, A., Berg, K., Hogset, A., Engebraten, O., Fodstad, O. *et al.* (2005) PCI-enhanced adenoviral transduction employs the known uptake mechanism of adenoviral particles. *Cancer Gene Ther.*, **12**, 439–448.

167. Folini, M., Berg, K., Millo, E., Villa, R., Prasmickaite, L., Daidone, M.G. *et al.* (2003) Photochemical internalization of a peptide nucleic acid targeting the catalytic subunit of human telomerase. *Cancer Res.*, **63**, 3490–3494.

168. Shiraishi, T. and Nielsen, P.E. (2006) Photochemically enhanced cellular delivery of cell penetrating peptide–PNA conjugates. *FEBS Lett.*, **580**, 1451–1456.

169. Boe, S. and Hovig, E. (2006) Photochemically induced gene silencing using PNA–peptide conjugates. *Oligonucleotides*, **16**, 145–157.

170. Oliveira, S., Fretz, M.M., Hogset, A., Storm, G., and Schiffelers, R.M. (2007) Photochemical internalization enhances silencing of epidermal growth factor receptor through improved endosomal escape of siRNA. *Biochim. Biophys. Acta*, **1768**, 1211–1217.

171. Selbo, P.K., Sivam, G., Fodstad, O., Sandvig, K., and Berg, K. (2000) Photochemical internalisation increases the cytotoxic effect of the immunotoxin MOC31-gelonin. *Int. J. Cancer*, **87**, 853–859.

172. Yip, W.L., Weyergang, A., Berg, K., Tonnesen, H.H., and Selbo, P.K. (2007) Targeted delivery and enhanced cytotoxicity of cetuximab-saporin by photochemical internalization

in EGFR-positive cancer cells. *Mol. Pharm.*, **4**, 241–251.

173. Weyergang, A., Selbo, P.K., and Berg, K. (2006) Photochemically stimulated drug delivery increases the cytotoxicity and specificity of EGF-saporin. *J. Control. Release*, **111**, 165–173.
174. Lou, P.J., Lai, P.S., Shieh, M.J., Macrobert, A.J., Berg, K., and Bown, S.G. (2006) Reversal of doxorubicin resistance in breast cancer cells by photochemical internalization. *Int. J. Cancer*, **119**, 2692–2698.
175. Keam, S.J., Scott, L.J., and Curran, M.P. (2004) Spotlight on verteporfin in subfoveal choroidal neovascularisation. *Drugs Aging*, **21**, 203–209.
176. de Leeuw, J., van der Beek, N., Bjerring, P., and Martino Neumann, H.A. (2010) Photodynamic therapy of acne vulgaris using 5-aminolevulinic acid 0.5% liposomal spray and intense pulsed light in combination with topical keratolytic agents. *J. Eur. Acad. Dermatol. Venereol.*, **24**, 460–469.
177. de Leeuw, J., de Vijlder, H.C., Bjerring, P., and Neumann, H.A. (2009) Liposomes in dermatology today. *J. Eur. Acad. Dermatol. Venereol.*, **23**, 505–516.
178. Ochsner, M. (1996) Light scattering of human skin: a comparison between zinc (II)-phthalocyanine and photofrin II. *J. Photochem. Photobiol. B*, **32**, 3–9.
179. Isele, U., van Hoogevest, P., Leuenberger, H., Capraro, H.-G., and Schieweck, K. (1994) Development of CGP 55847, a liposomal Zn-phthalocyanine formulation using a controlled organic solvent dilution method. *Proc SPIE.*, **2078**, 397–403.
180. Trachtenberg, J., Weersink, R.A., Davidson, S.R., Haider, M.A., Bogaards, A., Gertner, M.R. *et al.* (2008) Vascular-targeted photodynamic therapy (padoporfin, WST09) for recurrent prostate cancer after failure of external beam radiotherapy: a study of escalating light doses. *BJU Int.*, **102**, 556–562.
181. Kaplan, M.J., Somers, R.G., Greenberg, R.H., and Ackler, J. (1998) Photodynamic therapy in the management of metastatic cutaneous adenocarcinomas: case reports from phase 1/2 studies using tin ethyl etiopurpurin (SnET2). *J. Surg. Oncol.*, **67**, 121–125.
182. Schmidt, S. (1993) Antibody-targeted photodynamic therapy. *Hybridoma*, **12**, 539–541.
183. Schmidt, S., Wagner, U., Schultes, B., Oehr, P., Decleer, W., Ertmer, W. *et al.* (1992) Photodynamic laser therapy with antibody-bound dyes. A new procedure in therapy of gynecologic malignancies. *Fortschr. Med.*, **110**, 298–301.
184. Schmidt, S., Wagner, U., Oehr, P., and Krebs, D. (1992) Clinical use of photodynamic therapy in gynecologic tumor patients – antibody-targeted photodynamic laser therapy as a new oncologic treatment procedure. *Zentralbl. Gynakol.*, **114**, 307–311.

49 Tumor-Targeting Strategies with Anticancer Platinum Complexes

Markus Galanski and Bernhard K. Keppler

49.1 Introduction

The story of metal-based anticancer chemotherapy began in 1965, when Barnett Rosenberg accidentally discovered the cytotoxic properties of platinum complexes (Figure 49.1) [1–3]. In 1969, the first *in vivo* results in leukemia L1210- and sarcoma 180-bearing mice where published in *Nature* [4]. Out of four evaluated compounds, *cis*-diamminedichloroplatinum(II), today known as cisplatin, emerged to the most promising candidate. In 1971, cisplatin was investigated in cancer patients and finally received approval in 1978. Today, cisplatin, one of the few anticancer agents with real curative potential, is indispensable in the clinical routine. Cisplatin is used in testicular, ovarian, bladder, lung, head and neck, esophageal, cervical, and uterine cancer; it is also a second-line chemotherapeutic agent in most other advanced solid tumors. However, cisplatin therapy is accompanied by a set of severe side-effects, such as nephrotoxicity, nausea and vomiting, neurotoxicity, and ototoxicity. Additionally, some malignant tumors are inherently resistant to cisplatin chemotherapy or develop resistance after the first cycles of treatment.

Consequently, thousands of novel platinum complexes were synthesized in order to reduce the systemic toxicities and/or to broaden the spectrum of activity [5], resulting in the second-generation platinum drug, carboplatin (*cis*-diammine(1,1-cyclobutanedicarboxylato)platinum(II)), which was approved in 1989 (Figure 49.1). Carboplatin's chemical structure is similar to that of cisplatin and therefore it has not enlarged the spectrum of activity, especially not in cisplatin-resistant cancers. However, it is equipped with a lower general toxicity compared to cisplatin, being a reasonable and safer alternative. Carboplatin administration is not associated with a severe nephrotoxicity, it is less toxic to the nervous system, and causes nausea and vomiting; ototoxicity is milder [6].

Finally, in 2002, oxaliplatin ((1*R*,2*R*-cyclohexanediamine)oxalatoplatinum(II)), the third-generation platinum complex, was approved (Figure 49.1) [7]. Oxaliplatin was approved in 2004 for the first-line treatment of colorectal carcinoma in combination with 5-fluorouracil (5-FU) and leucovorin. It was among the first platinum-based agents showing no cross-resistance to *cis*- and carboplatin. Clinical

Drug Delivery in Oncology: From Basic Research to Cancer Therapy, First Edition.
Edited by Felix Kratz, Peter Senter, and Henning Steinhagen.

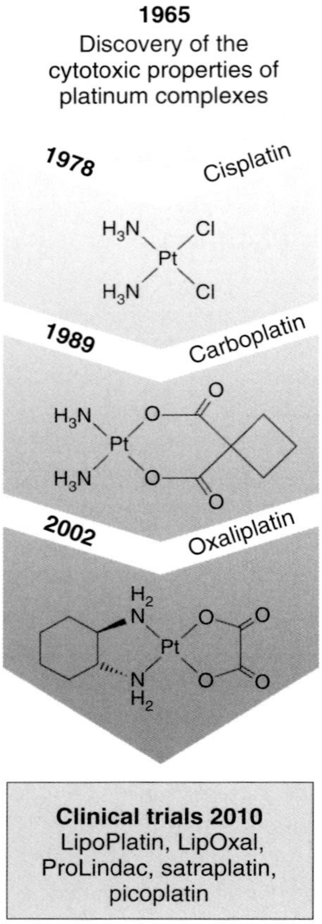

Figure 49.1 Milestones in platinum-based anticancer chemotherapy: cisplatin, carboplatin, and oxaliplatin received regulatory approval in 1978, 1989, and 2002, respectively. Currently, two liposomal platinum formulations (LipoPlatin and LipOxal), one polymeric platinum drug (ProLindac), and two novel low-molecular-weight platinum complexes (satraplatin and picoplatin) are being investigated in clinical trials.

trials based on different tumors of the gastrointestinal tract and breast and lung carcinomas are ongoing. Neurotoxicity – an initial transient peripheral sensory neuropathy and a long-term neuropathy – was found to be dose limiting. Nausea, vomiting, and nephrotoxicity are relatively mild.

Apart from cis-, carbo-, and oxaliplatin, three other platinum-based drugs have gained limited regional approval: nedaplatin (Japan), lobaplatin (China), and heptaplatin (South Korea). Currently, two liposomal formulations (LipoPlatin™ and LipOxal™) containing cis- or oxaliplatin, one polymer carrier loaded with the oxaliplatin fragment (ProLindac™), and two low-molecular-weight platinum complexes (satraplatin (Pt(IV) compound, oral administration) and picoplatin (sterically hindered)) are in clinical trials [8].

Looking back on the of development of platinum-based anticancer drugs, what was achieved and what is the perspective for the next decades? Several thousands of platinum complexes were synthesized and tested for their cytotoxicity and anticancer activity [9, 10]. In sum, nearly 40 complexes were evaluated in clinical trials and up to now three compounds have made their way into the clinics worldwide. Admittedly, it is a success story and represents a landmark in the development of anticancer chemotherapy with cisplatin as the queen of that type of complexes. However, we still fight with relatively low levels of specificity and high toxicity. It will become more and more difficult to find novel low-molecular-weight platinum complexes that will satisfy the needs of the cancer market [11].

Strategies to overcome these obstacles by focusing on drug delivery concepts are diverse, and basically dependent on the particular mechanism of action and chemistry of platinum complexes, which will be highlighted in Section 49.2.

49.2
Mode of Action of Platinum-Based Anticancer Drugs and Rationale for the Respective Drug Delivery Concept

Cisplatin is a square-planar metal complex, exhibiting four ligands (Figure 49.2). The two NH_3 ligands are *cis*-orientated (neighboring) and are nonexchangeable; they are the nonleaving or inert ligands. The two chloride ligands, however, are not so tightly bound; they are relatively labile and act as leaving groups. In pure water (absence of additives), cisplatin is not stable; it hydrolyzes to some extent to the respective compound with one aqua ligand under release of chloride. This reaction (aquation) can be reversed via increasing the concentration of chloride in solution. The formed aqua complex is an activated species and very reactive toward biologically relevant molecules. Nitrogen- and especially sulfur-containing

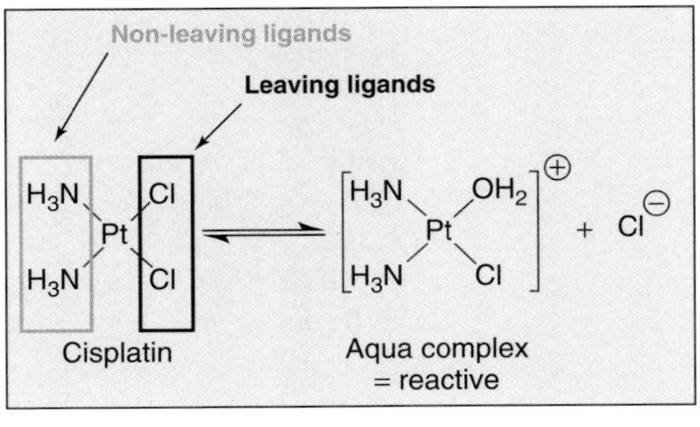

Figure 49.2 Equilibrium between cisplatin and the monoaqua complex in aqueous solution. Ammonia ligands are inert and therefore nonleaving; however, one or both chloro leaving ligands are exchangeable. In water, first the highly reactive monoaqua complex is formed under release of one chloride ligand. This reaction is usually called hydrolysis, although strictly speaking it is an aquation. In the presence of a high chloride concentration, the reaction is reversible under the formation of cisplatin.

compounds (like amino acids, peptides, or proteins) show a high tendency to react with cisplatin or its hydrolysis products [12], which can be explained by the $H_{ard}S_{oft}A_{cids}B_{ases}$ (HSAB) principle. (Due to the HSAB concept developed by Pearson, favored reaction products between metal ions (Lewis acids) and potential ligands (Lewis bases) can be predicted (e.g., Pt(II) is a soft metal ion and sulfur-containing ligands (thiols or thioethers) are prototypical soft bases. As a result, Pt(II) reacts preferentially with sulfur-containing biomolecules.) Consequently, it is not surprising that sulfur-based molecules have been investigated for their use as cytoprotective agents (antidotes) [13].

After intravenous infusion, cisplatin stays to some extent intact due to the high chloride ion concentration (100 mM) in the bloodstream. However, a large amount of cisplatin binds to proteins and it is assumed that these adducts do not serve as a reservoir with anticancer potential; it leads to detoxification.

Cisplatin is accumulated in the cells, normal or malignant (Figure 49.3), either via transporters, like the copper transporter Ctr1, or by passive diffusion [14]. Inside the cells, the chloride ion concentration is significantly lower (3–20 mM),

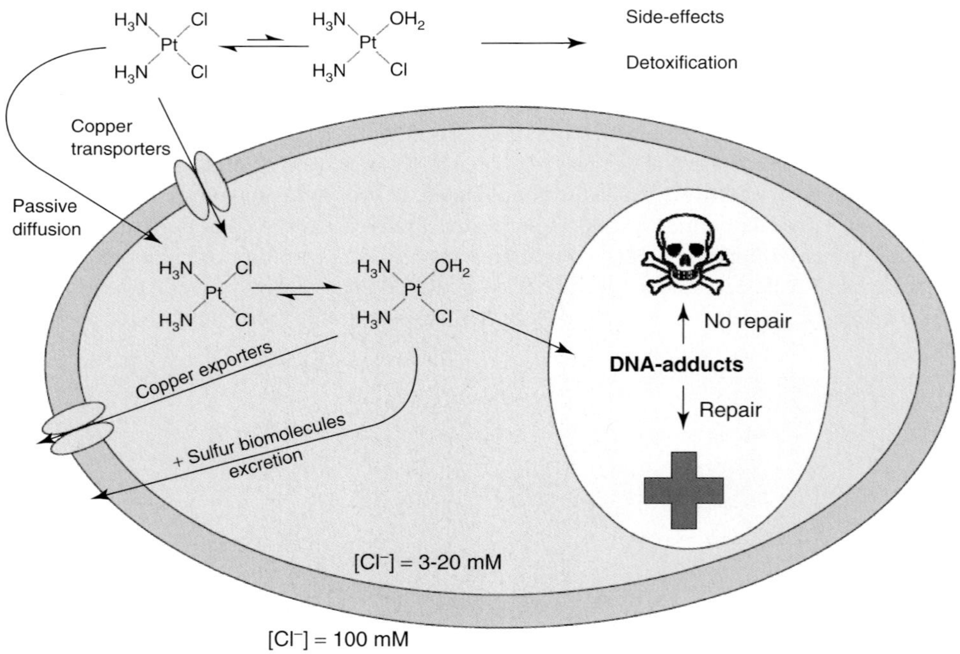

Figure 49.3 Mode of action of cisplatin: cisplatin enters the cell by passive diffusion or via transporters; inside the cell, it is aquated (hydrolyzed) due to the relatively low chloride ion concentration, forming species with one or two aqua ligands. Upon its way to the final target (i.e., the nuclear DNA) cisplatin is pushed out of the cells via copper exporters or reacts with sulfur-containing biomolecules (glutathione, metallothionein) and is excreted. Approximately 1% of the administered drug reaches the DNA. The DNA lesions lead to apoptosis or necrosis if they are not repaired by the cellular machinery.

shifting the equilibrium to the monoaqua complex. Different scenarios are now possible [15]: (i) the monoaquated species further releases one chloride ion, (ii) further degradation products are formed (e.g., hydroxo complexes), (iii) efflux of the complexes via copper exporters, (iv) reaction of the activated platinum species with sulfur-containing biomolecules and subsequent excretion (e.g., through the glutathione S-conjugate export pump), and eventually (v) reaction with the nuclear DNA.

It is astonishing that cisplatin actually reaches the final target in the presence of a plethora of biomolecules (platinophiles) with a high affinity for the central platinum ion; only approximately 1% of the administered dose ends up at the DNA. In accordance with the HSAB principle, platinum complexes react with nitrogen donor atoms of the nucleobases and not with the phosphate-sugar backbone. Overall, cisplatin binds to more than 90% at the N^7 position of guanine and preferentially (65%) at two neighboring guanine bases of one strand (Figure 49.4, cisplatin-d(GpG) adduct) [16]. This so-called intrastrand cross-link bends the DNA toward the major groove, and blocks replication and transcription, thereby inducing cell death. On the other hand, the cellular machinery has the ability to cope with cisplatin damage. Such adducts can be repaired, especially by nucleotide excision repair.

The mechanisms of action of carboplatin and oxaliplatin are very similar to cisplatin; again, the final target is DNA. In carboplatin, a bidentate dicarboxylato leaving ligand is bound to the platinum center; the nitrogen ligands are the same. The leaving ligand in carboplatin is not that labile as compared to the two chloride

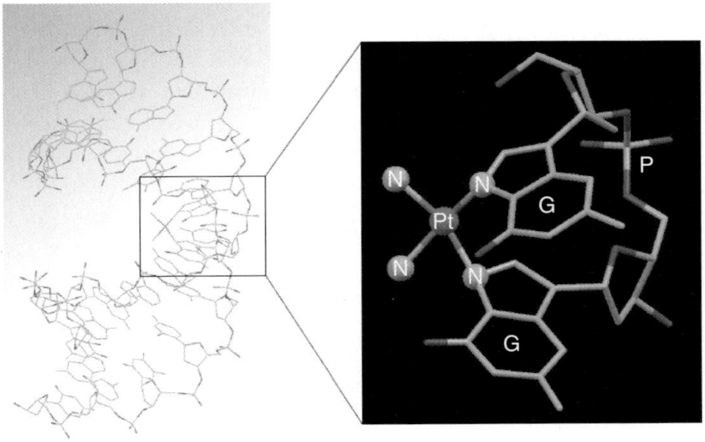

Figure 49.4 Crystal structure of double-stranded DNA containing the major adduct of the anticancer drug cisplatin [16]. The cytotoxic diammineplatinum(II) fragment $[Pt(NH_3)_2]^{2+}$ binds in the major grove to the N^7 positions of two neighboring guanine (G) bases of one strand (intrastrand d(GpG) adduct).

ions. As a result, carboplatin is not so reactive, can be administered at higher doses, and shows a different toxicity profile in comparison to cisplatin. Once carboplatin has reacted with the DNA, its adducts are identical to those deriving from cisplatin, explaining why carboplatin has no potential to be used in the case of cisplatin-resistant cancers. In oxaliplatin, the oxalate leaving group is also more inert than the chloro ligands in cisplatin. However, the diamine ligand is different in comparison to cis- and carboplatin; this does not only influence the lipophilicity of the drug (volume of distribution), it has a marked effect on the recognition and processing of oxaliplatin deriving DNA adducts [17]. Hence, oxaliplatin is active in colorectal carcinomas, which are inherently resistant to cis- and carboplatin.

The main objectives for developing novel anticancer platinum drugs are the reduction of side-effects and the activity in a broader spectrum of malignant tumors, especially those displaying intrinsic or acquired resistance. Resistance phenomena in platinum-based chemotherapy are multifactorial, including (i) reduced cellular drug uptake, (ii) increased drug efflux, (iii) drug inactivation by sulfur-containing biomolecules, (iv) enhancement of DNA repair, (v) decreased mismatch repair (futile mismatch repair of platinum–DNA adducts, thereby shielding the adduct from nucleotide excision repair), (vi) defective apoptosis, or (vii) modulation of signaling pathways.

Bearing in mind the mechanism of action of platinum drugs, their spectrum of activity as well as their systemic toxicities, what would be the strategies for the development of novel agents? Which innovative concepts do we need to be more successful in the fight against cancer?

The answer is relatively easy – we should find a platinum drug delivery concept selectively targeting the tumor cells. What we are searching for is something like a magic bullet for cancerous tissues. Of course this ideal is difficult to achieve; the following requirements build a basis for that approach: (i) significantly prolonged half-life in the bloodstream, (ii) decelerated metabolism and excretion, (iii) accumulation in the tumor tissue and tumor cells via active or passive drug targeting, (iv) activation/release of the drugs once they have been accumulated in the tumor tissue and cells, and (v) overall decreased reaction with platinophiles.

Further considerations are related to the particular chemistry of platinum complexes and to their mode of action. At the end of the drug delivery process, the platinum complex has to bind to DNA – the cytotoxicity is thereby dependent on the steric characteristics of the DNA adduct formation. When the ligand is too big, reaction with DNA may be inhibited, therefore cis- or oxaliplatin-like moieties should be released from the targeting group (of course it is also always favorable to use platinum fragments deriving from cis- or carboplatin, which have already proven anticancer activity). Advantageously, the targeting group could be attached to the leaving ligand (**I**, Figure 49.5). In that case, a cis- or oxaliplatin-like fragment is generated for attacking the DNA. Of importance is the fact that the targeting group must not be released from the metal center before reaching the tumor tissue. With respect to the latter requirement, it would be beneficial to couple the targeting group to the nonleaving ligand (**II**, Figure 49.5). However, this is only practicable when the targeting group is attached to platinum via a linker that can be cleaved

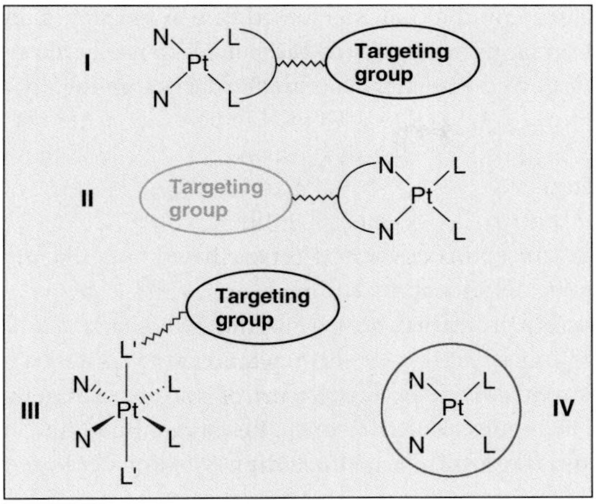

Figure 49.5 Different strategies for the drug targeting concept: (**I**) the targeting group is bound to the leaving ligands, (**II**) the targeting group is coupled to the nonleaving ligands, (**III**) the targeting group is attached to an axial ligand of an octahedrally configured Pt(IV) complex, or (**IV**) the platinum complex is incorporated into a liposome. N, nonleaving nitrogen donor ligands; L, leaving ligands; L′, ligands that will be released via reduction to the respective Pt(II) complex.

by enzymes or under slightly acid conditions (as found in many solid tumors). Otherwise, the construct is sterically too demanding to form cytotoxic adducts with the DNA.

A novel and very attractive approach takes advantage of octahedrally configured Pt(IV) complexes [18]. In these species the platinum center displays to extra ligands in the axial position (**III**, Figure 49.5). When the targeting group is attached to one of these ligands, it can be released together with the ligand under reducing conditions in the hypoxic tumor milieu, forming the respective Pt(II) complex. Last, but not least, the encapsulation of established platinum drugs in liposomes (**IV**, Figure 49.5) has emerged to be very successful and promising, although cisplatin, for example, is not really the prototypical agent for liposomal encapsulation. Cisplatin is sparely soluble in water and not soluble in common organic solvents typically used during the encapsulation process.

49.3 Examples

Drug targeting strategies with anticancer platinum complexes have emerged during recent years. They can principally be divided as (i) active and organ-specific targeting, and (ii) passive targeting. A rich series of complexes has been developed for active and organ-specific targeting; they share a common feature in most cases – they are small, low-molecular-weight platinum agents. None of these complexes has reached clinical trials so far. On the contrary, platinum agents intended for passive drug targeting are large molecules (bound to polymers, micelles, or entrapped in liposomes) or specifically build-up large molecules in the body. Currently, three representatives (LipoPlatin, LipOxal, and ProLindac) are in clinical evaluation.

49.3.1
Active and Organ-Specific Targeting

This strategy is mainly based on a receptor- or transporter-mediated targeting, or takes advantage of an organ-specific delivery approach.

Targeting the estrogen receptor is a promising strategy; besides endometrial and prostate tumors, mammary carcinomas express the estrogen receptor in 60–70% of cases. Estradiol derivatives as well as nonsteroidal antiestrogens and estrogens were in preclinical evaluation. One representative for that class of agents should be mentioned in which the oxaliplatin fragment was coupled to a tamoxifen derivative (Figure 49.6) [19]. Tamoxifen itself is currently used for the treatment of both early and advanced estrogen receptor-positive breast cancer. The novel complex showed *in vitro* satisfactory receptor binding and proved to be active in the MCF7 breast cancer cell line.

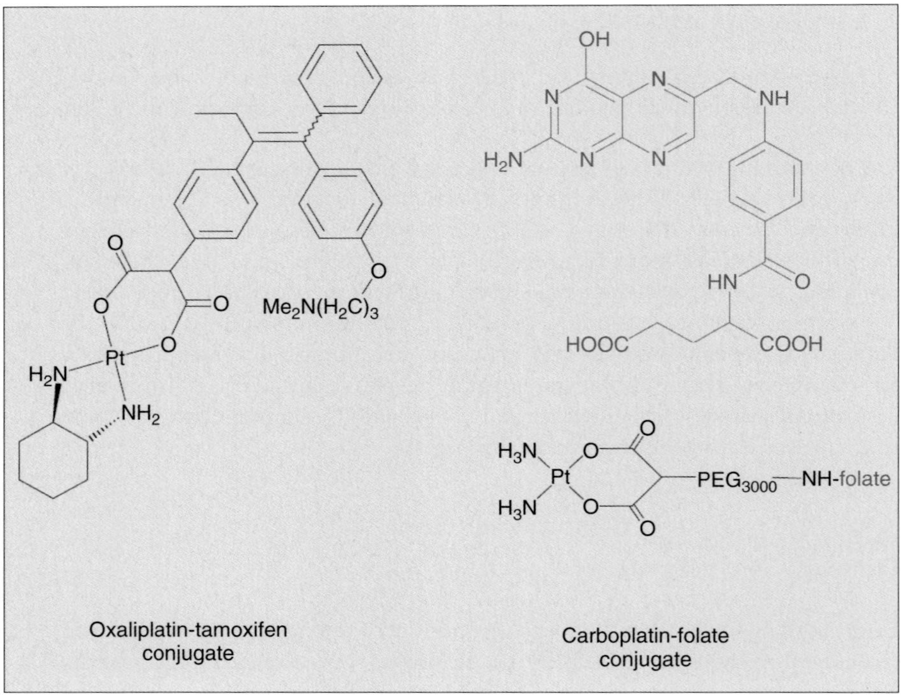

Figure 49.6 Oxaliplatin–tamoxifen and carboplatin–folate conjugates developed to target the estrogen and folate receptors, respectively.

A further route in the fight against cancer could be based on folate receptor-mediated endocytosis [20]. The expression of folate receptors in normal cells is low or absent; however, particularly ovarian and endometrial cancers use that pathway for internalizing folic acid. Consequently, a carboplatin-type folate conjugate (Figure 49.6) was developed, also displaying a poly(ethylene glycol) (PEG) spacer between the cytotoxic and the targeting moiety. Cellular uptake, cytotoxicity as well as DNA platination were investigated in a M109 murine lung carcinoma subline (M109 HiFR) expressing a high amount of folate receptor. Against expectations, the antiproliferative properties as well as platinum levels at the DNA were low. The authors concluded that the conjugates or the active moieties were neutralized or blocked during the endocytosis process and did not manage to reach the final target (i.e., the nuclear DNA) effectively [21].

Various types of saccharide constructs have been shown to be recognized on cellular surfaces. In particular, galactose receptors exclusively expressed by liver parenchymal cells are attractive targets for platinum-based delivery. In this context it should also be mentioned that binding to the receptors is enhanced by taking advantage of the so-called cluster effect (branched galactose units bind more effectively to the receptors in comparison to their unbranched analogs), which can be further optimized by varying the spatial distance as well as the flexibility of the galactose residues. In this way Gal4A-PEG-DA/CDDP was developed (Figure 49.7) [22]; the corresponding complex with an unbranched galactose as well as an analog completely without a galactose residue were not as cytotoxic as Gal4A-PEG-DA/CDDP in *in vitro* investigations in HepG2 human hepatoma cells, proving the importance of the targeting unit. However, subsequent promising *in vivo* results could not be presented.

Unfortunately, despite an innovative rationale, a real proof of concept for targeting the above-mentioned receptors in animal experiments is still missing. Convincing *in vivo* results of advanced preclinical trials have not yet been published.

Targeting the enterohepatic circulation (liver, bile duct, gall bladder) also seems to be an attractive approach. It takes advantage of a very efficient reuptake mechanism of bile acids synthesized in the liver. Bile acids are reabsorbed via ileal cells in the small intestine by specific transmembrane bile acid carrier proteins (also present in hepatocytes) assuring a low depletion of the bile acid pool and providing the basis for a marked organotropism toward the hepatobiliary system (enterohepatic circulation) [23]. For that purpose, bile acids were coordinated to the cytotoxic cisplatin fragment resulting in (beside others) Bamet-UD2 (Figure 49.7). In an orthotopically implanted mouse Hepa 1-6 hepatoma model in the liver of nude mice, Bamet-UD2 was superior compared to cisplatin and an analogous precursor Bamet-R2 with respect to survival time and body weight (Figure 49.8) [24].

Platinum levels in liver and tumor tissue were higher in Bamet-UD2-treated animals. Platinum accumulation in tissue and toxicity were investigated in cancer-free rats. Contrary to cisplatin, Bamet-UD2-treated rats accumulated lower platinum levels in the kidney, lung, heart, muscle, brain, bone marrow, and nerves. In the liver, however, the platinum content was significantly higher within the Bamet-UD2 group, demonstrating a good hepatic organotropism. It was found that organic

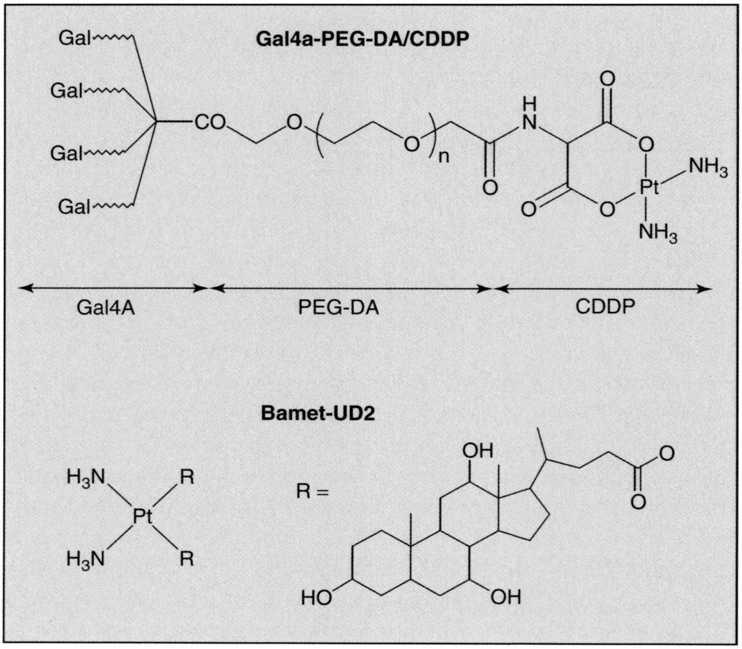

Figure 49.7 Chemical structures of Gal4A-PEG-DA/CDDP (a complex developed for galactose receptor targeting displaying a four-branched galactose unit (Gal4A), a PEG spacer (PEG-DA), and the cytotoxic cisplatin fragment (CDDP)) and a representative of the Bamet family (Bamet-UD2) having two ursodeoxycholate ligands.

anion and cation transporters expressed in the hepatocyte plasma membrane may account for these findings [25]. Additionally, Bamet-UD2-treated animals did not show any signs of severe toxicity as compared to the cisplatin group (neurotoxicity, bone marrow toxicity, and kidney damage). The promising *in vivo* anticancer activity is based on a strong proapoptotic and a weak pronecrotic effect [26]. In combination with the low toxicity, Bamet-UD2 seemed to be a promising candidate and further preclinical studies were announced. Up to now, it has not found its way into clinical trials.

More details and references about the targeting of estrogen, folate, and galactose receptors as well as of the enterohepatic circulation can be found in a series of recent review articles [27–30].

Osteosarcoma (primary bone tumors) and bone metastases are not easy to treat, since the blood supply of bone tissue is low and therefore bone targeting is really challenging. A serious problem display especially bone metastases taking into account that nearly 50% of tumors have the potential to metastasize to bones. Additionally, in the case of osteosarcoma, ossifying lung metastases (calcification of the lung tissue) are difficult to treat and life-threatening. For decades, bisphosphonates

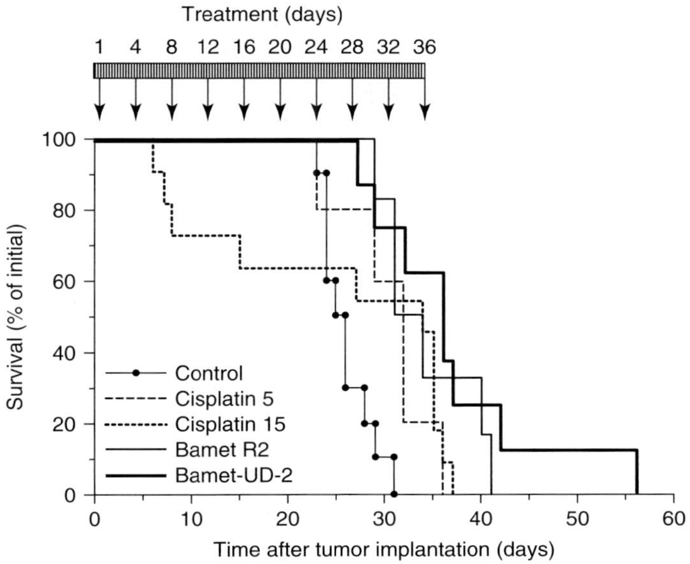

Figure 49.8 Kaplan–Meier curves for survival, as percentages of the initial number of animals per group, following orthotopic implantation of a fragment of approximately 1 mm^3 of mouse Hepa 1-6 hepatoma tumor in nude mice. The animals were treated intraperitoneally once every 4 days with either 15 nmol/g body weight of Bamet-R2 ($n = 6$), Bamet-UD2 ($n = 8$), or cisplatin ($n = 11$), or 5 nmol/g body weight of cisplatin ($n = 5$). The control group ($n = 10$) received only vehicle (sterile saline). Treatment was maintained for 5 weeks. (Reproduced with permission from [24].)

such as etidronate, clodronate, pamidronate, and zoledronate (among others) have been used for the treatment of Paget's disease, tumor-induced osteolysis, hypercalcemia, and postmenopausal osteoporosis. Furthermore, they have successfully been in use for the scintigraphy of bones. Due to their bisphosphonic residue, they show a high tendency to interact with calcium and therefore are equipped with remarkable osteotropic (bone-seeking) properties. Consequently, the cytotoxic diamineplatinum(II) fragments were coupled to a bis(phosphonic acid) function suitable to adsorb onto the bone surface (Figure 49.9) [31, 32].

In principal, the platinumphosphonato complexes showed a low cytotoxicity in the cisplatin-sensitive ovarian carcinoma cell line CH1 in the middle to high micromolar range. This is not surprising, taking into account that the complexes should be accumulated and activated at the tumor site [33]. However, *in vivo* the complexes were very active in a series of transplantable tumors such as MAC 15A colon adenocarcinoma, sarcoma 180, Ehrlich ascites, and Stockholm ascites with treatment to control (T/C) values of higher than 300%.

In a transplantable osteosarcoma induced by radioactive ^{144}Ce also displaying lung metastases, the platinumphosphonato complexes showed promising activity. In this respect it should be mentioned that an increase in lifespan can only be achieved when the development or growth of lung metastases is significantly

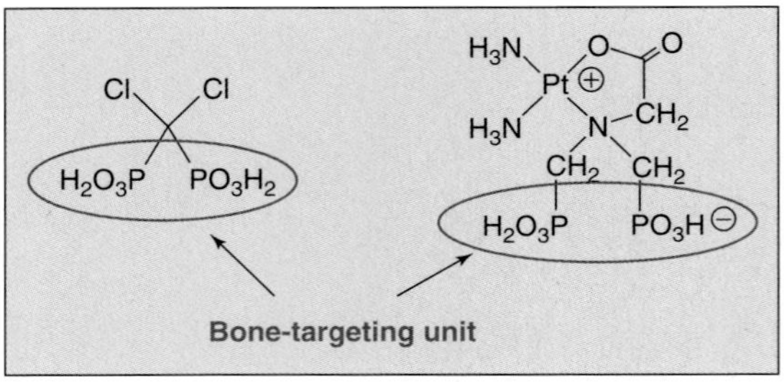

Figure 49.9 Chemical structure of clodronate (left) and a representative of platinumphosphonato complexes (right) both displaying an osteotropic bis(phosphonic acid) function.

inhibited. Both tumor growth as well as development of metastases in the lung could be blocked in comparison to untreated control animals (Figure 49.10).

Unfortunately, the patent situation of that highly promising compound class developed to be unfavorable, allowing further evaluation in clinical trials only as orphan drugs.

49.3.2
Passive Targeting

Tumor growth is accompanied by extensive angiogenesis in order to supply the tumor with nutrients. This process is rather uncontrolled and chaotic, leading to a defective architecture of tumor blood vessels (large gaps in endothelium cell–cell junctions). Moreover, lymphatic drainage is impaired and vascular permeability mediators are overexpressed. As a final consequence, this leads to an enhanced extravasation of macromolecular compounds, thereby opening up the possibility of accumulating cytotoxic agents in the tumor tissue via macromolecular constructs. This is known as the enhanced permeability and retention (EPR) effect ([34] and Chapter 3), and has emerged as a prominent option for attacking solid tumors.

49.3.2.1 Liposomal Drug Delivery – LipoPlatin and LipOxal

Liposomal encapsulation of cytotoxic agents has already proven to be a promising strategy in the fight against cancer. In these delivery vehicles (Figure 49.11), the drug is left unchanged; reactions (bond formation) with one of the liposome constituents are excluded. However, the process of liposomal entrapment is not in every case simple. In particular, cisplatin is not a prototypical agent, since it is sparely soluble in water and not soluble in organic solvents used for the process.

Some further prerequisites have to be taken into consideration when developing drug-loaded liposomes. The size of the liposomes should be in an optimal range in order to take advantage of the EPR effect. Moreover, naked liposomes (without a protective coating) can be detected by macrophages and destroyed, thereby releasing the drug before it reaches the tumor tissue. Last, but not least, improved

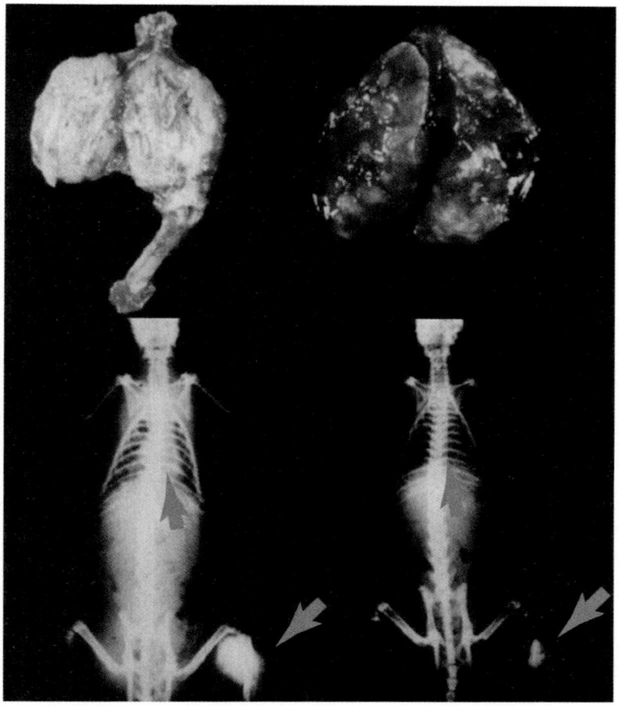

Figure 49.10 Transplantable $^{144}CeCl_3$-induced osteosarcoma of the rat is characterized by life-threatening dissemination in the lung. (a) Radiograph and dissected lung of a tumor-bearing animal taken 42 days after intratibial transplantation. (b) Radiograph and dissected lung of an animal treated with a platinumphosphonate 42 days after transplantation (lack of lung metastases, and dense and compact tumor). (Adapted from [32].)

cellular accumulation may also be a point to be envisaged during the design of novel liposomal formulations.

The first liposomes in clinical trials containing a platinum-based cytotoxic agent were SPI-77 loaded with cisplatin. In SPI-77, only neutral lipids were used and the ratio of lipids to cisplatin (mg of lipid/mg of cisplatin) was rather unfavorable at around 70 : 1 [35]. Efficacy in clinical evaluation was rather low. Improving the liposomal formulation finally resulted in LipoPlatin (Regulon; *www.regulon.org*) [36]. LipoPlatin (Figure 49.12) is composed of soy phosphatidylcholine (SPC-3), dipalmitoylphosphatidylglycerol (DPPG), cholesterol, and methoxyPEG–distearoylphosphatidylethanolamine (mPEG2000–DSPE). mPEG2000–DSPE was used for the protective coating; a half-life of 5 days was found in body fluids as compared to non-PEGylated liposomes (half-lives of only 20 min). The anionic lipid DPPG was further incorporated with the aim of facilitating cellular accumulation. DPPG and consequently also the DPPG-containing liposomes have fusogenic properties (i.e., the liposomes are

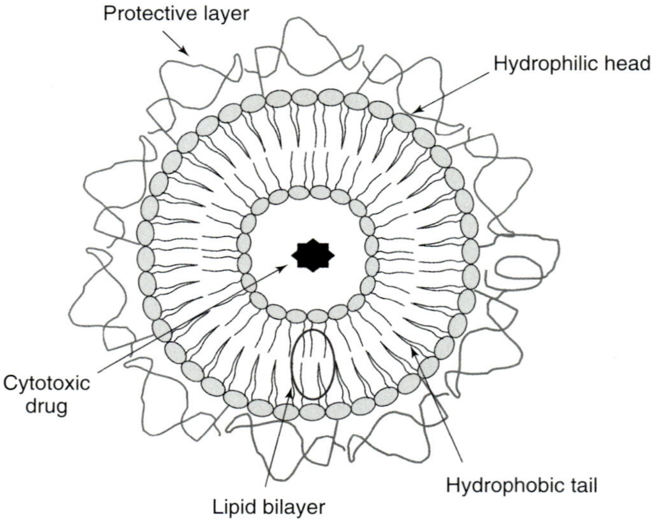

Figure 49.11 General composition of drug-loaded liposome additionally displaying a protective layer.

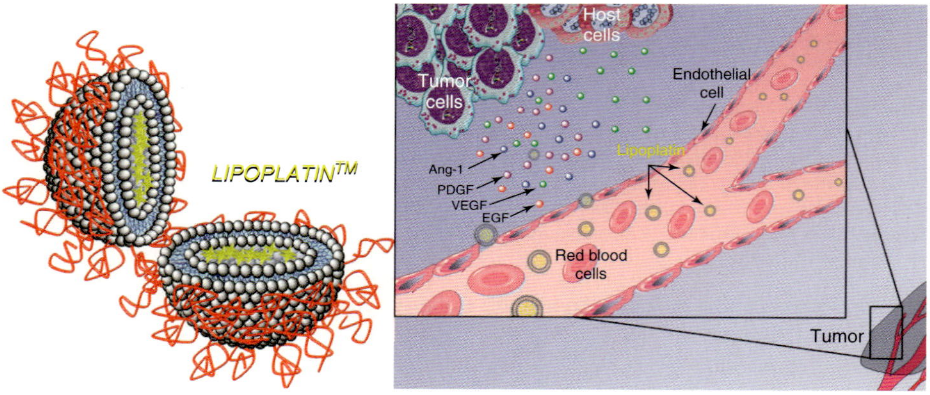

Figure 49.12 Cisplatin (yellow)-loaded liposomes (100 nm) are able to reach the tumor tissues via the EPR effect through the leaky vasculature. LipoPlatin's half-life in the bloodstream is long and recognition by macrophages is suppressed due to its protective coating with PEG (red). Ang-1, angiopoietin-1; PDGF, platelet-derived growth factor; VEGF, vascular endothelial growth factor; EGF, epidermal growth factor. (Reproduced with permission from [36].)

capable of fusing with the cell membrane and thereby easily crossing the cell membrane barrier). Very recently, a proof of principle was provided for the fusogenic pathway in MCF7 breast cancer cells *in vitro*. The liposomes were labeled with a fluorescent dye (fluorescein isothiocyanate) and fixed cells were visualized with confocal microscopy [37].

In addition to the different composition of SPI-77 and LipoPlatin, production of LipoPlatin was significantly changed and optimized. First, inverse micelles are now produced that are subsequently converted into liposomes, reaching entrapment efficiencies of up to 97%. The average liposome size is 110 nm. The lipid/cisplatin ratio could be significantly decreased by a factor of 10 to 7 : 1, which is of great interest since less lipid has to be injected into the patient.

Preclinical studies in mice, rats, and severe combined immunodeficient (SCID) mice revealed a generally lower toxicity of LipoPlatin, especially a lower nephrotoxicity. Treatment of rats with 5 mg/kg cisplatin or LipoPlatin resulted in differences in total platinum concentration in the kidneys (Figure 49.13) [38]. The maximum level of total platinum in the kidneys within the first 30 min after intraperitoneal bolus injection was the same. However, the steady-state platinum concentration in the kidneys in the following 6 days after injection was significantly different; platinum accumulation caused by cisplatin was 4 times higher in comparison to LipoPlatin. Presumably, the initial accumulation of LipoPlatin is not that effective in causing nephrotoxicity, which may be explained by an altered metabolism in comparison to cisplatin. In dogs, 150 mg/m^2 of LipoPlatin could safely be administered without a hydration protocol [39]. The clinical development of LipoPlatin will be discussed in Section 49.4.1.

Regulon also has a second platinum-based formulation in the pipeline – LipOxal, a liposomal encapsulated oxaliplatin. The clinical development of LipOxal will be discussed in Section 49.4.2.

49.3.2.2 **Polymeric Delivery Systems – ProLindac**

Contrary to LipoPlatin and LipOxal, platinum-containing polymeric delivery systems are real high-molecular-weight platinum derivatives, since the platinum center is coordinatively bound to the polymer backbone and not just entrapped in a larger construct without bond formation. Possible drug delivery systems include micelles, dendrimers, and natural or synthetic polymers, and have been reviewed recently [28–30].

One promising polymer bearing the cytotoxic oxaliplatin fragment is ProLindac (Access Pharmaceuticals; *www.accesspharma.com*). In ProLindac, the copolymer backbone is built of a hydroxypropylmethacrylamide (HPMA) monomer and a linker monomer in a ratio of 10 : 1 (Figure 49.14). HPMA is nonimmunogenic and nontoxic, and was one of the candidates to be used as a blood plasma expander for infusion solutions [40]. The linker monomer carries a triglycine spacer and at the end a chelating unit (aminomalonate unit) to which the cytotoxic oxaliplatin fragment is bound. Release of platinum from the chelator is pH dependent; at pH 5.4 it is 6.7 times greater in comparison to a pH of 7.4 [41]. The chelator binds to platinum via a nitrogen and an oxygen atom (*N,O*-chelation), which was proven by ^{195}Pt-nuclear magnetic resonance spectroscopy. Only in the beginning was the kinetically favored *O,O* chelate formed [42]. A second coordination side is also available at one of the glycine residues next to the aminomalonate unit. The average molecular weight of the platinum loaded polymer is 25 kDa. Platinum is

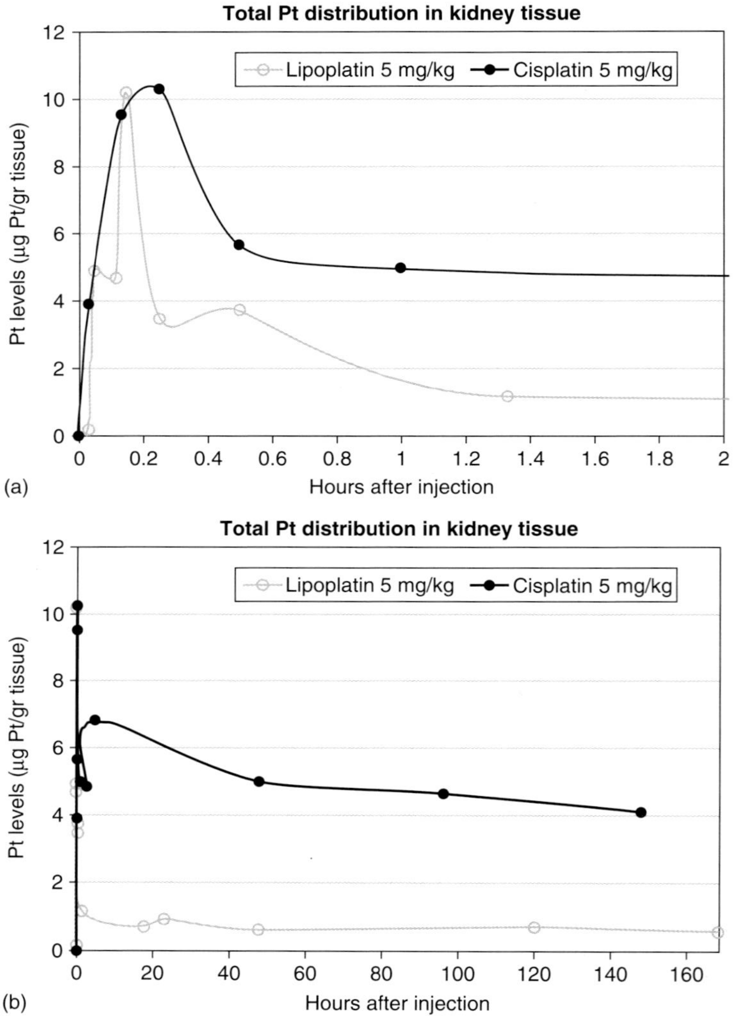

Figure 49.13 Treatment of rats with 5 mg/kg cisplatin or LipoPlatin. Administration of cisplatin or LipoPlatin results in the same maximum level of total platinum in the kidneys within 30 min after injection (a). However, the steady state of total platinum concentration is different for the two drugs in the following 6 days after injection (b). (Reproduced with permission from [38].)

released from the polymer to an amount of 1.5 or 4.5% after 3 or 24 h, respectively. Low-molecular-weight impurities are below 0.8%.

Anticancer activity was proven in a series of mouse tumor models, either syngeneic murine or human tumor xenografts. In all models, ProLindac was not less effective than oxaliplatin. For example, ProLindac was superior to oxaliplatin in L1210 murine leukemia and 0157 hybridoma or in three colon xenograft models

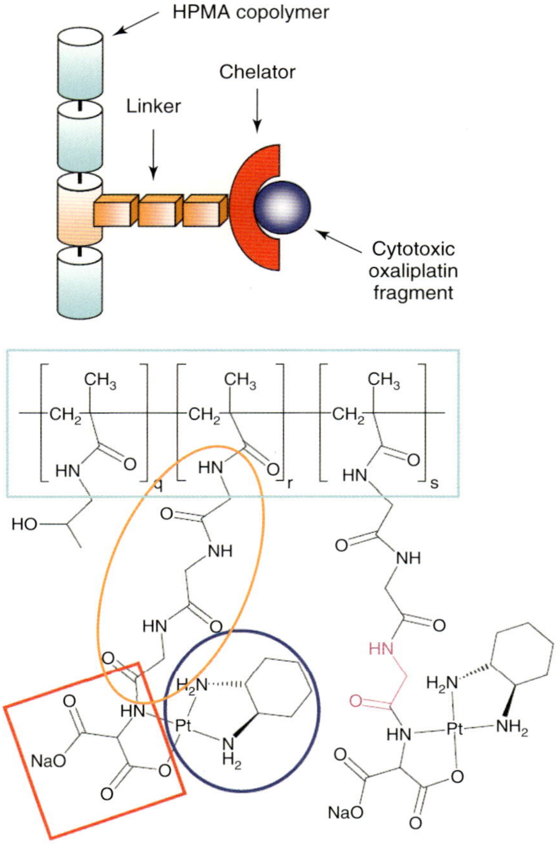

Figure 49.14 Partial structure of ProLindac: schematic presentation and chemical structure. HPMA copolymer backbone (light blue), triglycine spacer (orange), chelating unit (red), cytotoxic platinum fragment (blue), and further site for platinum coordination (magenta).

(Colo-26, Ht-29, and HCT116). *In vitro* studies in colon and ovarian cancer cell lines revealed a synergistic effect of ProLindac together with 5-FU, gemcitabine, and SN-38. Especially in M5076 sarcoma (cisplatin resistant), B16F10 melanoma, and 2008 ovarian xenograft, the efficacy of ProLindac was markedly superior compared to oxaliplatin [43]. The effect of equitoxic doses of ProLindac or oxaliplatin in mice on the growth of B16F10 melanoma is shown in Figure 49.15.

The maximum tolerated doses (MTDs) of ProLindac in two rodent models given intravenously once every 7 days for 3 weeks were: 106 mg Pt/kg (625 mg Pt/m^2) in male and female rats, 191 mg Pt/kg (573 mg Pt/m^2) in male mice, and 136 mg Pt/kg (408 mg Pt/m^2) in female mice. The clinical development of ProLindac will be discussed in Section 49.4.3.

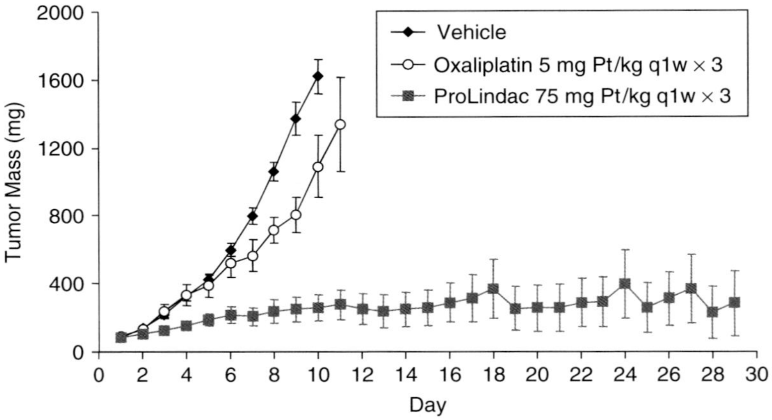

Figure 49.15 Antitumor activity of ProLindac in comparison to oxaliplatin in the subcutaneous murine B16F10 melanoma tumor model. Each agent was administered intraperitoneally at its respective MTD. (Reproduced courtesy of David Nowotnik, Access Pharmaceuticals.)

49.4
Clinical Development

49.4.1
LipoPlatin

An overview of the clinical development of LipoPlatin is summarized in Table 49.1. A phase I study in 27 patients at stage IV (19 pancreatic carcinomas) was conducted with doses ranging from 25 to 125 mg/m^2. The MTD was not reached. LipoPlatin was administered as second- or third-line treatment as an 8-h infusion repeated every 2 weeks. In sharp contrast to cisplatin chemotherapy, pre- or posthydration was not needed. Cisplatin's typical nephro-, neuro-, and ototoxicity were not seen; hematological and gastrointestinal toxicity were mild. Three patients showed a partial response and a stabilization of the disease was reported in 14 patients. Prescheduled surgery 20 h after LipoPlatin infusion revealed 10–50 times higher platinum levels in cancerous tissues in comparison to normal tissue. For example, in colon tumors accumulation was higher than in normal colon tissue by a factor of 200. However, the highest platinum level was found in gastric tumor specimens with 260 μg platinum/g tissue [44]. A further phase I study was performed in combination with gemcitabine in refractory or resistant non-small-cell lung cancer (NSCLC) patients with a recommended dose of 120 mg/m^2 cisplatin and 1000 mg/m^2 gemcitabine for phase II trials [45].

Recently, results of a phase I/II study of LipoPlatin together with 5-FU and radiotherapy for the treatment of locally advanced gastric cancer were published [46]. LipoPlatin at 120 mg/m^2 was given weekly in combination with 5-FU at

Table 49.1 Overview of the clinical development of LipoPlatin.

	LipoPlatin in combination with	Localization	In comparison to
Phase I	–	mainly pancreatic cancer	–
Phase I	gemcitabine	NSCLC	–
Phase I/II	5-FU + radiotherapy	gastric cancer	–
Phase II	gemcitabine	pancreatic cancer	–
Phase II	gemcitabine	NSCLC	–
Phase II	vinorelbine	breast cancer	–
Phase II	gemcitabine	cisplatin-pretreated NSCLC	–
Phase III	paclitaxel	NSCLC	cisplatin + paclitaxel
Phase III	gemcitabine	NSCLC	cisplatin + gemcitabine
Phase III	5-FU	SCCHN	cisplatin + 5-FU

400 mg/m^2 at day 1 per week; additionally the patients received 3.5-Gy fractions on days 2, 3, and 4. Apart from a mild toxicity, a high complete response rate was observed. Further testing of that setting for adjuvant postoperative or preoperative radio/chemotherapy in gastric cancer patients was recommended.

Series of phase II studies were conducted or are in progress [35]. A dose-escalation second-line treatment in pancreatic cancer patients who were refractory to previous chemotherapy was performed. Twenty-four patients were treated with a combination of 1000 mg/m^2 gemcitabine (60-min infusion) and 25–125 mg/m^2 LipoPlatin (8-h infusion on days 1 and 15). In this combination 100 mg/m^2 LipoPlatin was the MTD. No neuro- or nephrotoxicity was observed. It was recommended to change the schedule or increase the dose in order to enhance the efficacy. Weekly LipoPlatin (120 mg/m^2) together with gemcitabine (1000 mg/m^2; LipoGem arm) was investigated as first-line treatment in NSCLC patients in comparison to treatment with cisplatin (100 mg/m^2) plus gemicitabine (1000 mg/m^2; CisGem arm). Overall, LipoGem was better tolerated; nephrotoxicity was significantly reduced and myelotoxicity was the main side-effect. A promising response/stabilization rate in an adenocarcinoma histological subtype of NSCLC (83.3% in the LipoGem arm versus 54.2% in the CisGem arm) was found. In a further phase II trial, LipoPlatin (120 mg/m^2) in combination with vinorelbine (30 mg/m^2) in 20 patients with advanced or metastatic breast cancer (HER2/*neu*-negative) was investigated. Overall, promising activity and a good tolerance was found. A phase II trial in cisplatin-treated NSCLC cancer patients receiving LipoPlatin (120 mg/m^2) and gemcitabine (1000 mg/m^2) was also started. Again, a good response and tolerance were seen. This means nothing else than that the liposomal formulation of cisplatin is active in cisplatin-resistant tumors – a circumstance that is explainable by the different uptake in cancer cells.

Finally, in November 2007, LipoPlatin received orphan drug status from the European Medicines Agency (EMEA) for the treatment of pancreatic cancer (*www.ema.europa.eu/docs/en_GB/document_library/Orphan_designation/2009/10/WC500006089.pdf*). However, as noted by the EMEA, the following should be kept in mind: "Designated orphan medicinal products are still investigational products which were considered for designation on the basis of potential activity. An orphan designation is not a marketing authorization. As a consequence, demonstration of the quality, safety and efficacy will be necessary before this product can be granted a marketing authorization". A European multicenter phase II/III registrational study in 20 oncology centers for the first-line treatment of inoperable, locally advanced, or metastatic pancreatic cancer is in progress.

Three phase III studies have been initiated [35]. A first-line treatment of locally advanced or metastatic NSCLC comparing LipoPlatin (200 mg/m^2) and paclitaxel (135 mg/m^2, Lipo-Taxol arm) with cisplatin (75 mg/m^2) and paclitaxel (135 mg/m^2, Cis-Taxol arm) was successfully terminated. In total, 236 patients were enrolled in the treatment. Out of 229 patients evaluable, 114 received Lipo-Taxol and 115 were in the Cis-Taxol arm, respectively. Differences in median and overall survival as well as time to progression were not significant. However, patients receiving LipoPlatin showed a better quality of life and the toxicity profile was significantly different in both arms. Neurotoxicity, nausea and vomiting, myelotoxicity, and renal toxicity were lower in LipoPlatin-treated patients. In particular, nephrotoxicity was about 5-fold lower in the Lipo-Taxol arm. In a second phase III clinical trial, LipoPlatin (120 mg/m^2) in combination with gemcitabine (1000 mg/m^2, Lipo/gem arm) was investigated as first-line treatment in NSCLC patients in comparison to cisplatin (100 mg/m^2) plus gemcitabine (1000 mg/m^2, Cis/gem arm). Toxicities were lower in the Lipo/gem arm, especially neuro- and nephrotoxicity. It is also worthwhile mentioning that patients receiving LipoPlatin were treated on an outpatient basis without pre- and posthydration. The third phase III trial is investigating LipoPlatin (100 mg/m^2) in combination with 5-FU (1000 mg/m^2) in comparison to cisplatin (100 mg/m^2) plus 5-FU (1000 mg/m^2) in patients with squamous cell carcinoma of the head and neck (SCCHN). In the case of severe side-effects, dose reduction of cisplatin or 5-FU, but not of LipoPlatin, was performed. Neurotoxicity, mucositis, and nephrotoxicity were to a clinically relevant extent lower in the LipoPlatin arm. Taking into account an increased risk of renal toxicity in advanced SCCHN patients because of a poor hydration, LipoPlatin is an interesting option in these patients. With the aim of improving LipoPlatin's efficacy, an increased dose of LipoPlatin (120 mg/m^2) and a reduced infusion rate were recommended.

49.4.2 LipOxal

LipOxal has recently finished phase I clinical trials [47]. Twenty-seven patients suffering from stage IV gastrointestinal cancers, including colorectal, gastric, and pancreatic cancers, were enrolled in the studies. Patients were treated with LipOxal once weekly over 8 weeks with doses ranging between 100 and 350 mg/m^2. Treatment with 100–250 mg/m^2 LipOxal was not accompanied with serious side-effects. At doses of 300 and 350 mg/m^2, mild myelotoxicity, nausea, and neurotoxicity were observed. In all four patients treated with 350 mg/m^2 LipOxal, peripheral neuropathy was seen. Gastrointestinal tract toxicity was negligible and there was no renal toxicity, hepatotoxicity, cardiotoxicity, or alopecia. The MTD was set as 300 mg/m^2. Three patients out of 27 achieved partial response and 18 patients showed stable disease for 2–9 months. One of the responders had gastric cancer with bone metastasis. In the latter, reduction of bone metastasis and pain was observed. Overall, these results showed that LipOxal is capable of reducing side-effects and maintaining its effectiveness. Several phase II studies with LipOxal as first-line treatment of gastric cancer have been announced (*www.regulon.org*).

49.4.3 ProLindac

A dose-ranging open-label clinical phase I study was performed with ProLindac in Europe enrolling 26 patients [48]. ProLindac was administered intravenously in a 1-h infusion on days 1, 8, and 15 of a 4-week cycle. Doses ranged from 40 to 1280 mg Pt/m^2; the MTD was 640 mg Pt/m^2. Gastrointestinal toxicity (nausea, vomiting, diarrhea, or anorexia) was frequent (92%). Renal toxicity was observed in 35% of cases (elevation of serum creatinine or decreased creatinine clearance), myelosuppression was moderate, three patients had a sensory neuropathy of 1 day duration, and ototoxicity was not reported. Response to treatment was evaluable in 16 patients, two of them obtained a partial response (melanoma and ovarian cancer), three showed disease stabilization (melanoma, esophageal, and ovarian cancer), and one ovarian cancer patient had normalization of the CA-125 biomarker (established specific tumor marker for ovarian cancer).

A phase II clinical trial in Europe has recently been completed with the aim of optimizing dosing and scheduling [41] (*http://www.accesspharma.com/product-programs/prolindac/*). Twenty-six patients with late-stage and multiply pretreated recurrent ovarian cancer with metastases with a platinum-free period of more than 6 months were enrolled. Dose regimens between 900 and 1680 mg Pt/m^2 every 2 or 3 weeks (q2w or q3w) were studied. In patients receiving the highest dose, disease stabilization was observed in 66% of cases; overall 42% of patients showed a significant stabilization. Significant reduction of the CA-125 biomarker in many patients was documented. In contrast to Eloxatin® (oxaliplatin), there was no evidence for acute neurotoxicity. In a number of cases, chronic neurotoxicity was observed. An additional group of eight patients was treated with a new batch of ProLindac originating from an improved scalable production process, proving similar safety and efficacy.

A European multicenter study of ProLindac in combination with paclitaxel in late-stage ovarian cancer patients was announced by Access Pharmaceuticals.

Additionally, together with Asian partners from South Korea and China, further combination clinical studies are in the pipeline and should focus on other indications, such as hepatocellular, pancreatic, and endometrial cancer (among others).

49.5
Conclusions and Perspectives

For decades, platinum complexes have proven to be highly valuable anticancer drugs in clinical routine all over the world. However, platinum-based chemotherapy is accompanied by a set of severe side-effects. Moreover, tumors are inherently resistant or acquire resistance during treatment. During the last 40 years, several thousands of platinum complexes have been synthesized, and investigated with respect to their cytotoxic and tumor inhibiting properties. Since their mode of action (i.e., reaction with nuclear DNA) is in principle very similar, it will be very difficult to find novel candidates for evaluation in clinical trials. One strategy for overcoming these limitations is based on the concept of drug targeting, thereby conserving the cytotoxic properties, but reducing systemic toxicity. A rich series of complexes developed for receptor- or transporter-mediated targeting, or taking advantage of an organ-specific delivery approach has been investigated preclinically. *In vitro* results in cancer cell lines were promising, but unfortunately none of them have yet found their way into clinical trials. However, passive targeting due to the EPR effect has emerged as a delivery approach with great potential. This circumstance is reflected by the successful introduction of LipoPlatin, LipOxal as well as ProLindac into clinical evaluation. In all three cases, established anticancer agents (i.e., cisplatin or oxaliplatin) form the basis as the cytotoxic moiety. In LipoPlatin and LipOxal, cisplatin or oxaliplatin are encapsulated in liposomes; therefore, these agents cannot be classified as novel derivatives. Generally speaking, they are cis- or oxaliplatin formulations. Phase I–III clinical trials have demonstrated that LipoPlatin can be regarded as a safe alternative to cisplatin with markedly reduced adverse effects. In particular, nephrotoxicity was significantly lower during LipoPlatin chemotherapy, allowing an outpatient treatment without pre- and posthydration. In analogy, it was shown in phase I clinical trials that LipOxal is capable of reducing side-effects and, in parallel, maintain its effectiveness. In the case of ProLindac, the cytotoxic moiety of oxaliplatin is bound to a polymer – it is a real oxaliplatin derivative. The requirements for such macromolecular constructs are more challenging, since the platinum fragment has to be released from the polymer via breaking of chemical bonds. One phase II clinical trial was completed; further clinical investigations are announced.

Looking back on these results one might deduce that passive targeting is the strategy of choice with respect to the drug targeting concept. At first sight this seems to be true. However, it would not be the appropriate tactics only to focus on passive targeting. We are convinced that there is enough space for innovative approaches in the arena of active drug targeting.

Acknowledgments

The authors are indebted to the FFG – Austrian Research Promotion Agency (**811591**), the Austrian Council for Research and Technology Development (**IS526001**), the FWF (Austrian Science Fund), and COST D39.

References

1. Rosenberg, B., VanCamp, L., and Krigas, T. (1965) Inhibition of cell division in *Escherichia coli* by electrolysis products from a platinum electrode. *Nature*, **205**, 698–699.
2. Rosenberg, B. (1978) Platinum complexes for the treatment of cancer. *Interdiscip. Sci. Rev.*, **3**, 134–147.
3. Alderden, R.A., Hall, M.D., and Hambley, T.W. (2006) The discovery and development of cisplatin. *J. Chem. Educ.*, **83**, 728–734.
4. Rosenberg, B., VanCamp, L., Trosko, J.E., and Mansour, V.H. (1969) Platinum compounds: a new class of potent antitumour agents. *Nature*, **222**, 385–386.
5. Jakupec, M.A., Galanski, M., and Keppler, B.K. (2003) Tumour-inhibiting platinum complexes – state of the art and future perspectives. *Rev. Physiol. Biochem. Pharmacol.*, **146**, 1–53.
6. O'Dwyer, P.J., Stevenson, J.P., and Johnson, S.W. (2000) Clinical pharmacokinetics and administration of established platinum drugs. *Drugs*, **59** (Suppl. 4), 19–27.
7. Galanski, M., Jakupec, M.A., and Keppler, B.K. (2005) Oxaliplatin and derivatives as anticancer drugs – novel deign strategies in *Metal Compounds in Cancer Chemotherapy* (eds J.M. Pérez, M.A. Fuertes and C. Alonso), Research Signpost, Trivandrum, pp. 155–185.
8. Wheate, N.J., Walker, S., Craig, G.E., and Oun, R. (2010) The status of platinum anticancer drugs in the clinic and in clinical trials. *Dalton Trans.*, **39**, 8113–8127.
9. Galanski, M. (2006) Recent developments in the field of anticancer platinum complexes. *Recent Pat. Anticancer Drug Discov.*, **1**, 285–295.
10. Galanski, M., Jakupec, M.A., and Keppler, B.K. (2005) Update of the preclinical situation of anticancer platinum complexes: novel design strategies and innovative analytical approaches. *Curr. Med. Chem.*, **12**, 2075–2094.
11. Kelland, L. (2007) The resurgence of platinum-based cancer chemotherapy. *Nat. Rev. Cancer*, **7**, 573–584.
12. Reedijk, J. (1999) Why does cisplatin reach guanine-N7 with competing S-donor ligands available in the cell? *Chem. Rev.*, **99**, 2499–2510.
13. Jakupec, M.A., Galanski, M., and Keppler, B.K. (2004) The effect of cytoprotective agents in platinum anticancer theraphy in *Metal Complexes in Tumor Diagnosis and as Anticancer Agents*, Metal Ions in Biological Systems, Vol. **42** (eds A. Sigel and H. Sigel), Dekker, New York, pp. 179–208.
14. Arnesano, F. and Natile, G. (2009) Mechanistic insight into the cellular uptake and processing of cisplatin 30 years after its approval by FDA. *Coord. Chem. Rev.*, **253**, 2070–2081.
15. Wang, D. and Lippard, S.J. (2005) Cellular processing of platinum anticancer drugs. *Nat. Rev. Drug Discov.*, **4**, 307–320.
16. Takahara, P.M., Rosenzweig, A.C., Frederick, C.A., and Lippard, S.J. (1995) Crystal structure of double-stranded DNA containing the major adduct of the anticancer drug cisplatin. *Nature*, **377**, 649–652.
17. Dufrasne, F. and Galanski, M. (2007) The relation between stereochemistry and biological activity of platinum(II) complexes chelated with chiral diamine ligands: an intricate problem. *Curr. Pharm. Des.*, **13**, 2781–2794.
18. Hall, M.D., Mellor, H.R., Callaghan, R., and Hambley, T.W. (2007) Basis for design and development of platinum(IV)

anticancer complexes. *J. Med. Chem.*, **50**, 3403–3411.

19. Top, S., Bachir Kaloun, E., Vessières, A., Leclercq, G., Laïos, I., Ourevitch, M., Deuschel, C., McGlinchey, M.J., and Jaouen, G. (2003) Tamoxifen derivatives for delivery of the antitumoral (DACH)Pt group: selective synthesis by McMurry coupling, and biochemical behaviour. *ChemBioChem*, **4**, 754–761.
20. Xia, W. and Low, P.S. (2010) Folate-targeted therapies for cancer. *J. Med. Chem.*, **53**, 6811–6824.
21. Aronov, O., Horowitz, A.T., Gabizon, A., and Gibson, D. (2003) Folate-targeted PEG as a potential carrier for carboplatin analogs. Synthesis and *in vitro* studies. *Bioconjug. Chem.*, **14**, 563–574.
22. Ohya, Y., Nagatomi, K., and Ouchi, T. (2001) Synthesis and cytotoxic activity of macromolecular prodrug of cisplatin using poly(ethylene glycol) with galactose residues or antennary galactose units. *Macromol. Biosci.*, **1**, 355–363.
23. Marin, J.J.G., Romero, M.R., Vallejo, M., and Monte, M.J. (2005) Targeting of cytostatic bile acid derivatives toward tumours of the enterohepatic circuit. *Cancer Ther.*, **3**, 57–64.
24. Dominguez, M.F., Macias, R.I.R., Izco-Basurko, I., de la Fuente, A., Pascual, M.J., Criado, J.M., Monte, M.J., Yajeya, J., and Marin, J.J.G. (2001) Low *in vivo* toxicity of a novel cisplatin-ursodeoxycholic derivative (Bamet-UD2) with enhanced cytostatic activity versus liver tumors. *J. Pharmacol. Exp. Ther.*, **297**, 1106–1112.
25. Briz, O., Angeles Serrano, M., Rebollo, N., Hagenbuch, B., Meier, P.J., Koepsell, H., and Marin, J.J.G. (2002) Carriers involved in targeting the cytostatic bile acid-cisplatin derivatives *cis*-diammine-chlorocholylglycinate-platinum(II) and *cis*-diammine-bisursodeoxycholateplatinum(II) toward liver cells. *Mol. Pharmacol.*, **61**, 853–860.
26. Monte, M.J., Ballestero, M.R., Briz, O., Perez, M.J., and Marin, J.J.G. (2005) Proapoptotic effect on normal and tumor intestinal cells of cytostatic drugs with enterohepatic organotropism. *J. Pharmacol. Exp. Ther.*, **315**, 24–35.
27. Ott, I. and Gust, R. (2007) Preclinical and clinical studies on the use of platinum complexes for breast cancer treatment. *Anticancer Agents Med. Chem.*, 7, 95–110.
28. Galanski, M. and Keppler, B.K. (2007) Searching for the magic bullet: anticancer platinum drugs which can be accumulated or activated in the tumor tissue. *Anticancer Agents Med. Chem.*, **7**, 55–73.
29. Gabano, E., Ravera, M., and Osella, D. (2009) The drug targeting and delivery approach applied to Pt–antitumour complexes. A coordination point of view. *Curr. Med. Chem.*, **16**, 4544–4580.
30. Harper, B.W., Krause-Heuer, A.M., Grant, M.P., Manohar, M., Garbutcheon-Singh, K.B., and Aldrich-Wright, J.R. (2010) Advances in platinum chemotherapeutics. *Chem. Eur. J.*, **16**, 7064–7077.
31. Klenner, T., Wingen, F., Keppler, B.K., Krempien, B., and Schmaehl, D. (1990) Anticancer-agent-linked phosphonates with antiosteolytic and antineoplastic properties: a promising perspective in the treatment of bone-related malignancies? *J. Cancer Res. Clin. Oncol.*, **116**, 341–350.
32. Klenner, T., Valenzuela-Paz, P., Amelung, F., Muench, H., Zahn, H., Keppler, B.K., and Blum, H. (1993) Platinum phosphonato complexes with particular activity bone malignancies. Evaluation of an experimental tumor model highly predictive for the clinical situation in *Metal Complexes in Cancer Chemotherapy*, (ed. B.K. Keppler), Wiley-VCH Verlag GmbH, Weinheim, pp. 85–127.
33. Galanski, M., Slaby, S., Jakupec, M.A., and Keppler, B.K. (2003) Synthesis, characterization and *in vitro* antitumor activity of osteotropic diam(m)ineplatinum(II) complexes bearing a *N,N'*-bis(phosphonomethyl)glycine ligand. *J. Med. Chem.*, **46**, 4946–4951.
34. Matsumura, Y. and Maeda, H.A. (1986) New concept for macromolecular therapeutics in cancer chemotherapy: mechanism of tumoritropic accumulation of proteins and the antitumor agent SMANCS. *Cancer Res.*, **46**, 6387–6392.

35. Boulikas, T. (2009) Clinical overview on Lipoplatin™: a successful liposomal formulation of cisplatin. *Expert Opin. Investig. Drugs*, **18**, 1197–1218.
36. Boulikas, T., Pantos, A., Bellis, E., and Christofis, P. (2007) Designing platinum compounds in cancer: structures and mechanisms. *Cancer Ther.*, **5**, 537–583.
37. Regulon (2009) *LipoPlatin as a Trojan Horse for Cancer: Evidence that LipoPlatin Nanoparticles Fuse with, and Enter also by Phagocytosis through, the Cell Membrane [Press Release]*, Regulon, Mountain View, CA.
38. Devarajan, P., Tarabishi, R., Mishra, J., Ma, Q., Kourvetaris, A., Vougiouka, M., and Boulikas, T. (2004) Low renal toxicity of Lipoplatin compared to cisplatin in animals. *Anticancer Res.*, **24**, 2193–2200.
39. Boulikas, T. (2007) Molecular mechanisms of cisplatin and its liposomally encapsulated form, Lipoplatin™. Lipoplatin™ as a chemotherapy and antiangiogenesis drug. *Cancer Ther.*, **5**, 349–376.
40. Rihova, B. (2007) Biocompatibility and immunocompatibility of water-soluble polymers based on HPMA. *Composites B*, **38**, 386–397.
41. Nowotnik, D.P. and Cvitkovic, E. (2009) ProLindac (AP5346): a review of the development of an HPMA DACH platinum polymer therapeutic. *Adv. Drug Deliv. Rev.*, **61**, 1214–1219.
42. Sood, P., Bruce Thurmond, K., Jacob, J.E., Waller, L.K., Silva, G.O., Stewart, D.R., and Nowotnik, D.P. II (2006) Synthesis and characterization of AP5346, a novel polymer-linked diaminocyclohexyl platinum chemotherapeutic agent. *Bioconjug. Chem.*, **17**, 1270–1279.
43. Rice, J.R., Gerberich, J.L., Nowotnik, D.P., and Howell, S.B. (2006) Preclinical efficacy and pharmacokinetics of AP5346, a novel diaminocyclohexane-platinum tumor-targeting drug delivery system. *Clin. Cancer Res.*, **12**, 2248–2254.
44. Boulikas, T., Stathopoulos, G.P., Volakakis, N., and Vougiouka, M. (2005) Systemic lipoplatin infusion results in preferential tumor uptake in human studies. *Anticancer Res.*, **25**, 3031–3039.
45. Froudarakis, M.E., Pataka, A., Pappas, P., Anevlavis, S., Argiana, E., Nikolaidou, M., Kouliatis, G., Pozova, S., Marselos, M., and Bouros, D. (2008) Phase 1 trial of lipoplatin and gemcitabine as a second-line chemotherapy in patients with nonsmall cell lung carcinoma. *Cancer*, **113**, 2752–2760.
46. Koukourakis, M.I., Giatromanolaki, A., Pitiakoudis, M., Kouklakis, G., Tsoutsou, P., Abatzoglou, I., Panteliadou, M., Sismanidou, K., Sivridis, E., and Boulikas, T. (2010) Concurrent liposomal cisplatin (Lipoplatin), 5-fluorouracil and radiotherapy for the treatment of locally advanced gastric cancer: a phase I/II study. *Int. J. Radiat Oncol. Biol. Phys.*, **78**, 150–155.
47. Stathopoulos, G.P., Boulikas, T., Kourvetaris, A., and Stathopoulos, J. (2006) Liposomal oxaliplatin in the treatment of advanced cancer: a phase I study. *Anticancer Res.*, **26**, 1489–1493.
48. Campone, M., Rademaker-Lakhai, J.M., Bennouna, J., Howell, S.B., Nowotnik, D.P., Beijnen, J.H., and Schellens, J.H.M. (2007) Phase I and pharmacokinetic trial of AP5346, a DACH–platinum–polymer conjugate, administered weekly for three out of every 4 weeks to advanced solid tumor patients. *Cancer Chemother. Pharmacol.*, **60**, 523–533.

Index

Drug Delivery in Oncology: From Basic Research to Cancer Therapy, First Edition.
Edited by Felix Kratz, Peter Senter, and Henning Steinhagen.

acute lymphoblastic leukemia (ALL) 3
acute lymphocytic leukemia (ALL) 105
acute myeloid leukemia (AML) 96
acyclization-based SIL 556
acyl hydrazone-based conjugates 1299
acyl tail dynamics
– lipid 999
adaptors
– chemical 573
ADC (apparent diffusion coefficient) 35, 54
ADCC (antibody-dependent cellular cytotoxicity) 47, 292
ADCs 108
addition
– Michael-type 559
adducts
– platinum–DNA 1035
adeno-associated virus (AAV) 1426, 1433
adenocarcinomas 1457
adenovirus serotype 5 (Ad5) 1500
adenoviruses 1392, 1400
– oncolytic 1431
ADEPT (antibody-directed enzyme prodrug therapy) 6, 16, 17, 34, 951
– two-phase clinical trials 25
adhesion molecule
– epithelial cell 960
adjuvant bisphosphate therapy 807
administration 951
– antibody-targeted liposomal drugs 951
– combination chemotherapy 1022
adrenocortical tumors
– imaging 279
AEC 18
aerosolized liposomal paclitaxel 970
AEZS-108 1235
affinity
– antibodies 21
AFM13 469
agents 1013
– alkylating 34
– amphipathic 1041
– anti-MDR 1026
– antiangiogenic 599
– anticancer 45, 747, 763
– antineoplastic 276
– bifunctional chelating 92
– chain transfer 266
– chemically incompatible 1026
– complexation 253
– contrast 276, 1063
– conventional anticancer 7
– DNA-damaging 94
– hydrophobic 1040
– intravenously injected 328
– microtubule-stabilizing 24
– molecularly targeted 808
– NO-releasing 78
– radioimmunoscintigraphy 417
– radionuclide delivery 423
– reactive 1033
– surface stabilizing 1041
– therapeutic 443
aggregation
– liposomes 1005
aglycone functionality
– enediyne 95
AGM (aminogluthetimine) 820
AIDS-related Kaposi's sarcoma 919, 922
AIF (apoptosis-inducing factor) 1453, 1470
alanine transaminase 1542
albondin 792
albumin 747, 1099
– bovine serum 566, 1123
– carrier 786
– cationized 1501
– CBSA 1138, 1504
– cross-linked matrix 1136
– drug conjugates 772
– Evans blue– 73
– human serum 750, 862, 1133, 1323
– lactosaminated 1532
– microspheres 761
– mouse serum 90
– nab technologies 895, 1136
– nanoparticles 895, 1133, 1150
– serum 85
– synthetic approaches 759
– transcytosis 1134
– zzz 763
albumin-based nanoparticles
– clinical studies 1152
albumin-binding domain (ABD) 107
albumin-conjugated PEGylated nanoparticles
– cationic 1149
alemtuzumab 292
alendronate (ALN) 823, 825
alginate–drug conjugates 730
aliphatic anchors 1043
aliphatic systems
– releasable PEG linkers 649
alkylating agents 34
alkylating lysines 298
alkylation
– reductive 633
alkylator
– DNA 1336
ALL (acute lymphoblastic leukemia) 3

ALL (acute lymphocytic leukemia) 105, 107
alternative scaffolds 431
amides 1219
– amide/amino-derived linkages 646
– aromatic 1340
– spontaneous ring-closure 557
amino acids 12
– ω-amino fatty acids 1249
– metabolism 37
– transport imaging 257
– zwitterionic residue 77
amino groups
– lysine 1578
aminoacyl-tRNAs 1459
aminogluthetimine (AGM) 820
aminolysis 258
aminopeptidase P2 (APP2) 342
aminopolysaccharides 717
amiRNA 1421
AML (acute myeloid leukemia) 400
amlodipine 1026
ammonia ligands 1607
amphipathic drugs 909
amphipathic peptides
– Pep-3 1197
amphipathic surface stabilizing agents 1041
amphiphilic block copolymers 1103
amphiphilic polymers 627
– self-assembly 1078
AN-152 1235
– chromophore-labeled 1227
– fluorophore-labeled 1227
– structure 1224
AN-162 1239
AN-238 1238
analysis 1283
– analytical completeness 337, 338
– biodistribution 343
– retro-synthetic 1288
– western 339
anastomosis
– vessel 591
anatomic information
– coregistration 282
anatomy of BBB 1490
anchors
– aliphatic 1043
anemia 52
angiogenesis 36
– basic principles 34
– cytotoxic somatostatin analogs 1237
– imaging 260
– liver cancer 1551
– schematic representation 592
– tumors 13, 65, 591
angiogenic cascade 34
angiogenic factors 1419
angiogenic markers 1443
– dual targeting 616
– potential 596
angiogenic proteins 35
angiogenin 1453
angiographic arterial infusion 71
angiotensin II 75
angiotensin II-converting enzyme (ACE) 79
angiotensin-converting proteins 341
animal studies
– albumin-based nanoparticles 1139
anionic phospholipids 1373
AnnA1 knockout mice 65
Annexin-A1 (AnnA1) 344
antagonistic analogs
– GHRH 1249
antagonists 1219
– bombesin/GRP 1219
– GHRH 1247
Antennapedia protein
– Drosophila 1189
anthracycline-based regimen 12
anthracyclines 929, 933
anthrax toxin 1450, 1465
anti-ASNase antibodies 631
anti-CEA monoclonal antibody
– murine 25
anti-CEA scFv–Fc variants 99
anti-HER2 liposomes
– Fab¢ fragments 958
anti-HER2 mAb 957
anti-MDR agent
– amlodipine 1026
anti-mouse antibody
– human 111
anti-murine antibody
– human 455
anti-PEG Ig-mAb 79
antiangiogenesis 617
antiangiogenic agents 599
antiangiogenic approved therapies 593
antiapoptotic proteins 1228
antibiotics 1519
– benzoquinone ansamycin 605
– chromophore dienediyne 1543
antibodies 5
– ADCs 110
– ADEPT 19
– affinity 21, 100
– anti-ASNase 631

antibodies (*contd.*)
– anti-PEG Ig-mAb 79
– antibody–toxin conjugates 14
– antienzyme 22
– binding 7
– BsAbs 430, 483
– caveolae-dependent trafficking 329
– chimeric 292, 444
– clinical trials of ADCs 14
– conjugated 449
– delivery agents 423
– DiBi mini- 459
– dimeric domain 457
– effector functions 291, 293
– empowered 49
– engineered fragments 424, 425
– fluorescently labeled 331
– HAMA 455
– hetero-oligomeric 455
– human anti-mouse 111
– humanized 414, 444
– indirect photosensitizer-linker-mAb conjugates 1580
– intact 424, 425
– loaded 111
– marketed therapeutic 445
– monoclonal 24
– neutralizing 1459
– nucleosome-specific 961
– photosensitizer targeting 1575
– radiolabeled 412
– radionuclide delivery 411
– TandAb 469
– targeting ligands 1381
– targeting moieties 1205
– therapeutic agents 443
– "two-in-one" 453
antibody fragments
– PEGylated 634
antibody-based macromolecular systems 37
antibody-dependent binding 1203
antibody-dependent cellular cytotoxicity (ADCC) 38, 432
antibody-directed enzyme prodrug therapy (ADEPT) 17
antibody-mediated long-circulating liposome 955
antibody-modified liposomes 962
antibody-targeted chemotherapy 94
antibody-targeted liposomal drugs 968
antibody-targeted liposomes 954, 956
antibody–drug conjugates (ADCs) 450
– auristatin-based 305, 309
– calicheamicin-based 94, 253
– cancer therapy 295
– cytotoxic 72
– linker technologies 69
– most successful 86
– pharmacokinetics 300
antibody–maytansinoid conjugates (AMCs) 375
– activation 385
– clinical trials 384
– structure 378
anticancer agents 1013
– carriers 747
– complexation 253
– extravasation 45
– LDL 763
– serum albumin 763
– structure 7
– transferrin 763
anticancer combination therapy
– fixed ratio 1014
anticancer drugs
– categories 5
anticancer formulations
– liposomal 1007
anticancer liposomal drugs 954
anticancer platinum complexes 1605
antienzyme antibodies 22
antiestrogens 1612
antifolates 4
antigen 1163
– carcinoembryonic 19, 99, 425, 1167
– CD19 958
– hematopoietic 95
– prostate-specific 562
– PSMA 295
– target 295
antigen presentation
– FcRn 93
antigen-binding domain 86, 1447
antigen-mediated processing 385
– efficiency 387
antimetabolites 34
antineoplastic activity
– inherent 1195
antineoplastic agents 275
antineoplastic cargo 1192
antineoplastic platinum complexes 853
antinuclear autoantibodies (AnA) 961
– nucleosome interachtion 964
antiproliferative effect 952
– Bac-ELP-p21 688
– Pen-ELP-H1 686
antiretroviral therapy
– HAART 921

antisense oligonucleotides 543
antisense strand phosphorylation 1365
antitumor activity
– paclitaxel and TXP 1340
antitumor drugs
– pH dependence 56
antiviral approach 1419
APA-AST microcapsules 1088
APN 598
APN-targeted polymer therapeutics 613
apoptosis 43, 1445
– assays 269
– CD20 cells 268
– IAP 1200
– inhibitor of 1330
– liver cancer 1551
apoptosis-inducing factor (AIF) 1453, 1470
apoptotic sensor
– PhiPhiLux 259
APP2 (aminopeptidase P2) 342
apparent diffusion coefficient (ADC) 35, 45
applications 1263
– aptamer conjugates 1263
– biologic 1164
– CPPs 1190
– drug delivery systems 1022
– in vivo 1275
– PEGylated liposomes 939
– RNAi 1415
– SPECT/CT and PET/CT 272
– theranostic 1180
– therapeutic 1383
approved therapies
– antiangiogenic 593
aptamer conjugates 1263
– applications 1269
– toxicology 1276
aptamer–chimeric RNA 1274
aptamer–DOX conjugates 1270
aptamer–siRNA chimeras 1379
aptamers 1448
– isolation 1265
– secondary structure 1264
– targeted delivery 1266
– targeting ligands 1381
Ara-C (cytosine arabinoside) 651
– PEG– 652, 653
arabinogalactan–drug conjugates 732
arabinoside
– cytosine 651
architectures
– supramolecular 735
area under the time–plasma concentration curve (AUC) 891
arming
– CNTs 1167
aromatic amides 1339
aromatic systems
– releasable PEG linkers 646
arterial infusion
– angiographic 71
arteriovenous shunt perfusion 37
artificial microRNA 1421
artificial red blood cells 1062
ASGP (asialoglycoprotein) 1524
asialoglycoprotein (ASGP) 232, 730, 1524
asparagine (ASN) 630
aspartate transaminase 1542
aspergillins 1453
assays 1053
– apoptosis 269
– micropanning 16
– molecular imaging 52
assemblies
– block copolymer 1060
astrocytes 1491
astrocytomas
– temozolomide therapy 37
athymic nude mice 1229, 1247
ATP-binding cassette (ABC) transporters 1493, 1494
AUC (area under the time–plasma concentration curve) 891
Auger electrons 419
– emitters 423
Aureobasidium pullulans 730
auristatin 258
auristatin E 73, 79
– trigger group 583
auristatin-based ADCs 305, 309
autoantibodies
– antinuclear 961, 964
autophagy 1445
Au–Ag nanorods 1272
avascular growth phase 34
Avastin 473
azomethine ylides 1166

b

b emitters 421
B lymphocytes 413
b-glycerophosphat 1079
b-lactamase 828
b-lactamase–peptide fusion ligands 5
B-lymphoma xenografts 103
Bac-ELP-p21 685
– polypeptides 688

Bac-ELP1-H1 693
– rhodamine-labeled 695
Bac-ELP1-p21 689
backbone degradable polymer carriers 263
bacterial toxins 1462, 1464
bacterial vectors 1398, 1401
bacteriochlorin 1592
bacteriophages 3
Bamet-UD2 1613, 1614
barrier 887
– biological 887
– blood–brain 534
– to cancer development 53
– endothelial 1140
– steric 992
base pairing
– Watson–Crick 1415
BBB (blood–brain barrier) 534
– albumin–drug nanoparticles 1138
– alterations in brain tumors 1495
– anatomy 1490
– CNS targeting 1489
– CPPs 1193, 1208
– drug transporters 1492
BCAs (bifunctional chelating agents) 68
Bcl-2 1200
beacon
– photodynamic molecular 1588
benign tumors 272
benzoquinone ansamycin antibiotic 605
benzyl elimination 559
– amide/amino-derived linkages 646
– thiophenol derivatives 567
β-ligand conjugates
– releasable 1301
bevacizumab 1145
bidirectional transport
– IgG 91
Bifidobacterium 1401
bifunctional chelating agents (BCAs) 68
bilayer membrane structures
– closed 990
bilayers
– concentric 890
bilirubin
– serum 102
binding 1189
– antibody-dependent 7, 1203
– CD30-specific 1470
– cross-species 111
– drugs to polymer carriers 250
– FcRn 95
– nucleosome 964
– nucleotide 542
– specificity 961
binding pockets
– hydrophobic 1264
biocatalytic activation 564
bioconjugation properties 281
biodegradability 1163
– CNTs 1163
– hydrogels 1072
– micelles 1113
– polymers 739, 844
biodistribution 951
– analysis 343
– Fab4D5 108
– IT-101 736
– liposomes 970
– PEG-coated SWNTs 1176
– pretherapy 434
– trastuzumab 108
bioengineering
– molecular 695
biologic applications
– CNTs 1164
biologic persistence
– CNTs 1169
biological barriers 888
biological half-life
– targeted toxins 1459
biology
– cancer 13
bioluminescence 35, 51
biomarker imaging 41
biomarkers 1359
– cancer 33
– common 43
– hematological 33
– imaging 34
– PET/CT 250
– prognostic potential 273
– SPECT/CT 258
biopanning 6
biopolymers
– elastin-like 678
biorecognition 99
– molecular 268
biosynthesis
– eicosanoids 1326
biotin 1121
– structure 1304
biotin–drug conjugate design 1304
biotin–streptavidin linker 33
biotinylation 333
biotransformation
– CNTs 1177

biphasic elimination 738
Bis-AzoPC 1004
bispecific antibodies (BsAbs) 450, 483
– clinical trials 464, 465
– dual action 452, 471
– radionuclide delivery 430
– recombinant IgG-like 460
– single-chain 457
bispecific molecules
– recombinant 457
bispecific targeted toxins 1450
bispecific T-cell engager (BiTE) 464
bisphosphate therapy
– adjuvant 807
bivalent binding 453
bivatuzumab mertansine 297
BL22 1477
bladder cancers 1219
– cytotoxic somatostatin analogs 1219
– urinary 1231
bleeding tendency 19
bleomycin 921
block copolymers 1099
– amphiphilic 1099
– assemblies 1060
– micellar structures 1053
– MPEG–HPAE 1106
– PEO/PPO 675
– self-assembly 1054
blocking of FcRn-recycling 102
blood 951
– activity curves 97
– composition 748
– high pressure 75
– pharmaceutical nanocarriers 952
– proteins 747
– vessels 34, 911
blood cells
– artificial 1062
blood flow
– tumors 37
blood pH 1100
blood-borne delivery 43
blood–brain barrier (BBB) 534
– albumin–drug nanoparticles 1138
– anatomy 1490
– CNS targeting 1489
– CPPs 1193, 1208
– drug transporters 1492
BMC (methyl-β-cyclodextrin) 1141
BODIPY-ivermectin 1494
bolus 915
bombardment
– particle 1371, 1401
bombesin-releasing peptide 1244
– receptors 1244
bombesin/GRP antagonists 1244
bonds 1361
– cis double 1361
– cleavable 247
– disulfide 1002
– hydrazone 258
– thioether 258, 273
– unsymmetrical disulfide 1295
bone marrow 96
bone marrow-derived myeloid cells 34
bone metastases
– SPECT/CT 277
bone tumors
– primary 1614
boron neutron capture therapy (BNCT) 276, 538
boronated PAMAM dendrimer 538
bortezomib 908
bovine serum albumin (BSA) 566, 1123
– cationic 1138, 1504
bow-tie dendrimer 526
BR96–doxorubicin 95
bradykinin 79
brain metastases 432
brain tumors 1489
– BBB alterations 1489
– cytotoxic somatostatin analogs 1241
branched elimination linkers 573
branched galactose units 714
branched subunits 278
branching 275
– aberrant 693
– structural motif 514
breaking point
– predetermined 555, 874
breast cancer 929
– cytotoxic somatostatin analogs 1238
– LHRH cytotoxic analogs 1229
– metastatic 930
– PLD 916, 930
brentuximab vedotin 259
BSA (bovine serum albumin) 566, 1123
BsAbs (bispecific antibodies) 450, 464, 483
– clinical trials 465
– dual action 452, 471
– formats 454
– radionuclide delivery 430
– recombinant IgG-like 460
– single-chain 457
budding
– vesicular 329

building blocks 573
– NIPAAm 671
bypass
– BBB 1509
bystander effect 1397
– antigen-mediated processing 388

c
c-Myc inhibtor 684, 687
C-terminal tail
– cytoplasmic 1222
C-type lectins 596
cachexia 753
cadherin
– vascular endothelial 1179
Caenorhabditis elegans 1416
calcium phosphate
– lipid-coated 1379
calicheamicin 1283
– ADCs 93, 248
– discovery 95
– prodrug 75
camelids 463
camptothecin (CPT) 251, 762, 1305, 1334
– analogs 641
– MAG–CPT 852
– PEG–CPT 855, 856
– polymer-based combination therapy 809
– polysaccharide–drug conjugation 713
CanAg antigen 382
canalization 35
cancer 952
– biology 13
– biomarkers 33
– breast 929
– development barriers 38
– drug categories 5
– hormone-dependent 807
– human experimental 1228
– limits of conventional chemotherapy 34
– liver 1520
– metabolism and proliferation 36
– neuroendocrine 271
– NSCLC 27, 851, 1623
– ovarian 854, 925
– polymer-based combination therapy 805
– pre-antibody era 442
– progression and control 1324
– prostate 65
– PUFAs cell lines 1331
– staging 273
– thyroid 278
– zzz 278
cancer chemotherapy
– tumor-targeted liposomes 955
cancer gene therapy
– vectors 1398
cancer stem cells (CSCs) 95
cancer therapeutic agents
– molecularly targeted 808
cancer therapy 1163
– ADCs 295
– CNT constructs 1168
– empowered antibodies 46
– hyperthermia 668
– poloxamers 676
– targeted 1263
cancer-targeting ligands 3, 14
cancer-targeting ligand–drug conjugates 27
cancer-targeting peptides 6
– cell-penetrating 1189
capan-1 human pancreatic tumor xenograft model 1034
capillaries
– cerebral 1491
caplostatin 822
carbodiimides 708, 760
carbohydrate-based spacers 1293
carbon nanotubes (CNTs) 546, 1163, 1180
– arming 1167
– biodegradability 1169
– biologic applications 1164
– biotransformation 1177
– cancer therapy constructs 1168
– chemistry 1164
– drug delivery systems 896
– environmental concerns 1171
– interactions with cells and tissues 1168
– MWNT 546, 896, 1165
– PEGylation 1173
– pharmacokinetics 1170, 1173
– properties 1163
– SWNT 896, 1165
– toxicity 1170
carboplatin 829, 860, 1344, 1605
carboplatin–folate conjugates 1612
carboxy groups
– activated 1312
carboxylic groups
– immunoglobulins 969
carboxymethyl-Dex (CM-Dex) 713
carboxymethyl-pullulan (CM-Pul) 730
carboxypeptidases 34
– G2 (CPG2) 4, 20
carcinoembryonic antigen (CEA) 18, 425, 1167
– anti-CEA scFv–Fc variants 99

– monoclonal antibodies 24
carcinogenesis
– siRNA/miRNA 1361
cardiotoxicity 20, 608, 918
care
– supportive 25
carriers 1099
– albumin 786
– anticancer agents 747
– colloidal 1099
– hepatotropic 1532
– macromolecular 684
– multifunctional polymeric 249
– nanoparticulate 952
– nanosized 1523
– passive 1575
– polymeric 99, 264, 812, 839, 841
– reduced folate 1284
– site-specific 951
– temperature-sensitive 674
– thermo-responsive ELP 692
cascade
– angiogenic 34
cascade polymer 540
catabolism
– maytansinoids 303
cathepsin 40, 554
cathepsin B 876, 877
catheter
– PICC 6
cationic albumin-conjugated PEGylated nanoparticles 1149
cationic BSA 1138, 1504
cationic lipids/liposomes 1371
cationic polymers 1373
cationized albumin 1501
caveolae 329
caveolae-dependent trafficking of antibodies 329
caveolae-mediated transcellular delivery 1057
caveolar transport 1134
caveolin-1 knockout mice 330
cavities
– dendritic 256
CBI (cyclopropabenzindol-4-one) 67
CBR (clinical benefit rate) 932
CC531 960
CD13 613
CD19 antigen 958
CD20 cells
– apoptosis 269
CD22 102
CD30-specific binding 1470
CD33
– hematopoietic antigen 96
CD44 598, 724
CDC (complement-dependent cytotoxicity) 291
CDDP (cisplatin) 714, 829, 939, 1035, 1605, 1608
CDK (cyclin-dependent kinase) 1201
cDNA 1418
CDP (cyclodextrin-containing polycation) 1375
CEA (carcinoembryonic antigen) 18, 425
– anti-CEA scFv–Fc variants 99
– monoclonal antibodies 24
CEA (carcinogenic embryonic antigen) 1167
CED (convection enhanced delivery) 538
cell adhesion molecule (EpCAM) 464
cell cycle 11
– modulation 1198
– phases 11
cell delivery 1087
cell penetration 995
– triggerable 995
cell-based SELEX 1265
cell-binding domain 1447
cell-penetrating peptides (CPP) 1189
– applications 1189
– cancer targeting 1189
– cell cycle modulation 1198
– cellular uptake 681
– delivery vectors 1208
– internalization routes 1190
– intracellular delivery 680
– oncogenic signaling 1198
– RNA inteference 1365
– sequences 1191
– targeted toxins 1443, 1456
– targeting 1202, 1381
– TAT 1113
cell-penetrating small molecules 534
cell-targeting reactivity 993
cells 1053
– artificial 1053
– bone marrow-derived myeloid 34
– cancer stem 95
– CD20 269
– Daudi 470
– death 1445
– dividing 17
– endothelial 66, 332, 591
– hematopoietic 93
– hypoxic 267
– interactions with CNTs 1168
– Kupffer 1366

cells (*contd.*)
– living 1265
– log/fractional cell kill 14
– MX-1 1135
– neoplastic 236
– neovasculature 595
– NK 449
– proteome 336
– triggered targeting 995
– tumor-initiating 111
cellular cytotoxicity
– antibody-dependent 291
cellular proliferation 35, 685
cellular structure
– MRI 44
cellular transport 1300
cellular uptake 1133
– CPPs 681
– macromolecules 112
cell–cell contacts 35
cell–cell junction
– endothelial 72
central nervous system (CNS) 1138
– liposomal drug delivery 1502
– polymer nanoparticles 1505
– targeting 1489
cerebral capillaries 1491
cervical tumor hypoxia 41
CEUS (contrast enhanced ultrasound) 49
CFPAC-1 tumor xenograft 1348
chain reaction 1415
– dendritic 570
– polymerase 1416
chain transfer agent (CTA) 266
chains
– surface-grafted 992
chaotic microcirculation
– tumors 43
chaotic microvasculature 65
charged dendrimers 535
chelate-functionalized SWNTs 1176
chelating agents
– bifunctional 92
chelators 421
chemical adaptors 573
chemical conjugation 1271
chemical cross-linking 1074
chemical modification strategies 1362
chemical stability
– siRNA/miRNA 1365
chemical vectors 1371
chemical warfare 3
chemically incompatible agents 1026
chemically labile linkers 72
chemistry 1163
– and architecture 278
– CNTs 1164
– cross-linking 70
– linkage site 70
– polysaccharide–drug conjugation 707
chemoembolization
– transarterial 1521
chemotherapeutics 325
– cytotoxins 3
– growth factor targeted delivery 1311
– platinum-based combination 37
– PUFAs 1323
– temperature-sensitive carriers 674
chemotherapy 951
– calicheamicin ADCs 94
– combination 806, 1013
– cytotoxic 4, 121
– first-line/second-line 13
– HCC 1522
– limits 34
– proliferation imaging 266
– tumor hypoxia 51
– tumor-targeted liposomes 955
CHEMS (cholesteryl hemisuccinate) 998, 1377
chimeras 1361
– aptamer–siRNA 1361
– fiber/knob 1432
chimeric (mouse/human) mAb 239
chimeric antibodies 444
chimeric anti-CD52 antibody 292
chimeric RNA
– aptamer– 1274
chitin 717
chitosan 1079, 1084, 1374
chitosan-coated nanoparticles 894
chitosan–drug conjugates 717
– N-succinyl-chitosan derivatives 722
chlorambucil 1336
cholesterol 889, 1371, 1580
– conjugation 1275
– plasma 753
cholesterol paclitaxel prodrug nanoparticles 1042
cholesteryl hemisuccinate (CHEMS) 968, 1377
cholesterylhexadecyl ether (CHE) 1041
CHOP regime 442
choroid plexus epithelium 1503
chromophores 1178
– chromophore-labeled AN-152 1227
– dienediyne antibiotic 1543
chronic hepatitis 1519

chylomicrons 751
cilengitide 603
cintredekin besudotox 1479
circulating half-life
– aptamer conjugates 1275
circulating time
– liposomes 956
circulation
– enterohepatic 1613
circulation lifetime
– hydrophobic drugs 1041
cirrhotic livers 1542
cis-aconityl linkage 721
cis-double bonds 1372
cisplatin (CDDP) 714, 829, 1035
– discovery 1605
– mode of action 1608
– PEGylated liposomal formulations 939
cisplatin/irinotecan 1021, 1035
cleavable bond 101
cleavable conjugates 387
cleavable linkers 299
– intracellularly 79
– on-demand 26
cleavable prodrugs 951
– enzymatically 527
– half-lives 562
cleavage 951
– enzymatic 25
– glycosidase-based 71
– reductive 26
– thiol–disulfide exchange 379, 388
"click chemistry" 263
clinical applications 951
– liposomes 951
– local jet-injection 1407
– self-immolative linkers 582
– SPECT/CT and PET/CT 272
clinical benefit rate (CBR) 932
clinical development 1219
– GHRH antagonistic analogs 1219
– LHRH cytotoxic analogs 1235
– LipoPlatin 1622, 1623
– liposome formulations 1006
– LipOxal 1624
– liver tumor targeting 1550
– PDT 1591
– polymer-based combination therapy 816
– ProLindac 1625
– radioimmunoimaging 431
– RIT 434
– serum proteins 788
– targeted toxins 1472
clinical experience
– drug–polymer conjugates 839
clinical oncology 35
clinical practice
– imaging techniques 23
clinical studies 1133
– albumin-based nanoparticles 1133
– CombiPlex® formulations 1036
– CPX-1/CPX-351 1036, 1038
clinical trials 951
– ADCs 14
– ADEPT 16
– AMCs 384
– anticancer liposomal drugs 954
– BsAbs 464, 465
– drug–polymer conjugates 847, 848
– effector function-enhanced antibodies 293
– gene therapy 1402
– "Gene Therapy Clinical Trials Worldwide" 1431
– INNO-206 864
– liver tumors 1550
– local gene delivery 1395
– micellar structures 1055
– PEG prodrugs 855
– PEG–drug conjugates 653, 654
– PGA 858
– phase I 1038
– phase II 1039
– Pseudomonas aeruginosa exotoxin A 1474
– recombinant bispecific molecules 464
– RIP 1475
– RNAi 1384, 1417
– siRNA/miRNA 1383
– targeted diphtheria toxin 1473
– targeted protein toxins 1476
– two-phase 26
clinical tumor imaging 247
cloaking 536
clodronate 1616
clonal selection 49
closed bilayer membrane structures 990
Clostridium 1401
CLRX101 866
cluster effect 1613
CM-Chit (carboxymethyl-chitin) 719
CM-Dex (carboxymethyl-Dex) 713
CM-Pul (carboxymethyl-pullulan) 730
CMC (critical micelle concentration) 892
CMC-544 102, 107
– clinical development 110
CMDA 25
CMV (cytomegalovirus) promoter 1424

CNS (central nervous system) 1138
– liposomal drug delivery 1502
– polymer nanoparticles 1505
– targeting 1489
CNTs (carbon nanotubes) 546, 1163
– arming 1167
– biodegradability 1169
– biologic applications 1164
– biotransformation 1177
– cancer therapy constructs 1168
– chemistry 1164
– drug delivery systems 896
– environmental concerns 1171
– interactions with cells and tissues 1168
– PEGylation 1173
– pharmacokinetics 1170, 1173
– properties 1163
– theranostic applications 1180
– toxicity 1170
coated CNTs 1173
cobalamin 1300
coding tag 23
coencapsulation 940
coformulation
– in liposomes 1043
coil conformation
– random 247
colbalamin–cochicine conjugates 1302
colloidal carriers 1099
colloidal silica particles 333
COLO205 382, 389, 390
colon tumor xenograft
– DLD1 1346
colorectal cancer 1219
– cytotoxic somatostatin analogs 1219
– LHRH cytotoxic analogs 1234
– xenografts 645
comb polymer
– self-immolative 580
combination therapy 805, 1013
– administration strategies 1022
– combination chemotherapy 1020
– drug ratios 812
– fixed ratio 1014
– nab-rapamycin/perifosine 1147
– physicochemical characterization 816
– platinum-based 37
– polymer-based 805
– preclinical models 815
– target sites 811
– targeted protein toxins 1445, 1446
combinatorial peptide libraries
– OBOC 3, 12, 13, 16
CombiPlex® formulations 805
– hydrophobic agents 1040
– liposome-based 1029
– nanoparticle 1040
– reactive agents 1033
combotox 1480
compartmentalization 414
competition assay 1228
complement-dependent cytotoxicity (CDC) 291
complete response (CR) duration 1036
completeness
– analytical 337, 338
complex proteomes 337
complex self-immolative architectures 573
complexation
– anticancer agents 253
compromised microcirculation 43
computed tomography (CT) 887
– contrast agents 42
– SPECT/CT and PET/CT 247
– tumor imaging 34, 46
concentric bilayers 890
conditional RNA systems 1422
confocal microscopy
– xzy 1378
conjugated antibodies 449
conjugated pyrrolic ring systems 1571
conjugates 1519
– (un-)cleavable 387
– acid-activated PEG–drug 651
– acid-sensitive 772, 1536
– acyl hydrazone-based 1299
– ADCs 295
– albumin 772
– alginate–drug 730
– AMCs 378
– antibody–maytansinoid 375
– antibody–toxin 16
– aptamer 1263, 1269
– aptamer–DOX 1270
– arabinogalactan–drug 732
– biotin–drug 1304
– cancer-targeting ligand–drug 27
– carboplatin–folate 1612
– chitosan–drug 717
– clinical experience 839
– colbalamin–cochicine 1302
– combination therapy 810
– cyclodextrin–drug 735
– DCM-Dex-Gal4A-CDDP 718
– Dex-based drug 711
– Dex-peptide-MTX 719
– disulfide-linked trastuzumab 383

- drug–albumin 789
- drug–polymer 275, 1529
- enzyme-cleavable photosensitizer 1586
- FA–fluorescein 1300
- Fleximer–camptothecin 845
- folic acid–drug 27
- gadolinium–dendrimer 540
- growth factor–drug 1283, 1579, 1581
- HA–drug 724
- heparin–drug 727
- hydrolyzable drug–PEG 844
- LHRH 1223
- ligand–drug 3
- mAb–maytansine 85
- mAb–photosensitizer 1577
- natural polymer–drug 730
- nonantibody proteins 1580
- paclitaxel–PGA 840
- pectin–drug 732
- PEG–drug 627
- PEG–lipid 955
- PEG–phospholipid 1001
- PEG–TSCA 610
- peptide hormone–drug 105
- peptide ligand–drug 101
- pH-sensitive 731
- polygalactosamine–drug 735
- polymer peptide–drug 150
- polymer-based combination therapy 818
- polymer–drug 34, 93, 707, 830
- polymer–photosensitizer 1584, 1586
- polypeptide–drug 671
- polysaccharide-based 747
- protein–photosensitizer 1583
- PUFA–drug 1359
- PUFA–taxoid 1346
- pullulan–drug 729
- releasable β-ligand 1301
- releasable dual-drug 1295
- RGD-based polymer–drug 601
- second-generation taxoid 1332, 1345
- selectin-targeted polymer–drug 612
- small-molecule–photosensitizer 1588, 1589
- stable 1287
- synthetic approaches 759
- TAT–polymeric micelles 1114
- transferrin 772
- trastuzumab–maytansinoid 384
- vitamin–drug 1283
- water-soluble 272, 1298
- xyloglucan–drug 734

conjugation 1263
- bioconjugation properties 281
- chemical/physical 1271
- cholesterol 1275
- covalent 248
- doxorubicin (DOX) 75
- DOX–CPP 1193
- drug 1125
- lysine and cysteine residues 92, 93
- polysaccharide–drug 707
- PUFAs/cytotoxic drugs 1332
- SC-PEG 632
- SS-PEG 630
- strategies 376
- streptonigrin 66
- technologies 297

Consortium for Resourcing and Evaluating AMS Microdosing (CREAM) 36

contrast agents 276
- CT 47
- MRI 1063

contrast enhanced ultrasound (CEUS) 49

control
- cancer 1324

controlled drug delivery 1099

convection enhanced delivery (CED) 538

conventional anticancer agents
- structure 7

conventional chemotherapy 1071
- limits 34
- side-effects 16

conventional drugs
- ELP-delivery 689

conventional hybridoma production 414

convergent synthesis
- dendrimers 516

copolymers 1071
- acrylic 1071
- amphiphilic block 1103
- block 675, 1053
- block assemblies 1060
- fluorescently labeled HPMA 247
- long-circulating 272
- triblock 1061

core
- multifunctional 278

core/membrane lipid-based nanoparticles 1376

coregistration 1361
- anatomic information 282
- image 257

core–shell structure 1058

corona (shell) 1103

cotyledones 90

coupling
- transmural 42, 46

covalent conjugation 248
– DOX–CPP 1193
covalent modification
– CNTs 1166, 1178
CPG2 (carboxypeptidase G2) 20
– inactivation 7
CPP (cell-penetrating peptides) 1189
– applications 1189
– cancer targeting 1189
– cell cycle modulation 1198
– cellular uptake 681
– delivery vectors 1208
– internalization routes 1190
– intracellular delivery 680
– oncogenic signaling 1198
– RNA inteference 1365
– sequences 1191
– targeted toxins 1443, 1456
– targeting ligands 1381
– tumor targeting 1202
CPT (camptothecin) 528, 641, 762, 1305, 1334
– MAG-CPT 852
– PEG–CPT 855, 856
– polymer-based combination therapy 809
CPX-1 1032
– clinical studies 1038
– efficacy 1034
– phase I clinical trials 1038
– phase II clinical trials 1039
– preclinical pharmacology 1033
CPX-351 1013
– clinical studies 1036
– preclinical pharmacology 1030
CPX-351 liposomes 1030
CPX-571 1033
– efficacy 1036
– preclinical pharmacology 1035
cracking pattern 582
CREKA peptide 1149
Cremophor micelles 1592
Cremophor-paclitaxel 1141, 1153
Cre–loxP system 1423
critical micelle concentration (CMC) 892
critical solution temperature 668, 672
cross-linked albumin matrix 1136
cross-linked knedel
– shell 892
cross-linked micelles
– virus-mimetic 1122
cross-linked polymer network 1071
cross-linkers 887
– diacid-derivatized 887
– self-immolative 556
– sulfhydryl-reactive 1137
– thiophilic heterobifunctional 1289
cross-linking 85
– glutaraldehyde 1137, 1145
cross-reactive determinants 961
cross-species binding 111
crystallizable
– fragment 85
CSCs (cancer stem cells) 95
CT (computed tomography) 805
– contrast agents 42
– SPECT/CT and PET/CT 247, 805
– tumor imaging 34, 46
CTA (chain transfer agent) 250
culture
– endothelial cells 332
cutaneous contaminations 276
cutaneous T-cell lymphoma (CTCL) 1472
CVX-241 471
cyclic oligosaccharides 735
cyclic RGD-based vehicles 608
cyclin-dependent kinase (CDK) 1201
cyclization
– strategies 556
cyclodextrin 867
cyclodextrin-containing polycation (CDP) 1375
cyclodextrin–drug conjugates 735
cyclophosphamide 938
cyclopropabenzindol-4-one (CBI) 66
cyclosporine 1210
cylindrical micelles 1054
cynomolgus monkeys 99
Cys34 777
– in situ binding 779
cysteine 1001
– dicysteine-β-cyclodextrin 735
– SPARC 1135, 1155, 1323
– thiol–disulfide exchange cleavage 388
cysteine residues
– conjugation 92, 93
cytarabine 1030
cytochrome P450 enzyme 1349
cytokines 3
– pro-inflammatory 894
cytomegalovirus (CMV) promoter 1424
cytoplasmic C-terminal tail 1222
cytoplasmic signaling region 88
cytosine arabinoside (Ara-C) 651
– PEG– 652, 653
cytosolic drug release 1121
cytosolic pH 53
cytotoxic ADCs
– linkers 72

cytotoxic analogs
– LHRH 1221
cytotoxic bombesin analogs 1245
cytotoxic chemotherapy 3, 21
cytotoxic drugs 11
– molecular weight 1287
– PUFA synergy 1331
cytotoxic peptide analogs
– targeted 1220
cytotoxic somatostatin analogs 1219
– structure 1219, 1239
– targeted 1236
cytotoxic T-lymphocyte (CTL) 451
cytotoxicity 951
– 2C5-modified liposomes 965
– antibody-dependent cellular 291
– complement-dependent 291
– dendrimer-related 536
– dendritic architecture 535
– doxorubicin/vincristine 1029
cytotoxins
– chemotherapeutic 3

d

D-amino acid oxidase (DAO) 822
– structure 824
D-amino acids 1224
DAC (Drug Affinity Complex) 103
DAPK2 1471
DAR (drug-to-antibody ratio) 72
database "Gene Therapy Clinical Trials Worldwide" 1431
Daudi cells 470
Daudi lymphoma disease 1454
daunorubicin 1030
DAVLBH 1293
DC-SPION (dendrimer-coated superparamagnetic iron oxide nanoparticles) 266
DCM-Dex-Gal4A-CDDP conjugate 718
deblocking 564
decay products
– radioactive 420
decoding
– phage-display libraries 6
degradation domain
– oxygen-dependent 1205
deleterious drug–drug interactions 1033
delivery 1026, 1495
– agents 423
– aptamer isolation 1265
– aptamers 1266
– blood-borne 43
– caveolae-mediated transcellular 1057
– cell 1087
– controlled 1099
– convection enhanced 538
– conventional drugs 689
– CPP vectors 1208
– delivery platforms 1263
– EPR effect heterogeneity 72
– extracellular 1365
– gene 542, 1085
– growth factor targeted 1311
– HCC treatment 1522, 1530
– hepatotropic systems 1528
– heterogeneous 1008
– hormone-mediated nuclear 261
– hydrophobic small-molecule drugs 1139
– in vivo studies 390
– interstitial barriers 46, 47
– intracavitary 422
– intracellular 680
– intranasal 1509
– ligand-based systems 1189
– lipid-like molecules 1373
– liposomal 1502, 1616
– local gene 1391
– magnetically controlled 1507
– micellar structures 1053
– multiagent drug vehicles 1022
– nanoparticle 1271
– nanoscale systems 887, 1013
– nucleic acids 1195
– oligonucleotides 1150, 1195
– oral 721
– pathophysiological characteristics 65
– peptide receptors 1220
– peptide-mediated 610
– peptides 682
– pH-triggered micelles 1099
– photosensitizer 1571
– polymeric systems 1619
– proteins 1150, 1151
– radionuclide delivery vector 1207
– radionuclides 411
– respective 1446, 1607
– RNA approaches 1361, 1368
– serum proteins 752
– site-specific 1054
– small-molecule 1270
– tailor-made hydrogels 1071
– targeted drug 1284
– toxins 1455
– uniformity 989
– vascular characteristics 65
– vehicles 1573
DENA (diethylnitrosamine) 1538

dendrimer phthalocyanine-encapsulated polymeric micelle (DPc/m) 537
dendrimer-coated superparamagnetic iron oxide nanoparticles (DC-SPION) 266
dendrimer-related cytotoxicity 536
dendrimers 1489
– boronated PAMAM 538
– bow-tie 526
– brain targeting 1508
– charged 535
– cytotoxicity 535
– diagnostic application 539
– divergent/convergent synthesis 516
– end-group functionality 248
– functional groups 270
– gene delivery 542
– glycopeptide 24
– intracellular trafficking 535
– MTX-loaded 534
– nanoglobular platform 609
– pharmacokinetics 535
– polyplexes 1374
– self-immolative 575, 577
– targeting moiety 251
– therapeutic application 545
– translocation 535
– water-soluble 579
dendritic architectures
– complexation of anticancer agent 254
dendritic cavities
– doxorubicin (DOX) 255
dendritic chain reaction 570
dendritic compound
– YEE(GalNAcAH)3 1525
dendritic end-groups
– cloaking/masking 536
dendritic polyglycerol 527
dendritic polyglycerolamine 543
dendritic polymers 1443
– drug conjugation 1443
– drug encapsulation 1121
– oncology 274
– targeting modalities 530
dendritic scaffold
– drug–polymer conjugates 275
dendritic structures
– drug-conjugated 271
denileukin diftitox 1472
depolymerization 577
depression of the immune system 18
derivatization
– PEGylated liposomes 955
deshielding 1115
– pH-dependent 1203
design 1283
– biotin–drug conjugates 1283
– drug-encapsulated nanoparticles 1527
– drug-free macromolecular therapeutics 273
– LHRH cytotoxic analogs 1223
– PET 275
– polymer–drug conjugates 97
– targeted protein toxins 1443
desolvation
– ethanol 1145
detection of recurrence 274
development
– drugs 51
Dex-based drug conjugates 711
Dex–MMC 712
Dex-peptide-MTX conjugate 719
dexamethasone 917, 933
dextran (Dex) 711
DHA (docosahexaenoic acid) 1324
DHA–10-hydroxycamptothecin 1334
DHA–EPA–propofol 1335
DHA–illudin M 1336
DHA–LNA–DOX 1334
DHA–methotrexate 1338
DHA–paclitaxel (TXP) 1338
– antitumor activity 1340
– pharmacokinetics 1339
DHA–SB-T-1214 1347
DHAD 1547, 1553, 1554
diabodies 887
– diabody chains 456
– PSCA-specific 430
– single-chain 105
diacid-derivatized cross-linker 893
diacyl lipids 1580
diagnostics 1605
– dendrimers 539
– modern 14
diammineplatinum(II) fragment 1609
DiBi mini-antibodies 459
1,5-dichloro-3-thiapentane 4
dicysteine-β-cyclodextrin 735
dienediyne antibiotic
– chromophore 1543
diethylenetriaminepentaacetatic acid (DTPA) 270, 1303
diethylnitrosamine (DENA) 1538
diferric transferrin 749
differential accumulation/internalization 1263
differential regulation of gene expression 47
differentiation
– benign/malignant tumors 272

diffuse large B-cell lymphoma (DLBCL) 110
diffusion 33
diffusion coefficient
– apparent 38, 54
diffusion-weighted imaging (DWI) 46
dimeric domain antibodies 457
dimethylformamide 1166
diode
– light-emitting 693
1,2-dioleoyl-sn-glycero-3-phosphoethanolamine (DOPE) 998, 1371
dipalmitoylphosphatidylcholine (DPPC) 1574
dipalmitoylphosphatidylglycerol (DPPG) 1617
diphtheria A chain 1310
diphtheria toxin 1083, 1448
– targeted 1473
direct mAb–photosensitizer conjugates 1578, 1579
directional placental transport 90
disease control 1039
disialoganglioside GD2 958
diskoidal porous silicon microparticles 899
disorder band 1165
disorganized microcirculation 43
dispersed SWNTs 1172
dispersions
– phospholipid 889
distearoylphosphatidylcholine (DSPC) 908
distribution
– ADME 1173, 1175
disulfide bonds 989
– reduction 989
– unsymmetrical 1295
disulfide bridge 457
disulfide formation 24
disulfide linkers 78
– trastuzumab conjugates 383
disulfide-based linkers 376, 1288
divergent synthesis
– dendrimers 516
DLBCL (diffuse large B-cell lymphoma) 111
DLD1 human colon tumor xenograft
– P-gp+ 1346
DLT (dose-limiting toxicity) 991, 1032
DM1 376
DNA 1605
– adduct formation 1605
– inhibition of synthesis 235
– LPD 1376
– plasmid 1367, 1407
– platinum complexes 1609
– RACE 1418
– recombinant 27
DNA adducts
– platinum– 1035
DNA alkylator 1336
DNA intercalators 806
DNA-damaging agent 94
DNA/polymer complexes 1085
DNM 732
docetaxel 3, 675, 1345
– polysorbate-based 1141, 1154
docetaxel-loaded micelles 675, 677
dock-and-lock system 431
docosahexaenoic acid (DHA) 1324
dodecapeptides 4
domains 1443
– functional 1443
– organization 443
– targeted protein toxins 1447
DOPE (1,2-dioleoyl-sn-glycero-3-phosphoethanolamine) 998, 1371
dose
– maximum tolerated 1013, 1032, 1037
dose-dependent efflux 389
dose-escalation study 25
dose-finding
– CNTs 1171
dose-limiting toxicity (DLT) 991, 1032
dosing
– PLD 912
dosing platform
– ratiometric 1040
double bonds
– cis 1372
double-prodrug concept 556
DOX-DEX 817, 820
DOXO-EMCH 780, 784
– hepatotropic delivery 1536
– pharmacokinetics 790
DOXO-HYD 777
doxorubicin (DOX) 299
– aptamer–DOX conjugates 1270
– conjugation 75
– covalent conjugation with CPP 1193
– dendritic cavities 255
– Dex–DOX conjugates 713
– DHA–LNA–DOX 1334
– encapsulated 914
– fluorescent properties 608
– hydrazone-bound DOX moiety 613
– hydrogel-based therapy 1081
– hypoxic regions 45
– LHRH cytotoxic analogs 1224
– L-HSA–DOX 1536, 1540

doxorubicin (DOX) (*contd.*)
– ligand-assisted vascular targeting 605
– liposomes 809
– micelle formulation 676
– molecular structure 1270
– nanogels 1125
– nanoparticles 809
– PEG-liposomes 953
– PEGylated liposomal 909
– perivascular distribution 17
– pH-sensitive pullulan–DOX conjugate 731
– pH-triggered drug release 1112
– pharmacokinetics 790
– polyglycerol–DOX prodrugs 536
– polysaccharide–drug conjugation 711
– 2-pyrrolino-DOX 1225, 1246
– self-immolation 562
– toxicity profile 915
– transdrug 1546, 1553
– transferrin conjugates 772
– VAD 918, 933
doxorubicin/vincristine 1029
doxorubicin–HSA nanoparticles 1147
DPc/m (dendrimer phthalocyanine-encapsulated polymeric micelle) 537
DPPC (dipalmitoylphosphatidylcholine) 1574
DPPG (dipalmitoylphosphatidylglycerol) 1617
Drosophila
– antennapedia protein 1189
Drug Affinity Complex (DAC) 103
drug and linker selection 93
drug approval 53
drug carriers 989
– macromolecules 100
– multifunctional polymeric 249
drug complexes
– synthetic approaches 759
drug conjugates 627
– acid-sensitive 1536
– albumin 772
– conjugation strategies 298
– dendritic structures 271, 1123
– Dex-based 711
– growth factor– 1308
– polysaccharide-based 747
– polyunsaturated fatty acids (PUFAs) 1359
– synthetic approaches 759
– transferrin 772
– vitamin– 1283
drug delivery 1489
– brain targeting 1489
– controlled 1099
– EPR effect heterogeneity 72
– HCC treatment 1522, 1530
– hepatotropic systems 1528
– interstitial barriers 46, 47
– liposomal 1502, 1616
– macromolecular systems 36
– magnetic nanoparticles 47
– magnetically controlled 1507
– molecularly targeted 238
– multiagent vehicles 1022
– nanoparticle-based 346
– pathophysiological characteristics 65
– RNA approaches 1361
– serum proteins 752
– site-specific 1054
– strategy 599
– targeted 1284
– vascular characteristics 65
– vehicles 1573
drug delivery systems 1013
– applications 1013
– dual- 1026
– ligand-based 1189
– micellar structures 1053
– MSV 896
– nano- and microparticulate 887
drug design 1013
– FcRn 85
– IgG 85
– PET 275
– serum albumin 85
drug development
– imaging techniques 21
drug encapsulation 1133
– dendritic polymers 1133
– nab technologies 1137
– nanoparticles 1527
drug entrapment
– supramolecular 520
drug nanoparticles
– synthetic approaches 759
drug ratios 1014
– combination therapy 812
drug release 1099
– cytosolic 1099
– kinetics 814
– pH-triggered 1104
– self-immolative dendrimers 577
– two-step mechanism 555
drug-free macromolecular therapeutics 267
– design 273
drug-loaded liposomes 28, 954
drug-to-antibody ratio (DAR) 72

drugs 989
– actual delivery 989
– albumin–drug nanoparticles 1133
– amphipathic 909
– antibody-targeted liposomal 968
– anticancer liposomal 954
– bacterial toxins 1462, 1464
– BBB transporters 1492
– categories 5
– circulation lifetime 1041
– cytotoxic 15
– development and validation 51
– EPR effect 68
– export pumps 1493
– externally activated release 1001
– human proteins 1468
– hydrophilic 1081
– hydrophobic 719, 909
– LDL–drug complexes 786, 792
– lipophilic 761
– liposomal 890
– modification with CPPs 1191
– peptides 1082
– pH dependence 56
– plant toxins 1464, 1466
– polymer carrier binding 250
– and prodrugs 20
– protein-based 103, 1082
– release from polymersomes 1061
– respective delivery concept 1446, 1607
– RNAi 1384
– safety 257
– site-specific attachment 91
– small-molecule 1079
– solubility 840
– solubilizers 867
– targeting 951, 1489
– vector-coupled 1499
drug–albumin conjugates
– clinical development 789
drug–drug interactions 1015, 1349
– deleterious 1033
drug–polymer conjugates 839
– clinical experience 839
– clinical trials 847, 848
– dendritic scaffold 275
– derivatives 861
– hepatotropic delivery 1529
– HPMA 842
– second generation 865
– stable 871
drug delivery vehicles
– PDT 1576
DSPC (distearoylphosphatidylcholine) 908
DTPA (diethylenetriaminepentaacetatic acid) 270, 1303
DTX 4
DTX-encapsulated nanoparticle–aptamer (DTX-NP-Apt) 1271
dual action BsAbs 452, 471
dual formulation 1023
dual targeting
– angiogenic markers 616
dual-acting prodrugs 784, 878
– structure 787
dual-color screening method 20
dual-drug conjugates
– releasable 1295
dual-drug delivery systems
– dual systems 1026
dual-phase release mechanism 844
dual-targeted microbubbles 38
dual-variable-domain immunoglobulins (DVD-Igs) 461
dviding cells 17
DWI (diffusion-weighted imaging) 46
DX-8951 862
dye
– Nile Red 581
dynamic g-scintigraphy 85, 343
dynamics
– lipid acyl tail 999

e
E-selectin-mediated endocytosis 959
E1B-55K protein 1432
EC145 1289, 1290, 1293
ECF (extracellular fluid) 19
ECM (extracellular matrix) 724
– integrin ligands 603
– integrins 596
economic analysis 936
ectopic RNA 1368
Edman chemistry 20
effector function-enhanced antibodies 293
efficiency 951
– CPP cellular uptake 681
– polymer carriers 104
efflux effect
– P-glycoprotein 965
EGF (epidermal growth factor)
– CNTs 1167
EGFR (epidermal growth factor receptor) 533, 1313
– immunoliposomes 958
– liposomes 940
EGF–polylysine-β-amanitin 1311

eicosanoids
– biosynthesis 1326
eicosapentaenoic acid (EPA) 1324
elastin-like biopolymers 678
elastin-like polypeptide (ELP) 678
– intracellular delivery 680
– purification 680
– synthetis 678
electrons
– Auger 419, 423
electrophoretic techniques 748
electroporation 1370
electropores 1405
electrostatic repulsion 996
elimination 1013
– benzyl 646
– biphasic 738
– paclitaxel prodrugs 1042
– plasma 1043
– strategies 558
– thiophenol derivatives 567
elimination linkers 1071
– branched 573
– multiple 575
elimination-based trigger groups 564
elongated spacers 257
embolic microbeads 1080
embolization 1089
embryonic antigen
– carcinogenic 1167
emerging delivery platforms 1263
empowered antibodies
– cancer therapy 44
encapsulated doxorubicin 914
encapsulation 1163
– CNTs 1163
– drug 1122
– liposomal 1616
ϕ-end chemical phosphorylation 1365
end-groups
– dendritic 248, 536
endocrine approaches 1221
endocrine therapy 807
endocytic pH-triggered drug release 1106, 1115
endocytic vesicles 991
endocytosis 107
– E-selectin-mediated 959
– folate receptor-mediated 1284
– receptor-independent 1122
– receptor-mediated 1115, 1269
endogenous silencing pathway
– saturation 1368
endohedral filling 1165
endometrial cancer 1230, 1240
endonucleases
– fungal 1453
endopeptidase
– thermostable human 23
endosomal escape 247
endosomal pH 1059
endosomal release 1367
endosomes 296, 1100
endothelial barrier 1140
endothelial cadherin
– vascular 1179
endothelial cell membranes
– luminal 334
endothelial cell-targeted polymer therapeutics 597
endothelial cells 1189
– activation 591
– in culture 332
– neovasculature 595
– proliferating 592
– proteins 66
– proteome 336
endothelial cell–cell junction 72
endothelial expression 618
endothelial growth factor
– vascular 34, 261, 539, 637, 1198, 1330, 1416
endothelial sprouting 34
endothelium 1189
– fenestrated 328
– sinusoidal 328
– vascular 327
enediyne aglycone functionality 95
energy-independent membrane translocation 1189
engineered antibody fragments 424, 425
engineering 1189
– IgG 95, 96
– IgG half-life 101
enhanced mutagenesis 51
enhanced permeability and retention (EPR) 259, 326
– CPPs 1194, 1203
– drug–polymer conjugates 877
– heterogeneity 72
– PEG–drug conjugates 639
– pharmaceutical nanocarriers 952
– polymer-based combination therapy 810
– tumor targeting 85
enterohepatic circulation 1613
envelope-type nanodevice
– multifunctional 1377
environmental concerns
– CNTs 1171

enzymatic activation 564
enzymatic cleavage 25
enzymatically cleavable peptide linker 784
enzymatically cleavable prodrugs 527
– half-lives 562
enzyme prodrug systems 29
enzyme-cleavable photosensitizer conjugates 1586
enzyme-labile linkers 79
enzyme-related targeted protein toxins
– human 1469
enzymes 1359
– ADEPT 20
– cytochrome P450 1349
– ERK1/2 1329
– GDEPT 1397
– innate 1000
– PDEPT/PELT 812
– tumor-associated 250
– tumor-specific 1056
EORTC (European Organization for Research and Treatment of Cancer) 937
eosin-stained femurs 1032
EPA (eicosapentaenoic acid) 1324
EpCAM (cell adhesion molecule) 464
epidemiology of HCC 1519
epidermal growth factor (EGF)
– CNTs 1167
epidermal growth factor receptor (EGFR) 533, 1313
– immunoliposomes 958
– liposomes 940
epidermal necrolysis 297
epigenetic mechanisms 592
epigenetic suppression 1423
epirubicin 24, 824
epithelial cell adhesion molecule (EpCAM) 960
epithelium
– choroid plexus 1503
EPR (enhanced permeability and retention) 259, 326
– CPPs 1194, 1203
– drug–polymer conjugates 877
– heterogeneity 72
– PEG–drug conjugates 639
– pharmaceutical nanocarriers 952
– polymer-based combination therapy 810
– tumor targeting 85
ErbB2 1206
Erbitux 453
ERK1/2 (extracellular signal-regulated kinase) 1329
erythrocytes 52
erythrodysesthesia
– palmar–plantar 915, 916, 934
ester linkage 608, 638
esters
– spontaneous ring-closure 557
estradiol 829
estrogen receptor 807
estrogens 1612
ethanol desolvation 1145
European Organization for Research and Treatment of Cancer (EORTC) 937
Evans blue 66, 70, 756
Evans blue–albumin 73
excretion
– ADME 1173, 1178
exopolysaccharide 730
experimental cancers
– human 1228
exponential enrichment
– SELEX 1264, 1265
export proteins
– ABC 1497
Exportin-5 1435
expression
– endothelial 618
externally activated drug release 1001
externally activated targeting 1001
extracellular acidity
– tumors 1100
extracellular delivery
– siRNA/miRNA 1365
extracellular fluid (ECF) 19
extracellular matrix (ECM) 724
– integrin ligands 603
– integrins 596
extracellular pH-triggered drug release 1104
extracellular signal-regulated kinase 1/2 (ERK1/2) 1329
extravasation 23, 33
– anticancer agents 45
– Evans blue–albumin 73
– nanocarriers 991
– tissue 535
EZN-2208 642, 655, 866, 868
– preparation 643

f

Fab (fragment of antigen binding) 86
Fab4D5
– biodistribution 108
Fab¢ fragments 272
– anti-HER2 liposomes 958
FAM™-siRNA 1379
fatigue 19

fatty acid binding protein (FABP) 1325, 1326
fatty acids 1219
– ω-amino 1219
– polyunsaturated 1359
FA–fluorescein conjugate 1300
Fc fusion technology 95
Fc receptor
– neonatal 85
FcRn–ligand interactions 89
FcRn-mediated recycling 92
– blocking 102
FcRn-mediated transport 93
FcRn (neonatal Fc receptor) 85
– altered binding 95
– antigen presentation 93
– discovery 87
– kidneys 94
– liver 95
– structure 88, 89
FDA approval 53
18F-FDG 250
– radioimmunotherapy 266
FDG (fluorodeoxyglucose) 1102
Fe-transferrin 754
femurs
– eosin-stained 1032
fenestrated endothelium 328
Ferumoxtran-10 229
fetal neonatal immune thrombocytopenia (FNIT) 91
fetuin 1532
18F-FLT 250, 257, 266
FGF 533, 727
fiber/knob chimeras 1432
fibroblast growth factor 533, 727
fibroblasts
– stromal 46
filling
– endohedral 1165
first-generation PEG linker 630
first-line chemotherapy 13
FITC (fluorescein isothiocyanate) 110
fixed ratio anticancer combination therapy 1014
flavoprotein
– mitochondrial 1470
flexibodies 460
– tetravalent 458
Fleximer–camptothecin conjugate 845
flip-flop process 1325, 1326
flippase 1422
floxuridine/irinotecan 1032
fluid 1099
– extracellular 19
– intracellular 41
fluid pressure
– interstitial 36, 37, 39, 40, 41
fluid-phase pinocytosis 1114
fluorescein 249
– FA–fluorescein conjugate 1300
fluorescein isothiocyanate (FITC) 110, 965
– -labeled proteins 757
fluorescence 35, 49
fluorescence resonance energy transfer (FRET) 247
fluorescent liposomes 1003
fluorescent nab-paclitaxel 1140
fluorescent probes
– tumor detection 541
fluorescent properties
– DOX 608
fluorescent protein 1189
– GFP 262, 1198, 1421
fluorescently labeled antibodies 331
fluorescently labeled HPMA copolymers 107
fluorinated pyrimidine 1032
5-fluoro-2'-deoxyuridine 1534
5-fluorocytosine 1406
fluorodeoxyglucose (FDG) 1102
fluorogenic monomer units 580
fluorophore-labeled AN-152 1227
fluorophores 1178
5-fluorouracil (5-FU) 806
– toxicity profile 915
fluorouridine (FURD) 1147
FMISO 268
FNIT (fetal neonatal immune thrombocytopenia) 91
focused ultrasound
– high-intensity 669, 670
focused ultrasound treatment 1499
folate conjugates
– carboplatin– 1612
folate receptor 235
folate receptor-mediated endocytosis 1284
– preclinical pharmacology 1289
folate receptor-targeted liposomes 1001
folate receptor-targeted micelles 1119
folate-conjugated micelles 1057
folate-modified liposomes 967
folding
– head-to-tail 459
FOLFIRI regimen 1038, 1039
FOLFOX regimen 1039
folic acid 1283
– dendrimers 259

– heparin–folic acid–PTX 729
– structure 1284
folic acid–drug conjugates 27
formaldehyde 558
formulations
– liposome-based 1013
four-arm PEG 645
FR-targeted immunotherapy 1298
fractional cell kill 14
fragment crystallizable 85
fragment of antigen binding (Fab) 86
freeze-drying
– liposomes 970
FRET (fluorescence resonance energy transfer) 249
frustrated phagocytosis 1172
5-FU (5-fluorouracil) 806
functional domains 1446
functional groups
– dendrimers 270
functional imaging 249
functional lymphatics 37
functionality
– end-group 248
functionalized lipids 996
functionalized nanotubes 1168
fungal endonucleases 1453
FURD (fluorouridine) 1147
fusion
– vesicular 329
fusion ligands
– b-lactamase–peptide 5
fusion proteins 1443
– nonglycosylated 23
– recombinant 1457
fusion technology 1519
– Fc 95
– serum albumin 102, 104
Fv
– single-chain 452, 459

g

g emitters 417
g-scintigraphy 952
– dynamic 85, 343
– planar 85
gadolinium–dendrimer conjugates 540
galactosamine 1529, 1551
galactose units
– branched 714
gangliosides 910
gastric cancers
– cytotoxic somatostatin analogs 1243
gastrin-releasing peptide (GRP) 1244
– antagonists 1245
– receptors 1244
gastroduodenal artery 1559
gastrointestinal distress 19
gastrointestinal toxicities 1037
GCIG (Gynecologic Cancer Intergroup) 929
GD2 958
gel-phase membranes 992
gelation
– in situ 1077
geldanamycin 605
Gelonium multiflorum 1270
gel–solid transition region 998
gels
– hydro- 1072
gemcitabine 1043
gemtuzumab ozogamicin 75, 275
– calicheamicin ADCs 95
GEM–DOX 824
– structure 827
gene correction therapy 1392
gene delivery 1058
– dendrimers 542
– hydrogel-based therapy 1084
– intratumoral 1404
– local 1391
– locoregional 1405
– technologies 1404
gene expression 1328
– differential regulation 47
– long-term 1399
gene suppression 1397
gene therapeutic strategies 1391
gene therapy 1391
– clinical trials 1392
– nanoparticles 237
– vectors 1398
"Gene Therapy Clinical Trials Worldwide" database 1431
gene transfer 1399
gene vectors 346
gene-directed enzyme prodrug therapy (GDEPT) 1397
general toxicity 1461
genetic heterogeneity
– tumors 65
genome-wide libraries 1429
genomic instability 51
genomics approaches
– tissue-specific targets 335
GFP (Green Fluorescent Protein) 262, 1198, 1421
– plasmids encoding 995

GHRH (growth hormone-releasing hormone) 1220
– antagonistic analogs 1249
– antagonists 1247
– structure 1248
Gliadel wafers 1479
glioblastoma multiforme 1490, 1496
gliosis 40
GLP toxicology studies 1038
glucocorticoids 1559
glucopyranose 711
glucosamine 727
glucose analog tracer 1102
glucose oxidase (GOD) 1085
glucose pathway 38
glucosylation 534
glutaraldehyde 760
– cross-linking 1137, 1145
glutathione 86, 1504
glycopeptide dendrimers 24
glycopeptide library 20
glycoprotein
– α1-acid 1341
glycosidase-based cleavage 71
glycoside clusters
– synthetic 1525
glycosylation pattern 292
GM-CSF (granulocyte macrophage colony-stimulating factor) 1083
GOD (glucose oxidase) 1085
Golgi apparatus 775
Good Manufacturing Practice (GMP) 1174
– standards 27
gp60 receptor 792, 1134
gp60-mediated transcytosis 1324
GPCR superfamily 1244
gradient
– manganese sulfate 1028
granulocyte macrophage colony-stimulating factor (GM-CSF) 1083
granuloma formation 1171
granzyme B 1453, 1468
Green Fluorescent Protein (GFP) 262, 1198
– plasmids encoding 995
– viral vectors 1421
groove
– peptide-binding 88
growth
– repetitive 275
growth curve
– tumors 15
growth factor 1219
– fibroblast 533, 727
– insulin-like 1249
– vascular endothelial 34, 261, 539, 637, 1198, 1330, 1416
growth factor conjugates 1579, 1581
growth factor receptor
– epidermal 533, 940, 958, 1313
growth factor targeted delivery
– delivery of chemotherapeutics 1311
growth factor–drug conjugates 1283
growth hormone-releasing hormone (GHRH) 1220
– antagonistic analogs 1249
– antagonists 1247
– structure 1248
growth phase
– pre-/avascular 34
GRP (gastrin-releasing peptide) 1244
– antagonists 1245
– receptors 1244
gutless adenovectors 1431
Gynecologic Cancer Intergroup (GCIG) 929

h

H2-clearance technique 39
H460 human tumor xenograft 1349
HA (hyaluronic acid) 707
HA22 1462, 1477
HA22-LR 1463
HAART (highly active antiretroviral therapy) 921
hair loss 20, 915
hairpin RNA
– short 1392, 1406, 1415, 1418, 1425
half-life 1443
– biological 1443
– cytotoxic drugs 15
– enzymatically cleavable prodrugs 562
– IgG 101
– serum albumin 107
HAMA (human anti-murine antibody) 111, 455
hand/foot syndrome 860
HA–drug conjugates 724
HC homodimerization 461
HCC (hepatocellular carcinoma) 871, 1243
– chemotherapy/targeted therapy 1522
– epidemiology and incidence 1519
– multinodular 873, 1557
HDAC (histone deacetylase) 27
head-to-tail folding 459
heat activation 1001
heat map
– synergy 1021
heat-sensitive liposomal formulation 1554

heating system
– ultrasound-based 669
hematological biomarkers 33
hematological malignancies 924
hematopoietic antigen CD33 95
hematopoietic cells 93
hematopoietic progenitor cells 209
hematoxylin 1032
heparan sulfate proteoglycan (HSPG) 1503
heparin–drug conjugates 727
heparin–folic acid–PTX 729
hepatic cancers
– LHRH cytotoxic analogs 1233
hepatic clearance 629
hepatic micrometastases 1534
hepatitis
– chronic 1519
hepatobiliary clearance 1178
hepatocellular carcinoma (HCC) 871, 1243
– chemotherapy/targeted therapy 1522
– epidemiology and incidence 1519
– multinodular 873, 1557
hepatocytes 1524
hepatoma 71
hepatotoxicity 21
hepatotropic drug delivery systems
– preclinical development 1528
HepDirect™ prodrugs 1527, 1529
HER2-mediated processing 388
HER2-positive tumors 428
Herceptin 29, 239, 310, 444, 453, 473
herpes simplex virus-thymidine kinase (HSV-tk) 1397, 1402
hetero-oligomeric BsAbs 455
heterobifunctional cross-linker
– thiophilic 1289
heterobifunctional reagents 72
heterodimerization 462
heterogeneity 989
– EPR effect 72
– genetic 65
4D heterogeneity 42
heterogeneous delivery 1008
heterogeneous microcirculation 33
HFT nanoparticles
– self-assembled 729
HIF (hypoxia-inducible factor) 65, 1416
high blood pressure 75
high-intensity focused ultrasound (HIFU) 669, 670
highly active antiretroviral therapy (HAART) 921
highly ordered nanoarchitectures 1054
hind-leg paralysis 1341
Hippel
– von Hippel-Lindau protein 65
histamine-succinyl-glycine (HSG) 431
histidine moieties
– protonation 1125
histidine-derived polymers 1105
histocompatibility complex
– MHC 88
histone deacetylase (HDAC) 27
historic approaches 1189
– conventional chemotherapy 3
– targeted therapy 26
– vascular mapping 333
HIV treatment 1430
HIV-1 1189
HMPA–paclitaxel 852
13-HODE 1329
homing peptides 1203, 1207
homodimerization
– HC 461
hormonal approaches 1221
hormonally responsive tumors 26
hormone 1219
– growth hormone-releasing 1219, 1247
– luteinizing hormone-releasing 533, 1220
hormone receptor
– steroid 262
hormone-dependent cancers 807
hormone–drug conjugates
– peptide 150
hormone-mediated nuclear delivery 261
hormone-releasing hormone
– luteinizing 533
HPAE (poly(β-amino esters)) 1106
HPMA (N-(2-hydroxypropyl)methacrylamide) 66, 108, 110
– chemical structure 600
– DOX-DEX 817, 820
– drug–polymer conjugates 842
– fluorescently labeled copolymers 247
– hydrogel-based therapy 1081
– ligand-assisted vascular targeting 599
– liver tumor targeting 1551
– long-circulating copolymer 270
– multiblock polyHPMAs 267
– polymer-based combination therapy 814
– prodrugs 851
– trigger group 574
HSA (human serum albumin) 750, 1133, 1323
– doxorubicin–HSA nanoparticles 1147
– MTX conjugates 773
– MTX–HSA 862
– structure 86

HSAB concept 1608
HSG (histamine-succinyl-glycine) 431
HSPG (heparan sulfate proteoglycan) 1503
HSV-tk (herpes simplex virus-thymidine kinase) 1397, 1402
5-HT3 inhibitors 20
human anti-mouse antibody (HAMA) 111
human anti-murine antibody (HAMA) 455
human blood
– composition 748
human colon tumor xenograft
– DLD1 1346
human endopeptidase
– thermostable 23
human enzyme-related targeted protein toxins 1469
human experimental cancers 1228
human ovarian tumor xenograft
– A121 1348
human pancreatic tumor 1034
human proteins
– targeted toxins 1468
human serum albumin (HSA) 750, 1133, 1323
– doxorubicin–HSA nanoparticles 1147
– MTX conjugates 773
– MTX–HSA 862
– structure 86
human serum proteome 747
human telomerase reverse transcriptase (hTERT) 1591
human tumor xenografts
– pH 1101
humanized antibodies 414, 444
hyaluronic acid (HA) 707
hyaluronic acid (HA) binding receptor 598
hybrid imaging modalities 248
hybrid MRI/PET scanner 248
hybrid PET/CT 249
hybrid SPECT/CT 252
hybridoma production
– conventional 414
hybridoma technology 26
hydrazone bonds 258
hydrazone linker 1112
– AcBut 86
– acid-labile 86, 267
hydrazone-bound DOX moiety 613
hydrodynamic injection 1369
hydrodynamic radius 629
hydrogel networks
– polymer 1073
hydrogel-based therapy 1071
hydrogels 1071
– biodegradability 1071
– formation 1074
– gene delivery 1085
– injectable formulations 1076
– PDT 1087
– radiotherapy 1088
– siRNA 1085
– small-molecule drugs 1079
– tailor-made 1071
hydrolysis 558
– polymers 840
– unspecific 571
hydrolyzable drug–PEG conjugates 844
hydrophilic drugs
– hydrogel-based therapy 1081
hydrophilic linkers 74
hydrophilic molecular tails 1574
hydrophilicity/hydrophobicity balance 1116
hydrophobic agents
– CombiPlex® formulations 1040
hydrophobic binding pockets 1264
hydrophobic drugs 719, 909
– circulation lifetime 1041
hydrophobic polyglycerol–paclitaxel complex 522
hydrophobic side-chains 272
hydrophobic small-molecule drugs
– delivery 1139
10-hydroxycamptothecin 1334
hydroxyl groups
– polysaccharides 711
hyperosmotic solutions 1499
hypersensitivity reactions 1152
hyperstabilizing microtubules 895
hyperthermia 1088
– cancer therapy 668
– thermo-responsive polymers 670
hypoalbuminemia 752
hypomethylation 1016
hypothalamic LHRH1 1221
hypoxia 49
– cervical tumor 42
– chemotherapy 49
– imaging 41
– molecular imaging 258
– treatment resistance 49
hypoxia-inducible factor (HIF) 65, 1416
hypoxia-selective radiotracers 267
hypoxic cell fraction 267

i

IAP (inhibitor of apoptosis protein) 1200
identification
– tissue-specific targets 334
IFN (interferon) 632, 761, 1303, 1403, 1422
IFP (interstitial fluid pressure) 42, 43, 46
Ig-mAb
– anti-PEG 79
IGF (insulin-like growth factor) 1249
IgG 1359
– bidirectional transport 91
– domain organization 443
– engineered variants 95, 96
– Fc fusion technology 95
– intravenous 102
– pharmacokinetics 85
– zzz 85
IgG Fc
– structure 86
IgG-like BsAbs 460
iliac vessels 4
illudin M 1336
image coregistration 257
imaging 1053
– adrenocortical tumors 279
– amino acid transport 257
– biomarkers 33, 41
– clinical practice 24
– diffusion-weighted 46
– drug development 24
– functional 249
– hybrid modalities 248
– hypoxia 36
– hypoxic cell fraction 267
– lymphangiography 25
– microautoradiography 759
– microPET 428, 429
– molecular 42, 249, 258, 270
– MRI 34, 44, 50, 248, 1062
– near-IR 38
– neoangiogenesis 260
– noninvasive molecular 253
– optical 35
– photoacoustic 1180
– preclinical 258
– preclinical and clinical 247
– prognostic potential of biomarkers 273
– proliferative activity 264
– protein biosynthesis 257
– radionuclides 415
– radiopharmaceuticals 251, 259
– receptor expression 269
– targeted agents 233
– tracers 251, 259
– tumor 17
– ultrasound 34, 49
imaging assays
– molecular 52
imaging modalities 1178
imaging-guided surgery 1062
imatinib 38
imidazole-containing polymers 1119
imidazolidinones 557
immolation
– self- 591
immune stimulation 1367
immune system
– depression 18
immune therapy targeting 68
immune thrombocytopenia
– FNIT 91
immune-privileged sites 94
immunoconjugates 151
– radioactive 68
immunodeficiency disorder
– severe combined 1429
immunogene therapy 1394
immunogenicity 970, 1082
– targeted toxins 1460
immunoglobulin receptor
– polymeric 91
immunoglobulins 951
– carboxylic groups 951
– dual-variable-domain 461
– naked 449
– pharmacokinetics 85
– zzz 85
immunohistochemistry 1479
immunohistochemistry-based
microenvironment signature 1155
immunoliposomes 940, 951
immunologic responses 1169
immunoPET 418, 431
immunoproteins
– small 424
immunosuppressed status 472
immunotherapy
– FR-targeted 1298
immunotoxins 16, 649, 1444
– targeting moieties 1448
in situ albumin technology 784
in situ binding
– prodrugs 779
in situ gelation 1077
in situ molecular biology 1064
in situ radiolabeling 333
in vitro selection
– tumor cell-targeting phages 3

in vitro studies
– albumin-based nanoparticles 1139
in vivo applications
– aptamer conjugates 1275
in vivo selection
– tumor cell-targeting phages 14
in vivo studies
– thermo-responsive ELP carriers 692
in vivo tissue targeting
– lungs 341
inactivation
– CPG2 4
incidence of HCC 1519, 1520
incompatible agents
– chemically 1026
indirect photosensitizer-linker-mAb conjugates 1580
indolequinone 6
infertility 25
inflammatory tissues 72
infusion 1489
– angiographic arterial 71
– hyperosmotic solutions 1499
infusion reactions 918
inherent antineoplastic activity 1195
inhibition 1489
– ABC export proteins 1489
– DNA synthesis 235
– P-glycoprotein 1498
inhibitor of apoptosis protein (IAP) 1200, 1330
inhibitors 805
– 5-HT3 20
– c-Myc 684, 687
– topoisomerase I 67, 817
inhibitory response 774
injectable formulations
– hydrogel-based 1076
injection
– hydrodynamic 1369
innate enzymes 1000
INNO-206 789, 791, 863, 864
– clinical trials 864
inorganic nanoparticles 1272
inotuzumab ozogamicin 251
insoluble CNTs 1171
insulin-like growth factor (IGF) 1249
intact antibodies 424, 425
integrins 235, 596, 604
– $\alpha v \beta 3$ integrin 1150
– ECM ligands 603
– radiolabeled antagonists 262
intercalators
– DNA 806
interfacial defects
– pH-triggered 998
interfacial poly(L-histidine) 1121
interference
– RNA 1197, 1415, 1417
interferon (IFN) 632, 761, 1303, 1403, 1422
interleukins 761
– IL-12 1083
– IL-2 1477
interlipidic particle formation 1005
internal pH 53
internalization 1263
– differential 1263
– nontarget 1208
– photochemical 1589, 1590
– routes 1190
interpenetrating polymer network (IPN) 1081
interstitial barriers
– drug delivery 46, 47
interstitial compartment 33
interstitial fluid pressure (IFP) 41, 43, 46
interstitial/vascular interface 1102
interstitium
– tumor 41, 994
intestinal peptide
– vasoactive 968
intra-arterial therapy 1558
– SMANCS/Lipiodol 1558
intracavitary delivery 422
intracellular acidic compartments 92
intracellular delivery 680
intracellular fluid 42
intracellular release
– FA–drug conjugates 1286
intracellular trafficking 887
– dendritic architecture 535
– MSVs 900
intracellularly cleavable linkers 78
intranasal delivery 1509
intrathecal/intraventricular injection 1498
intratumoral gene delivery 1404
intravenous immunoglobulin G (IVIG) 102
intravenously injected agents 328
intravital microscopy (IVM) 340
intussusception 34, 36
inverse thermal cycling 680
inverted terminal repeats (ITR) 1433
ionizable lipids 1372
IR LED applicator 694
IR-activated release 1003
iRGD peptide 1057
irinotecan 809, 1032

irinotecan/cisplatin 1035
– synergy heat map 1021
iron oxide
– superparamagnetic 56
irreversible systems 1422
isolation 1263
– aptamers 1263
– maytansinoid metabolites 385
isothiocyanate
– fluorescein 757, 965
isozymes 1349
IT-101 738
– biodistribution 736
ITR (inverted terminal repeats) 1433
IVIG (intravenous immunoglobulin G) 102
IVM (intravital microscopy) 340

j
J774.1 macrophages 714
Jablonski diagram 1570
jet-injection 1405
– clinical applications 1407
junction
– endothelial cell–cell 72
juxtamembrane 1309
JV-1-38 1250

k
K-ras shRNAs 1433
Kaplan–Meier survival curve 1118, 1501, 1615
Kaposi's sarcoma 919, 922
KB cells 1293
keratinocytes
– skin 297
kidneys
– FcRn 94
kinase
– targeted 1471
kinetics of drug release 814
knedel
– shell cross-linked 892
knob chimeras
– fiber/- 1432
"knob-into-hole" mutations 457
knockout mice 1361
– AnnA1 65
– caveolin-1 330
Kupffer cells 1366

l
L-HSA 1534
– synthesis 1533
L-HSA–DOX 1536, 1540
LA/LNA–second-generation taxoids 1349
labile linkers
– chemically 72
lactosaminated albumin 1532
lactose residues 1540
ladder synthesis method 21
LC mispairing 461
LCP (lipid-coated calcium phosphate) 1379
LCST (lower critical solution temperature) 668
– PNIPAAm 672
LDL (low-density lipoprotein) 747, 1580
– anticancer agents 763
– LDL–drug complexes 786, 792
– radiolabeled 757
– receptor-mediated uptake 751
– synthetic approaches 759
– tumor cells 754
leakage
– vascular 66
lectins
– C-type 596
LED (light-emitting diode) 693
left ventricular ejection fraction (LVEF) 918, 1236
lentiviral vectors 1392, 1430
LET (linear energy transfer) 418
leukemia
– acute lymphoblastic 3
leukemic blasts 96
Lewis lung tumors 913
LHRH (luteinizing hormone-releasing hormone) 533, 1220
– conjugates 1223
– cytotoxic analogs 1221
– radioiodinated 1225
libraries 1415
– genome-wide 1415
– glycopeptide 20
– phage-display 3, 335, 1313
library design
– OBOC 18
lifetime
– circulation 1041
ligand optimization 22
ligand-assisted vascular targeting 591
ligand-based drug delivery systems 1189
ligand-based nanocarriers 1524
ligand-targeted approach 531
ligands 1605
– ammonia 1605
– b-lactamase–peptide fusion 5
– cancer-targeting 3, 14
– ECM 603

ligands (*contd.*)
– FcRn–ligand interactions 89
– nonantibody 967
– peptidomimetic 23
– SELEX 1264, 1265
– small-molecular-weight 1382
– targeting 1366, 1381
– ursodeoxycholate 1614
ligand–drug conjugates 3
– cancer-targeting 27
ligation
– Staudinger 571
light-emitting diode (LED) 693
Lindau
– von Hippel-Lindau protein 65
linear energy transfer (LET) 418
linkage 1099
– acid-cleavable 1099
– acid-sensitive 5, 738
– amide/amino-derived 646
– cis-aconityl 721
– ester 638
– hydrazone 1112
– succinate 722
linkage site chemistry 69
linker technologies 66
linkers 24
– AcBut hydrazone 86
– acid-labile hydrazone 107, 250
– acid-sensitive 25
– biotin–streptavidin 34
– branched elimination 573
– chemically labile 72
– chemistry 271
– cleavable 299
– cytotoxic ADCs 72
– disulfide 78
– disulfide-based 376, 1288
– enzymatically cleavable 784
– enzyme-labile 79
– ester 608
– first-generation PEG 630
– hydrophilic 74
– intracellularly cleavable 79
– macromolecular 1578
– multiple elimination 575
– noncleavable 71
– noncleavable thioether 272
– nondegradable 602
– on-demand cleavable 26
– optimal 381
– PEG-aldehyde 632
– peptidic 79
– peptidyl 717
– pH-responsive systems 1298
– photosensitizer-linker-mAb conjugates 1580
– releasable PEG 646
– second-generation PEG 631
– selection 95
– self-immolative 553, 1288
– tailor-made 793
– U-PEG-Lys-NHS 635
lipid acyl tail dynamics 999
lipid-based systems 887
lipid-coated calcium phosphate (LCP) 1379
lipidoids 1373
lipids 989
– functionalized 989
– ionizable 1372
– PEG-derivatized 1372
– self-assembled 990
– solid nanoparticles 1508
– tri-/diacyl 1580
Lipiodol 77, 871, 873, 1545, 1555
lipophilic drugs 761
lipophilicity
– small molecules 1287
LipoPlatin 1617
– clinical development 1622, 1623
lipoplexes 1371
– nonviral vectors 1401
– schematic formation 1372
lipopolyplexes 1376
lipoproteins 751
– low-density 747, 754, 1580
liposomal doxorubicin
– PEGylated 909
liposomal drug delivery 1502
liposomal drug delivery
– platinum complexes 1616
liposomal drugs 890
– anticancer 954
– preparation and administration 968
liposomal encapsulation 1616
liposomal formulations 1007
– heat-sensitive 1554
liposomal siRNA 900
liposome targeting
– nonantibody ligands 967
liposome-based formulations 889
– CombiPlex® 1029
– CPX-351 1013
liposome-membrane-incorporated synthetic polymers 966
liposomes 888
– 2C5-modified 965
– aggregation 1005

– anti-HER2 958
– antibody-mediated long-circulating 955
– antibody-modified 962
– antibody-targeted 956
– behavior affecting factors 908
– cationic 1371
– circulating time 956
– clinical applications 953
– coformulation in 1043
– CPX-351 1030
– DOX 809
– drug delivery vehicles 1573
– drug-loaded 29
– dual-drug delivery systems 1026
– fluorescent 1003
– folate receptor-targeted 1001
– folate-modified 967
– formation 907
– freeze-drying 970
– immuno- 951
– non-PEGylated 907
– nonviral vectors 1401
– nucleosome-specific antibodies 961
– PEGylated 891, 952
– PEGylated CPP– 1205
– PELT 812
– protein-coupled 1504
– responsive 989
– sterically stabilized 909, 913
– structure 907, 908
– targeted 955, 1502
– targeting 3
liposome–polycation–DNA (LPD) 1376
LipOxal
– clinical development 1624
liver 95
– X/myc transgenic 1548
liver resection 1521
liver toxicity 102
liver tumors 1519
– clinical developments 1519
– nanoparticles 1546
– reticuloendothelial system 1527
– targeting 1519
living cells 1265
LLP2A
– peptidomimetic ligand 24
LNA–DOX
– DHA– 1334
loaded antibodies 111
loading
– noncovalent 248
loading capacity 815
local ablative therapy 1521
local gene delivery 1391
– clinical applications 1407
– clinical trials 1395
– physical methods 1404
– technologies 1404
localization 1569
– SLN 276
– specific 420
– subcellular 683, 1573
localization signal
– nuclear 423
locked nucleic acid (LNA) 1364
locoregional gene delivery 1405
log cell kill 14
logP value 1079
long-circulating copolymer 270
– HPMA 270
long-circulating liposomes
– antibody-mediated 955
long-circulating polymer carriers 264
long-term gene expression 1399
longevity
– pharmaceutical nanocarriers 952
low-density lipoprotein (LDL) 747, 1580
– radiolabeled 757
– receptor-mediated uptake 751
– synthetic approaches 759
– tumor cells 754
lower critical solution temperature (LCST) 668
– PNIPAAm 672
LPD (liposome–polycation–DNA) 1376
luciferase 1503
luminal endothelial cell membranes 334
lung cancer
– non-small-cell 27, 851, 1623
lung targeting 341, 343
lung tumors
– Lewis 913
luteinizing hormone-releasing hormone (LHRH) 533, 1220
– conjugates 1223
– cytotoxic analogs 1221
– radioiodinated 1225
LVEF (left ventricular ejection fraction) 918, 1236
lymph nodes 14
lymphangiogenesis 37
lymphangiography 22
lymphatic drainage 591
lymphatic vessels 17

lymphatics
– functional 46
lymphoblastic leukemia
– acute 3
lymphocytes
– B 413
lymphoma
– non-Hodgkin's 38, 103, 294, 449, 1233, 1243
lymphotropic nanoparticles 227
– MRI 229
LyP-1 1195, 1208
lysine amino groups 1578
lysine modification 86
lysine residues
– conjugation 92, 93
lysines
– alkylating 298
lysis 292
– redirected 451
lysomotropic effect 270
lysosomal activation 387
lysosomal membrane 250
lysosomes 296, 1100

m

M-components
– urine 934
mAb 176
mAb–maytansine conjugates 85
mAb–photosensitizer conjugates 1577
– indirect 1580
macromolecular carrier 684
macromolecular drug delivery systems 35
macromolecular drugs
– EPR effect 68
macromolecular linkers 1578
macromolecular photosensitizers 1585
macromolecular prodrugs 271, 782
– serum 755
macromolecular therapeutics
– drug-free 267
macromolecules 1361
– drug carriers 99
– polysaccharides 701
– structural factors 101
macrophages 546
– J774.1 714
– splenic 1366
macropinocytosis 1060
MAG (methacryloyl-glycine) 852
magnetic field-activated release 1006
magnetic nanoparticles 44
magnetic resonance imaging (MRI) 34, 44
– cellular structure 46
– hybrid MRI/PET scanner 248
– lymphotropic nanoparticles 229
– magnetic nanoparticles 47
– metabolic response 46
– theranostic micelles 1062
magnetically controlled CNS delivery 1507
magnetofection 237
major histocompatibility complex (MHC) 88
MALDI-TOF 22
maleimide group 784
maleimide-carrying phospholipids 969
malignancies
– hematological 924
malignant diseases 14
malignant melanomas 1219
– cytotoxic somatostatin analogs 1219
– LHRH cytotoxic analogs 1233
malignant tumors 1443
– differentiation 272
– microvasculature 38
mammalian toxins 1480
manganese sulfate gradient 1028
manufacturing
– GMP 1174
MAPG (melanoma-associated proteoglycan NG2) 460, 468
mapping 1189
– accessible vascular targets 430
– historic approaches 333
– proteome 336
– validation 339
markers 1189
– angiogenic 596, 616
– tumor-labeling 1192
marketed therapeutic antibodies 445
masking
– dendritic end-groups 536
mass spectrometry (MS) 1053
– data quantification and normalization 338
– proteome mapping 336
matrix 1053
– extracellular 596, 724
– remodeling 35
matrix metalloprotease (MMP) 554, 1056
– CPPs 1204
– matrix remodeling 35
– MT1 959
– PDT 1588
maurocalcine 1194
maximum tolerated dose (MTD) 1013
– CombiPlex® formulations 1032
– CPX-351 1037

maytansine
– structure 376
maytansinoids 99, 310
– accumulation of metabolites 391
– AMCs 375
– catabolism 303
– isolation of metabolites 385
– trastuzumab conjugates 384
MB07133 1531
MDA435/LCC6 tumors 1028
MDR (multidrug resistance) 34, 1026
– conventional chemotherapy 16
– CPPs 1194
– multifunctional pH-sensitive micelles 1117
– PUFAs 1345
MDR-1 protein 1221
MDX-447 464
measles virus 1404
medical sciences
– nanotechnology 887
medicinal mushrooms 19
medicine
– personalized 793
melamine polymers 536
melanoma-associated proteoglycan NG2 (MAPG) 460, 468
melanomas
– malignant 1233, 1243
membrane transfer domain 1447
membrane type-1 matrix metalloproteinase (MT1-MMP) 959
membranes 1189
– endothelial cell 334
– energy-independent translocation 1189
– fusion 1005
– gel-phase 992
– lipopolyplexes 1376
– lysosomal 252
– PUFA–drug conjugates 1325
– rigidity 993
MEND (multifunctional envelope-type nanodevice) 1377
– structure 1378
mesochlorin 821
metabolic response
– MRI 46
metabolism 1163
– ADME 1163, 1177
– cancer 36
– tumors 65
metalloprotease
– matrix 35, 554, 1056, 1204, 1588
metastases 952
– bone 277
– brain 432
– pretherapeutic detection 275
– spontaneous 35
metastatic breast cancer 930
metastatic micronodule 74
methacryloyl-glycine (MAG) 852
methide
– quinone 559
methotrexate (MTX) 4, 259
– clinical development 789
– DHA– 1338
– HSA conjugates 773
– MTX-loaded dendrimers 534
– MTX–HSA 862
– serum proteins 762
methoxy poly(ethylene glycol) (mPEG-OH) 628
methyl PEG (MPEG) 1106
methyl-β-cyclodextrin (BMC) 1141
MFECP 27
MHC (major histocompatibility complex) 88
mi interfering RNA (miRNA) 1361, 1421
– therapeutic applications 1383
mice 1219
– athymic nude 1219, 1247
– knockout 66, 330
– nu/nu 1297
– SCID 105, 472, 1348
micellar nanodevices
– multifunctional 1064
micellar structures 1053
– drug delivery systems 1053
– self-assembled 611
micelle-based polymer systems 892
micelles 1099
– biodegradable 1099
– CMC 892
– Cremophor 1592
– cylindrical 1054
– docetaxel-loaded 675, 677
– DOX 676
– DPc/m 537
– drug delivery vehicles 1573
– dual-drug delivery systems 1027
– folate receptor-targeted 1119
– folate-conjugated 1057
– hydrophilicity/hydrophobicity balance 1116
– multifunctional pH-sensitive 1114
– pH-sensitive polymeric 1054
– pH-triggered 1099, 1113
– polyion complex 1058

micelles (*contd.*)
– polymeric 1508
– smart polymeric 1054
– SMA–pirarubicin 75
– stable 673
– surface charge 1113
– TAT-functionalized 1121
– theranostic 1062
– unimolecular 258
– virus-mimetic cross-linked 1122
Michael-type addition 559
– retro-aldol–retro-Michael tandem reaction 566
microautoradiography 759
microbeads
– embolic 1080
microbubbles 34, 49
– dual-targeted 38
microcapsules 581
– APA-AST 1088
– self-immolative polymers 581
microcirculation 1133
– chaotic 44
– disorganized 44
– heterogeneous 33
microdosing 36
microenvironment 1133
– immunohistochemistry-based signature 1133
– pathophysiological 48
– tumor 251
microflow rate 41
micrometastases
– hepatic 1534
Micromonospora echinospora 95
micronodule
– metastatic 74
micropanning assay 14
microparticles
– diskoidal porous silicon 899
microparticulate drug delivery systems 887
microPET imaging 428, 429
microPET/CT 254
microprojectiles 1371
microscopic tumors 33
microscopy 1163
– intravital 340
– xzy confocal 1378
microsequencing 19, 21
microspheres
– albumin 761
microtubule-stabilizing agents (MTSA) 24
microtubules 247
– hyperstabilizing 895
– staining 272
microvascular networks 1003
microvasculature 1361
– chaotic 65
– normal tissues and malignant tumors 38
microvessels 1361
– formation 34, 36
– functional irregularities 38
– structural irregularities 38
– tumor 331
mimetic peptide
– p21 685
mimicry
– vascular 34, 36
mini-antibodies
– DiBi 459
minibodies 424
minimal residual disease (MRD) 466
miRNA (mi interfering RNA) 1361, 1421
– therapeutic applications 1383
mispairing
– LC 461
mitochondrial flavoprotein 1470
mitochondrial targeting 260, 273
mitomycin 676
mitomycin C 722, 932
– PUFA–mitomycin C 1336
mitoxantrone-loaded nanoparticles 1547, 1553
MM-111 469
MMAE (monomethyl auristatin E) 73, 79
– trigger group 583
MMC 722
MMP (matrix metalloprotease) 554, 1056
– CPPs 1204
– matrix remodeling 35
– MMP-2 1464
– MT1 959
– PDT 1588
modern diagnostics 14
modification 1163
– covalent 1163, 1178
– CPP drugs 1191
– noncovalent 1167
2C5-modified liposomes 965
– cytotoxicity 965
modulation
– micelle surface functionality 1113
modulators
– vascular 79
moieties
– targeting 258

molecular adapter
– multifunctional 1466
molecular beacon
– photodynamic 1588
molecular bioengineering 695
molecular biology
– in situ 1064
molecular biorecognition 268
molecular imaging 249
– assays 52
– hypoxia 258
– noninvasive 253
– probes 43
– SSTR 270
molecular structure
– repetitive growth 513
molecular weight 1283
– cytotoxic drugs 1283
– polymer carriers 108
molecularly targeted agents 808
molecularly targeted drug delivery 238
molecules 1361
– cell-penetrating small 534
– lipidoids 1373
– recombinant bispecific 457
– tandem 468
monoaqua complex 1607
monoclonal antibodies (mAb) 239
– anti-HER2 mAb 957
– chemotherapeutics 326
– clinical activities 38
– clinical development 431
– conventional chemotherapy 6
– murine anti-CEA 24
– peptide receptors 1219
– radionuclide delivery 411
monomeric tracer labeling 262
monomethyl auristatin E (MMAE) 73, 79
– trigger group 583
monopalmitoylphosphatidylcholine (MPPC) 1002
MOPP therapy 25
motif
– structural 514
mouse serum albumin (MSA) 90
MPEG (methyl PEG) 1106
mPEG-OH (methoxy poly(ethylene glycol)) 628
MPEG–HPAE block copolymer 1106
MPPC (monopalmitoylphosphatidylcholine) 1002
MRD (minimal residual disease) 466
MRI (magnetic resonance imaging) 34, 44
– cellular structure 46
– hybrid MRI/PET scanner 248
– lymphotropic nanoparticles 229
– magnetic nanoparticles 47
– metabolic response 46
– theranostic micelles 1062
MS (mass spectrometry) 887
– data quantification and normalization 338
– proteome mapping 336
MSA (mouse serum albumin) 90
MSV (multistage vector) 888, 896
– intracellular trafficking 900
– schematic illustration 898
MT1-MMP (membrane type-1 matrix metalloproteinase) 959
MTD (maximum tolerated dose) 1013
– CombiPlex® formulations 1032
– CPX-351 1037
MTSA (microtubule-stabilizing agents) 24
MTX (methotrexate) 259, 1312
– clinical development 789
– DHA– 1338
– HSA conjugates 773
– MTX-loaded dendrimers 534
– MTX–HSA 862
– serum proteins 762
MUC1 1199
mucosal surfaces 91
multiagent drug delivery vehicles 1022
multiagent therapies 808
multiarm PEG 867
– structure 844
multiblock polyHPMAs 267
multicenter trial 1343
multidrug resistance (MDR) 34
– conventional chemotherapy 16
– CPPs 1194
– multifunctional pH-sensitive micelles 1117
– PUFAs 1345
multidrug-resistant (MDR) tumors 1026
multifunctional core 278
multifunctional envelope-type nanodevice (MEND) 1377
– structure 1378
multifunctional micellar nanodevices 1064
multifunctional molecular adapter 1466
multifunctional pH-sensitive micelles 1114
multifunctional polymeric drug carriers 249
multilayer
– polyelectrolyte 725
multimerization 1501
multinodular HCC 873, 1557
multiple elimination linkers 554

multiple myeloma 933, 936
– PLD 935
multistage vector (MSV) 888
– intracellular trafficking 900
– schematic illustration 898
multivalency 1382
multiwalled carbon nanotube (MWNT) 546, 1165
– ADME 1176
– drug delivery systems 896
murine γ-retroviruses 1429
murine anti-CEA monoclonal antibody 24
murine tumors 3
mushrooms
– medicinal 19
mustard gas 4
mustine 3
mutagenesis
– enhanced 51
mutations
– "knob-into-hole" 457
MX-1 cells 1135
myeloid cells 36
– bone marrow-derived 34
myeloma 952
– multiple 933, 935, 936
myelosuppression 18, 1342
– reversible 25
Mylotarg® 75, 102, 278, 297
– calicheamicin ADCs 95
– New Drug Application 102

n

N-(2-hydroxypropyl)methacrylamide (HPMA) 66, 108, 110
– chemical structure 600
– DOX-DEX 817, 820
– drug–polymer conjugates 842
– fluorescently labeled copolymers 247
– hydrogel-based therapy 1081
– ligand-assisted vascular targeting 599
– liver tumor targeting 1551
– long-circulating copolymer 270
– multiblock polyHPMAs 267
– polymer-based combination therapy 814
– prodrugs 851
– trigger group 574
N-isopropylacrylamide (NIPAAm) 671
N-succinyl-chitosan derivatives 722
nab-docetaxel 1145
nab-paclitaxel 1139
– clinical studies 1152
nab-rapamycin/perifosine 1147
naked immunoglobulins 449
Nano-PICsomes 1062
nanoarchitectures
– highly ordered 1054
nanocapsules
– photosensitizers 538
nanocarriers 887
– ligand-based 1524
– pH-sensitive 257
– solid tumor targeting 1523
nanodevices 1361
– multifunctional envelope-type 1361
– multifunctional micellar 1064
– theranostic 1062
nanoemulsions
– dual-drug delivery systems 1027
nanogels 1072, 1078, 1122
nanoglobular dendrimeric platform 609
nanomolar range 1287
nanoparticle albumin bound (nab) technologies 761, 895, 1136
– drug encapsulation 1137
– product pipeline 1148
– small-molecule drugs 1139
nanoparticles 887
– active targeting 232
– albumin 895
– albumin-conjugated PEGylated 1149
– albumin–drug 1133
– cationic lipid 1371
– chitosan-coated 894
– clinical studies 1152
– CombiPlex® formulations 1040
– core/membrane lipid-based 1376
– DC-SPION 266
– delivery 346, 1271
– DOX 809
– doxorubicin–HSA 1147
– drug delivery vehicles 1573
– drug-encapsulated 1527
– gene therapy 237
– inorganic 1272
– liver tumors 1546
– lymphotropic 68, 229
– magnetic 44
– mitoxantrone-loaded 1547, 1553
– passive targeting 55
– polymer 1505
– Polysorbate 80-coated 1506
– prodrug 1042
– SCK 893
– self-assembled HFT 729
– siRNA 545
– solid lipid 1508

– SPION 43, 899, 1089, 1548
– synthetic approaches 759
– targeted therapy 236
– targeting liposomes 124
– transferrin–USPIO 233
– tumor-targeting 16
nanoparticulate drug delivery systems 887
– combination chemotherapy 1013
nanoparticulate pharmaceutical carriers 952
nanopharmaceuticals 814
nanorods
– Au–Ag 1272
nanosized hydrogels 1072
nanotechnology
– medical sciences 887
nanotubes 887
– carbon 546, 896, 1163
– covalent modification 1166, 1178
– functionalized 1168
– MWNT 546, 896, 1165
– noncovalent modification 1167
– SWNT 896, 1165
natural killer (NK) cells 449
natural polymer–drug conjugates 730
NCT (neutron capture therapy) 539
NDA (New Drug Application)
– Mylotarg® 102
near-IR imaging 38
necrolysis
– epidermal 297
necrosis 1445
necrosis factor
– TNF 96
necrotic areas 16
needle injection 1405
neoangiogenesis
– imaging 260
neocarzinostatin (NCS) 772, 871
– hepatotropic delivery 1543, 1555
neonatal Fc receptor (FcRn) 85
– altered binding 95
– antigen presentation 93
– discovery 87
– kidneys 94
– liver 95
– structure 88, 89
neonatal immune thrombocytopenia
– fetal 91
neoplasms
– secondary 25
neoplastic cells 236
neovasculature endothelial cells 595
nephrotoxicity 22
nervous system 281
networks 1071
– cross-linked 1071
– hydrogel 1073
– interpenetrating 1081
– microvascular 1003
– signaling 11
neuroendocrine cancers 271
neuroendocrine tumors 270, 281
neurological side-effects 24
neurovascular unit 1490
neutralizing antibodies 1459
neutron capture therapy (NCT) 539
– boron 277, 538
neutropenia 1344
neutrophil
– polymorphonuclear 451
New Drug Application (NDA)
– Mylotarg® 102
NHL 103, 203, 294
– cytotoxic somatostatin analogs 1243
– immune therapy targeting 449
– LHRH cytotoxic analogs 1233
Nile Red 581
nitric oxide synthase (NOS) 67
2-nitroimidazole 268
nitroglycerin 78
nitrosylcobalamin 1302
NK (natural killer) cells 449
NKTR-102 645, 868
NKTR-105 639, 655
NLS (nuclear localization signal) 423
NO-releasing agents 78
non-Hodgkin's lymphoma 38, 102, 294
– cytotoxic somatostatin analogs 1243
– immune therapy targeting 449
– LHRH cytotoxic analogs 1233
non-PEGylated liposomes 907
non-small-cell lung cancer (NSCLC) 27, 851, 1343, 1349, 1403
– LipoPlatin 1623
nonantibody ligands
– liposome targeting 967
nonantibody proteins 1580
noncleavable linkers 71
noncleavable thioether linkers 269
noncovalent associations 456
noncovalent loading 282
noncovalent modification
– CNTs 1167
nondegradable linker 602
nonenveloped viruses 1433
nonglycosylated fusion protein 22
noninvasive molecular imaging 253
nonlactosaminated albumin 1540

nonmetabolizable CHE 1041
nontarget internalization 1208
nonviral vectors 1058, 1398, 1401
– subcellular trafficking pathways 1060
normal tissues
– microvasculature 38
normalization
– MS data 338
NOS (nitric oxide synthase) 67
NPC (nuclear pore complex) 247
NSCLC (non-small-cell lung cancer) 27, 851, 1343, 1349, 1403
– LipoPlatin 1623
nu/nu mice 272, 1297
nuclear delivery
– hormone-mediated 261
nuclear localization signal (NLS) 423
nuclear pore complex (NPC) 247
nuclease resistance 1275
nucleic acids 1189
– delivery 1189
– locked 1364
– site-specific delivery 1055
nucleobase modification 1364
nucleosome binding 964
nucleosome-specific antibodies 961
nucleosomes
– interaction with AnAs 964
nucleotide binding 542
nude mice
– athymic 1229, 1247

o

O-glycan-peptide signatures 1271
O2-sensitive CPP systems 1204
oasireotide 1237
OATP (organic anion transporting polypeptide) 1493
obinutuzumab 449
OBOC (one-bead/one-compound) lbraries 3, 11, 14, 16
octanol/water partition coefficient 1079
ODD (oxygen-dependent degradation domain) 1205
oligomeric BsAbs
– hetero- 455
oligonucleotides 542
– albumin nanoparticle delivery 1150
– antisense 543
– delivery 1195
– PEGylation 656
– vectorization 1196
oligosaccharides
– cyclic 735
"On"/"Off" systems 1423
on-demand cleavable linkers 26
oncaspar 655
ONCOFID 866
ONCOFID-P 725, 726, 871
oncogenes 1199
oncogenic signaling 1198
oncology 1415
– clinical 35
– dendritic polymers 274
oncolytic adenoviruses 1431
Onconase®
– ranpirnase 1480
oncoproteins 1199
one-bead/one-compound (OBOC) lbraries 4, 12, 14, 16
Ontak® 1472
ONYX-015 1400, 1403
Opaxio 830, 857
– structure 810
– tumor uptake 842
optical imaging 200
optimal dose schedule
– PLD 938
optimal linker selection 381
optimization
– ligand 22
oral delivery 721
ordered nanoarchitectures 1054
organ-specific targeting
– platinum complexes 1612
organic anion transporting polypeptide (OATP) 1493
organs
– penetration 415
osteosarcoma 1614
osteosclerotic bone metastases 278
ovarian cancer 925
– cytotoxic somatostatin analogs 1240
– LHRH cytotoxic analogs 1230
– PLD 927
– ProLindac 854
ovarian tumor xenografts 1467
overexpression
– SPARC 1144
oxaliplatin 1605
– liposomal encapsulated 1619
– oxaliplatin–tamoxifen 1612
oxidative activation 569
oxycarbonyl group 558
oxygen species
– reactive 1328, 1331, 1569

oxygen-dependent degradation domain (ODD) 1205
oxygenation
– pretherapeutic 268
ozogamicin
– gemtuzumab 276

p

P-glycoprotein 1493
– inhibition 1498
P-glycoprotein (P-gp) 612
P-glycoprotein efflux effect 965
P-gp+ DLD1 human colon tumor xenograft 1346
p16 1201
p21 1202, 1207
p21 mimetic peptide 685
p27 1202
P450
– cytochrome 1349
p53 1200
PACA (polyacrylcyanoacrylate) 1527
paclitaxel 258
– aerosolized liposomal 970
– antitumor activity 1340
– brain targeting 1497
– DHA– 1338
– ester linkage 638
– heparin–folic acid–PTX 729
– HMPA– 852
– hydrogel-based therapy 1079
– ligand-assisted vascular targeting 606
– nab- 1139
– PEG–Gly–paclitaxel 641
– PEG–paclitaxel derivatives 640
– poly(glutamic acid)-bound 554
– polyglycerol–paclitaxel complex 522
– polymer-based combination therapy 807
– polysaccharide–drug conjugation 713
– prodrug nanoparticles 1042
– PUFAs 1332
– second-generation taxoid conjugates 1345
– transcytosis 1140, 1141
paclitaxel prodrugs
– elimination 1042
paclitaxel/gemcitabine 1043
paclitaxel–PGA conjugate 840
palliative treatment 13
palmar–plantar erythrodysesthesia (PPE) 915, 916, 934
PAMAM (poly(amidoamine)) 270, 279
– boronated 538
– diagnostic application 541
Panc-1 pancreatic tumor xenograft 1348
pancreatic cancers 1219
– cytotoxic somatostatin analogs 1219
– LHRH cytotoxic analogs 1234
pancreatic tumor
– human 1034
particle bombardment 1371, 1401
particle formation
– interlipidic 1005
PAsp(DET) (poly(N-(N-(2-aminoethyl)-2-aminoethyl)aspartamide)) 1059
passive carriers 1575
passive targeting 639
– CPPs 1203
– nanoparticles 55
– platinum complexes 1616
pathophysiological characteristics
– solid tumors 65, 667
pathophysiological microenvironment 48
pathophysiology 952
– receptor 33
– tumors 782
patient self-assessment questionnaire 921
PBAVE 1376
PBCA (poly(butyl cyanoacrylate)) 1505
PBS (phosphate-buffered saline) vehicle control 468
PCI (photochemical internalization) 1589, 1590
PCL (poly(3-caprolactone)) 612
PCR (polymerase chain reaction) 1416
PDEPT (polymer-directed enzyme prodrug therapy) 812, 813
pDNA (plasmid DNA) 1367, 1407
PDP (pyridyldithiopropionate) 956
PDT (photodynamic therapy) 277, 537, 1149
– clinical developments 1591
– drug delivery vehicles 1576
– growth factor targeted delivery 1311
– hydrogel-based 1087
– targeting and delivery 1569, 1573
PDZ 1459
PE (Pseudomonas aeruginosa exotoxin A) 34
– clinical trials 1474
– targeted 1448, 1460
pectin–drug conjugates 732
PEG (poly(ethylene glycol)) 1053
– palisade 1053
– pH-triggered micelles 1103
– prodrugs 855
– surface-grafted chains 992
– toxicity profile 628
– U-PEG 633
PEG dilemma 79
PEG-aldehyde linker 632

PEG-coated SWNTs
– biodistribution 1176
PEG-derivatized lipids 1372
PEG-detachable systems 1059
PEGA (poly(ethylene glycol) acrylamide) 19
pegfilgrastim 633
peginterferon-a2a 634
PEGylated antibody fragments 634
PEGylated CPP–liposomes 1205
PEGylated liposomal doxorubicin (PLD) 909
– breast cancer 916, 930
– economic analysis 936
– multiple myeloma 935
– optimal dose schedule 938
– ovarian cancer 927
– pharmacokinetics 912
– radiolabeled 920
– targeting 910
PEGylated liposomes 891
– brain targeting 1502
– cisplatin 939
– derivatization 955
– development 952
– doxorubicin (DOX) 953
– dual-drug delivery systems 1026
– EGFR 940
– newer applications 939
– radiolabeled 920
– targeting 910
– toxicity profile 915
PEGylated nanoparticles
– albumin-conjugated 1149
PEGylation 627
– CNTs 1173
– oligonucleotides 656
– permanent 630
– polyplexes 1059
– releasable 638
– site-specific 628
– targeted toxins 1460
PEG–Ara-C 652, 653
PEG–camptothecin analogs 641
PEG–drug conjugates 627
– acid-activated 651
– clinical trials 653, 654
– hydrolyzable 844
– pharmacokinetics 636
PEG–Gly–paclitaxel 641
PEG–lipid conjugates 955
PEG–paclitaxel derivatives 640
PEG–phospholipid conjugates 1001
PEG–TSCA conjugates 610
PEI (polyethyleneimine) 615
PEI (polyethylenimide) 1373
PEI (polyethylenimine) 1137
PELT (polymer enzyme liposome therapy) 812
PEM (polyelectrolyte multilayer) 725
Pen-ELP-H1 989
– antiproliferative effect 686
– c-Myc inhibtor 687
Pen-ELP1-H1 685
penetration 989
– cell 989
– nanocarriers 991
– rapid 1276
– triggerable 995
pentaheptad peptides 268
PEO (poly(ethylene oxide)) 673
Pep-3 1197
peptide conjugates
– PDT 1579, 1581
peptide hormone–drug conjugates 150
peptide ligand–drug conjugates 4
peptide linker
– enzymatically cleavable 784
peptide nucleic acid (PNA) 1591
peptide receptor radionuclide therapy (PRRT) 272
peptide-based spacers 1288
peptide-binding groove 88
peptide-mediated delivery 610
peptides 5
– amphipathic 1197
– bombesin/gastrin-releasing 1244
– cancer-targeting 3
– cell penetrating 1113
– cell-penetrating 680, 1189, 1443, 1456
– CREKA 1149
– delivery 682
– drugs 1082
– homing 1203, 1207
– iRGD 1057
– p21 mimetic 685
– pentaheptad 268
– PHSCN 545
– radiolabeling 418
– receptors 1219
– RGD 102, 255, 262, 263
– RGD4C 1117
– targeted cytotoxic analogs 1220
– targeting ligands 1382
– TAT 995
– therapeutic 684
– Trojan 1447
– tumor-homing 1149
– vasoactive intestinal 968
peptidic linkers 79

peptidomimetics 4
– ligand LLP2A 23
peptidyl linker 708
perfusion 1489
– arteriovenous shunt 37
– tumors 46
pericytes 1491
perifosine 1147
peripherally inserted central catheter (PICC) 6
perivascular distribution
– doxorubicin 17
permanent linkages 628
permanent PEGylation 630
permeability 951
– EPR 85, 251, 326, 639, 952, 1194, 1203
– liposomes 999
– vascular factors 66
peroxidation
– PUFAs 1331
peroxynitrite 72
persistence
– biologic 1169
personalized therapeutics 16, 793
PET (positron emission tomography) 28
– CNTs 1179
– drug design 275
– functional and molecular imaging 249
– image generation 416
– immunoPET 418, 431
– radiation treatment planning 275
– radionuclide delivery 414, 415
– radiopharmaceuticals 251
– tracers 251
– tumor imaging 34
PET/CT 247
– biomarkers 250
– clinical applications 272
– preclinical imaging 258
PFS (progression-free survival) 1039, 1154
PGA (poly(glutamic acid)) 3
– clinical trials 858
– drug–polymer conjugates 839, 857
– prodrugs 857
pGHRH-R 1248
pH
– human tumor xenografts 1101
pH dependence
– antitumor drugs 56
pH-dependent activation 569
pH-dependent deshielding 1203
pH-responsive linker systems 1298
pH-sensitive copolymer 1205
pH-sensitive CPP systems 1204
pH-sensitive micelles 1099
– multifunctional 1099
– polymeric 1054, 1108
– tumor delivery 1099
pH-sensitive nanocarriers 257
pH-sensitive pullulan–DOX conjugate 731
pH-triggered drug release 1104
– endocytic 1115
pH-triggered exposure of TAT 1113
pH-triggered interfacial defects 998
pH-triggered modulation
– micelle surface functionality 1113
phage-display libraries 3
– growth factor targeted delivery 1313
– tissue-specific targets 335
phages
– tumor cell-targeting 12, 14
phagocytosis
– frustrated 1172
pharmaceutical carriers 951
– nanoparticulate 951, 952
– site-specific 951
pharmacokinetics 36, 85
– ADCs 300
– AMCs 379
– AN-152 1235
– CNTs 1170, 1173
– combination chemotherapy 1020
– dendrimers 249
– dendritic architecture 535
– DOX 790, 914
– DOXO-EMCH 790
– FcRn 95
– liposomes 970
– nab-paclitaxel 1152
– PEG–drug conjugates 636
– PLD 912, 914
– sterically stabilized liposomes 913
– TXP 1339
pharmacology
– preclinical 1030, 1033, 1035, 1289
phase I trials 1013
– CPX-1 1013
– TXP 1342
phase II trials
– CPX-1 1039
phase II/III trials
– TXP 1343
phase transition
– temperature-triggered 672
PHEMA (poly(hydroxyethyl methacrylate)) 1072, 1089
phenyl ring 560
phenylazides 567

PhiPhiLux 532
phosphate-buffered saline (PBS) vehicle control 468
phosphatidylcholine–cholesterol–PEG2000–DSPE liposomes 1026
phosphatidylinositol 3-kinase 1416
phospholipid dispersions 889
phospholipids 1361
– anionic 1361
– maleimide-carrying 969
– PEG–phospholipid conjugates 1001
– photoisomerizable 1004
– PUFAs 1326
– synthesis 250
phosphorylation 1365
phosporamidate prodrugs 560
photoacoustic imaging 1180
photochemical activation 572
photochemical internalization (PCI) 1589, 1590
photochemistry 1569
photodynamic molecular beacon (PMB) 1588
photodynamic therapy (PDT) 277, 537, 1149
– clinical developments 1591
– drug delivery vehicles 1576
– growth factor targeted delivery 1311
– hydrogel-based 1087
– targeting and delivery 1569, 1573
photoimmunoconjugate (PIC) 1577
photoisomerizable phospholipid 1004
photomultiplier tubes (PMTs) 258
photophysics 1569
photopolymerization 1077
photosensitizer-linker-mAb conjugates
– indirect 1578
photosensitizers 247, 1080, 1087, 1149, 1571
– enzyme-cleavable conjugates 1586
– ideal 1571
– mAb–photosensitizer conjugates 1577
– macromolecular 1585
– nanocapsules 538
– polymer–photosensitizer conjugates 1584, 1586
– protein–photosensitizer conjugates 1583
– small-molecule–photosensitizer conjugates 1588, 1589
– structure 1572
– targeting via antibodies 1575
PHSCN peptide 545
phthalocyanine-encapsulated polymeric micelle
– dendrimer 537
phthalocyanines 1571
physical conjugation 1271
physical cross-linking 1074
physicochemical characterization
– combination therapy 816
physiological pH 1059
PIC (polyion complex) micelles 1058
PICC (peripherally inserted central catheter) 6
PICsomes 1061
pIgR (polymeric immunoglobulin receptor) 91
PIHCA 1546, 1547, 1553
pinocytosis
– fluid-phase 1114
PIONEER 859, 876
pirarubicin 73
pirarubicin micelles
– SMA– 75
PK1 843
PK2 1551
– hepatotropic delivery 1529
– structure 1532
placental transport
– directional 90
planar g-scintigraphy 85
plant RIPs 1451
plant toxins 1464, 1466
plasma cholesterol 753
plasma clearance 379
plasma elimination 1043
plasma proteins 748
plasmid DNA (pDNA) 1367, 1407
plasmid expression
– shRNA 1418
plasmid-derived shRNAs 1420
plasmids encoding GFP 995
plasmon resonance
– surface 112
platinophiles 1609
platinum complexes 839
– antineoplastic 839
– liposomal drug delivery 1616
– targeting strategies 1605
platinum-based combination chemotherapies 37
platinum-refractory tumors 928
platinumphosphonato complexes 1615
– structure 1616
platinum–DNA adducts 1035
PLD (PEGylated liposomal doxorubicin) 909
– breast cancer 916, 930
– economic analysis 936
– multiple myeloma 935
– optimal dose schedule 938

- ovarian cancer 927
- pharmacokinetics 912
- radiolabeled 920
- targeting 910
PLLA (poly(L-lactic acid)) 674, 1105
Pluronics 675
PMB (photodynamic molecular beacon) 1588
PMN (polymorphonuclear neutrophil) 451
PMTs (photomultiplier tubes) 258
PNA (peptide nucleic acid) 1591
PNiPAAm 1077
Pol III promoter 1419
poloxamers 675, 676
poly(β-amino esters) (HPAE) 1106
poly(3-caprolactone) (PCL) 612
poly(amidoamine) (PAMAM) 270, 279
- boronated 538
- diagnostic application 541
poly(butyl cyanoacrylate) (PBCA) 1505
poly(e-caprolactone) spacer 257
poly(ethylene glycol) (PEG) 1053
- drug conjugates 1053
- palisade 1059
- PEG-aldehyde linker 632
- PEGylation 627, 628
- PEG–camptothecin analogs 641
- PEG–CPT 855, 856
- pH-triggered micelles 1103
- polymer-based combination therapy 817
- SC-PEG 631
- SS-PEG 630
- surface-grafted chains 992
- toxicity profile 628
- U-PEG 633
poly(ethylene glycol) acrylamide (PEGA) 19
poly(ethylene oxide) (PEO) 673
poly(glutamic acid) (PGA) 839
- clinical trials 839
- drug–polymer conjugates 839, 857
- prodrugs 857
poly(glutamic acid)-bound paclitaxel 554
poly(hydroxyethyl methacrylate) (PHEMA) 1072, 1089
poly(L-glutamic acid) (PGA) 3
poly(L-histidine)
- interfacial 1121
poly(L-lactic acid) (PLLA) 674, 1105
poly(N-(N-(2-aminoethyl)-2-aminoethyl) aspartamide) (PAsp(DET)) 1059
poly(N-isopropylacrylamide) (PNIPAAm) 671, 1077
- chemotherapeutics 674
poly(organophosphazene) (PPZ) 677
poly(propylene oxide) (PPO) 673
polyacetal polymers
- biodegradable 844
polyacids 1103
polyacrylcyanoacrylate (PACA) 1527
polyarginine 1210
polybases 1103
polycation
- cyclodextrin-containing 1375
polyconjugates
- schematic formation 1376
polyelectrolyte multilayer (PEM) 725
polyethyleneimine (PEI) 615, 1137, 1373
polygalactosamine–drug conjugates 735
polyglycerol
- dendritic 527
polyglycerolamine 544
- dendritic 543
polyglycerol–DOX prodrugs 536
polyglycerol–paclitaxel complex
- hydrophobic 522
polyion complex (PIC) micelles 1058
polylysine backbone 1587
polymer carriers 99
- backbone degradable 263
- drug binding 250
- efficiency 104
- long-circulating 264
polymer enzyme liposome therapy (PELT) 812
polymer nanoparticles 1505
polymer peptide–drug conjugate 150
polymer therapeutics 262, 591, 701
- APN-targeted 613
- endothelial cell-targeted 597
- targeted 599
polymer vesicles 1054
polymer-based combination therapy 805
- clinical development 816
- EPR effect 810
- preclinical development 817
- target sites 811
polymer-based systems 89, 1053
polymer-directed enzyme prodrug therapy (PDEPT) 812, 813
polymerase chain reaction (PCR) 1416
polymeric carriers
- polymer-based combination therapy 812
polymeric delivery systems 1619
polymeric immunoglobulin receptor (pIgR) 91
polymeric micelles 892, 1054
- brain targeting 1508

polymeric micelles (*contd.*)
– dendrimer phthalocyanine-encapsulated 537
– dual-drug delivery systems 1027
– pH-sensitive 1054, 1108
– smart 1054
– TAT-conjugated 1114
polymeric photosensitizer prodrug (PPP) 1587
polymers 1071
– amphiphilic 627, 1078
– biodegradable 739, 844
– carriers 839, 841
– cascade 540
– cationic 1373
– cross-linked network 1071
– dendritic 274
– histidine-derived 1105
– hydrogel networks 1073
– hydrogel-based prodrugs 1081
– hydrolysis 840
– imidazole-containing 1119
– interpenetrating network 1081
– liposome-membrane-incorporated 966
– mAb–photosensitizer conjugates 1578
– melamine 536
– protective 955
– self-immolative comb 580
– smart 1074
– stimuli-sensitive 668, 1074
– synthetic 671, 953
– thermo-responsive 667
– titratable 999
polymersomes 1054, 1061
– drug release 1061
polymer–drug conjugates 34, 707
– combination therapy 810
– combined with radiotherapy 830
– design 89
– natural 730
– polymer-based combination therapy 818
– RGD-based 601
– selectin-targeted 612
– water-soluble 272
polymer–photosensitizer conjugates 1584, 1586
polymorphoneutrophils 1570
polymorphonuclear neutrophil (PMN) 451
polypeptides 1071
– Bac-ELP-p21 688
– elastin-like 678
– polypeptide–drug conjugate 671
polyphosphazene 1082
polyplexes 1373
– PEGylation 1059
– schematic formation 1374
polysaccharide-based drug conjugates 747
polysaccharides 1133
– Chemical structure 702
– hydroxyl groups 711
polysaccharide–drug conjugates
– synthesis 708
polysaccharide–drug conjugation 707
Polysorbate 80-coated nanoparticles 1506
polysorbate-based docetaxel 1141, 1154
polyunsaturated fatty acids (PUFAs) 1359
– internalization 1325
– second-generation taxoid conjugates 1345
POMP regimen 12
pop-up mechanism
– versatile tumor targeting 1121
pore complex
– nuclear 247
pores 989
– transbilayer 989
– transmembrane 1000
porosification of silicon 897
porous silicon microparticles
– diskoidal 899
positron emission tomography (PET) 27
– CNTs 1179
– drug design 275
– image generation 416
– immunoPET 418, 431
– PET/CT 247
– radiation treatment planning 275
– radionuclide delivery 414, 415
– radiopharmaceuticals 251
– tracers 251
– tumor imaging 34
positron emitters 417
– immunoPET 418
postcapillary venules 69
PPD modification 1378
PPE (palmar–plantar erythrodysesthesia) 915, 916, 934
PPO (poly(propylene oxide)) 673
PPP (polymeric photosensitizer prodrug) 1587
PPZ (poly(organophosphazene)) 677
PrAgU2 1465
Prato reaction 1166
pre-antibody era 442
preclinical development 1219
– bombesin/gastrin-releasing peptides 1219
– CombiPlex® formulations 1030
– cytotoxic somatostatin analogs 1236

– GHRH antagonists 1247
– hepatotropic drug delivery systems 1528
– LHRH cytotoxic analogs 1221
– PDT 1573
– polymer-based combination therapy 817
– responsive liposomes 994
– targeted toxins 1462
preclinical evaluations 1359
– cross-species binding 112
– TXP 1338
preclinical imaging 805
– SPECT/CT and PET/CT 258
– tumors 247
preclinical models
– combination therapy 815
preclinical pharmacology 1013
– CPX-1 1033
– CPX-351 1030
– CPX-571 1013
– FA–drug conjugates 1289
preclinical studies 1053
– micellar structures 1053
– second-generation taxoid conjugates 1345
precontrast 230
predetermined breaking point 555, 874
preparation
– antibody-targeted liposomal drugs 968
pretargeting 429
– receptors 541
pretherapeutic detection
– metastases 275
pretherapeutic tumor oxygenation 268
pretherapy biodistribution 434
prevascular growth phase 34
primary bone tumors 1614
pristine SWNTs 1175
pro-inflammatory cytokines 894
pro-prodrugs 556
proapoptotic proteins 1228
probes 1489
– fluorescent 541
– molecular imaging 44
prodrugs 1163
– and drugs 20
– brain targeting 1495
– calicheamicin 75
– cholesterol paclitaxel 1042
– dual-acting 784, 787, 878
– enzymatically cleavable 527, 562
– enzyme prodrug systems 4
– GDEPT 1397
– HepDirect™ 1527, 1529
– HPMA 851
– hydrogel-based 1081
– in situ binding 779
– macromolecular 251, 755, 782
– paclitaxel 1042
– PDEPT 812, 813
– PEG 855
– PGA 857
– phosporamidate 560
– polyglycerol–DOX 536
– polymeric photosensitizer 1587
– site-specific activation 591
– tripartate 556
product pipeline
– nab technologies 1148
products
– double-prodrug concept 556
progenitor cells
– hematopoietic 1430
progeny virus 1426
prognostic potential
– imaging biomarkers 273
progression
– cancer 1324
progression-free survival (PFS) 1039, 1154
progressive acidification 991
proliferating endothelial cells 592
proliferation 35
– cellular 35, 685
– liver cancer 1551
proliferative activity 264
proliferative factors 1419
ProLindac 1619
– clinical development 1625
– drug–polymer conjugates 853
– partial structure 1621
promoter
– Pol III 1419
propofol 1335
prostate cancer 11
– cytotoxic somatostatin analogs 1240
– LHRH cytotoxic analogs 1230, 1232
prostate-specific antigen (PSA) 562
prostate-specific membrane antigen (PSMA) 295, 1265
– siRNA 1274
protamine 1198
proteases 79, 1586
– protease-dependent activation 1203
– upregulation 554
protective polymers 955
protein toxin 1310
protein transduction domain (PTD) 1381, 1447
– TAT 1456
protein-based delivery system 1151

protein-based drugs 103
protein-coupled liposomes 1504
proteins 1489
– ABC export 1489
– albumin nanoparticle delivery 1150
– angiogenic 35
– angiotensin-converting 341
– Antennapedia 1189
– antiapoptotic 1228
– ASGP 730
– biosynthesis imaging 257
– conjugation with SC-PEG 632
– conjugation with SS-PEG 630
– drugs 1082
– E1B-55K 1432
– FABP 1325, 1326
– fluorescein isothiocyanate-labeled 757
– GFP 262, 1198, 1421
– human 1468
– IAP 1200
– MDR-1 1221
– nonantibody 1580
– nonglycosylated fusion 22
– plasma 748
– proapoptotic 1228
– purified 1265
– radiolabeling 418
– recombinant fusion 1457
– reductive alkylation 633
– RIP 1451, 1452, 1475
– serum 747
– targeted toxins 1443
– targeting ligands 1382
– tumor suppressor Rb 687
– vitamin B12-binding 1300
– von Hippel-Lindau 65
protein–photosensitizer conjugates 1583
proteoglycan NG2 460, 468
proteolytic activation 564
proteolytic degradation 92, 96
proteome 337
– alterations 49
– human serum 747
– vascular endothelial cells 336
proton sponge effect 1059, 1118, 1375
protonation of histidine moieties 1125
PRRT (peptide receptor radionuclide therapy) 272
PSA (prostate-specific antigen) 562
PSCA-specific diabodies 430
Pseudomonas aeruginosa exotoxin A (PE) 111
– clinical trials 1474
– targeted 1448, 1460
Pseudomonas toxin 13
PSMA (prostate-specific membrane antigen) 295, 1265
– siRNA 1274
PTD-DRBD 1198
PUFA–chlorambucil 1336
PUFA–drug conjugates 1359
– gene expression 1328
– PUFA peroxidation 1331
– signal transduction pathways 1328
– structure 1333
PUFA–mitomycin C 1336
PUFA–taxoid conjugates 1346
PUFA–tegafur 1337
pullulan–drug conjugates 729
pulmonary side-effects 22
pumping
– transvascular 329
purification of ELPs 680
purified proteins 1265
pyridoxine 1307
pyridyldithiopropionate (PDP) 956
pyrimidine
– fluorinated 1032
pyrolidine 1176
2-pyrrolino-DOX 1225
– structure 1246
pyrrolic ring systems
– conjugated 1571

q

QD–photosensitizer hybrids 1575
quantification
– MS data 338
quantum dots (QD) 1574
quenching
– self- 1587
quercetin 1027
quinone methide elimination 559

r

radiation treatment planning 275
radioactive decay products 420
radioactive immunoconjugates 77
radioactive nonmetabolizable CHE 1041
radiofrequency tumor ablation 971
radioimmunoconjugate 27
radioimmunoimaging
– clinical development 431
radioimmunoscintigraphy agents 417
radioimmunotherapy (RIT) 266, 411, 1206
– clinical development 434
radioiodinated LHRH 1225
radiolabeled antibodies 412

radiolabeled bombesin analogs 1245
radiolabeled CNTs 1176
radiolabeled integrin antagonists 262
radiolabeled LDL 757
radiolabeled PEGylated liposomes 920
radiolabeled PLD 920
radiolabeled transferrin 753
radiolabeling
– in situ 333
radiometals 421
radionuclides 1189
– delivery 411, 1189
– g imaging 417
– imaging 415
– PRRT 272
– theranostics 435
– therapeutic 418, 419
radiopeptide therapy 271
radiopharmaceuticals 251, 259
radiotherapy 805
– combined with polymer–drug conjugates 805
– growth factor targeted delivery 1311
– hydrogel-based 1088
– polymer-based combination therapy 812
– targeted 414, 1238
radiotracers 34, 36
– hypoxia-selective 267
random coil conformation 247
ranpirnase
– Onconase® 1480
rapamycin 1432
rapid amplification of cDNA ends (RACE) 1418
rapid penetration 1276
ratio-dependent synergy 1016, 1031
– In vitro evidence 1017
ratiometric dosing platform 1040
ratios
– drug 1014
rats
– Sprague-Dawley 693
Rb (tumor suppressor protein) 687
RCC (renal cell carcinoma) 1223
– cytotoxic somatostatin analogs 1241
– LHRH cytotoxic analogs 1232
reactive agents
– CombiPlex® formulations 1033
reactive oxygen species (ROS) 1328, 1331, 1569
reactivity
– cell-targeting 993
realizing 759
receptor-independent endocytosis 1122
receptor-mediated endocytosis 1115, 1269
receptor-mediated uptake of LDL 751
receptors 1519
– ASGP 840
– bombesin/gastrin-releasing peptides 1244
– epidermal growth factor 533, 940, 958, 1313
– estrogen 807
– expression imaging 269
– folate 235, 1119, 1284
– GHRH 1247
– gp60 792, 1134
– hyaluronic acid binding 598
– LHRH 1221
– neonatal Fc 85
– pathologies 33
– peptides 1219
– pIgR 91
– pretargeting 541
– PRRT 272
– receptor/antigen targeting 786
– RHAMM 724
– somatostatin 34, 270, 1236
– steroid hormone 261
– toll-like 1277, 1367
– transferrin 960, 966
– tumor-specific 1444
– tumoral 1222
– VEGF 261
recombinant AAV vectors 1434
recombinant bispecific molecules 457
– clinical trials 464
recombinant DNA techniques 27, 88, 695
recombinant factor VIIa 103
recombinant fusion proteins 1457
recombinant IgG-like BsAb 460
recurrence 274
recycling 1053
– blocking 102
– FcRn-mediated 92
red blood cells
– artificial 1062
redirected lysis 451
reduced folate carrier (RFC) 1284
reduction of disulfide bonds 1002
reductive activation 566
reductive alkylation 633
reductive cleavage 25
reductive environment 1291
reductive release 1306
regioisomers 1312
regulation of gene expression
– differential 49
releasable β-ligand conjugates 1301

releasable dual-drug conjugates 1295
releasable linkages 628
releasable PEG linkers 1099
– aliphatic systems 649
– aromatic systems 646
releasable PEGylation 638
release 1099
– cytosolic 1099
– dual-phase mechanism 844
– endocytic 1115
– endosomal 1367
– from polymersomes 1061
– intracellular 1286
– IR/UV-activated 1003
– magnetic field-activated 1006
– pH-triggered 1104
– reductive 1306
– responsive 994
– slow-release mechanism 1341
– triggered 996
– ultrasound-activated 1005
remodeling
– matrix 35
renal cell carcinoma (RCC) 1223
– cytotoxic somatostatin analogs 1241
– LHRH cytotoxic analogs 1232
renal clearance 629
– threshold 94, 856
repetitive growth
– molecular structure 274
replication of viruses 1432
repulsion
– electrostatic 996
resistance
– multidrug 16, 34, 1117, 1194, 1345
– nuclease 1275
resonance energy transfer
– fluorescence 249
respective delivery concept 1446, 1607
respiratory distress syndrome 23
response 989
– inhibitory 774
– metabolic 46
– RECIST 34
– to therapy 274
responsive liposomes 989
– preclinical development 989
– solid tumor therapy 989
responsive release 994
restaging 274
retargeting 450
– T-cell 464
retention
– EPR 85, 251, 326, 639, 952, 1194, 1203
retention time in target tissue 1276
reticuloendothelial system 909
reticuloendothelial system (RES) 992
– liver tumors 1527
retro-aldol–retro-Michael tandem reaction 566
retro-synthetic analysis 1288
retroviral vectors 1392, 1400
– shRNA delivery 1428
γ-retroviruses
– murine 1429
reverse transcriptase
– human telomerase 1591
reversible myelosuppression 177
reversible systems 1423
RGD peptides 148, 262, 263
– structure 255
RGD sequence 1382
RGD-based polymer–drug conjugates 601
RGD-based vehicles
– cyclic 608
RGD4C 1117
RHAMM (receptor for hyaluronic acid-mediated motility) 724
rhodamine-labeled Bac-ELP1-H1 695
ribosomal display technologies 423
ribosome-inactivating protein (RIP) 1452
– clinical trials 1475
– plant 1451
ricin 1453
rigidity
– membranes 993
ring
– phenyl 560
ring closure
– spontaneous 557
ring systems
– conjugated pyrrolic 1571
RIT (radioimmunotherapy) 266, 411
– clinical development 434
rituximab 444
RNA 1263
– aptamer–chimeric 1263
– artificial micro- 1421
– chemical vectors 1371
– conditional systems 1422
– delivery 1361, 1368
– ectopic 1368
– micro- 1361, 1421
– small interfering 542, 545, 609, 899, 1058, 1085, 1273, 1361, 1379
RNA interference (RNAi) 1197
– clinical trials 1417
– viral vectors 1415

RNAi drugs
– clinical trials 1384
Rnase
– targeted 1470
ROS (reactive oxygen species) 1328, 1331, 1569
RRM2 1385

s
safety
– drug 251
safety pharmacology assessment 109
safety studies
– CNTs 1171
Salmonella 1401
saponinum album 1468
saporin-based targeted toxins 1456
SAR (structure–activity relationship) 18
sarcomas 952
– Kaposi's 919, 922
– soft-tissue 937
– Yoshida 54
saturation of endogenous silencing pathway 1368
SC-PEG (succinimidyl carbonate PEG) 631
scaffolds 1415
– alternative 310
– dendritic 275
SCC (squamous cell carcinomas) 40
scDb (single-chain diabodies) 105
scFv (single-chain Fv) 452, 459
scFv–Fc fragments 425, 426
SCID (severe combined immunodeficiency disorder) 1429
– SCID mice 105, 472, 1348
SCK (shell cross-linked knedel) 892
– nanoparticles 893
screening 1359
– drug–drug interaction 1349
– dual-color method 20
– phage-display libraries 6
– virtual 1313
second generation drug–polymer conjugates 865
second-generation PEG linker 631
second-generation taxoid conjugates 1332, 1345
– LA/LNA– 1349
second-line chemotherapy 13
secondary neoplasms 25
secondary structure
– aptamers 1264
secreted protein, acidic and rich in cysteine (SPARC) 782, 1135, 1323
– nab-paclitaxel 1155
– overexpression 1144
selectin 596
selectin-targeted polymer–drug conjugates 612
selection
– optimal linkers 381
SELEX (systematic evolution of ligands by exponential enrichment) 1264, 1265, 1381
self-assembly 1071
– amphiphilic polymers 1071
– block copolymers 1054
– HFT nanoparticles 729
– lipids 990
– micellar structures 611
self-assessment questionnaire
– patient 921
self-immolation 591
– complex architectures 573
self-immolative comb polymer 580
self-immolative dendrimers 575
– drug release 577
self-immolative linkers (SILs) 553, 1288
– acyclization-based 556
– clinical application 582
self-immolative polymers
– microcapsules 581
self-immolative spacers 5, 25
self-quenching 1587
sensor
– apoptotic 532
sentinel lymph node (SLN) mapping 247
– SPECT/CT 276
sequence variation 444
sequential transcytosis 342
serum albumin 85
– anticancer agents 763
– bovine 566, 1123
– half-life 107
– human 750, 862, 1133, 1323
– mouse 90
– structure 86
– targeting 102, 105
– zzz 763
serum albumin fusion technology 102, 104
serum bilirubin 99
serum proteins 747
– clinical development 788
serum proteome
– human 747
serum testosterone level 1086
severe combined immunodeficiency disorder (SCID) 1429
– SCID mice 103, 472, 1348

shell
– core–shell structure 1058
shell (corona) 1103
shell cross-linked knedel (SCK) 892
– nanoparticles 893
shielding/deshielding mechanism 1115
short hairpin RNA (shRNA) 1391, 1406
– plasmid expression 1418
– plasmid-derived 1420
– steric hindrance 1425
SHR (steroid hormone receptor) 261
shunt perfusion
– arteriovenous 40
sialoglycoprotein 96
side-chains
– hydrophobic 272
side-effects 1359
– conventional chemotherapy 16
– neurological 24
– pulmonary 22
– vascular 23
signal transduction pathways 1328
signaling 1189
– cytoplasmic region 88
– networks 24
– oncogenic 1198
– PUFA–drug conjugates 1325
silencing pathway
– endogenous 1368
silica particles
– colloidal 333
silicon
– porosification 897
silicon microparticles 899
SILs (self-immolative linkers) 553
– acyclization-based 556
– clinical application 582
single formulation 1023
single-chain diabodies (scDb) 105
single-chain Fv (scFv) 452, 459
single-photon emission computed tomography (SPECT) 805
– radionuclide delivery 411, 415, 433
– radiopharmaceuticals 259
– SPECT/CT 247
– tracers 259
– tumor imaging 34, 35
single-type therapy 806
singlewalled carbon nanotube (SWNT) 896, 1165
– biodistribution 1176
– dispersed 1172
– PEG-coated 1176
– structure 35
sinusoidal endothelium 328
SIP (small immunoproteins) 424
siRNA (small interfering RNA) 542, 1197, 1361
– aptamer conjugates 1273
– aptamer–siRNA chimeras 1379
– hydrogel-based therapy 1085
– ligand-assisted vascular targeting 609
– MSV 899
– nanoparticles 545
– PIC micelles 1058
– therapeutic applications 1383
site-specific drug attachment 90
site-specific drug delivery 1054
site-specific PEGylation 628
site-specific pharmaceutical carriers 951
site-specific prodrug activation 591
size fractionation 232
size-dependent targetability 281
skin keratinocytes 297
SLN (sentinel lymph node) mapping 247
– SPECT/CT 276
slow-release mechanism 1341
small immunoproteins (SIP) 424
small interfering RNA (siRNA) 542, 1197, 1361
– aptamer conjugates 1273
– aptamer–siRNA chimeras 1379
– hydrogel-based therapy 1085
– ligand-assisted vascular targeting 609
– MSV 899
– nanoparticles 545
– PIC micelles 1058
– therapeutic applications 1383
small molecules 1283
– cell-penetrating 534
– lipophilicity 1287
small-animal hybrid scanners 249
small-molecular-weight ligands 1382
small-molecule delivery 1270
small-molecule drugs 1079, 1139
small-molecule–photosensitizer conjugates 1588, 1589
SMANCS 65, 67, 70, 871
– hepatotropic delivery 1543, 1555
– postmarketing survey 1558
– structure 872, 1544
SMANCS/Lipiodol 77, 1558
smart polymeric micelles 1054
smart polymers 1074
SMA–pirarubicin micelles 75
SOD (superoxide dismutase) 1084
soft-tissue sarcomas 937
solid lipid nanoparticles 1508

solid tumors 1391
– accessible vascular targets 415
– local gene delivery 1391
– pathophysiological characteristics 65, 667
– responsive liposomes 989
– serum proteins 752
– targeting 1523
– vascular characteristics 65
solubility 577, 840
solution temperature
– lower critical 668, 672
somatostatin 269
– receptors 1236
– targeted cytotoxic analogs 1236
somatostatin receptor (SSTR) 34
– molecular imaging 270
spacers 1283
– carbohydrate-based 1283
– elongated 257
– peptide-based 1288
– poly(e-caprolactone) 257
– self-immolative 6, 25
SPARC (secreted protein, acidic and rich in cysteine) 782, 1135, 1323
– nab-paclitaxel 1155
– overexpression 1144
specific localization 420
specificity
– binding 961
specifier (trigger) 556, 564
SPECT (single-photon emission computed tomography) 1053
– functional and molecular imaging 249
– radionuclide delivery 411, 415, 433
– radiopharmaceuticals 259
– tracers 259
– tumor imaging 34, 35
SPECT/CT 247
– adrenocortical tumors 279
– biomarkers 258
– bone metastases 277
– clinical applications 272
– neuroendocrine tumors 281
– preclinical imaging 258
– SLN mapping 276
– thyroid cancer 278
Spectral Index 339
spherical micelles 1054
SPIO (superparamagnetic iron oxide) 56
– active targeting 232
SPION (superparamagnetic iron oxide nanoparticles) 44, 899
– dendrimer-coated 270
– hydrogel-based 1089
– YCC-DOX 1548
splenic macrophages 1366
split-mix synthesis method 17
sponge effect
– proton 1059, 1118, 1375
spontaneous metastasis 85
spontaneous ring-closure
– esters/amides 557
Sprague-Dawley rats 693
sprouting
– endothelial 34
squamous cell carcinomas (SCC) 40
SS-PEG (succinimidyl succinate PEG) 630
SS1P 649, 650, 1479
SSTR (somatostatin receptor) 34, 269
– molecular imaging 270
stability
– chemical 1365
stable conjugates 871, 1287
stable micelles 673
staging of cancer 273
staining 1013
– microtubules 272
– tissue 339
standards
– GMP 27
Staudinger ligation 571
"stealth" type liposomes 1026
stealth effect 79
STELLAR 859
stem cells
– cancer 95
steric barrier 992
steric hindrance
– shRNA expression 1425
sterically stabilized liposomes 909
– pharmacokinetics 913
– structure 908
steroid hormone receptor (SHR) 261
stimuli
– tumor-intrinsic 994
stimuli-sensitive polymers 668, 1074
strategy
– drug delivery 599
streptadivin 34
streptonigrin 66
stromal fibroblasts 46
structural and functional irregularities
– tumor microvessels 38
structural factors
– macromolecules 112
structural motif
– branching 514

structure
– molecular 275
structure modification 1365
structure–activity relationship (SAR) 18
structure–function analysis 1014
subcellular fate of macromolecules 101
subcellular localization 1573
– CPP-ELPs 683
subcellular organelles
– pH variations 1100
subcellular targeting 258
subcellular trafficking pathways
– nonviral vectors 1060
subunits
– branched 278
succinate linkage 722
succinimidyl carbonate PEG (SC-PEG) 631
succinimidyl succinate PEG (SS-PEG) 630
sugar modification 1364
suicide gene therapy 1397
suicide substrates 566
sulfhydryl-reactive cross-linkers 1137
sulfo-NHS-LC-biotin 532
super-stealth property 1063
superoxide dismutase (SOD) 1084
superparamagnetic iron oxide (SPIO) 56
– active targeting 232
superparamagnetic iron oxide nanoparticles (SPION) 43, 899
– dendrimer-coated 258
– hydrogel-based 1089
– YCC-DOX 1548
supportive care 6
suppression
– epigenetic 1423
supramolecular architectures 735
supramolecular drug entrapment 520
supramolecular voids 275
surface charge
– micelles 1113
surface functionalities
– micelles 1113
surface plasmon resonance 112
surface stabilizing agents
– amphipathic 1041
surface-grafted chains 992
surgery
– imaging-guided 1062
survival
– progression-free 1039, 1154
survival curve
– Kaplan–Meier 1118, 1501, 1615
SWNT (singlewalled carbon nanotube) 896, 1165
– biodistribution 1176
– dispersed 1172
– PEG-coated 1176
– structure 1164
sympathetic nervous system 281
synergy 1099
– endocytic release/endocytosis 1099
– heat map 1021
– In vitro evidence 1017
– PUFAs/cytotoxic drugs 1331
– ratio-dependent 1016, 1031
synthesis 1219
– cytotoxic somatostatin analogs 1219
– L-HSA 1533
– ladder method 22
– LHRH cytotoxic analogs 1223
– phospholipids 250
– polysaccharide–drug conjugates 707
– split-mix method 17
synthetic glycoside clusters 1525
synthetic ligands 1526
synthetic polymers 953
– liposome-membrane-incorporated 966
– thermo-responsive 671
synthetis
– elastin-like polypeptide 678
systematic evolution of ligands by exponential enrichment (SELEX) 1264, 1265, 1381
systemic FcRn-mediated recycling 92
systemic toxicity 1610
systems biology approach 1015

t

T-cell engager
– bispecific 464
T-cell response 28
T-cell retargeting 464
T-cell targeting 110
T-lymphocytes
– cytotoxic 451
tag
– coding 23
tailor-made hydrogels 1071
tailor-made linkers 793
tails 1219
– cytoplasmic C-terminal 1219
– hydrophilic molecular 1574
TandAb antibodies 469
tandem molecules 468
tandem reaction
– retro-aldol–retro-Michael 566

target antigen selection 295
target cell activation
– (un-)cleavable AMCs 389
target cell metabolites 386
target cell specificity 1366
target identification
– drugs 52
target space
– transvascular pumping 329
target tissue
– retention time in 1276
targetability
– size-dependent 281
targeted cancer cells 385
– bystander effects 388
targeted cancer therapy 1263
targeted cytotoxic peptide analogs 1220
targeted cytotoxic somatostatin analogs 1236
targeted delivery 1263
– aptamer isolation 1263
– aptamers 1266
– folate receptor-mediated endocytosis 1284
targeted diphtheria toxin 1473
targeted imaging agents 233
targeted kinase 1471
targeted liposomes 1502
targeted polymer therapeutics 599
targeted protein toxins 1443
– clinical trials 1443
– combination therapy 1445, 1446
– domains 1447
– enzyme-related 1469
– schematic overview 1444
targeted radiotherapy 414, 1238
targeted RIP variants 1475
targeted Rnase 1470
targeted therapy 26
– HCC 1522
– nanoparticles 236
– thermo- 1272
targeted toxins 1443
– biological half-life 1459
– bispecific 1443
– clinical development 1472
– immunogenicity 1460
– preclinical development 1462
– saporin-based 1456
– tumor penetration 1461
targeting 1053
– active 1053, 1205, 1612
– anticancer platinum complexes 1605
– cell-penetrating peptides 1189
– central nervous system 1489
– CPPs 1202
– dendritic polymers 513
– drug 951
– dual 616
– EPR 85
– externally activated 1001
– folate receptor-targeted micelles 1119
– FR-targeted immunotherapy 1298
– immune therapy 483
– in vivo 341
– LHRH conjugates 1223
– ligand-assisted vascular 591
– liposomes 3, 967
– liver tumors 1519
– lung tumors 343
– mitochondrial 260, 273
– nanosized carriers 1523
– organ-specific 1612
– passive 56, 639, 1203, 1616
– PDT 1573
– PEGylated liposomes 910
– peptide receptors 1219
– pH-dependent 1205
– photosensitizer 1569
– polysaccharide-based drug conjugates 747
– pop-up mechanism 1121
– pre- 429
– pre-antibody era 442
– principles 34
– protein toxins 1443
– receptor/antigen 786
– serum albumin 105
– subcellular 260
– TcRn 102
– tissue 282
– to T-cells 110
– triggered cell 995
– using transferrin 773
– vascular 327
– vitamin 1308
targeting ligands 1366
– immunoliposomes 966
– siRNA/miRNA 1381
targeting moieties 258
– antibodies 1205
– dendrimers 251
– immunotoxins 1448
targets 1099
– tissue-specific 334
– vascular 411
– xenograft 26
TAT (protein transduction domain) 1456
TAT (transactivator of transcription) 1113, 1189
TAT peptide 995

TAT-conjugated polymeric micelle 1114
Tat-ELP-GFLG-DOX complex 689, 692
TAT-functionalized micelles 1121
TATA box 1424
taxanes 12, 909, 930, 1145
taxoid conjugates
– second-generation 1332, 1345
Taxol 1142
Taxotere 1154
tegafur 1337
temozolomide 830
– astrocytomas 37
temperature 1361
– LCST 668, 672
– temperature-sensitive carriers 674
– temperature-triggered phase transition 672
terminal modification 1365
terminal repeats
– inverted 1433
testosterone level
– serum 1086
Tet-inducible systems 1424
TetR 1426
Δ8-tetrahydrocannabinol 1134
tetrasulfoindotricarbocyanine (TSCA) 608
– PEG–TSCA conjugates 610
tetravalent flexibodies 458
Tf-CRM107 773, 788
TfR (transferrin receptor) 960, 966
theranostics 1062
– CNTs 1180
– radionuclides 435
therapeutic agents
– molecularly targeted 808
therapeutic antibodies 443
– marketed 445
therapeutic applications 1361
– dendrimers 545
– siRNA/miRNA 1383
therapeutic peptides 684
therapeutic radionuclides 419
therapeutic strategies
– gene 1391
therapeutics 805
– APN-targeted polymer 613
– drug-free macromolecular 267
– personalized 16
– polymer 263, 591, 701
– targeted polymer 599
therapy 805
– adjuvant bisphosphate 805
– antiangiogenic approved 593
– boron neutron capture 276, 538
– cancer 295
– combination 1013
– empowered antibodies 46
– endocrine 807
– gene 237, 1394
– HAART 921
– hydrogel-based 1071, 1075
– hyperthermia 668
– immunogene 1394
– intra-arterial 1558
– local ablative 1521
– local gene delivery 1391
– multiagent 808
– neutron capture 539
– PDEPT 812
– PELT 812
– photodynamic 278, 537, 1087, 1149, 1311
– polymer-based combination 805
– PRRT 272
– radioimmunotherapy 1206
– radionuclides 418
– radiopeptide 271
– response to 274
– responsive liposomes 989
– single-type 806
– suicide gene 1397
– targeted 236
– targeted thermotherapy 1272
– temozolomide 39
– vectors 1398
– viro- 1397
thermal ablation 898
thermal cycling
– inverse 680
thermo-responsive ELP carriers 692
thermo-responsive polymers 667
– hyperthermia treatment 670
– synthetic 671
thermocouple 694
ThermoDox 1554
thermosensitive gelation 1077
thermostable human endopeptidase 23
thermotherapy 1088
– targeted 1272
thioether bonds 258, 272
thioether linkers
– noncleavable 273
thiol-binding moiety 784
thiolation reagents 93
thiol–disulfide exchange cleavage 379, 388
thiophenol derivatives
– benzyl eliminations 567
thiophilic heterobifunctional cross-linker 1289

thrombocytopenia
– FNIT 91
thymidine analogs
– structure 256
thymidylate synthase 1534
thyroid cancer 278
TICs (tumor-initiating cell) 111
time–plasma concentration curve 891
tissue-specific targets 1163
– genomics approaches 335
– identification 334
tissues 1163
– damage 23
– extravasation 535
– interactions with CNTs 1168
– microvasculature 38
– pH variations 1100
– retention time in 1276
– staining 339
– targeting 281, 341
– ulceration 24
titratable groups 1103
titratable polymers 999
TML (trimethyl lock) 647
TNF (tumor necrosis factor) 96
TNF-α-expressing vector 1406
TNF-related apoptosis-inducing ligand (TRAIL) 1454
TNP-470 822
α-tocopherol 1307
toll-like receptor (TLR) 1277, 1367
tomography
– computed 34, 47
topoisomerase I inhibitor 67, 817
topotecan 928
toxic moieties 1452
toxic payload 34
toxicity 1163
– cardio- 20
– CNTs 1170
– dose-limiting 991, 1032
– gastrointestinal 1037
– general 1461
– hepato- 21
– liver 102
– nephro- 22
– systemic 1610
toxicity profile 952
– PEG 628
– PEGylated liposomes 915
toxicology 1013
– aptamer conjugates 1013
– GLP 1038
toxins 1443
– anthrax 1443, 1465
– bacterial 1462, 1464
– biological half-life 1459
– delivery 1455
– diphtheria 1448
– mammalian 1480
– plant 1464, 1466
– protein 1310
– Pseudomonas 13
– targeted 1443, 1460
tracers 1099
– glucose analog 1099
– labeling 262
– PET imaging 251
– SPECT imaging 259
TRAIL (TNF-related apoptosis-inducing ligand) 1454
transactivator domain
– VP16 1425
transactivator of transcription (TAT) 1113, 1189
– TAT-functionalized micelles 1121
transaminases 102
transarterial chemoembolization 1521
transbilayer pores 1000
transcellular delivery
– caveolae-mediated 1057
transcription factors 1328
transcriptome 49
transcytosis 1507
– albumin 1134
– gp60-mediated 1324
– paclitaxel 1140, 1141
– sequential 85
transdrug
– DOX 1546, 1553
transducers
– HIFU 670
transfection ability 1058
transfection efficiency
– electroporation 1370
transferrin 747, 1584
– anticancer agents 763
– diferric 749
– DOX conjugates 772
– drug conjugates 772
– radiolabeled 753
– synthetic approaches 759
– targeting strategies 773
– X-ray structure 749
transferrin cycle 750
transferrin receptor (TfR) 960, 966
transferrin-based therapeutics 1463

transferrin-conjugated PEGylated liposomes
– brain targeting 1502
transferrin–USPIO nanoparticles 233
transgenes 1393
transgenic livers
– X/myc 1548
transillumination 1003
translocation
– dendrimers 535
transmembrane glycoprotein 1309
transmembrane pores 1000
transmembrane sialoglycoprotein 96
transmural coupling 43, 47
transvascular pumping target space 329
trastuzumab 239, 310, 933, 1151
– biodistribution 108
trastuzumab conjugates
– disulfide-linked 383
trastuzumab emtansine 384
trastuzumab–maytansinoid conjugates 384
treatment planning
– radiation 275
triacyl lipids 1580
trials 1359
– clinical 1343
– phase I 1342
– phase II/III 1343
triblock copolymers 1061
trigger (specifier) 556
– elimination-based groups 564
triggerable cell penetration 995
triggered cell targeting 995
triggered release 996
trimethoxybenzylidene acetals 1112
trimethyl lock (TML) 647
tripartate prodrugs 556
triple body 460
Trojan peptides 1447
tropoelastin 678
TSCA (tetrasulfoindotricarbocyanine) 608
– PEG–TSCA conjugates 610
tube formation 35
tumor cell-targeting phages 12
– in vivo selection 14
tumor extracellular pH-triggered drug release 1104
tumor microvessels 331
– functional irregularities 38
– structural irregularities 38
tumor necrosis factor (TNF) 96
tumor suppressor protein Rb 687
tumor targeting 1099
– EPR 85
– nanoparticles 16
– passive 639
– polysaccharide-based drug conjugates 747
– pop-up mechanism 1121
tumor therapy
– responsive liposomes 989
tumor xenografts
– colorectal 645
tumor-associated enzymes 249
tumor-homing peptides 1149
tumor-initiating cell (TICs) 111
tumor-intrinsic stimuli
– activation 994
tumor-labeling markers 1192
tumor-promoting eicosanoid biosynthesis 1326
tumor-specific activation 564
tumor-specific enzymes 1056
tumor-specific receptor 1444
tumor-targeted liposomes
– cancer chemotherapy 955
tumoral receptors
– LHRH 1222
tumoritropic accumulation 65
tumors 951
– ablation 951
– acidosis 53, 55
– adrenocortical 279
– angiogenesis 65, 591
– blood flow 37
– brain 1241, 1495
– cell cycle modulation 1198
– cervical 42
– chaotic microcirculation 44
– extracellular acidity 1100
– fluorescent probes 541
– genetic heterogeneity 13
– growth curve 15
– HER2-positive 428
– hormonally responsive 26
– hypoxia imaging 40
– hypoxic cell fraction 267
– imaging 17
– in vivo delivery studies 390
– interstitium 41, 994
– Lewis lung 913
– liver 1519
– lung 343
– lymphangiogenesis 37
– MDA435/LCC6 1028
– MDR 1026
– metabolism 65
– microenvironment 251
– microscopic 33

– microvasculature 38
– murine 4
– neuroendocrine 270, 281
– pathophysiological microenvironment 48
– pathophysiology 65, 667, 782
– penetration by targeted toxins 1461
– perfusion 46
– pH-triggered micelles 1099
– platinum-refractory 928
– pretherapeutic oxygenation 268
– primary bone 1614
– proliferative activity 264
– RECIST 34
– recurrence 40
– solid 433, 752
– suppressor p16 1201
– suppressor p21 1202, 1207
– suppressor p27 1202
– suppressor p53 1200
– targeting 1202
– targeting principles 34
– types 6
– uptake of Opaxio 842
– vascular characteristics 65
– vascular targeting 327
– vascularity 37
– vascularized 990
– zzz 278
tunable dendrimers 535
"two-in-one" antibodies 453
two-phase clinical trials
– ADEPT 25
TXP (DHA–paclitaxel) 1338
– antitumor activity 1340
– pharmacokinetics 1339

u
U-PEG 633
U-PEG-Lys-maleimide-Fab¢ 637
U-PEG-Lys-NHS linker 635
ulceration
– tissue 24
ultra-small SPIO (USPIO) particles 227
ultrasound 1489
– contrast enhanced 49
– high-intensity focused 669, 670
– imaging 34, 48
– treatment 1499
ultrasound-activated release 1005
ultrasound-based heating system 669
uncleavable conjugates 387
uniformity
– delivery 989
unimers 1103
unimolecular micelles 257
unspecific hydrolysis 571
unsymmetrical disulfide bond 1295
upregulation
– proteases 554
uptake
– via targeting ligands 1366
urinary bladder cancers
– LHRH cytotoxic analogs 1231
urine M-components 934
uronic acid 727
ursodeoxycholate ligands 1614
US Food and Drug Administration 53
USPIO (ultra-small SPIO) particles 227
UV-activated release 1003

v
V-region 444
vacuolization 21
validation 1163
– drugs 51
– tumor mapping 339
variable domains 444
vascular characteristics
– solid tumors 65
vascular co-option 36
vascular endothelial cadherin 1179
vascular endothelial cell proteome 336
vascular endothelial growth factor (VEGF) 34, 539, 637
– CPPs 1198
– neoangiogenesis 261
– PUFAs 1330
– viral vectors 1416
vascular endothelium 327
vascular leakage 66
vascular mapping
– historic approaches 333
vascular mimicry 34, 36
vascular modulators 79
vascular permeability factors 66
vascular side-effects 23
vascular targeting 327
– ligand-assisted 591
vascular targets
– mapping 411
vascularity 37
vascularized tumors 990
vasculogenesis 34, 36
vasoactive intestinal peptide (VIP) 968
Vectibix 453

vector-coupled drugs 1499
vectorization of oligonucleotides 1196
vectors 1391
– bacterial 1391
– cancer gene therapy 1398
– chemical 1371
– lentiviral 1430
– nonviral 1401
– radionuclide delivery 1207
– recombinant AAV 1434
– retroviral 1428
– TNF-α-expressing 1406
– viral 1400, 1415
VEGF (vascular endothelial growth factor) 34, 539, 637
– CPPs 1198
– neoangiogenesis 261
– PUFAs 1330
– viral vectors 1416
VEGF receptor 261
vehicle control
– PBS 468
vehicles
– cyclic RGD-based 608
ventricular ejection fraction
– left 918
venules
– postcapillary 69
versatile tumor targeting 1121
vesicles
– endocytic 991
vesicular budding and fusion 329
vessels 952
– anastomosis 591
– iliac 4
– lymphatic 20
vinblastine 932
vincristine 917, 921, 933, 1029
vincristine/quercetin 1027
VIP (vasoactive intestinal peptide) 968
viral vectors 1398, 1400
– main properties 1428
– production 1428
– RNAi 1419
– shRNA delivery 1426
virotherapy 1397
virtual screening 1313
virus 1415
– adeno-associated 1415, 1433
– herpes simplex 1397, 1402
– measles 1404
– nonenveloped 1433
– replication 1432
virus-mimetic cross-linked micelles 1122
vitamin B12-binding proteins 1300
vitamin B9 1284
vitamin E 1331
vitamin repositioning 1122
vitamin targeting 1308
vitamin–drug conjugates 1283
voids
– supramolecular 275
von Hippel-Lindau protein 65
VP16 transactivator domain 1425

w

wafers
– Gliadel 1479
water solubility 577
water-soluble conjugates 1298
water-soluble dendrimers 579
water-soluble polymer–drug conjugates 272
Watson–Crick base pairing 1415
weight
– molecular 108
western analysis 339
window chamber model 76
wortmannin 821, 822

x

X-ray tomography
– SPECT/CT and PET/CT 247
X-rays
– CT 34
X-rhodamine 249
X/myc transgenic livers 1548
Xeloda 860
xenobiotics
– brain targeting 1492
xenograft models 3, 12
– Capan-1 human pancreatic tumor 1034
xenograft targets 26
xenografts 1359
– A121 ovarian tumor 1348
– B-lymphoma 103
– CFPAC-1 1348
– colorectal tumor 645
– H460 human tumor 1349
– ovarian tumor 1467
– P-gp+ DLD1 human colon tumor 1346
– Panc-1 pancreatic tumor 1348
– pH 1101
xerostomia 25
XMT-1001 865, 866
xyloglucan–drug conjugates 734
xzy confocal microscopy 1378

y

z